Hypoxia

Into the Next Millennium

ADVANCES IN EXPERIMENTAL MEDICINE AND BIOLOGY

A Continuation Order Plan is available for this series. A continuation order will bring delivery of each new volume immediately upon publication. Volumes are billed only upon actual shipment. For further information please contact the publisher.

Hypoxia
Into the Next Millennium

Edited by

Robert C. Roach
Department of Life Sciences
New Mexico Highlands University
Las Vegas, New Mexico, USA

Peter D. Wagner
Department of Medicine
University of California San Diego
La Jolla, California, USA

and

Peter H. Hackett
University of Washington School of Medicine
and Emergency Department
St. Mary's Hospital and Medical Center
Grand Junction, Colorado, USA

Springer Science+Business Media, LLC

Library of Congress Cataloging-in-Publication Data

Hypoxia : into the next millennium / edited by Robert C. Roach, Peter D. Wagner, Peter H. Hackett.
   p. ; cm. -- (Advances in experimental medicine and biology ; v. 474)
  "Proceedings of the Eleventh International Hypoxia Symposium, held February 28-March 3, 1999, at Jasper Park Lodge, Edmonton, Alberta, Canada"--T.p. verso.
  Includes bibliographical references and index.
  ISBN 978-0-306-46289-4   ISBN 978-1-4615-4711-2 (eBook)
  DOI 10.1007/978-1-4615-4711-2
  1. Anoxemia--Congresses. I. Roach, Robert C., 1956- II. Wagner, P. D. (Peter D.) III. Hackett, Peter H. IV. International Hypoxia Symposium (11th : 1999 : Edmonton, Alta.) V. Series.
  [DNLM: 1. Anoxia--Congresses. WF 143 H99855 1999]
  RB150.A67 H96 1999
  616.07--dc21

          99-047777

ISBN 978-0-306-46289-4

Proceedings of the Eleventh International Hypoxia Symposium, held February 28–March 3, 1999, at Jasper Park Lodge, Alberta, Canada

© 1999 Springer Science+Business Media New York
Originally published by Kluwer Academic / Plenum Publishers in 1999

http://www.wkap.nl/

10 9 8 7 6 5 4 3 2 1

A C.I.P. record for this book is available from the Library of Congress

DR. HERB HULTGREN

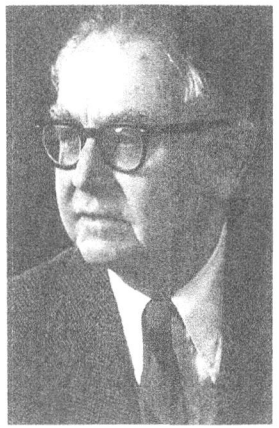

On October 18, 1997, Herbert N. Hultgren, MD, a pioneering researcher in the field of high altitude medicine and famed cardiologist, died at his home in Stanford, California at the age of 80. His hemodynamic investigations of patients with high altitude pulmonary edema (HAPE) in the Peruvian Andes and in Colorado were the defining studies demonstrating that HAPE was associated with pulmonary hypertension due to prominent hypoxic pulmonary vasoconstriction, and not due to heart failure. In a series of ingenious studies in dogs, he gradually reduced the volume of the pulmonary circulation demonstrating that high pressure and flow through a constricted vascular bed could result in alveolar edema. His resultant elaboration of the "overperfusion" theory of HAPE remains to this day the most widely accepted hypothesis of this elusive condition. Herb's fund of knowledge regarding high altitude medicine was legion, and it grew from his love of the mountains. Herb was an avid climber and medical advisor for the American Alpine Club. Herb considered the publication of his book, High-Altitude Medicine, a crowning achievement to his career in high altitude physiology and medicine (see details at *www.highaltitudemedicine.com*). We lost a friend and mentor with Herb's passing. We are honored to dedicate the 11th International Hypoxia Symposium and this book to the memory of Herb Hultgren.

PREFACE

Hypoxia is a constant threat throughout life. The International Hypoxia Symposia brings together international experts from many different fields, with clinicians, clinical researchers and basic scientists present to discuss the state-of-the-art regarding normal and abnormal (pathophysiological) responses to hypoxia. Representatives from 27 countries joined together for four days of intense presentations, interspersed with superb skiing on nearby Marmot Mountain. At the end of the millennium, many of the papers contained herein mentioned the frontiers yet to be explored in human and animal responses to hypoxia.

We continued the tradition of a mix of clinical and basic science presentations at the 11th International Hypoxia Symposium. Topics covered in great detail, most often with a clinical preparatory talk, included the broad area of visitors to high altitude, and the latest developments on high altitude cerebral and pulmonary edema. Many experts from outside the field contributed to an excellent and challenging session on the brain in hypoxia, including discussion of mechanisms of high altitude headache, and similarities between ischemic and hypoxic injury to the brain. The role of the blood brain barrier in hypoxia was covered in two excellent papers. The latest developments in our understanding of how humans and animals manage lactate during exercise and hypoxia was featured. The merging field of hypoxia interactions with vascular growth was covered in a fascinating series of papers covering the lung, the placenta and skeletal muscle. The final group of papers relates to how humans adjust to extreme hypoxia. Two special papers characterize the high quality of this session, one focused on the history of human experience in extreme hypoxia, and the other began a debate on what limits human exercise responses in extreme hypoxia. In addition to the plenary papers presented here, all abstracts submitted to the meeting are included in the book.

Another new beginning is our new relationship with Plenum/Kluwer Academic Publishing for rapid publication of this book. In addition to their professionalism and modern, computer assisted publishing techniques, *Hypoxia: Into the Next Millennium* will be indexed and readily accessible around the world.

We hope that this collection of papers prepared especially for this volume will allow us to share with a wider audience the special intellectual experience that is the International Hypoxia Symposia. The enthusiasm and excitement felt at the time of the conference is contained in these pages.

Robert C. Roach, Peter D. Wagner, Peter H. Hackett, Editors, May, 1999

ACKNOWLEDGMENTS

The 11th International Hypoxia Symposium was a resounding success due to the outstanding faculty and the lively participation of the largest-ever group of registrants. As our first Hypoxia Symposium as organizers we were most gratified to find that the unique blend of physicians, physiologists and molecular biologists that make up the Hypoxia audience could continue the great Hypoxia tradition in a new setting with many new colleagues. The *Hypoxia experience* that Charlie Houston, Geoff Coates and John Sutton created lives on, of its own accord, in the hearts and minds of hundreds of people that make the biennial pilgrimage to northern Alberta.

For 1999, Hypoxia moved from Lake Louise to Jasper. The fit between Hypoxia and Jasper Park Lodge was perfect. In the casual but elegant atmosphere by the shores of Lake Beuvert the meeting soon found its own life and rhythm. The many new faces added to the excitement of scientific exchange from dawn to well after dusk. At Jasper Park Lodge we must thank Mr. Dave Monteer and his staff in conference services for doing an excellent job to make our stay exceptional. The staff at Marmot Mountain deserve special appreciation for their warm welcome and friendly assistance.

Ms. Sharron Studd from the Office for Continuing Medical Education at McMaster University deserves a special thanks from us for doing an extraordinary job of holding our hands through our first year as organizers of Hypoxia. Her professionalism, dedication and good sense of humor made the Symposium possible.

The financing of the Hypoxia Symposia remains a challenge. This year we had the generous support of a number of individuals, including Drs. Annalisa Cogo, Allen Cymerman, Bengt Kayser and Lorna Moore. Thanks are also due to those members of the Advisory Committee of the International Hypoxia Symposium who paid their expenses so that funds were available to bring several young scientists from underdeveloped countries to the meeting. Special thanks are due the American Physiological Society for sharing their member mailing lists, and to New Mexico Highlands University. We are especially grateful to the US Army Medical Research Acquisition Activity and Medical Expeditions, Inc. (UK) for their generous financial support.

Please join us for the 12th International Hypoxia Symposium, planned for the full moon in early March, 2001 at Jasper Park Lodge, Alberta, Canada.

Robert Roach and Peter Hackett, Co-Chairmen
International Hypoxia Symposia, Internet: ***www.hypoxia.net***

CONTRIBUTORS

Peter Bärtsch
Department of Sports Medicine
Rupprecht Karls University
Heidelberg, Germany

George A. Brooks
Exercise Physiology Laboratory
Department of Integrative Biology
University of California
Berkeley, California, USA

Lester R. Drewes
Department of Biochemistry and
Molecular Biology
University of Minnesota School of
Medicine
Duluth, Minnesota, USA

Simon Gibbs
National Heart and Lung Institute
Imperial College of Science,
Technology and Medicine
London, UK

Peter Hackett
Affiliate Associate Professor
University of Washington
Seattle, Washington and Grand
Junction, Colorado, USA

George Heigenhauser
Department of Medicine
McMaster University
Hamilton, Ontario, Canada

Peter Hochachka
Department of Zoology
University of British Colombia
Vancouver, British Colombia, Canada

Hans Hoppeler
Department of Anatomy
University of Bern
Bern, Switzerland

Tom Hornbein
Department of Anesthesiology
University of Washington
Seattle, Washington, USA

Konstantin-A. Hossmann
Max-Planck-Institut für neurologische
Forschung
Köln, Germany

Charles Houston
Professor Summa Emeritus
Burlington, Vermont, USA

Daniel Jimenez
Compañia Minera Doña Ines de
Collahuasi
Iquique, Chile

John Kingdom
Maternal and Fetal Medicine
University of Toronto
Toronto, Ontario, Canada

John Krasney
Department of Physiology and
Biophysics
University at Buffalo
Buffalo, New York, USA

Ben Levine
Institute for Exercise &
Environmental Medicine
University of Texas Southwestern
Dallas, Texas, USA

Michael Moskowitz
Stroke and Neurovascular Regulation
Laboratory
Massachusetts General Hospital
Boston, Massachusetts, USA

Annabel Nickol
Medical Expeditions
Canton, Cardiff, UK

Susan Niermeyer
Section of Neonatology
University of Colorado School of
Medicine
Denver, Colorado, USA

Marcus E. Raichle
Department of Radiology and
Neurology
Washington University School of
Medicine
St. Louis, Missouri, USA

John T. Reeves
Department of Medicine
University of Colorado Health
Science Center
Denver Colorado, USA

Drummond Rennie
Deputy Editor West JAMA and
University of California San Francisco
San Francisco, California, USA

Jean-Paul Richalet
A.R.P.E. UFR de Medecine
Bobigny Cedex, France

Robert Roach
Department of Life Sciences
New Mexico Highlands University
Las Vegas, New Mexico, USA

Urs Scherrer
Department of Internal Medicine
Centre Hospitalier Universitaire
Vaudois
Lausanne, Switzerland

Lothar Schilling
Neurochirurgische Klinik
Ruprecht-Karls-Universitat
Heidelberg
Klinikum Mannheim
Mannheim, Germany

Brownie Schoene
Division of Respiratory
Disease/Harborview Medical Center
University of Washington
Seattle, Washington, USA

John Severinghaus
Department of Anesthesiology
UCSF, San Francisco, California,
USA

Kurt Stenmark
Division of Pediatric Critical Care and
Developmental Lung Biology
University of Colorado Health
Science Center
Denver, Colorado, USA

Fabiola Leon Velarde
A.R.P.E. UFR de Medecine
Bobigny Cedex, France and Lima,
Peru

Peter Wagner
Department of Medicine
University of California at San Diego
La Jolla, California, USA

John West
Department of Medicine
University of California at San Diego
La Jolla, California, USA

CONTENTS

MOUNTAIN MEDICINE

HIGH ALTITUDE PULMONARY EDEMA

HYPOXIA AND REGULATION OF VASCULAR GROWTH

HUMAN PHYSIOLOGY IN EXTREME HYPOXIA

CHRONIC MOUNTAIN SICKNESS CONSENSUS GROUP

TRIBUTE TO NIELS LASSEN

ABSTRACTS

Chapter 1

Herb Hultgren in Peru: What Causes High Altitude Pulmonary Edema?

Drummond Rennie

Deputy Editor (West), JAMA.and Institute for Health Policy Studies, University of California, San Francisco, USA

Key words: history, Peru, high altitude pulmonary edema

Abstract: Herbert Hultgren, a cardiologist who kept a careful diary all his career, arrived in Peru at the beginning of 1959 to study the occurrence of pulmonary hypertension in children at high altitude with patent ductus arteriosus. There, he was told about a strange condition, high altitude pulmonary edema (HAPE), and found that to Peruvian physicians looking after mine employees and their families, its occurrence was almost routine. With his Peruvian colleagues, Herb immediately began a systematic study of the condition, including catheter studies. Though the absence of left ventricular enlargement suggested a non-cardiac form of pulmonary edema, and though this is what he suggested in his first publication, in two subsequent papers, one written with Charles Houston, who contributed cases occurring in mountaineers, Herb wrote that the most probable cause was left ventricular failure. What is extraordinary is that before he finally submitted the two papers, he had certain knowledge that in one case of HAPE at least, left atrial pressure had been shown to be normal. Herb's contributions, then and later, to the elucidation of HAPE were enormous.

Hypoxia: Into the Next Millennium,
Edited by R. C. Roach, *et al.* Kluwer Academic/Plenum Publishing, New York, 1999.

1

1.   INTRODUCTION

In the spring of 1962, I began work as a resident at The Brompton Hospital in London, a well-known post-graduate center dedicated to the investigation and treatment of people with lung and heart conditions. One of my fellow residents, John Verrier Jones, who had the previous year been on an RAF expedition to K6 in the Karakorum, told us about a fellow climber who had suddenly gone into apparent left ventricular failure at 19,000 feet altitude (5,790m) 15. The climber had just as rapidly recovered with descent and rest. Jones, who later published his experience 15, referred to the report by Charles Houston 6, and to two reports by a man called Herbert Hultgren. 11, 12. As a climber, I was naturally interested because Houston's name was well known to me from the 1936 Nanda Devi expedition, and his expeditions to K2. The first thing I did was to get hold of the September 8th issue of the New England Journal of Medicine to see what the fuss was about 6. I was not ashamed that I'd missed his account: after all, it had come out during the first week of my internship at Guy's Hospital in London.

Charlie's article, entitled *"Acute Pulmonary Edema of High Altitudes"* contained two chest x-rays: severe pulmonary edema on January 1st, 1959, and complete clearing on January 4th. They were utterly convincing and I was entranced.

It was the purest coincidence that later I should become interested in the renal function of children with cyanotic congenital heart disease. Later still, after moving to the States, in order to investigate the healthy analogs of such hypoxic patients, I would conduct several investigations of well-acclimatized Quechua Indians in Peru from 1968 to 1972. At the same time, I would come to work with Charlie on Mt. Logan, from 1969 to 1975. So it was inevitable that I would meet Herb Hultgren to discuss high altitude problems. Though Herb and I were never to work together, I always knew him to be a giant in the field.

When Herb died in 1997, his widow, Barbara, asked me to say a few words about him at his memorial service. Thereafter, Barbara was generous in sharing information about him. In particular, Barbara gave me access to Herb's diaries. My own experiences in the same parts of Peru a few years after Herb's visits made it easy for me to relate to, and assess, his work there. Here I shall concentrate on only three years in a long, busy, and productive life to illuminate the first steps in the elucidation of the pathophysiology of HAPE. I shall not touch on Herb's climbing, or his teaching, and shall mention only briefly his major contributions to cardiology.

2. HERB'S STORY

Born in 1917, in Santa Rosa, an hour north of San Francisco, Herb graduated from Stanford in 1939. He went on to medical school at Stanford, the clinical part of the training being in San Francisco. He received his MD degree in 1943, and did a year's residency at Stanford before serving in the US Army in Europe from 1944 to 1945. He later published a scientific account of his studies on the starved prisoners who had been released from concentration camps and whom he had treated at the end of the war 4.

Returning to Stanford and a year's residency in pathology, he applied for a fellowship in hematology at Harvard, under William Castle at the Thorndike Memorial Laboratory, at Boston City Hospital. Castle could not give him a position, but Laurence Ellis could, so in 1947 Herb became a cardiologist. As Hancock has noted, this was just when "cardiac catheterization was being introduced into clinical practice, and the surgical treatment of mitral stenosis was beginning". 4. He returned west in 1948 (a cross-country journey he made by car in the company of Phil Lee, later assistant secretary for health to both Presidents Johnson and Clinton). Herb joined the faculty of Stanford, at its San Francisco campus, married Barbara, founded the Division of Cardiology, and set up the first cardiac catheterization laboratory west of the Mississippi. Cardiology had suddenly become interesting because the clinician, with access to pressures and flow rates, could become a physiologist, and, together with the surgeon, could do something about that pathology. From 1948 until 1959, Herb, a consummate physiologist, concentrated on valvular and congenital heart disease. These were the areas cardiology itself concentrated upon, and together with Frank Gerbode, the cardiac surgeon, Herb made Stanford into a prominent cardiological center. He became particularly interested in the consequences of severe pulmonary hypertension in patent ductus arteriosus, with a consequent right-to-left shunt and cyanosis 10.

3. HERB'S DIARIES

Herb's diaries are terse, practical and unemotional. His handwriting is clear and easy to read, with almost no corrections. Each and every day carries an entry, usually about five lines long. They are professional, factual, with little in the way of speculation. He frequently mentions his small children, whose progress obviously interests him greatly. There are occasional references to current events, the Kennedy-Nixon debates, Sputnik, but I looked in vain for agonizing dilemmas, deeply explored; for lengthy and subtle analyses; for character sketches of those he met, Hecht,

Leutold, Luft, Shumway, Tenney, Houston. The entries that cover weekend trips carry calculations of distances covered, and the time taken, and when they got there. But almost nothing about the effort, the view, the sense of the place, the pleasure of camping, or teaching the kids to fish. Only once does he expand, and that is in the little diaries of his visits to Peru, the first in February, 1959. Indeed, much of that diary seems to have been incorporated in the *Stanford Medical Bulletin* article 8. So much so that it seems as though the efficient Herb had written his diary with that end in view. Reading the diaries, it is impossible not to be moved by his humility, his hard work, his ability to keep the problem always before him, and his dogged determination to solve it.

It is clear that Herb himself customarily worked with astonishing efficiency on several projects at once. Being a practical man, in the garden, in the house or in the lab, he admired practical abilities in his assistants and often noted it with approval. He may find others tedious, but rarely criticizes their science in his diaries.

4.   HERB'S FIRST VISIT TO PERU

I was particularly interested in Herb's account of his first visit to Peru, where he learned of the existence of high altitude pulmonary edema. Thirty-six years later, Herb told John West that in 1954, Lewis Dexter had advised him to look into the occurrence of patent ductus arteriosus in children born at high altitude who might have pulmonary hypertension. 7.

"Friday January 9, 1959 A big day! Received notice this morning that the NIH will let me use the perfusion grant money for the Peru trip." This was to study the effect of altitude on patent ductus arteriosus. Herb received a check for $1600 for the Peru trip on Feb 1st. He took his Boards in Atlanta. Then Herb, with his closest friend from medical school and climbing companion, Warren ("Spick") Spickard, flew to Lima, a 19 pound ECG machine in Herb's case, arriving on February 10th, 1959.

In Lima he made sure he met all the excellent physicians such as Dante Peñaloza, Javier Arias-Stella, the pathologist, and, of course, *"Carlos Monge Jr. we had a delightful lunch at the Savoy. Carlos is a goldmine and we will learn a lot from him."* They also had *"dinner at Toscana - fine Peruvian restaurant. During dinner the curse of the Incas struck me down with violent force - chills, nausea & cramps. What lousy luck."* Herb notes: *"So far we have met only laboratory workers who have had excellent training in the USA"*. Later, Herb met Dr. Alberto Hurtado, but the latter was too busy to pay him any attention.

On February 12th, 1959, within two days of arrival, Herb was introduced to the syndrome of pulmonary edema occurring at high altitude by Dr Victor Alzamora, at Dos de Mayo Hospital in Lima. Herb wrote: *"He has seen 3 instances of death at high altitude due to pul. edema in previously normal people - one with a normal exercise ECG - he developed marked bradycardia in the mountains & since 2 of his cousins died suddenly there he stays in Lima."* (Dr Alzamora died of an acute myocardial infarction at the age of 48 in 1961, during Herb's third visit).

Heavy rains had washed away the railroad tracks and the road, as well as some small towns, something that occurs regularly at this time of year, and makes it the worst possible season for the investigator. The restless Spickard took a trip to Cuzco, and the two filled in time with a visit to Huaras, Yungay and the Quebrada de Yanganuco to look at the Cordillera Blanca. But 13 days passed before the road becomes passable and they are able to drive up to La Oroya, via Ticlio and Morococha on February 23.

Herb's diary for February 23, 1959 reads: " *Many rockfalls on the road but no crews cleaning them...Ticlio and Morocha-huge mines with dismal buildings-slag piles-concrete workers houses-snow and glaciers on adjacent peaks and outside each village huge graveyards. Life is cheap up here. A dismal-god-forsaken area! A serious problem at present is a huge strike against the Cerro de Pasco Corporation involving 15,000 men. They want a 50% wage increase and the company has offered 22%. Everything is at a standstill and American families have been moved down to near Lima to avoid 'incidents.' ...Finally reached La Oroya - buildings - workers houses and stores crowded along a street in a deep canyon. Then out to the Chulec Gen. Hosp. - a modern looking stone building overlooking a rolling river and many nice homes of American mine workers."* He meets the head of Chulec Hospital, *"Dr. Kurt Hellriegel - an active - polite - enthusiastic slightly elderly German surgeon."* The very day of arrival, after an exhausting drive on washed out roads, and over a 4,754 m pass, and down to 3,726 m, *"Had a long talk with Kurt largely about acute pulmonary edema in soroche. This has been seen many times here at the hospital and we will try to go over the clinical records on these cases."*

The very next day, Feb 24. *"Have started to review cases of acute pul. edema with soroche - making an English abstract of each case and reviewing the films."* Feb 25. *"Today we worked hard going through lots of cases with soroche and acute pulmonary edema. There is no doubt about the existence of this clinical entity and the x-ray films are dramatic. Why no cardiac enlargement?"* He had already identified the chief conundrum, and is already planning a systematic study: Feb 27. *"I will make up a study protocol for the doctors here so that if they see any cases of pulmonary edema in my absence they can carry out these studies and send me the data".*

Spickard left for the United States early the next morning, after 3 days at La Oroya. Herb's diary shows the pace with which he worked: *"Mar 2. "Worked hard all day-rolled and labeled ECGs from San Cristobal (4,710 m) Not all showed RVH-some were entirely normal. Reviewed exercise tests done on Spick and me in Lima and La Oroya. Neither were positive. Started to graph B.P. responses to hypervent. and exercise. Red. 35mm negative of 38 x-rays showing all stages of acute pul. edema with soroche. Began reviewing Morla's thesis on the subject ....Dr. Ortega says that pul. edema and death in burros at high altitude is common and is called la veta."* (Morla was Dr Leoncio Lizarraga Morla) 23.

He himself, despite the strike, saw cases of pulmonary edema. For example:*Mar 10. "Saw James Mitlon - a boy* (with) *clear x-ray evidence of pulmonary edema - no râles - tachycardia - heave over outflow tract and loud P2. (send for data). Had Zevallos do a VP & CT."* To the locals, it was a well-known phenomenon: *"All families here are very afraid of pul. edema in their children and they give these kids O2 on the way up and after arrival. In most cases this is not necessary but Lundberg sets a poor example by doing the same and also putting 2 of his kids (he has 2 b and 1 g - 7 - 6) in the hospital as a precaution. Therefore all other families do the same and are upset when there are not enough O2 tents to go around."* [Lundberg] *"Knows that many cases of acute pul. edema did strenuous exertion before they became ill."*

Meanwhile he did an astonishing amount of work on patent ductus.

Feb 28 at San Cristobal (4,710m). *"...- he* [Dr. Contreras] *had 40 kids waiting for me. I worked fast and did complete ECGs on 11 between the ages of 4 and 10 yrs. All had cold hands - small pulses - very reddish blue cheeks and hands. No true clubbing but a hard prominence at the base of the nails. I worked fast but soon became quite dyspneic and tired - had to sit down a lot and found myself making many mental errors hence I had to very carefully check every mental operation. Finished at 11:30 and then a huge lunch..."*

But his acclimatization improved: Mar 1. *"Last night I played 4 games of volleyball. I am accepted by the staff as a good player now."* And his diary is peppered with observations about animals and Indian folklore about the effects of altitude on cows, brisket disease and so on.

What is even more astonishing is that within 10 days of arrival at high altitude, Herb has started writing papers: Mar 3. *"Today I wrote out nearly 3/4 of the paper on pul. edema! Will have about 17 cases total and will review the data in the paper by Bardales and the thesis by Lizarraga making a total of 43 cases with 2 deaths."*Mar 4. *"Finished the final rough draft of the paper today and now I am going over it to fill in factual details."* Mar 7. *"This morning I reviewed all the x-rays and ECGs on the 44 cases of* *pulmonary edema and soroche and completed the first draft of the paper. It can be typed as soon as I arrive home."*

Herb returned to Lima on March 11th, 16 days after reaching La Oroya. Before he left La Oroya he had almost finished his paper on HAPE, had made a huge start on his study of patent ductus at altitude, was beginning a study of animal and human hearts at altitude, and made detailed plans for his next visit. Moreover, he did this essentially alone, Spickard being there for the first 3 days only. Reading his diary and his Stanford paper convinces me that he wrote the latter single handed. I am in awe.

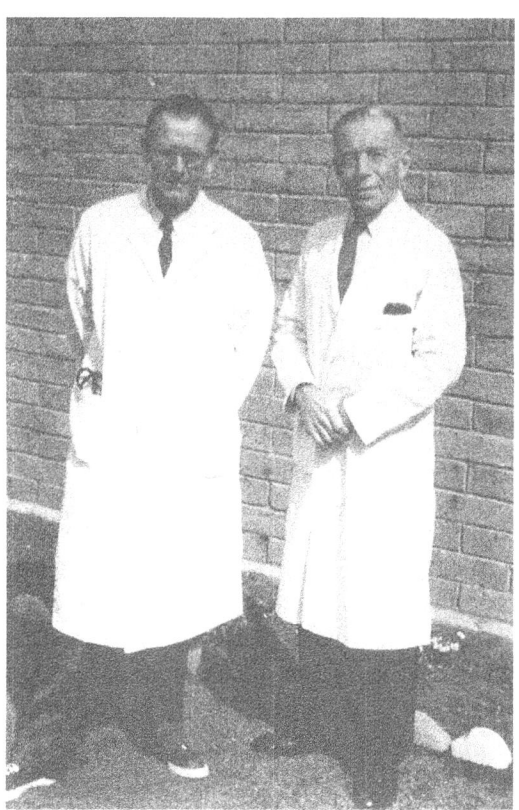

Figure 1. Herb Hultgren and Kurt Hellriegel at Chulec Hospital, La Oroya, Peru, 1960.

5. WRITING THE PAPERS

Herb was home by March 15th, 1959, and 2 days later rewrote portions of the pulmonary edema paper, noting that on Wednesday, March 18, 1959:

" Started a paper which will summarize the work I did in Peru for the Stanford Medical Bulletin ." Over the next few months, he keeps talking about these two papers, and his diary gives the impression that they are progressing fast, the second draft of the Stanford Medical Bulletin being complete on March 29th, 1959. But it wasn't published for 13 months 8. *"Sunday, August 9, 1959 Slowly working on the Peruvian papers."* The pulmonary edema paper became the large amalgamated paper that went to Medicine, and was published in 1961 11.

So why did it take him so long to publish? And why did he bury the first paper in such a journal?

First, he had to close down the Stanford operations in San Francisco on July 1, 1959, then move his lab to Stanford, and set up the cardiac catheter laboratory at Stanford, hiring and training assistants. For four months, he had to commute to Stanford from Mill Valley, 2 1/2 hours a day. Then, when he and Barbara had completed the sale of his house in Mill Valley, and they had moved out, they had to live in a small apartment in Palo Alto because the building of his house at Stanford, which he oversaw and which started in May, was not complete until the end of the 1959. In December, he wrote:. *"The apt. walls are closing in more and more!...All 3 boys have burns from the heater .."*

At the same time, Herb had to build up a new practice from scratch, and, when this proved highly successful, deal with the patient load, as well as the teaching, while trying to negotiate space and duties with his new colleagues. And he had to keep the research going, secure grants for the lab and plan further studies in Peru. In addition, there were epic family weekend journeys, say, to Shasta with the Spickards.

So it's not surprising to see, on Thanksgiving Friday, 1959, that the Peruvian papers, apparently almost ready to submit to journals in March, 8 months earlier, are still incomplete *"Spent the afternoon at the new house leveling fill with a shovel. Although this puts me in good shape and saves money it is a boring - long job...More work in the lab - for the first time I spent a quiet morning working on the paper on Medical Experiences in Peru again."*

Herb ends the year: *December 28, 1959. "A dog in Shumway's lab has survived 4 days after a heart transplant from another dog. ... 1st open heart here will be done next week - ...Bills are piling up but fortunately checks are coming in also."*

6.　　SALT LAKE CITY

1960 started well. February 6, 1960. *"Hans Hecht invited me to a symposium on high altitude at Salt Lake at the end of the month."*

Tuesday, February 23, 1960. *"Worked on material for high altitude symposium in Salt Lake City this weekend. Received sections of a cow with Brisket Disease from Peru."* February 26, 1960. *"Asked for a leave of absence for June and July for Peru."* At least he was now planning to go at the best time of year.

On February 28, 1960, he flew to Salt Lake City. *"Hans met us at 9:30 and we drove to Alta to ski but the road was blocked by an avalanche...to The Carriage House for an excellent dinner with the Hechts and Bill and Liz Ann Carnes. Had to bring our own cocktails and no wine due to Utah's primitive liquor laws."*

The program for the "Symposium on Altitude Physiology" in the cardiovascular division of the University of Utah, is glued into Herb's diary. Apart from Herb, the visiting speakers were Charles S Houston, Aspen Institute, and Ulrich C. Luft of the Lovelace Clinic, Albuquerque, New Mexico. Houston was due to to speak on "Altitude stresses and altitude tolerance" and wrap up the symposium on a second day devoted to Brisket disease, with "Experiences on K2". Herb was down to speak on "The normal cardiovascular state at altitude" and, with Luft, "Acute mountain sickness".

"Monday, February 29, 1960. Cardiac Conference in Hans' lab at 8:30.....to the amphitheater to meet Charlie Houston (How ston) and his wife. Ulrich Luft who skied with us yesterday was a disappointment. Houston has a good collection of pulmonary edema cases from mountaineering journals and personal correspondence and Leuthold has heard of some via the Indian government. We should probably pool our cases and write them up as a separate report? Lunch at an excellent cafeteria in the new Prudential Insurance Building. Drinks with the Carnes before dinner and then to the Hecht's for a fine party and a buffet supper listening to many interesting yarns about mountaineering by Houston and Leuthold. Luft knew of no cases of altitude pulmonary edema from airforce experience or literature."

Of the second day of the meeting, March 1, Herb writes: *"The day was largely devoted to Brisket Disease with a good review of the problem by both the Salt Lake and Denver groups. Concluding talks by Houston on his experience on K2 was a gem."*

Bob Grover and Jack Reeves were both in the audience (they were part of the "Denver group"), and neither has any recollection of Herb's talk.

Herb returned to Stanford: *"Sunday March 6, 1960. Worked on pul. edema paper in AM - started putting in a vegetable garden in the afternoon."*

A week later: *"March 14, 1960. Read Mosso's Life of Man on the High Alps...2 cases of high altitude pul. edema reported in this book published in 1898."* On March 17th: *"Working on pulmonary edema paper and beginning to get things together for Peru."* Two days later: *"Saturday March 19, 1960. A letter from Houston who will join us in the pul. edema paper."*

"Friday March 25, 1960. A lot of catching up to do. Rita getting out the 1st draft of the pul. edema paper. I hope Houston will join us and include his case report." Worries about his lab continued: *"Training grant reduced 1/2 and will be reconsidered in June."*

Herb had for the first time met Alberto Hurtado in Lima on March 12, 1959. It had not been a satisfactory meeting. *"He apologized profusely for not leaving more time to meet me."* A year later, Herb fared no better. He notes: *"April 7, 1960. Yesterday I drove to SF in the afternoon to hear Hurtado give the Lilly Lecture* (at the American College of Physicians meeting) - *not much new - only mentioned pulmonary edema. Tried to talk with him after the lecture but he was in a hurry. He certainly doesn't seem interested at all in me or my projects I should write him - meet him in Lima and send him a copy of the paper."* Though Herb was well aware of the importance of HAPE, others were apparently more skeptical. He wrote on May 1, 1960 in Atlantic City: "*Cardiology papers not very interesting and I am even more disappointed on not getting the pulmonary edema work on.*"

Still, his practice was growing fast and he was practicing for his next visit to Peru: *"Monday May 30, 1960. Practicing Van Slyke technic - doing correction factors and dissecting hearts for R and L vent. wts."* Shortly after, he signed a petition for Stevenson for President.

Another visit to Peru, on June 8, 1960, delayed the papers further. This time, he was accompanied by Jack Kelly, whom he had trained in his laboratory. And this time, Herb came at the best season of the year. After a brief stay in Lima (Herb carefully records how to make a Pisco Sour) they reached Chulec on June 14, to a warm reunion with the staff. Uncharacteristically, Herb suffered from severe Cheyne-Stokes respirations: "*I seemed to recall every hyperpneic period and really felt dyspneic - this is what congestive failure must be like*". Then, June 17, 1960: "*I found my BCG [ballistocardiograph] after smoking looks terrible while it is fairly normal before smoking so I have given up the whole business. This is a good place to start.*" Despite that, he was soon playing volley ball every evening. The two dissected the hearts of lambs, cows, horses and llamas to measure right ventricle/ total heart weight ratios. He also performed cardiac catheterizations on patients with chronic mountain sickness, and normals, in the evenings or very early when the lab was clear. Emilio Marticorena came down from Cerro de Pasco to help him. There were delays because the Van Slyke was broken, (replacement parts did not arrive until July 18, a month later) or the electric power supply unreliable. Meanwhile, they dissected the hearts of numerous animals. Herb records reading numerous books, and at weekends, Herb would go fishing. No mention was made of pulmonary edema. Herb returned home on July 24, 1960.

Herb did not record the appearance of Charlie Houston's paper in the New England Journal of Medicine on September 8, 1960, just as he had failed to remark that of his own paper in the Stanford Medical Bulletin four months before. In that curious paper, part travel diary, and part science, Herb seems to favor the idea that HAPE is non-cardiogenic. *"The mechanism of this syndrome is unknown. The normal cardiac size and the absence of murmurs or gallop sounds during the acute stage suggests that left ventricular failure is absent. Constriction of the pulmonary venules distal to the capillaries and a shift of blood volume from the periphery to the lungs due to peripheral vasoconstriction may be important contributory mechanisms."* 8. The very strangeness of the format of the paper explains why Herb sent it to the Stanford Medical Bulletin.

Herb's diary continues: *"Sunday November 6, 1960. Finished final review of Pul. Edema paper. Wednesday December 21, 1960. Finished 2nd pul. edema paper...(Harry) Miller doing a fine job on the heart dissections."* Yet this was against a background of increasing worries about grant support: *"Monday November 21, 1960. The grant app. for high altitude work has been turned down so now I must start all over again and apply for other grant support." "Tuesday November 29, 1960. Our lab financial situation for the coming year is grim because our Chronic Hypoxia grant was turned down...Talked to the House Staff on Peru. Our paper on pul. circ. in the altitude is on the West. Soc. Program."*

"Monday December 5, 1960. Cardiac patients continue to be referred in large numbers. Checks come in and we may make it through this month with heaviest expenses ever without cashing bonds. P.Edema paper on WAPs program and Pul. Circ. paper on West. Soc. Program."

Friday January 27, 1961 (at Carmel.) *"I gave the Pul. Edema paper in the afternoon and it was well received. Should give rabbits pneumonitis and then see if this enhances their ability to develop pul. edema due to saline infusions and elev. of L.A. pressure."*

"Tuesday March 14, 1961. Have done 3 papers in the past 4 months - two on high altitude pul. edema and one on errors in cardiac catheterization with a bit of work done on the effect of high altitude on man and animals (two papers) which I will hold until Fall since I can collect more related data this summer."

Then came an entry that one would have expected would change everything:

"Friday April 7, 1961. Heard Boris Surawicz talk today at 1:00 re electrolytes and the EKG. He had just come from Salt Lake where he brought a fascinating story. A doctor Bates of Monterey - a pediatrician -

got severe acute pulmonary edema at Alta and came down to Salt Lake General Hospital where he volunteered for a cardiac catheterization. The PA pressure was 70 and the LA pressure via a foramen ovale was 7! He was not supposed to have any heart disease. This is amazing and I hope it is confirmed."

Talcott Bates developed HAPE at Alta, 3,125 m and was catheterized the next day. He survived to be a co-author of the 1962 paper by Fred et al. 3

Herb uses exclamation marks sparingly and never again uses the word "amazing" in this 3 year period, so his excitement is apparent. He immediately recognized the significance of the observation of a normal left atrial pressure in HAPE. Indeed, he, a cardiac physiologist, must surely already have discussed with his friend Hans Hecht the possibility of chancing on just such a patient as Talcott Bates with his patent foramen ovale. It was now clear that the cause of HAPE could not possibly be any temporary failure of the heart, but must lie in the lungs or pulmonary vasculature.

"Saturday April 29, 1961. Finished proof reading the first pul. edema paper and sent it off to Medicine - it will appear in the May issue." This is the famous paper that was published in <u>Medicine</u> in September, 1961 11.

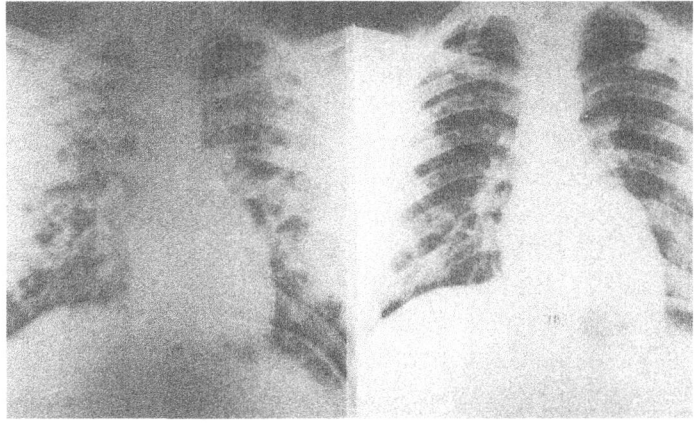

Figure 2. Why is the heart not enlarged? High altitude pulmonary edema, Chulec Hospital

"Tuesday May 2, 1961. Revised pul. edema paper #2 in light of comments by Will Siri and will send it off to the Brit. M. J." (Herb must have meant the <u>British</u> <u>Heart</u> <u>Journal</u>, which is where it eventually appeared 12.

7.   THE THIRD VISIT TO PERU

Charlie and Herb met again on Saturday June 10, 1961. (In Tulsa) where Herb met Dave Rytand, Marsh Tenney and Hans Hecht: "*Up early to go over my talks - visited with Tenney and Dave. ..The morning program which I presided over went fairly well but Clapper insisted on all discussants going to a microphone and the projector jammed in the middle of Houston's talk. Did not have a chance to visit much with Houston unfortunately.*"

Herb paid his third visit to Peru from June 28 to August 23, 1961. He went with Harry Miller, and worked first at La Oroya and then Cerro de Pasco. Though on the previous visit, Herb made almost no mention of HAPE, on this occasion he saw several cases. *July 14, 1961:* "*Pul. Edema very common in the kids - rare in adults*". "*July 19, 1961. A very important day for this expedition ..Lopez said he had an 8 year old in the hospital with acute pul. Edema. An excellent case - typical history - cough & x-rays.*" Two hours later they had cancelled their trip to Cerro de Pasco and the catheter study was underway. "*This turned out to be a very tough job .I could not get into the brachial artery - abandoned it. Fluoro worked poorly - catheter plugged - venospasm but finally got RA - PA & PAw pressures before & after O2 & PA bloods before and after O2. Later in the afternoon I got a BA sample - dark - & after O2 a second one bright red. Remarkable drop in PA pressure & slowing of heart rate on O2.*" Herb found this boy's sister had "*a tachycardia - no symptoms but definite mild pul. edema by x-ray - a good example of subclinical pul edema*". They did another catheter study on another 8-year old Caucasian boy with pulmonary edema on August 2, making a lengthy journey from Cerro de Pasco to La Oroya to do so; another on August 7, on a Peruvian worker, and the last on August 8 in a 12 year-old Caucasian girl. HAPE had become routine.

Herb took a trip to climb above Hauras, and returned to Stanford on August 23rd to bad news.

8.   SPICKARD'S DEATH:

"*August 24, 1961. At noon the letter from Don Hall telling of Spick's death. What a blow! I could do little the rest of the day. Finally in the evening we sent Jo a telegram .*" Spickard had fallen to his death on August 20th. There is a newspaper article stuck into Herb's diary titled "Body of Dr. Spickard May Remain on Whatcom Mountain." "*August 25, 1961. Talked to Bud Tensley about Spick who said they were roped - descending - Spick last when he fell and rope was cut on a sharp rock.*"

Six weeks later: "Friday October 6, 1961. Pul. edema paper finally out - Spick's name misspelled on the front page". The next day: *"Saturday October 7, 1961. Worked on high altitude paper."*

9.   CHARLIE HOUSTON

Meanwhile, and in another part of the forest, what of Charlie Houston, and the case he described in the New England Journal of Medicine in September, 1960 6? This was of a 21 year old cross country skier whom Charlie rescued, and who was a naturally a great puzzle to Charlie on New Year's Day, 1959. He noted pulmonary edema on x-ray, with a normal cardiac silhouette and an ECG that 5 physicians interpreted in 5 ways. Just over 4 months later, May 11, 1959, the man, Ron Cox, was examined by a cardiologist, Dr. Gil Blount in Denver, who considered his heart normal and did not know what to make of the episode, a milder version of which had occurred before.

A month later, after Ron had been seen by Blount, Charlie wrote to Mrs Cox. I am indebted to Dr Robert Grover for the following two letters:

Letter to Mrs. Harriet Cox from Charles S. Houston on May 22, 1959.

"Dear Mrs. Cox,

Let me say once more-and you may read this to Ron. Ron definitely had congestive failure in December, and the cause was probably extreme exertion at high altitude under extreme conditions. Just what the contribution of work, cold and height were respectively, will not be known. He can go into failure again given the same or similar conditions, and he must recognize this fact ."

By the end of August, 1959, Charlie's thinking had not really changed, though Charlie had sought a very august opinion, a year before Charlie's paper appeared in the New England Journal of Medicine.

Letter to Mrs. Harriet Cox from Charles Houston, dated August 27, 1959.

"Dr. Paul Dudley White visited me a few days ago, and spent some time reviewing Ron's case and his cardiograms. He too was very puzzled, but finally felt that the most probable state of affairs was that Ron did not have any heart disease but had had a temporary failure of the left ventricle causing his symptoms. ..His case will be written up probably in the fall or the winter rather than at once, since Dr. White wanted another cardiologist in the East to review the tracings before he made a final decision."

Charlie felt it urgent to warn climbers of a new danger and he did so in Summit, dated April 1960 5 shortly after the Salt Lake City meeting. The article is entitled "Pneumonia or Heart Failure?" He concludes that a previously health athlete can go into heart failure under certain conditions, and this may occur at high altitude and be mistaken for pneumonia.

Charlie then went on to write the famous article "Acute Pulmonary Edema of High Altitude", to which I referred at the start 6. In the paper, Ron Cox's case is described in detail, and brief sketches of four others, including "LBM", who turned out to be my friend, Bruce Meyer, an orthopedic surgeon from Carmel. Charlie gives an admirably terse account. But it is a quite unclear at the end whether he thinks HAPE was a cardiogenic edema or not. Arguing that Charlie was tipped off that HAPE was non-cardiogenic first of all depends on proof that Charlie knew it was, and put that fact into his New England Journal of Medicine paper. He didn't.

Why didn't Herb write up his Peruvian cases without including Charlie's? My guess, from the diary, is that Herb was a little in awe of Charlie. Herb, mostly a weekend climber, was well aware of Charlie's climbing deeds. And the Medicine article suggests that they both had to satisfy themselves that the "pneumonia" of climbers was the same as the HAPE affecting Peruvians and Westerners in the Andes.

10.   PRIORITY?

A controversy has recently arisen over who deserves priority in descriptions of HAPE. Who first described HAPE? As West has well shown, 23 and as Herb was the first to acknowledge, the condition was described by several physicians in South America, including Ravenhill 19, Crane (at the very hospital at Chulec where Herb later worked) 2, Lizarraga 16, Bardalez 1 and others. Who first described it in English? Ravenhill, who called it a cardiac form of puna, or altitude disease 19, and then, in a letter to The Practitioner in 1955, Irvine 14.

Finally, who first put the lesion squarely in the lungs? That is a more complex question, and the controversy is of other people, not the protagonists. Charlie has denied ever claiming priority, and I believe him. We know from Herb's extensive diaries and his behavior over 38 years that he did not claim priority either. Though Herb twice expressed frustration that his paper on pulmonary edema was not accepted for the young Turks meeting at Atlantic City in 1960, (Diary, March 31, 1960, May 1, 1960), never did he express any envy, nor any feeling about being scooped. "*I have never made an issue of priority since I believe it is a somewhat selfish policy*".(Herb Hultgren to Jack Reeves, 1995) The reason in his case is simple: he was always conscious that he had been shown HAPE by the Peruvians.

I think that we would do better to think in terms of individual contribution. The contributions of each have been immense.

First, Charlie. He was an experienced climber, a researcher and physician, when, at the age of 45, he organized and carried out a strenuous rescue, saving Ron Cox's life on New Year's Day, 1959. Charlie at once realized there was something very strange. The man was superbly fit, and recovered rapidly. Throughout 1959, and after Ron Cox's case had been reviewed by Paul Dudley White, even until the New England Journal of Medicine article a full year later, he believed that HAPE was due to left ventricular failure. White encouraged Charlie to send the paper to the New England Journal of Medicine, but the evidence seems to be that White did not indicate that Cox had non-cardiogenic edema. Charlie writes: "*This particular type of acute pulmonary edema in the presence of a normal heart has been reported rarely if at all in the medical literature*". "*The mechanism of this type of pulmonary congestion is not clear*" 6. He rejects cold injury of the lung, pulmonary embolism, pneumonia, coronary disease, myocarditis, arrhythmia, mitral stenosis or pericarditis. Charlie wrote at the end "*recent observations indicate that both acute and chronic anoxia may cause striking elevation of pulmonary artery pressure, failure of the left ventricle and pulmonary edema. Since exercise and severe cold, together with anoxia, might have cumulative effects, this explanation seems to be the most probable. One may thus describe this type of pulmonary edema as almost physiologic.*" (He cited Hecht H. Discussion. Proceedings of High Altitude Symposium, University of Utah, Salt Lake City, March 6, 1960) 6.

Charlie's article became a classic, and it received immediate world-wide attention. Charlie already had an extensive acquaintance of climbers, indeed, the other 4 cases in the article show this. There is little doubt that Charlie's article was a big stimulus to research and saved lives. He referred to Herb's cases as only a "personal communication", when they had both been at Salt Lake City together, had corresponded and had agreed to aggregate their cases for what became the Medicine article. But one cannot blame him for not citing Herb's Stanford Medical Bulletin article. Indexing services were a good deal less efficient back then.

Herb had an easier time of it. He didn't meet the problem up to his waist in powder snow, in gathering darkness, faced by a moribund patient, and a long way from safety. And then with no cardiologist on hand.

On February 12, 1959, 6 weeks after Charlie rescued Ron Cox, Herb, who was a superbly trained cardiologist and physiologist, in Peru to study patent ductus arteriosus, was told about the condition, HAPE, in the civilized circumstances of Lima by Dr. Alzamorra, as if its existence were a well-known fact. He then reviewed many cases, already documented by people who had looked after patients with the syndrome.

Hans Hecht held the Salt Lake City meeting, which first brought Charlie and Herb together, to discuss brisket disease. Herb knew Hecht well. In reply to Bob Grover, 35 years later, Herb wrote about the Salt Lake City meeting ..."*Did I tip Charlie off that HAPE was a non-cardiac pulmonary edema? I am sure I did...When I returned I wrote Charlie re the cases I had seen hence his reference #8 Hultgren - personal communication...*" (Herb Hultgren to Bob Grover, February 7, 1995.) But the evidence from their papers suggests that Herb misremembered.

By the end of 1961, what Herb Had done was remarkable enough. Working unacclimatized at altitude, and almost entirely without help from Spickard, who had to return home, he rapidly added a systematic description of HAPE to an already busy research program on patent ductus. Before he left, he had set up a protocol for further studies. Despite enormous changes at work, he had written the major part of three papers submitted within about a year of his first Peru visit. He had started sketching out a series of lab experiments to find a good animal model. These experiments were later to provide the basis for his theory of overperfusion.

The Medicine paper is a classic. It was finished 7 1/2 months after Charlie's paper in the New England Journal of Medicine, and is in two parts: 15 cases from Chulec Hospital, and a review of 14 cases reported previously by Lizarraga 16 and 12 cases studied by Bardales 1. The second part consists of mountaineering cases, including Ron Cox, Bruce Meyer, Mosso's case (Pietro Ramella) and the case of Dr Jacottet who died on Mt Blanc at the turn of the century. Sandwiched between the two parts is a lengthy discussion of the cause. They authors exclude pneumonia, and note the numerous signs of pulmonary hypertension. The general causes, of course, are noted to be increased capillary pressure or increased capillary permeability. They then consider: redistribution of blood from systemic to pulmonary circuit; increased total blood volume; constriction of pulmonary veins or venules, all of which they say must be investigated further.

Finally, they consider "*Acute left ventricular failure. This is of course the most likely cause of the syndrome. Its exact nature and severity cannot be determined until studies have been made in patients with high altitude pulmonary edema*". They note that "*severe anoxia may produce left ventricular failure*" in experimental animals. "*The absence of consistent cardiac enlargement, the absence of other clinical signs of left ventricular failure and the absence of evidence of underlying heart disease, might suggest that acute left ventricular failure is not the* sole basis *for the pulmonary edema, and that other contributory factors are important.*" At the end of the article, the authors conclude that "*the most likely cause of the edema is acute left ventricular failure.*"

This paper was largely written by Herb. It was certainly proof read and sent off to <u>Medicine</u> by Herb, and this happened on April 29th, 1961, more than a year after the Salt Lake City meeting.

The next year, Herb, with Spickard and Lopez, published again on HAPE in the <u>British Heart Journal</u> 12. We know that paper was sent off to the journal in early May, 1961, about 3 days after the <u>Medicine</u> paper, or its proofs, (the diary is unclear) had been submitted. The <u>British Heart Journal</u> paper describes two US cases and 6 more Peruvian cases of HAPE, two of them fatal. The discussion, for a cardiological audience, states that the cause is unknown. The possibilities already mentioned in the <u>Medicine</u> paper (which is referenced in the printed version) are again run through. The authors note that "*In 2 instances rather obvious <u>increases</u> in heart size occurred upon recovery.*" Herb (and his co-authors) discuss the idea that this was not "*ordinary left ventricular failure*", but hypervolemia and increased work load alone raising left ventricular filling pressure, with normal myocardial function. "*In the majority of cases there is no evidence of an underlying pneumonia*". They discuss the confusing evidence on the effect of digitalis, and suggest that they, along with antibiotics, may be used for treatment ("despite the lack of evidence"). Herb, who was surely the dominant author, again suggests that "*pulmonary venous constriction induced by hypoxia may be the fundamental causative mechanism. This would result in elevation of pulmonary capillary pressure without elevation of left ventricular diastolic pressure.*"

This article, of which Charlie was not a co-author, seems to go further towards suggesting that HAPE might be a non-cardiogenic pulmonary edema. It is possible that Herb had been sending the proofs, rather than the manuscript, to <u>Medicine</u> on April 29, 1961, and his note on November 6, 1960. "*Finished final review of Pul. Edema paper.*" might have meant that he'd finished the <u>Medicine</u> paper nearly six months before, and had sent the manuscript off at around that time. This would have allowed time Herb to change his views about the cause of HAPE. But even if he did, neither paper states unequivocally that HAPE is non-cardiogenic, and Herb was first author of both. Furthermore, the first states that left ventricular failure is the most likely cause.

The biggest conundrum of all is the striking absence from both the <u>Medicine</u> and <u>British Heart Journal</u> articles of any reference whatsoever to the case of Talcott Bates, which Herb had known about for over 3 weeks. This case presented Herb with the clearest possible evidence from Salt Lake City that HAPE was not due to left ventricular failure. The Hecht group's catheterization results solved the problem: from thence forth, HAPE, was regarded as non-cardiogenic 3. But there isn't even a footnote added in proof.

This is an astonishing omission. So what was going on? I would suggest that the cautious Herb was reluctant to put hearsay into print, (and steal the thunder from the friends in Salt Lake City who'd made the discovery). I'd also suggest that the secret knowledge Herb had about the Salt Lake City findings emboldened him in his discussion in the <u>British</u> <u>Heart</u> <u>Journal</u> paper to return to his original theory that HAPE was non-cardiogenic, though once again, he made no mention of the Salt Lake City results.

But as to the Herb-Charlie priority question? There is no controversy. No one stole anything and everything that happened was in the best traditions of research. What we have here are a pair of physician researchers who both brought to the table ideas, brains, patients, keen eyes, and an obsession to advance knowledge and save lives. If Herb was far more of a cardio-physiologist, and Charlie far more of a general internist -climber, that made the mix the more powerful. And if, with the powerful help of hind-sight, we look back and blame one or the other for being so slow in getting the answers, or so tentative in acknowledging advances in thinking, we might remember how mountainous our own scientific questions were to us, and how hesitant we were to climb those mountains.

11.   POSTSCRIPT

In 1967, Herb moved his operations to the Palo Alto Veteran's Administration Hospital. Hancock has described how Herb had, in the early sixties, "already shifted his major cardiological interest to coronary artery disease." 4. He played a leading role in the famous Veterans Administration Cooperative Study of Coronary Artery Surgery. Randomized trials of surgery are still uncommon, and this study of CABG surgery was a landmark event, and set the stage for the later massive randomized trials of thrombolytic therapy 4. Indeed, when I was the deputy editor of the <u>New</u> <u>England</u> <u>Journal</u> <u>of</u> <u>Medicine</u>, I remember receiving the main paper from Herb 18. I also remember wondering for a moment why he was wasting a good altitude brain on such matters, though a more dispassionate observer might well call this Herb's greatest contribution to medicine.

Brownie Schoene tells us 21 that Herb's last paper on HAPE, written with Rod Wilson from Anchorage and Jon Kosek, a pathologist at Stanford, was in review the weekend he died at the age of 80. It was published in Wilderness and Environmental Medicine shortly thereafter, at the end of 1997 13.

Schoene wrote: "Herb Hultgren was the leading investigator in the field of HAPE in the 1960s and 1970s." 13 With his colleagues, especially Bob Grover, Herb demonstrated an abnormal circulatory response to high altitude, an accentuated pulmonary hypertension, in subjects with a previous history of high altitude pulmonary edema. 9 From the broncho-alveolar lavage experiments done by Schoene, Hackett and others on Denali 22, we know that the edema fluid is typical of a permeability edema. This is now being challenged by Maggiorini 17, who finds that the pulmonary capillary pressure, but not permeability, increases on exposure to altitude in HAPE susceptible subjects.

Herb's most interesting theory, built on his studies on patients with HAPE, and on his attempts to find a good animal model of HAPE, is his notion that HAPE is due to patchy vasoconstriction with overperfusion of the those capillaries that are left open, as may occasionally occur associated with acute pulmonary embolism in humans. Whether that is the case is still unknown, indeed, the uncertainties around the sequence of events that produce the edema 20, mean that there are still a myriad questions to answer. Forty years after Charlie rescued his skier and Herb first went to Peru, there are still rich prizes to be won.

12.   CHRONOLOGY

January 1, 1959. Charles Houston rescues Ron Cox (later Alex Drummond). Over the next few days, Charlie realizes that RC has something unusual.

February 12, 1959. Lima: Herb told of the existence of HAPE by Dr L Lizarraga, who had published on the subject in 1955.

February 25, 1959, at Chulec Hospital, he began reviewing case histories with Peruvian physicians to whom HAPE or "soroche with acute pulmonary edema", was commonplace. Herb immediately identified the lack of cardiac enlargement as crucial.

March 10, 1959, sees a case of HAPE at Chulec, 7 days after starting to write a paper on HAPE.

February 29 to March 1, 1960. Speaks at the "Symposium on Altitude Physiology" organized by Hans Hecht. Meets Charles Houston for the first time. Houston tells him of his mountaineering cases and Leuthold of cases he has heard of occurring "in India".

March 14, 1960, finds Mosso's description of a case of HAPE.

March 19, 1960, Charlie Houston accepts Herb's invitation to combine their cases.

May, 1960. Published "Medical experiences in Peru" in the Stanford Medical Bulletin 8. Herb clearly states that the edema is non-cardiogenic.

May 11, 1959, Charlie's patient, Ron Cox, found to have a normal heart.

Late August, 1959. Ron Cox's case reviewed by Dr Paul Dudley White, who thought Cox had had a temporary failure of the left ventricle.

April, 1960. Charlie warns climbers with his article in Summit.

September 8, 1960. Houston's article published in the New England Journal of Medicine. Left ventricular failure due to anoxia is stated to be the most probable cause of HAPE.

Sunday November 6, 1960. Herb finishes the final review of the paper on HAPE, of which Houston was last author. This was then presumably sent on by Herb to Medicine. This article states that acute left ventricular failure is the most likely cause of HAPE.

January 27, 1961: Herb was planning to "give rabbits pneumonitis and then see if this enhances their ability to develop pul. edema due to saline infusions and elev. of L.A. pressure". This means that at the least, Herb was still open to the idea that LA pressure is raised in HAPE.

April 7, 1961: Herb was told that the LA pressure in Talcott Bates was only 7mm Hg, while the PAP was 70 mm Hg, and he reacts: "This is amazing and I hope it is confirmed." Herb up to that point either thought HAPE was a temporary LV failure and was astonished to be proved wrong, or he was excited and gratified at the confirmation of his conjecture that HAPE was NOT due to left ventricular failure.

April 29, 1961. Herb "Finished proof reading the first pul. edema paper and sent it off to Medicine" thinking it would appear in the May issue.

No one else but Herb, the first author, sent in the proofs, and he checked them, and, despite what he knew about Talcott Bates' normal LA pressures, and despite what he sent off for publication in the British Heart Journal 3 days later, the article calls left ventricular failure the most likely cause. In 1995, Herb wrote to Jack Reeves: *"I wrote the whole paper and did all the data analysis and got the chest films reproduced and this was the paper in Medicine."*

May 2, 1961. Herb finished revising the British Heart Journal paper, which consists of further observations on HAPE. Increased left ventricular filling pressures is suggested as a cause, and hypoxic pulmonary venous constriction is suggested as the fundamental mechanism.

August 20, 1961. Warren Spickard killed in a climbing accident.

October 6, 1961. The Medicine article published.

REFERENCES

1. Bardalez, A. Algunoscasos de edema pulmonar agudo por soroche grave. *Anal Fac Med Lima* 38: 232-243, 1955.
2. Crane, H. L. I. Soroche-mountain sickness-anoxemia. *Anal Fac Med Lima* 11: 306-308, 1927.

3. Fred, H. L., A. M. Schmidt, T. Bates, and H. H. Hecht. Acute pulmonary edema at altitude. Clinical and psychological observations. *Circulation* 25: 929-937, 1962.

4. Hancock, E. W. Herbert N. Hultgren. *Clin Cardiol* 21: 695-697, 1998.

5. Houston, C. Pneumonia or Heart Failure? *Summit* 6: 2-3, 1960.

6. Houston, C. S. Acute pulmonary edema of high altitude. *N Engl J Med* 263: 478-480, 1960.

7. Hultgren, H. Letter to John West. In: *High Life. A History Of High-Altitude Physiology And Medicine*, edited by W. J. Oxford: Oxford University Press, 1998.

8. Hultgren, H., and W. Spickard. Medical experiences in Peru. *Stanford Medical Bulletin* 18: 76-95, 1960.

9. Hultgren, H. N., R. F. Grover, and L. H. Hartley. Abnormal circulatory responses to high altitude in subjects with a previous history of high altitude pulmonary edema. *Circulation* XLIV: 759-770, 1971.

10. Hultgren, H. N., A. Selzer, A. Purdy, E. Holman, and F. Gerbode. The syndrome of patent ductus arteriosus with pulmonary hypertension. *Circulation* 8: 15-35, 1953.

11. Hultgren, H. N., W. B. Spickard, K. Hellriegel, and C. S. Houston. High altitude pulmonary edema. *Medicine* 40: 289-313, 1961.

12. Hultgren, H. N., W. B. Spickard, and C. Lopez. Further studies of high altitude pulmonary edema. *Br Heart J* 24: 95-102, 1962.

13. Hultgren, H. N., R. Wilson, and J. C. Kosek. Lung pathology in high-altitude pulmonary edema. *Wilderness Environmental Medicine* 8: 218-220, 1997.

14. Irvine, G. Acute pulmonary edema and mountaineering. *The Practitioner* 174: 108-109, 1995.

15. Jones, J. V. Letters to the Editor. *Lancet* February 24: 426-427, 1962.

16. Lizarraga, L. Edema agudo del pulmon. *Anal Fac Med Lima* 38: 244, 1955.

17. Maggiorini, M. Evidence against a high permeability edema in early HAPE. *(Personal communication)*, 1999.

18. Murphy, M. L., H. N. Hultgren, K. Detre, J. Thomsen, T. Takaro, and and Participants in the Veterans Administration Cooperative Study. Treatment of chronic stable angina. *New Engl J Med* 297: 621-627, 1997.

19. Ravenhill, T. H. Some experiences of mountain sickness in the Andes. *J Trop Med Hygiene* 1620: 313-320, 1913.

20. Scherrer, U., C. Sartori, M. Lepori, Y. Allemann, H. Duplain, L. Trueb, and P. Nicod. High-altitude pulmonary edema: from exaggerated pulmonary hypertension to a defect in transepithelial sodium transport. In: *Hypoxia: Into the Next Millennium*, edited by R. C. Roach, P. D. Wagner and P. H. Hackett. New York: Plenum/Kluwer Academic Publishing, 1999, p. 93-107.

21. Schoene, R. B. High-altitude pulmonary edema; more lessons from the master. *Wilderness Environmental Medicine* 8: 202-203, 1997.

22. Schoene, R. B., P. H. Hackett, W. R. Henderson, E. H. Sage, M. Chou, R. C. Roach, W. J. Mills Jr, and T. R. Martin. High altitude pulmonary edema. Characteristics of lung lavage fluid. *JAMA* 256: 63-69, 1986.

23. West, J. B. *High Life. A History Of High-Altitude Physiology And Medicine*. New York: Oxford University Press, 1998.

Chapter 2

High Altitude Cerebral Edema and Acute Mountain Sickness
A Pathophysiology Update

Peter H. Hackett

University of Washington School of Medicine and Emergency Department, St. Mary's Hospital and Medical Center, Grand Junction, Colorado, USA

Key words: pathophysiology, altitude illness, vasogenic edema, cytotoxic edema, intracranial dynamics, intracranial pressure, ICP, blood-brain barrier, cerebrospinal fluid

Abstract: The diagnosis, treatment and prevention of high altitude cerebral edema (HACE) are fairly well established. The major unresolved issues are 1) the pathophysiology, 2) the individual susceptibility, and 3) the relationship of HACE to acute mountain sickness (AMS) and to high altitude pulmonary edema (HAPE).

In the context of the two types of cerebral edema, cytotoxic (intracellular) and vasogenic, a leaking of proteins and water through the blood-brain barrier (BBB), a recent MRI study in persons ill with HACE (16) suggested a predominantly vasogenic mechanism. Causes of increased BBB permeability might include mechanical factors (loss of autoregulation and increased capillary pressure), ischemia, neurogenic influences (adrenergic and cholinergic activation), and a host of permeability mediators. Once vasogenic edema develops, cytotoxic edema generally follows, and although likely in HACE, this is still unproven. Symptoms of HACE are related to increased intracranial pressure (ICP), and death is from brain herniation. Treatment is directed both to lowering ICP by reducing the volume of intracranial contents, and to stopping the vasogenic leak.

Hypoxia: Into the Next Millennium,
Edited by R. C. Roach, *et al.* Kluwer Academic/Plenum Publishing, New York, 1999.

Evidence is accumulating that established moderate to severe AMS is due to cerebral edema, but whether this is true for early AMS (headache) is unclear. New work suggests that the brain swells on ascent to altitude, but that this is unrelated to AMS. Preliminary data showing that those with less cerebrospinal fluid volume (a tighter fit of the brain in the cranium) were more likely to develop AMS supports the hypothesis of Ross that those with less ability to accommodate the increased brain volume are the ones that suffer AMS. The blood-brain barrier and intracranial hemodynamics are the two key elements in the pathophysiology of HACE and AMS.

1.   INTRODUCTION

Acute mountain sicknesses (AMS) and high altitude cerebral edema (HACE) are related neurological disorders that strike unacclimatized persons on ascent to high altitude. While the clinical aspects of diagnosis, treatment and prevention of AMS and HACE are well established, their pathophysiology remains elusive. Clinical findings, neuroimaging, and autopsy clearly reveal brain edema as the cause of HACE, but what type of edema and what triggers it in only certain individuals is far from clear. Because of the close clinical relationship between AMS and HACE, physicians have considered for decades that HACE is a severe from of AMS, implying that AMS is mild cerebral edema (13, 18, 49). Supporting this idea, an excellent animal model has demonstrated increased brain water and elevated intracranial pressure (ICP) in sheep with what appears to be AMS (29). On the other hand, very few people with AMS actually develop HACE, and HACE is most often associated with high altitude pulmonary edema (HAPE; 15). Do AMS and HACE truly share a common pathophysiology and represent the two clinical ends of a pathological spectrum? Convincing evidence in humans is incomplete. My purpose is to address the following questions: 1) what do we know of the pathophysiology of the brain in HACE? 2) is AMS a mild form of HACE? and 3) what explains the inherent individual susceptibility to these maladies? Finally, what therapeutic implications follow from current concepts of the pathophysiology?

2.   CEREBRAL OXYGENATION AND METABOLISM

Is HACE due to cerebral hypoxia and/or altered metabolism? Careful measurements of brain oxygen delivery and metabolism are not yet available in humans with altitude illness. Persons acclimatizing well to moderate altitude appear to maintain brain O_2 delivery and metabolism, as reflected by normal cerebral venous PO_2 and normal overall cerebral metabolic rate (30). This is accomplished through increases in ventilation, cerebral blood flow, and hemoglobin concentration, the latter due to the decline in plasma volume (17). Oxygen delivery, therefore, is the net result of multiple factors that vary among individuals: hypoxic ventilatory response, hypocapnic ventilatory sensitivity, cerebral vasoreactivity to both oxygen and carbon dioxide, and fluid balance responses (See Severinghaus for a recent review of this complex subject (46)). To date, attempts to correlate AMS/HACE with any of these variables, or with the degree of hypoxemia, has been relatively fruitless, with the exception of the extreme hypoxemia of HAPE, the setting in which HACE occurs most often. During HAPE, it is unlikely that cerebral oxygenation can be maintained; experiments in humans and animals show that brain O_2 delivery is maintained only down to SaO_2 in the range of 80%, a value higher than commonly seen in HAPE. An answer to the question of the role of brain oxygenation and metabolism in HACE awaits measurements in ill humans. Careful measurements done in the hypoxic sheep model of AMS/HACE, however, make it clear that brain edema can develop without cerebral hypoxia. Cerebral oxygen delivery was maintained at or above sea level values, the fraction of oxygen extracted by the brain stayed the same, and global cerebral consumption of oxygen was stable. Despite no overall brain oxygen deficit, sheep still became ill with AMS/HACE.

If, as in the sheep model, cerebral oxygenation and global metabolism were normal, then how could we explain these neurologic syndromes? One possible explanation is neurotransmitter dysfunction. Although oxygen delivery is sufficient to maintain overall metabolism and energetics (no depletion of ATP), other extra-mitochondrial cellular processes may be affected that are much more sensitive to hypoxia. Specifically, the synthesis or metabolism of serotonin, dopamine and acetylcholine are very oxygen-sensitive. The Km for oxygen of tryptophan hydroxylase is 37 Torr, for tyrosine hydroxylase is 7.6 Torr, and for cytochrome oxidase is 0.07 Torr. As a result, high-energy phosphates (ATP) remain unchanged at arterial PO_2 values as low as 20-25 torr. In contrast, serotonin synthesis is diminished in animals at high altitude (8). Further, a few studies have suggested that dopaminergic drugs such as amphetamine or even a diet rich in tyrosine can improve cognitive function and well-being in humans at high altitude (3, 7). More recent work showed that dopamine synthesis itself was actually enhanced during hypoxia, suggesting that changes in post-synaptic receptors and signal transduction might be the source of altered dopaminergic function (2). Depletion of acetylcholine is a candidate for causing the fatigue so common at altitude (8). Neurotransmitter dysfunction most likely explains the reversible cognitive deficits and mood changes at high altitude, but could they account for some symptoms of acute mountain sickness? This hypothesis has not yet been addressed, and it deserves attention.

3.   MECHANISMS OF BRAIN SWELLING AND CEREBRAL EDEMA

The fact that cerebral hypoxia *per se* may not explain AMS/HACE raises the question of whether it is the changes responsible for maintaining oxygenation that are also responsible for cerebral edema. First, a distinction between brain edema and brain swelling is worthwhile. Brain edema is defined as an abnormal accumulation of fluid within the brain parenchyma, producing a volumetric enlargement of the tissue (24). Thus, neither a shift of water from the extracellular space to the intracellular space, nor a volumetric enlargement based on an increase in cerebral blood volume (CBV) constitutes edema. Brain swelling refers to enlargement of the brain from any cause, including increased blood volume or CSF volume. Accumulation of CSF in AMS/HACE is ruled out on the basis of neuroimaging which has shown small ventricles (22, 37, 54) and reduced extracerebral CSF (54) on ascent to altitude, both in those with and without illness.

3.1   Cerebral blood volume (CBV)

In contrast to the numerous measurements of cerebral blood flow during various clinical states at high altitude, measurements of cerebral blood volume are quite limited. In monkeys, a CBF increase of 50% increased CBV by about 15%, and twice that much for a flow increase of 100% (10). An equivalent volume increase (15%) in a 1500 gm human brain would be 6 to 8 mls (with the recent advent of near-infrared-spectroscopy, quantified measurements of CBV, as well as oxygenation and flow, should be forthcoming). An increase in CBV of 6 to 8 mls would be sufficient to displace some CSF, and therefore could be detected by neuroimaging as smaller ventricles and less extracerebral CSF. Such an increase in volume is probably easily buffered by CSF dynamics, and is insufficient to raise intracranial pressure and cause symptoms by itself. In the presence of brain edema, however, the intracranial pressure-volume curve is shifted to the left, and small increases in blood volume will cause large increases in intracranial pressure (ICP; Figure 1). Reflecting this fact, reducing blood volume by hyperventilation is a common practice in the treatment of cerebral edema. Thus, while a high CBV may cause brain swelling, it would contribute to increased ICP only in the setting of increased brain water (or inability to accommodate the swelling by CSF dynamics). Increased cerebral blood volume does not cause cerebral edema.

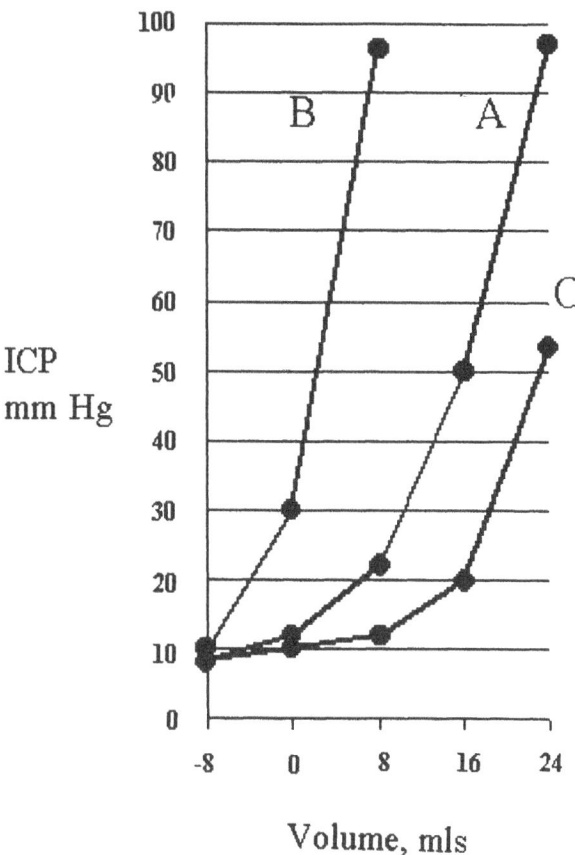

Figure 1. The relationship of pressure to volume in the cranium. Small increases in volume do not affect ICP until a threshold is reached, after which pressure rises exponentially (A). The initial flat part of the curve is due to accommodation by semi-elastic membranes and change in CSF dynamics. In the presence of edema (B), small changes in volume markedly impact CSF; the opposite is true in a dehydrated brain (C).

3.2   Fluid shifts and cytotoxic edema

Water accumulation in the brain can be due to cytotoxic edema
(intracellular), vasogenic edema (leak of the blood-brain barrier [BBB] with
extravasation of proteins), or both (the most common scenario) (25). Early
explanations of HACE (and AMS) invoked a cytotoxic mechanism, based on
the "normal" fluid shifts associated with successful acclimatization to high
altitude. Extracellular water declines (mostly due to the decrease in plasma
volume), and intracellular fluid (ICF) increases in most, but not all studies
(5, 6, 17, 20). Hannon showed an increase in total body ICF on the order of
0.25 liters, or 12% (17; see Figure 2). A mechanism for this shift into the
intracellular space was recently reported by Green et al., who found a down-
regulation of muscle Na+-K+ATPase in climbers to 6200 m (9). Although
fluid changes were not measured, the presumed decrease in cell membrane
ionic pumping could explain the increase in cell volume documented in the
previous studies. To what extent the normal brain at altitude or the "AMS
brain" participates in this shift is not known, but animal studies indicate such
a shift does take place in the brain (11). However, as mentioned, since no net
fluid gain results, this shift from the ECF does not cause edema. The
hypothesis that this "normal" shift of fluid into the ICF by itself causes
HACE (21) is therefore not tenable.

True cytotoxic edema generally develops from toxins affecting cell
membranes or from ischemia. In fact, with total ischemia, there is actually
no edema, merely a shift of fluid into the cells from the extracellular space.
However, with transient ischemia (cardiac arrest) or with partial reperfusion
(after ischemic stroke), water becomes available from the systemic
circulation, and it moves across the BBB into the extracellular space, first
because of the osmotic gradients resulting from tissue injury and interference
with cellular osmoregulation (with experimental ischemia, the cell swelling
can be detected by direct measurements within two to three minutes, and
increase in water content of the tissue within five minutes; 24). Secondly, an
opening of the BBB takes place that greatly influences the course and
outcome of the edema. At this stage, the edema becomes a combination of
cytotoxic and vasogenic, tissue damage is generally severe, and the edema is
more pronounced in gray matter than white matter. There are no data
supporting this scenario in response to the modest hypoxia of high altitude;
i.e., there is no evidence for a severe ischemic insult causing HACE. Once
HACE develops, however, cytotoxic edema may follow and worsen the
edema. This is because as extracellular fluid accumulates due to the
increased BBB permeability of vasogenic edema, the distance between the
capillary and the cell increases, and oxygen and nutrients cannot reach the
cells, rendering them ischemic (25). Hackett et al. argue that this situation

may well arise in the latter stages of HACE (16). (See vasogenic edema.) Severinghaus has also mentioned ischemia on this basis as a mechanism of HACE (47). Cytotoxic edema might develop as HACE progresses, but it does not explain AMS or the early stage of HACE.

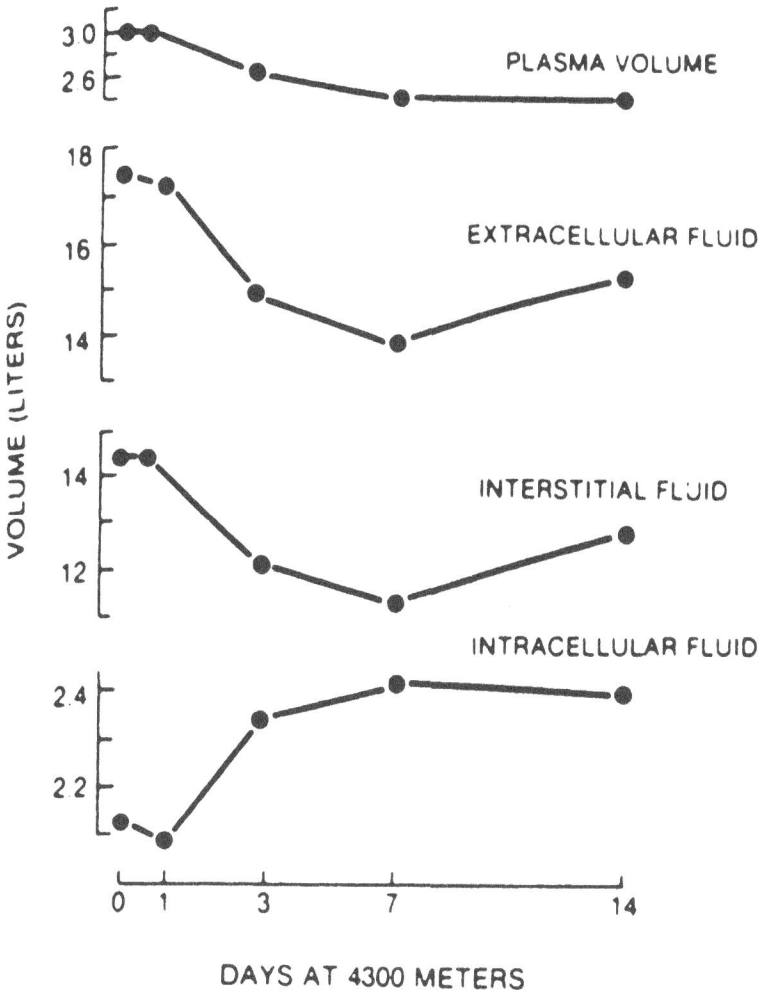

Figure 2. Changes in volume of body fluid compartments during successful acclimatization to 4300 m. The large decrease in extracellular fluid results from reductions in plasma volume, shift into the intracellular space, and diuresis. From (17).

3.3 Vasogenic edema

Recent evidence suggests that HACE is associated with vasogenic edema; i.e., a translocation of proteins and fluid from the vascular space across the BBB (16). Magnetic resonance imaging (MRI) in 7 of 9 men with HACE, 8 of whom also had HAPE, showed high T2 signal intensity in the white mater only, particularly in the corpus callosum (Figure 3). This pattern of reversible white matter edema without gray matter involvement indicates a vasogenic rather than cytotoxic mechanism, at least in the clinical stage when these scans were obtained. Gray matter consists of tightly packed, tangled cellular structures, whereas white matter has an orderly network of extracellular channels, is less dense, and offers less resistance to invasion by edema fluid. Vasogenic edema thus spreads preferentially through the white matter. Klatzo likens vasogenic edema to a river overflowing its banks; if it resolves prior to secondary ischemia, the brain tissue is left relatively undamaged (24). The clinical course supports this view, since all subjects made complete recovery, and the follow-up MRI scans were normal (16). Cytotoxic edema is not so benign (24). Other evidence for a vasogenic edema includes the time course of onset and resolution of HACE, animal experiments (27), the clinical response to steroids, the lack of neurologic sequelae, and tissue and cell experiments showing increased permeability of cerebral endothelium exposed to hypoxia.

What causes the vasogenic edema? As with HAPE, both mechanical factors (BBB failure equivalent to capillary failure in HAPE) (51) and biochemical mediators should be considered. Mayhan and Heistad (35) showed that acute, severe elevations of cerebral capillary pressure (Pcap) resulted in a mechanical vascular leak via disruption of cerebral veins. Abbott has demonstrated that stretching of brain endothelium induces increased BBB permeability (1). A number of authors have suggested that in the setting of hypoxic cerebral vasodilatation, autoregulation might be impaired (32), resulting in high cerebral capillary pressure (Pcap) and vasogenic edema (31, 50). Krasney and associates addressed this issue of cerebral vasodilatation, capillary pressure and brain edema in a series of sheep experiments. They first showed that cerebral Pcap rose from 20 to 50 mm Hg and remained elevated during 96 hours of hypoxia (28). This was accompanied by an increase in epidural pressure and increased filtration of plasma across the brain microcirculation; i.e., increased brain water, along with symptoms of AMS/HACE. To test whether the edema was due to the increased CBF and Pcap, they then subjected animals to CO_2 breathing and also to nitroglycerin infusion, both of which elevated CBF and Pcap to even greater levels than hypoxia, but neither of which produced as much brain edema as did hypoxia. They concluded that cerebral vasodilatation and elevated Pcap *per se* did not explain the edema (27, 53). It is important to note that there was no systemic hypertension or elevation of central venous pressure in these animal experiments, as there would be in humans at altitude during exercise. Nonetheless, these experiments indicate another factor besides vasodilatation is necessary to disrupt the BBB and cause AMS/HACE. Of course, as they comment, with any change in BBB conductance, flux of fluid will be greater in the presence of elevated capillary pressure. To state it another way, in the setting of elevated cerebral Pcap, only a small perturbation in BBB permeability is necessary to produce brain edema. Could chemical mediators induced by hypoxia or its consequences be the cause of vasogenic edema? Mediators identified to date include bradykinin, histamine, arachidonic acid, free radicals including oxygen and hydroxyl radicals, and nitric oxide. The role of nitric oxide (NO) is unclear. NO from endogenous (endothelial) NO synthase (eNOS) seems to be necessary for proper functioning of the BBB, (27, 45) while NO from inducible NO synthase (iNOS) appears to increase BBB permeability. Hypoxia strongly generates iNOS, and Clark has hypothesized that iNOS is a likely culprit to explain the edema of AMS/HACE, perhaps in an interaction with inflammatory cytokines (See p. 373 in this volume, (4)). Excellent recent reviews of vasogenic edema mediators are available. (See chapter 11 in this volume and 44, 45).

Other possible mechanisms of BBB permeability change also deserve consideration. Raichle, in an interesting study not yet repeated, demonstrated in monkeys a central noradrenergic mechanism that effected an increase in BBB permeability via innervation of the cerebral arterioles. Stimulation of the locus coeruleus prompted an immediate leak of the BBB (40). Others have suggested a general problem of endothelial dysfunction during hypoxia that produces leaky blood vessels (41). Increased permeability of the vascular bed of the brain, retina, lung, peripheral tissues, and kidney at high altitude support this notion, but data are presently insufficient to accept this hypothesis.

Severinghaus has proffered angiogenesis as a mechanism for HACE (47). A process well described in brain tumors and in neonatal development of the brain, angiogenesis produces new capillary growth in response to expression of vascular endothelial growth factor (VEGF). There is evidence that with acute hypoxia, even the adult brain will express VEGF secondary messengers, but no evidence yet that that this will actually increase BBB permeability as it does in tumors and neonates. Of interest is that this process is effectively blocked by dexamethasone (thus its effectiveness in shrinking brain tumors). Severinghaus also feels that angiogenesis explains the retinal hemorrhages (47); these hypotheses merit further investigation.

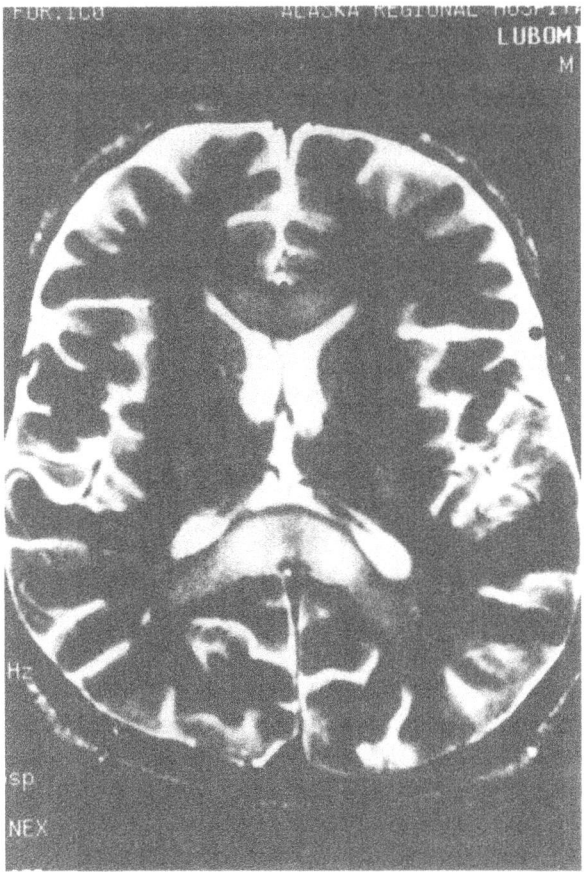

Figure 3. T-2 weighted magnetic resonance image of a mountain climber with high altitude cerebral edema, during acute illness (this page), and after recovery (top of next page). Note the markedly high signal in the area of the splenium of the corpus callosum.

4.   ACUTE MOUNTAIN SICKNESS

Is AMS due to mild cerebral edema? The clinical view of HACE as a severe form of AMS (14, 21, 49) implies that at some point in the illness of AMS, true brain edema develops, heralded clinically by elevated ICP, ataxia and altered mental status (encephalopathy), and demonstrable edema upon neuroimaging. However, HACE more commonly develops in persons with HAPE who often do not have a prodrome of AMS. This could reflect a different pathophysiology, but more likely, the severe hypoxemia of HAPE produces brain swelling rapidly, masking the earlier symptoms of AMS.

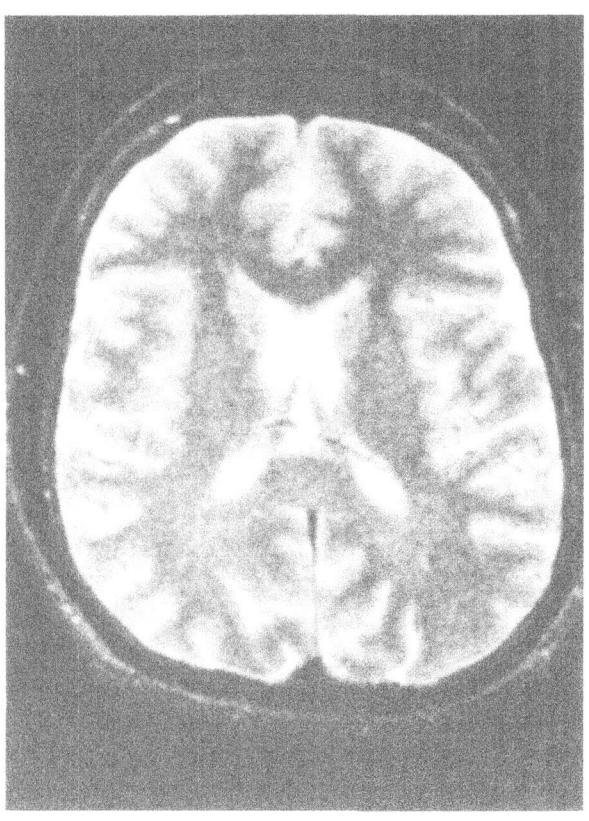

What is the evidence for brain edema in AMS? The model developed by Krasney and associates indicates that an AMS or HACE-like syndrome in sheep is associated with increased brain water and elevated intracranial pressure (29). Since they found evidence of severe edema, he labeled this a model of HACE. But the sheep exhibited symptoms similar to humans with moderate AMS: decreased appetite and marked lethargy, without unconsciousness, ataxia or death. The hazy line between AMS and HACE mirrors a common clinical situation in humans, and the term AMS/HACE reflects this overlap. The incidence of illness was similar to that reported for humans exposed to very high altitude (9 of 12 sheep exposed to 10% O_2 over 96 hrs), and control sheep exposed to the same hypoxia but without symptoms did not develop evidence of brain edema by wet-to-dry tissue ratios. This series of elegant studies is the best animal model to date, and compelling evidence that at least moderate to severe AMS is associated with brain edema. See Krasney for a recent review of this work (27).

Neuroimaging in humans has also provided evidence of brain edema in AMS, but inconsistently, in large part due to inconsistent definition of AMS and HACE. Kobayashi et al. performed head computerized tomography (CT) on 9 climbers with HAPE and "neurologic signs." (26). Four were in coma, 4 had drowsiness, and one had only a headache. Other signs such as ataxia were not reported. Eight of the 9 displayed clear cerebral edema. Without more details, whether some of these patients met the criteria for AMS, or whether all had clinical HACE is unknown. Levine et al. (33) reported diffuse low density on brain CT in the sickest of 5 subjects ill with AMS after a 48 hour altitude exposure, but did not mention specific signs and symptoms, and whether he had AMS or HACE is not clear. The report of Matsuzawa et al. (34) provides compelling evidence for brain edema in moderate to severe AMS. After a 24-hour simulated altitude exposure, T2 signal in the white matter was increased in the sickest 4 of 7 subjects with AMS, indicating vasogenic edema. These subjects met the criteria for AMS, and had no ataxia or altered mental status; i.e., they did not have clinical HACE. This study strongly suggests that moderate to severe AMS is an early stage of HACE.

Is there evidence for brain edema in the earliest stages of AMS? Two recent sophisticated MRI studies attempted to answer this question. Muza et al. demonstrated increased brain volume in men with and without AMS after 32 hours exposure to a simulated altitude of 4400 m (37). Post-exposure MRI was done with the subjects breathing hypoxic gas. Therefore, CBF and CBV were presumably still elevated. Though they could not differentiate blood from tissue volume, the 26 ml mean increase in volume is far more than expected from increased blood volume alone. All seven subjects had increased brain volume, unrelated to presence or severity of AMS, suggesting that the brain swells on ascent to altitude irrespective of AMS. Icenogle et al. and Kilgore et al. performed a similar study with 15 subjects (4 males) exposed to a simulated altitude of 4800 m for 8 to 12 hours (22). Subjects in this study were chosen on the basis of demonstrated susceptibility or resistance to AMS, and the ill subjects developed moderate to severe AMS (mean Lake Louise score = 6.8) They measured ventricular CSF rather than brain volume, and found a mean decrease of 12 ml (11%), with no difference between those who were well and those who were ill. Since the post-exposure MRI was done after at least 20 minutes of normoxia (the subjects were not kept hypoxic in the MR unit), CBF and blood volume might have returned to normal values, indicating that the decrease in CSF volume was reflecting an increase in brain water. As in the Muza study, however, without a way to subtract blood volume, the question of whether this represents an increase in blood or brain water is unsettled. Interestingly, Kilgore et al. did show a small but significant increase in T2 signal in the corpus callosum, hinting that vasogenic edema was starting (23). Those with AMS had twice the increase in signal of the non-AMS group, although the difference did not quite reach statistical significance. With a longer exposure, their results might have been similar to Matsuzawa; i.e., edema would have been more obvious in those with moderate to severe AMS. A third study also found brain swelling in early altitude exposure. Zavasky and Hackett reported that three subjects at simulated altitude for 8 to 10 hours had increased brain volume measured by MRI, without a relationship between volume change and AMS scores (54). As with the studies of Icenogle and Muza, these data imply that brain swelling occurs on ascent to altitude, it may or may not be edema, and it is not necessarily associated with AMS.

In summary, an animal model and neuroimaging studies with altitude exposure 24 hours or longer confirm vasogenic cerebral edema in moderate to severe AMS. In non-AMS, mild AMS, and in moderate to severe AMS groups with less than 24 hours altitude exposure, brain swelling is present, but whether this is due to increased blood volume or increased brain water requires further study. Although evidence is accumulating to support the hypothesis that AMS to HACE represents a continuum of mild to severe cerebral edema, sensitive non-invasive measurements of increased brain water and ICP are necessary to settle this issue in early AMS. Determining whether the initial headache is caused by cerebral vasodilatation, a migraine-like mechanism, brain edema and/or increased ICP will be particularly interesting and may lead to new therapies.

5. INTRACRANIAL PRESSURE

If all brains swell on ascent to altitude, could it be an incidental finding and have nothing to do with AMS? This might be true if the swelling were due merely to increased blood volume, but not if it is due to increased brain water. The sheep model clearly showed that increased brain water was associated with illness (28). If, as Hansen and Evans hypothesized (18), brain cell compression causes AMS, then we cannot answer the question of whether swelling is causing symptoms without measurements of ICP, preferably epidural pressure (27). Because of differences in volumetric buffering among individuals, the magnitude of the volume change does not predict the increase in ICP. The MRI's in AMS (33, 34) did not display compression of gyri or effacement of sulci suggestive of a severe elevation of ICP, but such gross changes would not be expected in those without frank clinical HACE. Symptoms could result, however, from a moderate elevation in ICP, or perhaps from transient episodes of raised ICP.

Direct measurements of ICP or CSF pressures in subjects with mild AMS are scarce. Hartig and Hackett did a pilot study with three subjects during simulated exposure to 5000 m altitude (19). CSF pressure measured by lumbar catheter while supine and at rest showed only a slight increase, without a relation to headache score. However, they also noted that CSF pressure became markedly elevated during moving about and during periodic breathing. One of their subjects with periodic breathing demonstrated a remarkable three-fold increase in ICP, from 10 to 30 mm Hg, in phase with the nadir of the oscillating SaO_2 (Hackett, unpublished observations). This suggested that brain compliance was altered, so that small changes in intracranial volume (blood) would markedly impact ICP. Measurements confirmed this: the change in CSF pressure for a given change in cerebral blood flow (induced by hypoxic gas breathing) was 43% higher at altitude than at sea level. Further, measures that objectively reduced ICP (oxygen and hyperventilation) improved symptoms, while increasing ICP by hypoxic gas or 7% CO_2 breathing (the latter which also raised SaO_2) made subjects considerably worse (12). These data are consistent with altered brain compliance due either to increased brain water or a large increase in blood volume. Cummins, a British neurosurgeon, noted a similar phenomenon in a climber who developed AMS at 4725 m. This man, who had an ICP telemetry device in place through a hole in his skull, had normal ICP values while lying still, but just turning his head nearly doubled his ICP, and it tripled with a "press up" done in the supine position. Upon descent to 3630 m, all values returned to normal after his symptoms of AMS resolved. The same measurements were normal in two others without AMS. Cummins considered this evidence for cerebral edema (B. Cummins, personal communication, 1991). One study that used an indirect measurement of ICP via tympanic membrane displacement and showed no increase of ICP in those with AMS is difficult to evaluate because of the questionable reliability of the technique (52). A fair summary is to say that despite the evidence for brain swelling and altered compliance in early AMS, limited data to date have not confirmed the presence of elevated intracranial pressure. Whether and at what point the ICP would be consistently elevated at rest in these AMS victims is unknown; continued monitoring of ICP as people become more severely ill would be unethical. A high research priority is for accurate non-invasive measurements of ICP across a spectrum of AMS severity in individuals undertaking their own altitude sojourns.

6. INTRACRANIAL HEMODYNAMICS, INDIVIDUAL SUSCEPTIBILITY AND THE "TIGHT FIT" HYPOTHESIS

The adult intracranial vault contains on average roughly 1500 ml of brain matter (1400 grams, 45 to 60 ml of blood, and approximately 60 ml of CSF, with another 60 ml CSF in the spinal canal. Since the brain is encased in a membrane with little elasticity inside a rigid skull, small increases in volume can increase intracranial pressure (Figure 1). Volume buffering within the cranium is accomplished through CSF dynamics: first a displacement of CSF through the foramen magnum into the available space in the spinal canal, then increased re-absorption of CSF at the arachnoid villi, and thirdly, decreased CSF production (36; Figure 4). When brain swelling is too great for successful accommodation by a change in CSF dynamics, pressure rises rapidly and exponentially, the brain compresses against fixed structures in the cranium, and the relatively elastic vascular compartment compresses and CBF diminishes, producing ischemia. Interestingly, the volume buffering capacity depends on the anatomy of the craniospinal axis. Brain swelling is better tolerated when a greater proportion of the neuroaxis is CSF, such as in the atrophic elderly or those of any age who happen to have a large spinal canal. The brain volume to intracranial volume ratio assesses the "tightness" of the brain in the cranial vault. This ratio is generally higher in children (.95 to .98), and tends to vary more in adults (.92 to .98) Primarily, it is a function of individual anatomy, with a small decline with increasing age. Another consideration in children, and particularly infants, is that immature cranial sutures and open fontanels also allow for some accommodation of brain swelling.

Secondly, a larger spinal canal affords greater volumetric buffering. Research in children with hydrocephalus and with animal mod s has led to the construct of the pressure volume index (PVI), a calculation that reflects the compliance of the system when all compartments are communicating, as is the case during hypoxia. Simply put, it is the volume required to raise the ICP tenfold. This number is variable, but on average, it is about 26 mls for the adult brain (48; Figure 5). The PVI is highly related to the diameter of the spinal canal; in particular, the sagittal subarachnoid space at the level of the 7th thoracic vertebra (38; Figure 6). Normal anatomical variation displayed in the figure explains the variation in the PVI. Ross, a neurologist in Edmonton, proposed in 1985 an explanation for the apparent random nature of AMS (43). He reasoned that since persons with smaller intracranial and intraspinal CSF capacity have less compliance, they would become more symptomatic from mild brain swelling, and develop AMS. This "tight fit" hypothesis, as I call it, could help explain the inherent individual susceptibility. An explanation invoking random anatomical differences might also explain the poor correlation of AMS with oxygen transport, CBF, hemoglobin, hypoxic ventilatory response, or any other physiological variable examined to date, including the brain swelling seen in mild AMS. Cummins tested part of this hypothesis with a pilot study about 10 years ago.

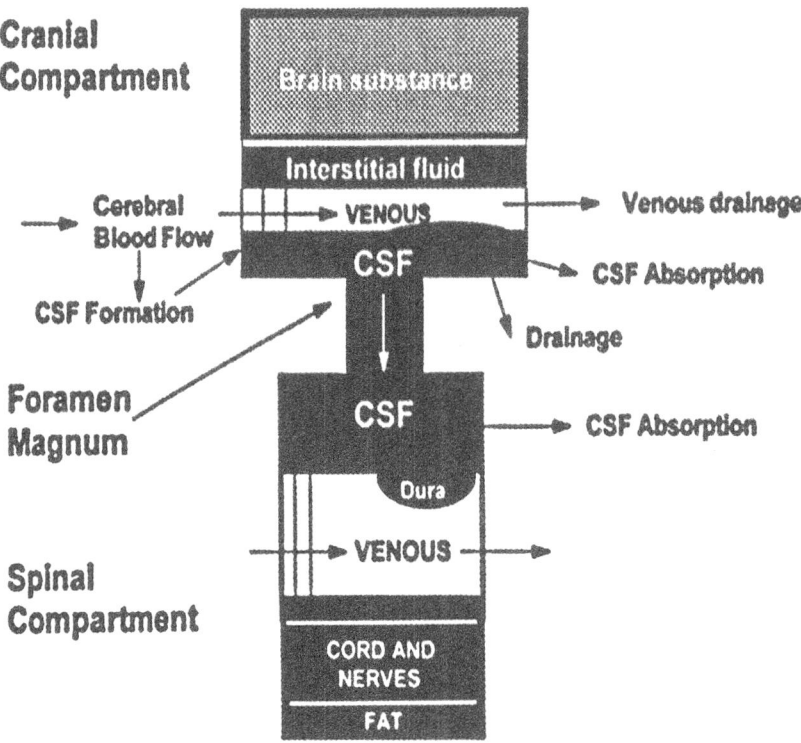

Figure 4. A schematic diagram of CSF dynamics. In response to an increase in brain volume, CSF is displaced into the spinal canal, CSF absorption increases, and CSF formation declines. Adapted from (42).

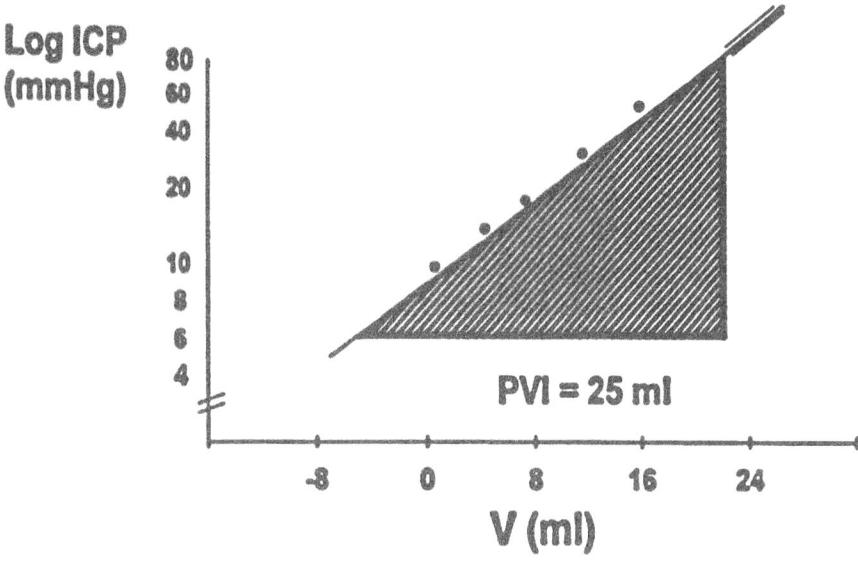

Figure 5. The pressure-volume index indicates the volume addition in the cranium required to raise the ICP tenfold. From 42).

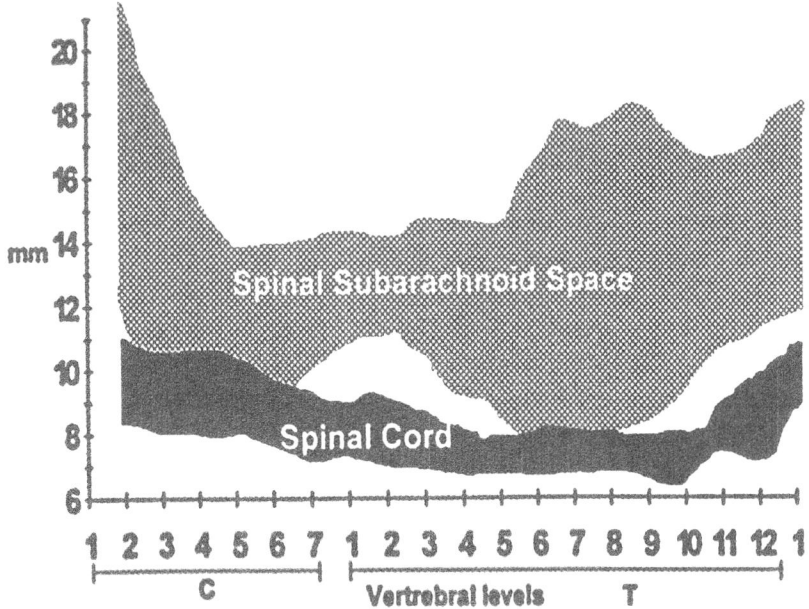

Figure 6. A diagram of the range of values of the sagittal diameter of spinal cord (lower lines) and subarachnoid space (upper lines) at various vertebral levels in age groups 18-88 years. From (38).

Using a five-point scale, he scored the brain ventricular volumes of 11 Himalayan climbers by CT scanning prior to the expedition, and then compared both an AMS score and a separate neurological score with ventricular size, and found a significant inverse correlation (B. Cummins, personal communication, 1991). Zavasky and Hackett did a similar analysis with MR measurement of brain volume to intracranial vault volume ratios in three subjects before and after simulated altitude exposure. Although too few subjects to analyze the data statistically, the ranking of the measured ratios exactly matched the ranking for symptoms and for age (inversely for age), supporting the hypothesis that a "tight brain" predisposed an individual to AMS (54). No one has yet attempted to correlate spinal canal volumes with AMS, nor examine the relationship of AMS to the combination of brain "tightness" and spinal diameter. This interesting idea supported by preliminary data certainly warrants further study. Figure 7 incorporates this concept into a schema of pathophysiology.

7.   IMPLICATIONS FOR THERAPY

Successful therapy of AMS/HACE should be directed to reducing brain volume and ICP and stopping the vasogenic leak. Increasing the inspired and alveolar PO_2 by oxygen, descent or hyperbaria immediately reduces CBF and blood volume, and therefore ICP. These measures also improve arterial oxygenation and stop the stimulus for brain edema formation. Hyperventilation at least transiently improves oxygenation and reduces CBF and CBV. Acetazolamide, while it does not reduce CBF and CBV, does increase oxygenation by increasing ventilation, reduces CSF formation, and forces a diuresis. Furosemide also reduces brain extracellular volume through its diuretic action, and was found to be very useful by the Indian Army (49). The osmotic diuretics (mannitol, urea and glycerol) are particularly effective, at least transiently, for vasogenic edema, but have not been tested in AMS/HACE. Dexamethasone is thought to reduce BBB leak by many different pathways; it blocks angiogenesis, blocks lipid peroxidation, stabilizes mast cells, and might affect iNOS production. Steroids also block the hypoxia-induced permeability increase in cerebral endothelial monolayer cultures (39). The fact that dexamethasone is so effective in treating and preventing AMS suggests that the pathophysiology must be related to a pathway or pathways influenced by the drug. As the molecular mechanism of AMS/HACE unfolds, even more specific and better therapeutic agents will become available.

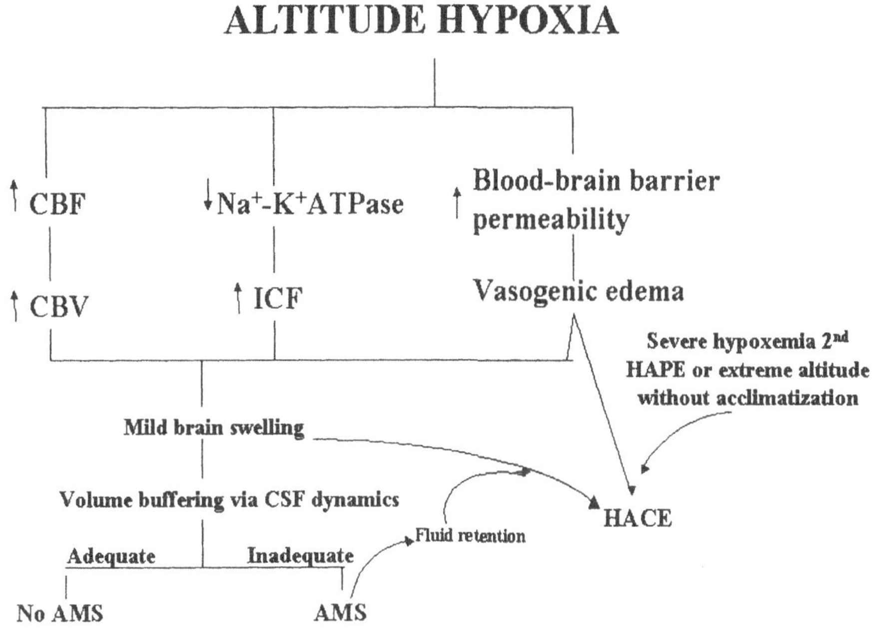

ALTITUDE HYPOXIA

Figure 7. A schema of pathophysiology of AMS and HACE. Symbols: CBF = cerebral blood flow, CBV = cerebral blood volume, ICF = intracellular fluid, BBB = blood-brain barrier. The primary mechanism of AMS/HACE is vasogenic edema, but increased blood volume and intracellular fluid volume will contribute to the altered brain compliance and increase in ICP as illness progresses. Mild edema remains asymptomatic if CSF volumetric buffering is successful. Once AMS develops, fluid retention aggravates edema formation.

8.   SUMMARY

Despite normal cerebral oxygenation and normal global cerebral metabolism, vasogenic edema develops in humans (and sheep) who become moderately ill with AMS during 24 hours or more of hypoxic exposure. The hypothesis that AMS is due to cerebral edema appears true for moderate to severe illness, but whether early AMS, especially the headache, is caused by edema is not known. Other mechanisms for the headache, perhaps similar to those of migraine need to be explored. Hypoxic cerebral vasodilatation appears to be a necessary ingredient, but does not *per se* explain the development of brain edema. HACE is predominantly a vasogenic edema, and a number of biochemical mediators as well as mechanical factors might play a role in the pathophysiology. Brain cell swelling (cytotoxic edema) likely has a role only in the later stages of HACE, and not in AMS. New data suggest that the brain swells upon ascent to high altitude regardless of AMS. Whether this is due to edema or engorgement with blood is not yet clear. The "tight fit" hypothesis proposes that individual anatomy of the craniospinal axis determines tolerance to mild brain swelling and might help explain individual susceptibility; preliminary studies support this notion. Therapy of AMS and HACE is directed to reducing brain volume and stopping the blood-brain barrier leak (i.e., oxygenation, diuretics and steroids), before secondary ischemia develops. New therapies directed specifically toward the defect in BBB permeability are likely to be successful and warrant investigation.

REFERENCES

1. Abbott, N., and P. Revest. Control of brain endothelial permeability. *Cerebrovasc Brain Metb Rev* 3: 39-72, 1991.
2. Akiyama, Y., K. Koshimura, T. Ohue, K. Lee, S. Miwa, S. Yamagata, and H. Kikuchi. Effects of hypoxia on the activity of the dopaminergic neuron system in the rat striatum as studied by in vivo brain microdialysis. *J Neurochem* 57: 997-1002, 1991.
3. Banderet, L. E., and H. R. Lieberman. Treatment with tyrosine, a neurotransmitter precursor, reduces environmental stress in humans. *Brain Res Bull* 22: 759-762, 1989.
4. Clark, I. Can excessive iNOS induction explain much of the illness of acute mountain sickness? (Abstract). In: *Hypoxia: Into the Next Millennium*, edited by R.C. Roach, P.D. Wagner and P.H. Hackett. New York: Kluwer Academic/Plenum Publishers, 1999.
5. Claybaugh, J. R., D. P. Brooks, and A. Cymerman. Hormonal control of fluid and electrolyte balance at high altitude in normal subjects. In: *Hypoxia and Mountain Medicine*, edited by J. R. Sutton, G. Coates and C. S. Houston. Burlington, VT: Queen City Press, 1992.
6. Consolazio, C. F., H. L. Johnson, and H. J. Krzywicki. Body fluids, body composition, and metabolic aspects of high-altitude adaptation. In: *Physiological Adaptations: Desert and Mountain*, edited by M. K. Yousef, S. M. Horvath and R. W. Bullard. New York, NY: Academic Press, 1972, p. 227-241.
7. Dill, D. B., O. O. Benson, W. H. Forbes, and F. G. Hall. Benzedrine sulphate (amphetamine) and acute anoxia. I. respiratory effects. *J Aviat Med* 11: 1-6, 1940.
8. Gibson, G. E., W. Pulsinelli, J. P. Blass, and T. E. Duffy. Brain dysfunction in mild to moderate hypoxia. Am J Med 70: 1247-1254, 1981.
9. Green, H., B. Roy, S. Grant, M. Burnett, C. Otto, A. Pipe, and D. McKenzie. Down-regulation in muscle Na-K ATPase concentration following a 21 day expedition to 6200 m (Abstract). In: *Hypoxia: Into the Next Millennium*, edited by R.C. Roach, P.D. Wagner and P.H. Hackett. New York: Kluwer Academic/Plenum Publishers, 1999
10. Grubb, R. L., M. E. Raichle, J. O. Eichling, and M. M. Ter-Pogossian. The effects of changes in PaCO2 on cerebral blood volume, blood flow, and vascular mean transit time. *Stroke* 5: 630-639, 1974.
11. Gwan, K., J. Gazendam, and A. K. Van Zanten. Influence of hypoxia on the composition of isolated edema fluid in cold-induced brain edema. *J Neurosurg* 51: 78-84, 1979.
12. Hackett, P., and G. Hartig. Cerebral blood velocity and cerebral spinal fluid pressure in acute mountain sickness. In: *Hypoxia and Mountain Medicine*, edited by J. Sutton, G. Coates and C. Houston. Burlington, Vermont: Quenn City Printers, 1991, p. 302.

13. Hackett, P. H., I. D. Rennie, R. F. Grover, and J. T. Reeves. Acute mountain sickness and the edemas of high altitude: A common pathogenesis? *Respir Physiol* 46: 383-390, 1981.

14. Hackett, P. H., I. D. Rennie, and H. D. Levine. The incidence, importance, and prophylaxis of acute mountain sickness. Lancet 2: 1149-1154, 1976.

15. Hackett, P. H., and R. C. Roach. High-altitude medicine. In: *Wilderness Medicine*, edited by P. A. Auerbach. St. Louis: Mosby, 1995, p. 1-37.

16. Hackett, P. H., P. R. Yarnell, R. Hill, K. Reynard, J. Heit, and J. McCormick. High-altitude cerebral edema evaluated with magnetic resonance imaging: clinical correlation and pathophysiology. *JAMA* 280: 1920-1925, 1998.

17. Hannon, J. P., K. S. Chinn, and J. L. Shields. Effects of acute high altitude exposure on body fluids. Fed Proc 28: 1178-1184, 1969.

18. Hansen, J. E., and W. O. Evans. A hypothesis regarding the pathophysiology of acute mountain sickness. *Arch Environ Health* 21: 666-669, 1970.

19. Hartig, G. S., and P. H. Hackett. Cerebral spinal fluid pressure and cerebral blood velocity in acute mountain sickness. In: *Hypoxia and Mountain Medicine*, edited by J. R. Sutton, G. Coates and C. S. Houston. Burlington, VT: Queen City Press, 1992.

20. Honig, A. Electrolytes, body fluid volumes and renal function in acute hypoxic hypoxia. *Acta Physiol Pol* 30: 93-125, 1979.

21. Houston, C. S., and J. G. Dickinson. Cerebral form of high altitude illness. *Lancet* 2: 758-761, 1975.

22. Icenogle, M., D. Kilgore, J. Sanders, A. Caprihan, and R. Roach. Cranial CSF volume (cCSF) is reduced by altitude exposure but is not related to early acute mountain sickness (AMS) (Abstract). In: *Hypoxia: Into the Next Millennium*, edited by R.C. Roach, P.D. Wagner and P.H. Hackett. New York: Kluwer Academic/Plenum Publishers, 1999

23. Kilgore, D., J. Loeppky, J. Sanders, A. Caprihan, M. Icenogle, and R. Roach. Corpus callosum (CC) MRI: Early altitude exposure (Abstract). In: *Hypoxia: Into the Next Millennium*, edited by R.C. Roach, P.D. Wagner and P.H. Hackett. New York: Kluwer Academic/Plenum Publishers, 1999

24. Klatzo, I. Pathophysiologic aspects of brain edema. *Acta Neuropath (Berl)* 72: 236-239, 1987.

25. Klatzo, I. Presidential address: Neuropathologic aspects of brain edema. *J Neuropath Exp Neurol* 26: 1-14, 1967.

26. Kobayashi, T., S. Koyama, K. Kubo, M. Fukushima, and S. Kusama. Clinical features of patients with high altitude pulmonary edema in Japan. *Chest* 92: 814-821, 1987.

27. Krasney, J. A. Cerebral hemodynamics and high altitude cerebral edema. In: *Hypoxia: Women at Altitude*, edited by C. S. Houston and G. Coates. Burlington: Queen City Publishers, 1997, p. 254-267.

28. Krasney, J. A. A neurogenic basis for acute altitude illness. *Med Sci Sports Exerc* 26: 195-208, 1994.

29. Krasney, J. A., D. C. Curran-Everett, and J. Iwamoto. High altitude cerebral edema: An animal model. In: *Hypoxia: The Adaptations*, edited by J. R. Sutton, G. Coates and J. E. Remmers. Philadelphia, PA: BC Dekker, 1990, p. 200-205.

30. Lassen, N. A. The brain: cerebral blood flow. In: *Hypoxia: Man at Altitude*, edited by J. R. Sutton, N. L. Jones and C. S. Houston. New York, NY: Thieme-Stratton, 1982, p. 9-13.

31. Lassen, N. A., and A. M. Harper. High-altitude cerebral oedema. *Lancet* : 1154, 1975.

32. Levine, B. Dynamic cerebral autoregulation at high altitude (Abstract). In: *Hypoxia: Into the Next Millennium*, edited by R.C. Roach, P.D. Wagner and P.H. Hackett. New York: Kluwer Academic/Plenum Publishers, 1999.

33. Levine, B. D., K. Yoshimura, T. Kobayashi, M. Fukushima, T. Shibamoto, and G. Ueda. Dexamethasone in the treatment of acute mountain sickness. *N Engl J Med* 321: 1707-1713, 1989.

34. Matsuzawa, Y., T. Kobayashi, K. Fujimoto, S. Shinozaki, and S. Yoshikawa. Cerebral edema in acute mountain sickness. In: *High Altitude Medicine*, edited by G. Ueda, J. T. Reeves and M. Sekiguchi. Matsumoto, Japan: Shinshu Univ Press, 1992, p. 300-304.

35. Mayhan, W., and D. Heistad. Role of veins and cerebral venous pressure in disruption of the blood-brain barrier. *Circ Res* 59: 216-220, 1986.

36. Miller, J. Volume and pressure in the craniospinal axis. Clin Neurosurg 22: 76-105, 1975.

37. Muza, S., T. Lyons, P. Rock, C. Fulco, B. Beidleman, S. Smith, I. Morocz, G. Zientaral, and A. Cymerman. Effect of altitude exposure on brain volume and development of acute mountain sickness (AMS) (Abstract). In: *Hypoxia: Into the Next Millennium*, edited by R.C. Roach, P.D. Wagner and P.H. Hackett. New York: Kluwer Academic/Plenum Publishers, 1999.

38. Nordqvist, L. The sagittal diameter of the spinal cord and subarachnoid space in different age groups: a roentgenographic post-mortem study. *Act Radiol Diagn (Stockh)* suppl 227: 1-96, 1964.

39. Ogawa, S., S. Koga, and R. Kuwabara. Hypoxia-induced increased permeability of endothelial monolayers occurs through lowering of cellular cAMP levels. *Am J Physiol* 262: C546-C554, 1992.

40. Raichle, M., B. Hartman, J. Eichling, and L. Sharpe. Central noradrenergic regulation of cerebral blood flow and vascular permeability. *Proc Nat Acad Sci* , 1975.

41. Richalet, J. P., A. Hornych, C. Rathat, J. Aumont, P. Larmignant, and P. Remy. Plasma prostaglandins, leukotrienes and thromboxane in acute high altitude hypoxia. *Respir Physiol* 85: 205-215, 1991.

42. Ropper, A. Raised intracranial pressure in neurologic disease. *Sem Neurology* 4: 397-407, 1984.

43. Ross, R. T. The random nature of cerebral mountain sickness. Lancet 1: 990-991, 1985.

44. Schilling, L. Mediators of vasogenic edema. In: *Hypoxia: Into the Next Millennium*, edited by R.C. Roach, P.D. Wagner and P.H. Hackett. New York: Kluwer Academic/Plenum Publishers, 1999.

45. Schilling, L., and M. Wahl. Brain edema: Pathogenesis and therapy. *Kidney Int* 51: S69-S75, 1997.

46. Severinghaus, J. Cerebral Circulation at Altitude. In: *High Altitude*, edited by T. Hornbein and R. Schoene. New York: Marcel Decker, 1999.

47. Severinghaus, J. W. Hypothetical roles of angiogenesis, osmotic swelling, and ischemia in high-altitude cerebral edema. *J Appl Physiol* 79: 375-9, 1995.

48. Shapiro, K., A. Marmarou, and K. Shulman. Characterization of clinical CSF dynamics and neural axis compliance using the pressure-volume index. I: The normal pressure-volume index. *Ann Neurol* 7: 508-514, 1980.

49. Singh, I., P. K. Khanna, M. C. Srivastava, M. Lal, S. B. Roy, and C. S. V. Subramanyam. Acute mountain sickness. *N Engl J Med* 280: 175-184, 1969.

50. Sutton, J. R., and N. Lassen. Pathophysiology of acute mountain sickness and high altitude pulmonary oedema: an hypothesis. *Bull Europ Physiopath Respir* 15: 1045-1052, 1979.

51. West, J. B., and O. Mathieu-Costello. High altitude pulmonary edema is caused by stress failure of pulmonary capillaries. *Intl J Sport Med* 13: S54-S58, 1992.

52. Wright, A. D., C. H. Imray, M. S. Morrissey, R. J. Marchbanks, and A. R. Bradwell. Intracranial pressure at high altitude and acute mountain sickness. *Clin Sci Colch* 89: 201-4, 1995.

53. Yang, S. P., and J. A. Krasney. Cerebral blood flow and metabolic responses to sustained hypercapnia in awake sheep. *J Cereb Blood Flow Metab* 15: 115-123, 1995.

54. Zavasky, D., and P. Hackett. Cerebral etiology of acute mountain sickness MRI findings. *Wilderness Environ Med* 6: 229-230, 1995.

Chapter 3

Lung Disease at High Altitude

Robert B. Schoene

Division of Pulmonary and Critical Care Medicine, University of Washington,
Providence/Seattle Medical Center, 500 17ᵗʰ Ave, Seattle, WA 98124, USA

Key words: pulmonary disease, asthma, COPD, emphysema, bronchitis

Abstract: The lungs are a delicate interface between the atmosphere and our bodies across which oxygen diffuses from the air we breathe to the blood which carries oxygen to the cells and mitochondria. In healthy lungs at sea level where there is a surfeit of oxygen, this process occurs easily, whereas, in lungs with disease it becomes a task which may not be fully successful and hypoxemia may ensue or worsen. At high altitude where the barometric pressure (Pb) and thus the supply of oxygen is lower, the job of getting oxygen to the blood, even in the healthy lung is more difficult, and in the diseased lung it may be impossible. This presentation will review the lungs' responses to high altitude, with emphasis on the abnormal. Both acute and chronic responses of patients with pre-existing lung disease will be reviewed. Pulmonary diseases encountered at high altitude in previously healthy people, such as high altitude pulmonary edema and chronic mountain sickness will be touched on only as they pertain to other patients. Pre-existing lung disease (with and without hypoxemia at sea level) such as obstructive lung diseases (asthma, COPD, emphysema), and restrictive lung diseases (sarcoid, asbestosis, interstitial pulmonary fibrosis) will be discussed in terms of gas exchange, lung mechanics, and treatment at high altitude. Disorders of ventilatory control; e.g., obesity-hypoventilation syndrome and sleep apnea, may present formidable problems, and guidelines for their treatment will be discussed. Infectious lung diseases; e.g., pneumonia, cystic fibrosis, and pulmonary vascular disorders such as chronic mountain sickness, primary pulmonary hypertension, and congenital absence of the pulmonary artery are important disorders that require special attention because of the accentuated hypoxic pulmonary vascular response encountered at high altitude. The purpose therefore, is to provide the medical practitioner with the insight into prevention, recognition, and treatment of pulmonary problems encountered specifically at high altitude, as well as guidance on how best to advise patients with lung disease who want to fly in airplanes and/or ascend to high altitude for work or pleasure.

1.   INTRODUCTION

On the journey of oxygen from the air to the mitochondria, the lung imposes the first and most formidable barrier. Even across the healthy lung, the greatest drop in the partial pressure of oxygen from atmospheric air to the cells occurs. This is imposed by the partial pressure of carbon dioxide in the alveolus as well as impairment of the diffusion of oxygen from the air to the blood across the alveolar-capillary membrane. In the healthy lung, this feat is achieved rather easily; but in a lung that has disease, especially at high altitude, an already decreased partial pressure of oxygen in the air encounters formidable obstacles on its route to the hemoglobin molecule in the blood. It will be the purpose of this paper, first to discuss briefly the lungs response to high altitude and the pulmonary pathophysiology that is unique to the high altitude environment, and then discuss more extensively the effect of high altitude upon individuals with pre-existing lung disease at low altitude.

2.   THE LUNG'S RESPONSE TO HIGH ALTITUDE

At high altitude the lung encounters air that is less dense than that at sea level; and although the fraction of oxygen is the same throughout Earth's atmosphere, this decreased density is a reflection of the lower barometric pressure and thus the lower content of oxygen in the air. Additionally, the air may be colder and drier.

Oxygen is transported from the air to the blood through the lung by both convection and diffusion. Convection is the transport of oxygen in the air through the conducting airways from the trachea to the smallest respiratory bronchioles. In order to carry out this task, the lung must generate differential pressures from the atmosphere to the alveoli, which is a function of lung mechanics. Air is drawn into the lung by the development of a pressure which is negative relative to the atmospheric pressures. This is perpetrated by the strength of the respiratory muscles and the compliance of the thorax. The density of air is less at high altitude conveying a lower resistive load to breathing than at sea level. This results in less work of breathing especially in patients with obstructive and restrictive lung disease although the clinical significance has never been quantified.

The quantity of oxygen in the alveolus is dependent upon the degree of alveolar ventilation that, by the law of mass balance, strikes a balance between the other main gases in the alveolus: carbon dioxide and nitrogen. The greater the degree of alveolar ventilation, the lower is the partial pressure of carbon dioxide, and the higher the partial pressure of oxygen. This partial pressure of oxygen plays a critical role in the next major step of the transport of oxygen from the air to the blood, which is by diffusion. Diffusion is critically dependent upon a drop in partial pressure of oxygen from the air to the blood, thus the greater the degree of alveolar ventilation, the higher is the partial pressure of oxygen in the alveolus and thus the greater driving pressure for oxygen to the blood. Any lung diseases, which impair alveolar ventilation, such as respiratory muscle weakness, fixation of the thoracic cage, or an increase in airway resistance such as in obstructive lung diseases, could minimize alveolar oxygen partial pressure. Of course, this is a critical factor at high altitude where the ambient partial pressure of oxygen decreases the higher one goes. The resultant partial pressure of oxygen in the alveolus and thus the driving pressure for diffusion are less.

Another important factor which is particularly critical at very high altitude is the drive to breathe which emanates from the central nervous system such that any impairment in this drive may lead to a less than optimal degree of alveolar ventilation and thus relative alveolar hypoxia. In patients with lung disease the ability to generate a greater degree of alveolar ventilation, in spite of the central drive, may be impaired which further accentuates the dilemma of attaining adequate oxygenation ultimately to he tissues.

3.   REACTION OF RESPIRATION TO HIGH ALTITUDE

The sequence of events of the ventilatory response to high altitude begins with an increase in alveolar ventilation stimulated by an increase in respiratory drive from the hypoxemia. Once oxygen is in the alveolus, the process of transfer of oxygen from air to the blood, as mentioned above, depends upon a diffusion gradient for oxygen. The alveolar-epithelial lining imposes very little resistance for diffusion of oxygen into the plasma through the capillary and endothelial layer. The next step requires some affinity of hemoglobin for binding oxygen which is augmented by a left-shift in the oxygen-hemoglobin disassociation curve, secondary to the respiratory alkalosis from the hypoxemic stimulus.

Another important response of the lung to high altitude is the rapid development of increased pressures in the pulmonary vasculature that are a result of the hypoxic pulmonary vasoconstrictive response (HPVR) initiated by alveolar hypoxia. The degree of this response may play an important role in the adaptation and maladaption of individuals to high altitude in that those with a brisk HPVR and accentuated degree of hypoxemia secondary to lung disease are particularly susceptible to marked pulmonary hypertension and right-heart failure.

4.   CLINICAL CONDITIONS SPECIFIC TO HIGH ALTITUDE

Little space will be dedicated in this chapter to conditions that are unique to high altitude. They will be discussed at length in a number of other places in this volume. The two entities though which are worthy of note are high altitude pulmonary edema (HAPE) and chronic mountain sickness (CMS). They are mentioned in the context of gaining insight into the physiologic responses to hypoxia which, when of a certain degree, are appropriate and beneficial and, when they are excessive, are clearly detrimental.

HAPE is a non-cardiogenic form of pulmonary edema that occurs in otherwise healthy individuals who have ascended too rapidly to high altitude without time for acclimatization. Although the disease can be fatal, it is easily treated with oxygen or descent to a lower altitude. Importantly, the lung architecture usually remains intact. Of particular interest is the association of HAPE with accentuated pulmonary artery pressures which may be the initiating stress on the pulmonary capillary epithelium which subsequently leaks from the intra- to extra-vascular space, including the alveoli. What is, therefore, usually a normal response to exposure to high altitude that improves ventilation and perfusion match and thus gas exchange, becomes excessive and thus may be deleterious.

CMS is another entity that is an example of an exaggerated physiologic response to the stress of hypoxia. In CMS, accentuated hypoxemia from inadequate alveolar ventilation and excessive erythrocytosis are the initiating culprits for the disease which then leads to accentuated pulmonary hypertension, cor pulmonale and subsequent right-heart failure. Extraordinary examples of secondary polycythemia occur primarily in the Andes and in some areas of North America, and it is interesting to speculate about why the signal of hypoxemia initiates such an extraordinary, abnormal response leading to high morbidity and mortality.

5. SEA LEVEL PULMONARY CONDITIONS AFFECTED BY HIGH ALTITUDE

An excellent treatise of pulmonary diseases affected by high altitude is presented by Hackett (8a), but the following will deal with a few further specific points.

5.1 Chronic Obstructive Pulmonary Disease

Obstructive lung disease is the most common clinical entity encountered in any practice of pulmonary medicine. Its main underlying pathophysiologic characteristic is high resistance to airflow in the airways, which leads to areas of low ventilation with respect to perfusion, which leads to hypoxemia. Thus , the hypoxemia of high altitude would be more profound. The lower density gas at high altitude, which should improve airflow, is not enough to overcome the increase in airway resistance from these diseases. Chronic bronchitis, emphysema and asthma are the major entities to be considered.

Smoking which is so common all around the world is the major culprit contributing to the high prevalence of COPD. From a physiologic standpoint, this category of obstructive airway disease is particularly affected by hypobaric hypoxia. As this disease fluctuates on a periodic basis, and as the patients operate on a very steep portion of the oxygen-hemoglobin dissociation curve, small changes in PaO_2 lead to much more profound changes in arterial oxygen saturation. Thus, Renzetti et al. (14) found that the death rate for COPD at some high communities in the United States was higher than that for a low altitude group during a two and half year follow up (50 versus 35 per cent). These findings were corroborated by other studies at high altitude areas in the United States (2, 10) and may have been the factor for many people with COPD leaving their high altitude homes for lower altitude communities (13). In COPD, the combination of smoking and living at high altitude can be a lethal combination; whereas, each factor can act independently on the increase in mortality (1). In some high altitude communities in South America and Asia, the lack of chimney ventilation in many houses where wood fires are used for cooking and heat can add a third co-morbid factor (15). Clearly, moving to a lower altitude where the barometric pressure is higher would improve longevity and lifestyle in many of these patients. In fact, an interesting study by Kramer (8) showed that moving patients with severe COPD to below sea level (the Dead Sea barometric pressure almost 800mm Hg) increased their PaO_2 from a precarious 54 mm Hg to 69 mm Hg.

The low altitude physician, therefore, must be aware of the effect of high altitude in patients with COPD, since a move to or a trip to visit relatives at even modest high altitude may have devastating effects upon the precariously hypoxemic low altitude COPD patient. Supplemental oxygen must be considered as a temporary therapeutic option in many patients whose oxygen saturations hover around 90% at low altitude; an increase in the amount of supplemental oxygen in patients already on it may be important. Furthermore, the same guidelines should be followed during air travel, where the commercial airline cabin pressure may vary anywhere from a comparable altitude of 6000 to 8500 feet. The average barometric pressure in airplanes of approximately 600 mm Hg results in even mild hypoxemia in normal individuals; in patients with hypoxemic COPD the PaO_2 may be precariously low (16).

A number of investigators (3-7) have issued guidelines on how to evaluate and treat patients with hypoxemia who are going to travel by air, but these methods are often tedious. It may be more efficacious merely to order low-flow oxygen to patients whose oxygen saturations linger anywhere from 88-92% at sea level, or increase the rate of flow in patients already on supplemental oxygen. A very difficult problem emerges, however, in patients with hypoventilatory, hypoxemic respiratory failure in whom a higher than usual PaO_2 may blunt their ventilatory response, such that the hypercapnia and hypoxemia may even worsen to precarious levels. In these cases, careful titration, as difficult as it may be to estimate, may be important.

The response, however, of patients with COPD to high altitude is not always predictable nor is it always a negative one. Graham and Houston (1978) studied eight patients with moderate COPD without cor pulmonale who ascended to a moderate altitude of 1920 meters. Their symptoms were surprisingly mild (fatigue and insomnia) in spite of the decline in PaO_2 from the low 60 to high 40 and low 50 mm Hg range. With several days of acclimatization at that altitude, they were able to increase their alveolar ventilation and improve their oxygenation. The authors, therefore, concluded that patients with moderate, non-hypercarbic COPD could do acceptably well upon ascent to a moderate altitude where recreation is common, but they did not extend their study nor comment on the long-term effects of such exposure important.

5.2   Asthma

The story in asthma is more unpredictable. Many patients with asthma and their physicians find that they actually improve their symptoms or just do not have any problem with their asthma during sojourns to high altitude.

This may seem surprising in light of the fact that cold, dry air is often an inciting factor for exercise-induced asthma. The anecdotal evidence, however, is surprisingly to the contrary. These findings may be secondary to fewer allergens and /or air pollutants encountered in many high altitude areas (11). The data on asthma at high altitude are primarily in the pediatric literature which have varied results. Some studies have shown improvement in children living at high altitudes (17) and some have shown worsening (12). These and other studies have concentrated on the relatively low concentration of allergens at high altitude. Further work is necessary to substantiate the claims of improvement at high altitude and pediatric asthma.

As for exercise-induced asthma (EIB), the reports are mostly anecdotal. It is this author's experience that most active individuals with EIB should not be discouraged from high altitude activities but should have careful counseling on what to do if their asthma worsens, have a full complement of their usual medications, and proceed with initial caution. As for the potential relationship between asthma and altitude illness, particularly HAPE, there are no data one way or the other. It would be reasonable to assume that individuals with airflow obstruction would develop more profound hypoxemia and thus predispose them to greater pulmonary hypertension and subsequently HAPE, but this is all just speculation at this point.

5.3   Miscellaneous Lung Diseases

There are essentially no data on the effect of high altitude on patients with restrictive lung disease. Anecdotal evidence suggests that regardless of their low altitude PaO_2, their usual level of dyspnea at low altitude is worsened at high altitude. These patients tend to have chronic stimulation of their mechanoreceptors and with assumed hypoxemia that they would incur at high altitude, the stimulation of their chemoreceptors would accentuate their dyspnea. This should probably be explained to them, and if necessary, a measurement of their pulse oximetry could be taken at high altitude to insure adequate oxygenation. Those patients with low altitude hypoxemia are particularly vulnerable to worsening hypoxemia and dyspnea, and thus need to be advised and treated.

As mentioned earlier, the more difficult patients to manage are those who have hypoxemic hypercapnic respiratory failure with or without restrictive or obstructive disease whose physiologic response to the ambient hypoxia might be quite unpredictable. Theoretically, the hypoxia of moderate altitude could stimulate their chemosensors and thus maintain adequate oxygenation in spite of the hypercapnia. On the other hand, the worsening hypoxemia may be such that they can't compensate because of impaired lung mechanics, and thus expose themselves to the potential complications of precariously low oxygenation. Supplementing them with oxygen ahead of time is also a dicey situation because of the unpredictability of the response of their alveolar ventilation to oxygen. It is this author's experience that many of these patients with alveolar hypoventilation who are able to generate an adequate voluntary increase in ventilation do quite well with respiratory stimulants such as Provera (20 mg po tid) both at low and high altitude. This intervention gives greater assurance that the delicate balance of hypoventilation and blunted chemosensitivity is not lost.

5.4   Sleep Disorders

Discussing sleep-disordered breathing at high altitude is like going to a congress of linguists with no common language to speak. In other words, there are no good clinical data available on the response of these patients upon ascending to high altitude. Here again, the physiology is quite varied and complicated in these patients, such that their response to greater ambient hypoxia is quite unpredictable. Kryger et al. (9) looked at chronic hypoventilation, sleep-disordered breathing and polycythemia. They studied the effects of the respiratory stimulants, acetazolamide and medroxyprogesterone acetate, on patients with polycythemia and periodic breathing during sleep and found some improvement with obliteration of their periodic breathing by acetazolamide, and higher oxygen saturations, but further studies to follow up on this finding are lacking.

As in patients with hypoxemic alveolar hypoventilation, to predict how patients with sleep-disordered breathing will react to high altitude is mere guesswork. For instance, it is conceivable (and this author has seen cases) that the hypoxia of moderate altitude may, in fact, stimulate the peripheral chemosensors such that dysrhythmic breathing (even with obstruction) is obliterated and the hypoxemia actually improves. On the other hand, if the periodic breathing persists and/or the obstruction in patients with obstructive sleep apnea continues, the hypopneic or apneic phases may be characterized by even more profound hypoxemia. It is conceivable then that these dips in oxygenation may lead to more severe pulmonary hypertension, polycythemia and cardiovascular complications. One way to predict this, which unfortunately is usually quite tedious, is to have patients repeat a sleep study while breathing hypoxic gas comparable to the altitude to which they are going. Many of these people are otherwise quite healthy and active and desire to have recreation at moderate altitude, and this kind of testing could elucidate or predict their response. Rarely is this done, however. This uncertainty again emphasizes the need for further clinical research in this arena.

6.   SUMMARY

It is frustrating that in clinical practice, information about the response of patients to moderate altitude is lacking or reduced to myth and anecdote. Common questions, as have been posed above, can't be answered with any degree of certainty in many cases. The practitioner, therefore, has to rely on a modicum of knowledge of pulmonary physiology, both gas exchange and lung mechanics, and common sense to advise the patient to do what is best for him or her. It is a fertile area for good clinical research that I hope some young investigators will become interested and take the baton with purpose in sight.

REFERENCES

1. Cote T., D. Stroup, D. Dwyer, J. Horan, D. Peterson Chronic obstructive pulmonary disease mortality: A rule for altitude. *Chest.* 103:54-59, 1993.
2. Coultas D.B., J.M. Samat, C.L. Wiggins Altitude and Mortality from chronic obstructive lung disease in New Mexico. *Arch Environ Health.* 39:355-359, 1984.
3. Dillard T., L. Moores, K. Bilello, Y. Phillips The pre-flight evaluation – a comparison of the hypoxia inhalation test with hypobaric exposure. *Chest.* 107:352-357, 1995.
4. Dillard T.A., B.W. Berg, K.R. Rajagopal, J.W. Dooley, W.J. Mehm Hypoxemia during air travel in patients with chronic obstructive pulmonary disease. *Ann Int Med.* 111:362-367, 1989.
5. Dillard T.A., Hypoxemia during altitude exposure. A meta analysis of chronic obstructive pulmonary disease. *Chest.* 103:422-425, 1993.
6. Gong H, D.P. Tashkin, E.Y. Lee, M.S. Simmons, Hypoxia-altitude simulation test. Evaluation of patients with chronic airway obstruction. *Am Rev Resp Dis.* 130:980-86, 1984.
7. Gong H. Air travel in oxygen therapy and cardiopulmonary patients. *Chest.* 101:1104-1113, 1992.
8. Graham W. G., C. S. Houston. Short Term Adaptation to Modern Altitude. *Patients with Chronic Obstructive Pulmonary Disease. JAMA. 240:1491-1494, 1978.*
9. Hackett P. H., High Altitude and Common Medical Conditions. In: *High Altitude,* Hornbein T. F. & R. B. Schoene, eds., *In Lung Biology and Health and Disease,* executive editor, Claude Lenfant, Marcel Dekker, publishers, New York (in press).
10. Kramer M.R., C Springer, N Berkman, M Glazer, M Bublil, E Bar-Yishay, S. Godfrey. Rehabilitation of hypoxemic patients with COPD at low altitude at the Dead Sea, the lowest place on earth. *Chest.* 113:571-575, 1998.
11. Kryger M., J.V. Weil, R.V. Grover. Chronic mountain polycythemia: a disorder of the regulation of breathing during sleep? *Chest.* 73:303-304, 1978.
12. Matsuta S., T. Onda, Y. Iikura. Bronchial Responses of Asthmatic Patients in an Atmosphere-Challenging Chamber. *Inter Arch Allergy Immunol.* 107:402-405, 1995.
13. Moore L., A. Rohr, J. Maisenbach, J. Reeves. Emphysema mortality is increased in Colorado residents at high altitude. *Am Rev Resp Dis.* 126:225-228, 1982.14. Peroni D.G., A.L. Boner, G. Vallone, I. Antolini, J.O. Warner. Effective allergen avoidance at high

altitude reduces allergen-induced bronchial hyperresponsiveness. *Am J Repir Crit Care Med.* 149:1442-46, 1994.

15. Platts-Mills T., R. Sporik, J. Ingram, R. Honsinger. Dog and cat allergens and asthma among school children in Los Alamos, New Mexico, USA: Altitude 7200 feet. *Inter Arch Allergy Immunol.* 107:301-303, 1995.

16. Regensteiner J.G., Moore L.G., Migration of the elderly from high altitudes in Colorado. *JAMA.* 253: 3124-3128, 1985.

16. Renzetti A.D., J.H. McClement, B.D. Litt. The Veteran's Administration cooperative study of pulmonary function. *Am J Med.* 41:115-139, 1966.

18. Saiyed H., Y. Sharma, Sadhu. Non-occupational pneumoconiosis at high altitude villages in central Ladakh. *Br J Ind Med.* 48: 825-829, 1991.

19. Schwartz J.S., H.Z. Beucowitz, K.M. Moser. Air travel hypoxemia with chronic obstructive pulmonary disease. *Ann Intern Med.* 100:473-77, 1984.

20. Simon H, M. Grotzer, W. Nikolaizik, K. Blaser, M. Shoni. High altitude climate reduces peripheral blood T lymphocyte activation, eosinophilia, and bronchial obstruction in children with house dust-mite allergic asthma. *Ped Pulmonol.* 17:304-311, 1994.

Chapter 4

Commuting to High Altitude
Recent Studies of Oxygen Enrichment

John B. West
Department of Medicine, University of California San Diego, La Jolla, California 92093-0623, USA

Key words: laboratory module, sleep apnea, control of ventilation, neuropsychological function

Abstract: Further studies have been carried out on the potential value of oxygen enrichment of room air for commuters to high altitude. Novel ways of providing oxygen-enriched spaces for working and sleeping are being tested at the California Institute of Technology where a radiotelescope is being designed for an altitude of 5,000 m in north Chile. The modules are containers such as those used on container ships, and they are fitted out in California and then sealed and transported to the telescope site in Chile. The result is a turn-key facility which shows promise for field studies. The oxygen is provided by oxygen concentrators, and different modules are used for sleeping, living, and laboratory quarters. Two extensive experiments on oxygen enrichment were carried out at the University of California White Mountain Research Station, altitude 3,800 m, in the summer of 1998. The first study was devoted to the mechanism for the increase in arterial oxygen saturation on the day after sleeping in an oxygen-enriched atmosphere compared with sleeping in ambient air (5). Possible mechanisms include less fluid accumulation in the lung associated with acute mountain sickness, or a change in the control of ventilation. A double blind study was therefore carried out of the effects of sleeping in oxygen enrichment on both the ventilatory response to hypoxia and to carbon dioxide. In a related study, subjects who had been at an altitude of 3,800 m for two days, and were therefore partially acclimatized, were studied at a simulated altitude of 5,000 both breathing ambient air and 27% oxygen. The studies were done at 3800 m altitude by enriching the atmosphere of the test room with appropriate amounts of nitrogen or oxygen. An extensive series of neuropsychological tests were carried out with the objective of determining

Hypoxia: Into the Next Millennium,
Edited by R. C. Roach, *et al.* Kluwer Academic/Plenum Publishing, New York, 1999.

57

which features of CNS function were improved by oxygen enrichment at an altitude of 5,000 m.

1.   INTRODUCTION

Increasingly, people are commuting from low altitudes to high altitudes to work. One of the best examples is the Collahuasi mine in north Chile, altitude 4,500 - 4,600 m, where up to 6000 workers have recently been employed at any one time. Many of these commute to the mine from sea level, spending 7 days at the mine, and then returning to sea level for 7 days to live with their families. Another example is the telescope site in north Chile, south-west of San Pedro de Atacama. Here the altitude is 5000 m and workers commute each day from San Pedro, which is at an altitude of 2,400 m. This pattern of commuting to a remote or hazardous environment is typical of the development of industries in many areas. Similar patterns occur for manning oil rigs in the North Sea, and mining exploration in remote north-western Australia.

2.   MODULAR FACILITIES PROVIDING OXYGEN ENRICHMENT IN THE FIELD

An interesting recent development has been the use of containers, such as those used in container ships, for providing oxygen-enriched living and laboratory quarters in the field. This approach has been used by Dr. Tony Readhead and his colleagues at the California Institute of Technology. This group is building a radiotelescope to be sited at an altitude of 5,000 m in north Chile. The containers are completely fitted out in California, where the oxygen enrichment can be tested, and the containers are then sealed and shipped to the field site, where they are opened and then fully operational. This type of turn-key arrangement clearly has great advantages for setting up facilities in remote areas.

Figure 1 shows a sketch of a possible design. In this instance, a standard shipping container of dimensions 20 feet (6.10 m) long, 8 feet (2.44 m) wide, and 8 feet high can be fitted out as living space with two beds, a laboratory, or a machine shop. A larger laboratory can be housed in a standard shipping container of dimensions 40 feet (12.19 m) long by 8 feet wide by 8 feet high.

A feature of the telescope site is that ample electric power is available from diesel generators because the radiotelescope itself needs a lot of power. Therefore, the oxygen can be generated using modular oxygen concentrators such as the AirSep New Life (AirSep Corporation, Buffalo, NY). A typical concentrator provides 5 liters per minute of 90 percent oxygen and requires 350 watts of electrical power. Figure 1 shows that the outputs of three concentrators are combined and mixed with ambient air to give an oxygen concentration of 27 percent. This is therefore an increase of oxygen concentration of 6 percent which will reduce the equivalent altitude by 1,800 m (7) to 3200 m.

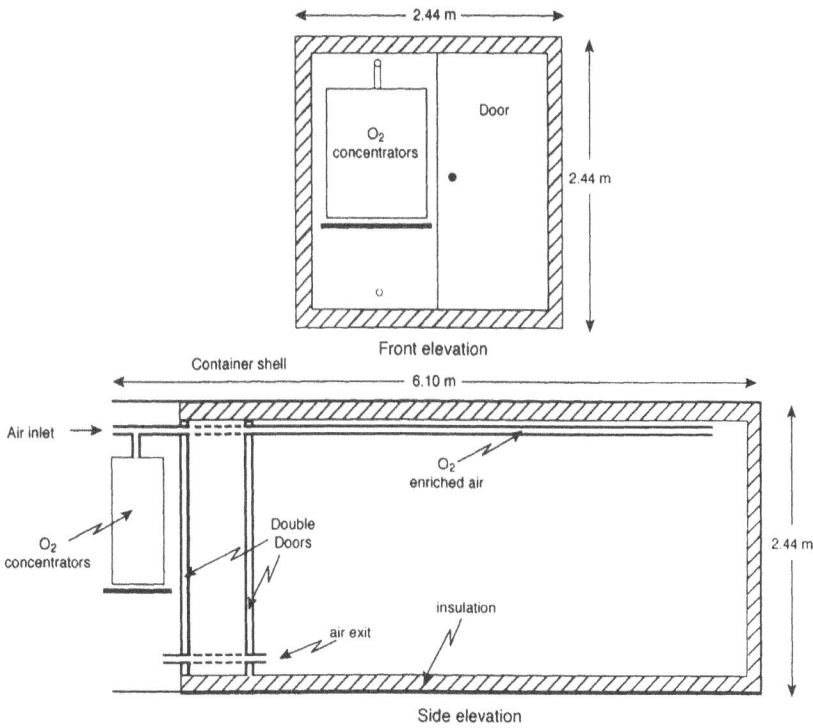

Figure 1. Sketch of a self-contained oxygen-enriched module suitable for field work at high altitude. The module uses a standard shipping container. This version is 20 feet (6 .10 m) long but standard containers 40 feet (12 .19 m) long are also available.

The oxygen concentrators are located outside the room itself which is entered through a double door forming a lock to reduce contamination of the air inside the room with outside air. The flow of enriched air (room ventilation) is equal to 300 liters per minute, and this is delivered by a pipe to the far end of the container. An exit port with a one-way flap valve is provided near the door. The walls, ceiling and floor of the container are well insulated against cold using extruded polyurethane insulation, and the container has an electrical heater. Oxygen and carbon dioxide analyzers continuously sample the composition of the air inside the room and the results are displayed both inside the room and outside the door.

In this setting where ample electrical power is available, oxygen concentrators are the preferred way of providing the oxygen enrichment. However, in sites where power is not available, the oxygen can be provided from liquid oxygen tanks. Typical tanks have a nominal capacity of 189 liters (Taylor-Wharton, XL 50, Theodore, AL) although the tank is never completely filled for safety reasons. Such tanks have been used to oxygen enrich dormitory rooms in mines in Chile. It is not difficult to find liquid oxygen in north Chile because there is a plant at the huge mine in Chuquicamata. However, because the tanks have to be refilled from time to time, oxygen concentrators are more convenient if electrical power is available. Also in most settings, using oxygen concentrators is the cheaper option.

3.   EFFECTS OF NOCTURNAL OXYGEN ENRICHMENT

During the summer of 1998, further studies of the effects of sleeping in an oxygen enriched environment were carried out at the Barcroft facility of the University of California White Mountain Research Station, altitude 3800 m.. The studies were spearheaded by Michele McElroy. Twenty-four volunteers drove from San Diego to the Barcroft facility in one day, and they were studied during the night of that day and the following night, either breathing ambient air or 24 per cent oxygen. The treatments were given in random order and neither the subjects nor the person responsible for the analysis of the data were aware of the treatment.

The oxygen enrichment was provided using a special room as previously described (5). The physiological measurements during the night included breathing movements with an inductance plethysmograph (Ambulatory Monitoring, Ardsley, NY), and arterial oxygen saturation using a pulse oximeter (Ohmeda, Madison, WI or Novametrix, Wallingford, CT). Subjective measurements of sleep were also obtained, and an assessment of acute mountain sickness was done using the Lake Louise acute mountain sickness scoring survey (1).

This study confirmed the results of our previous study (5) showing that sleep-disordered breathing was substantially reduced when subjects breathed 24 percent oxygen as opposed to ambient air. Both the number of apneas and the times spent in periodic breathing were significantly reduced. This study also confirmed the previous finding of a greater increase in arterial oxygen saturation from evening to morning in subjects who slept in oxygen enrichment compared with ambient air. (Of course both measurements of arterial oxygen saturation were made when the subjects were breathing ambient air.) In the present study, the arterial oxygen saturation was continuously monitored by the pulse oximeter over a period of 15 minutes, and the average values were automatically determined. This procedure gave more reliable results than the spot measurements of arterial oxygen saturation that had been made in the previous study. However, the results were almost identical.

An additional measurement of arterial oxygen saturation was made at midday following the night in oxygen enrichment or ambient air. Interestingly, much of the improvement in oxygen saturation was lost during the morning. Thus, the improvement in arterial oxygen saturation following one night of oxygen enrichment was transient.

Improvement in arterial oxygenation as a result of sleeping in an oxygen enriched atmosphere could result from at least two different mechanisms. One possibility is that the pathological changes associated with acute mountain sickness are lessened by sleeping in oxygen enrichment. For example, if the amount of subclinical pulmonary edema is reduced by the oxygen enrichment, this could result in a higher level of arterial oxygenation. Another possibility is that oxygen enrichment alters the control of breathing. It is known that the patients with sleep-disordered breathing at sea level who are treated with continuous positive airway pressure (CPAP) may have a higher daytime arterial PO_2 than a similar untreated group of patients (4). Furthermore, it has been shown that some patients with obstructive sleep apnea treated with CPAP develop an increased ventilatory response to carbon dioxide within one or two nights of treatment (3).

To test whether the control of ventilation was altered by a night of sleeping in oxygen enrichment, the subjects had their ventilatory responses to both oxygen and carbon dioxide measured in the evenings before sleeping and in the mornings after waking. The results of these tests are still being analyzed.

4. EFFECTS OF OXYGEN ENRICHMENT IN THE WORKPLACE ON NEUROPSYCHOLOGICAL PERFORMANCE

As indicated earlier, Cal Tech is planning to install a radiotelescope at an altitude of 5,000 m in north Chile. The same site has been chosen for another very large radiotelescope known as the millimeter array (MMA), which will be jointly designed and operated by a U.S. and European consortium. For both these facilities, the astronomers will live in San Pedro de Atacama, altitude, 2,400 m and commute daily to the 5,000 m site. Since the barometric pressure at the site is only 419 Torr, the inspired PO_2 is only 78

Torr, that is, 52 percent of its sea level value. It is well established that this altitude impairs neuropsychological function including visual sensitivity, attention span, short-term memory, arithmetic ability, and decision-making ability (6).

In order to determine what aspects of neuropsychological function are improved by oxygen enrichment at this altitude, an extensive study was carried out at the Barcroft facility of the University of California White Mountain Research Station (WMRS) in the summer of 1998. This was spearheaded by Andre Gerard. Since the altitude at this facility is only 3,800 m, it was necessary to simulate an altitude of 5,000 m by reducing the oxygen concentration of the test room by adding nitrogen. The oxygen concentration was reduced from 21 to 18 percent by nitrogen enrichment, and this gave the same inspired PO_2 as breathing ambient air at an altitude of 5,000 m.

To simulate the effect of oxygen enrichment at an altitude of 5,000 m, the oxygen concentration of the WMRS room at 3,800 m was increased from 21 to 23 percent. This gave the same inspired PO_2 as breathing 27 percent oxygen at 5,000 m altitude. Note that breathing a 6 percent oxygen mixture at this altitude reduces the equivalent altitude by 1,800 m, that is to 3,200 m (7). The oxygen enrichment was carried out using oxygen concentrators. In order to provide nitrogen enrichment, the oxygen concentrators were used in a reverse mode so that the effluent nitrogen-enriched air was pumped into the room, whereas the oxygen that was produced by the oxygen concentrator was led out to waste. This procedure was suggested by Dr. John Severinghaus.

The subjects spent two days acclimatizing to the altitude of 3,800 m before entering the room at a simulated altitude of 5,000 m. This partial acclimatization allowed a better model of the situation in Chile, where the astronomers will live at an altitude of 2,400 m and commute to the telescope site. In addition, exposing sea level subjects to an altitude of 5,000 m without any acclimatization could be hazardous. The subjects underwent the neuropsychological testing in the room on the third and fourth day at high altitude. For one of the sessions the subject breathed ambient air at a simulated altitude of 5,000 m, and for the other session they breathed a simulated oxygen-enriched atmosphere of 27 per cent at 5,000 m. The order of the measurements was randomized and neither the subjects nor the person analyzing the results was aware of the altering.

An extensive series of neuropsychological tests was developed in collaboration with Dr. Igor Grant of the Department of Psychiatry, UCSD Medical School. The tests came from packages developed by experimental psychologists and the technical details will not be given here. The tests included trails B, digit symbol, fingertapping rate, digit vigilance time, pegboard filling time, matrix reasoning, story learning, story recall, rapid visual information processing, mood assessment, reaction times, and cursor tracking accuracy. Some of the tests were from a computer package designed for measuring neuropsychological function during the NASA Neurolab mission. The results have not been fully analyzed but improvements were seen in reaction times, hand-eye coordination, and mood.

A problem with this experimental design is that the subjects are aware that they are being tested, and if they are very competitive (as most of our subjects were), they try very hard during the test itself. The result might be that they score better during this relative brief testing (about an hour long) than they would during the course of a typical working day. In other words, it is possible that the performance during a specific testing period does not accurately reflect neuropsychological function over the period of a whole day. Psychologists have been aware of this problem for a long time. During the International High Altitude Expedition to Cerro de Pasco, Peru in 1921-1922, Barcroft and colleagues (2), at an altitude of 4,330 m, were convinced that their mental efficiency was reduced, and that they were prone to make errors over the course of the day. However, they found that when they forced themselves to concentrate on a particular task, this could be accomplished. Thus it might be that the effects of oxygen enrichment are more valuable than can be demonstrated by formal neuropsychological testing.

REFERENCES

1. Anonymous. The Lake Louise Consensus on the definition and quantification of altitude illness. In: *Hypoxia and Mountain Medicine*, edited by J. R. Sutton, G. Coates and C. S. Houston. Burlington, VT: Queen City Press, 1992.

2. Barcroft, J., C. A. Binger, A. V. Bock, H. S. Forbes, G. Harrop, J. C. Meakins, and A. C. Redfield. Observations upon the effect of high altitude on the physiological processes of the human body carried out in the Peruvian Andes, chiefly at Cerro de Pasco. *Proc Roy Soc London (Series B)* 211: 352-480, 1923.

3. Berthon-Jones, M., and C. E. Sullivan. Time course of change in ventilatory response to CO_2 with long-term CPAP therapy for obstructive sleep apnea. *Am Rev Respir Dis* 135: 144 -147, 1987.

4. Leech, J. A., E. Onal, and M. Lopata. Nasal CPAP continues to improve sleep-disordered breathing and daytime oxygenation over long-term follow-up of occlusive sleep apnea syndrome. *Chest* 102: 1651-1655, 1992.

5. Luks, A. M., H. van Melick, R. Batarse, F. L. Powell, I. Grant, and J. B. West. Room oxygen enrichment improves sleep and subsequent day-time performance at high altitude. *Respir Physiol* 113: 247-258, 1998.

6. McFarland, R. A. Physiological implications of life at altitude and including the role of oxygen in the process of aging. In: *Physiological Adaptations: Desert and Mountain*, edited by M. K. Yousef, S. M. Horvath and R. W. Bullard. New York: Academic Press, 1972, p. 157-181.

7. West, J. B. Oxygen enrichment of room air to relieve the hypoxia of high altitude. *Respir Physiol* 99: 225-32, 1995.

Chapter 5

The Pregnant Altitude Visitor

Susan Niermeyer

University of Colorado School of Medicine: The Children's Hospital, Denver, Colorado, USA

Key words: pregnancy, altitude, hypoxia, placenta, fetus, exercise

Abstract: The human fetus develops normally under low-oxygen conditions. Exposure of a pregnant woman to the hypoxia of high altitude results in acclimatization responses which act to preserve the fetal oxygen supply. The fetus also utilizes several compensatory mechanisms to survive brief periods of hypoxia. While fetal heart rate monitoring data during air travel suggest no compromise of fetal oxygenation, exercise at high altitude may place further stress on oxygen delivery to the fetus. The limited data on maternal exercise at high altitude suggest good tolerance in most pregnancies; however, short-term abnormalities in fetal heart rate and subsequent pregnancy complications have been observed, as well. A survey of Colorado obstetrical care providers yielded consensus that preterm labor and bleeding complications of pregnancy are the most commonly encountered pregnancy complications among high-altitude pregnant visitors. Dehydration, engaging in strenuous exercise before acclimatization, and participation in activities with high risk of trauma are behaviors that may increase the risk of pregnancy complications. Medical and obstetrical conditions which impair oxygen transfer at any step between the environment and fetal tissue may compromise fetal oxygenation. Knowledge of the medical, obstetrical, and behavioral risk factors during pregnancy at high altitude can help the pregnant visitor to high altitude avoid such complications.

1.   INTRODUCTION

The lure of the mountains affects not only men; women now participate in nearly every aspect of work and sport in high mountain locations. Easy transportation and the development of resorts and conference centers have opened the mountains not only to those who live nearby, but to travelers who come from far away – often near sea level. Thus, opportunities for pregnant women to visit high altitude have increased, resulting in questions for women and their doctors. These questions are frequent among those who live near high-mountain communities, but they also arise in parts of the world far removed from high-altitude zones, where familiarity with altitude-associated problems may be limited. The questions relate not only to effects of the high-altitude hypoxia, but also to the effects of travel and exercise in the pregnant woman at high altitude. Although acute high-altitude exposure has obvious impact on a pregnant woman's cardiovascular and pulmonary performance, the most compelling issues are those of fetal well-being: threats of fetal hypoxia and/or ischemia or pregnancy complications of premature labor, premature rupture of membranes, placental abruption or bleeding from placenta previa.

After a brief review of the physiology of normal pregnancy at sea level, data will be presented regarding placental oxygen transport upon high-altitude exposure. Available human data from observations of pregnant women during air travel and exercise at high altitude will be summarized. The clinical factors that can complicate a pregnancy upon acute high-altitude exposure will be discussed with reference to the underlying physiology. Finally, general recommendations will be proposed regarding travel during pregnancy and avoidance of acute mountain sickness, as well as specific strategies to avoid exercise-related complications at high altitude.

2.   PHYSIOLOGY OF NORMAL PREGNANCY AT SEA LEVEL

Prior to considering the effect of high altitude, it is useful to review the anatomy of the placental circulation and the physiology of this organ of fetal respiration.

The fetus normally develops under low-oxygen conditions. Oxygen moves from the atmosphere to fetal tissues through a series of steps, alternating between bulk transport and diffusion of oxygen. The first step, bulk transport of oxygen from the atmosphere to the maternal alveoli, is enhanced by the progesterone-stimulated hyperventilation of pregnancy. A mother breathing room air at sea level has an arterial pO_2 of 85 to 100 mm Hg and a resting pCO_2 of 30 mm Hg (12). Oxygen diffuses across the maternal alveolar-capillary membrane, and is carried again by bulk flow (cardiac output) from the lungs to the placenta. A 40% increase in cardiac output (from 3.5 to 6.0 l/min) occurs early in pregnancy; at least two-thirds of the increase has occurred by the end of the first trimester (8). The increase occurs due to increased circulating blood volume and increased stroke volume, with only a minor (10%) increase in heart rate. Cardiac output rises still further on exertion and in labor; but, as pregnancy progresses, the increase of cardiac output with exercise diminishes, probably due to limitation of venous return (22). The uterine artery, one of many branches of the internal iliac artery, delivers systemic arterial blood to the placental circulation. Other branches of the iliac artery supply the large muscles of the hip and lower extremity, which exert completing demands for blood flow during exercise.

Within the human hemochorial placenta, oxygen transport occurs by diffusion from maternal blood in the intervillous space to fetal blood in capillaries of the terminal villi (Figure 1). Maternal spiral arteries penetrate the myometrial wall and convert into flaccid, sac-like uteroplacental vessels which dilate to accommodate the greatly augmented blood flow. Maternal blood enters the intervillous space via arterial inlets in the basal plate and flows toward the chorionic plate as a funnel-shaped stream "much as water from an actively flowing brook penetrates a reed filled marsh" (26). After percolating through a fetal lobule, maternal blood drains through basal venous outlets into the uterine vein (10). Oxygen diffuses across the placental microvillus into the superficial capillary network of the fetal circulation. Fetal blood converges through the villous stem veins and cotyledonary veins of the placenta, to the umbilical vein, which delivers oxygenated blood from the placenta to the fetus.

Flow through the intervillous space probably represents a combination of concurrent, countercurrent, cross-current and pool flow; however, the observed oxygen and carbon dioxide gradients correspond best to a concurrent model, with umbilical vein oxygen tensions slightly lower than those in the uterine vein (5,20). At sea level, with a maternal arterial pO_2 of 90 mm Hg and uterine vein pO_2 of 40 mm Hg, the observed fetal pO_2 rises from 24-25 mm Hg in the umbilical artery to 35-40 mm Hg in the umbilical vein.

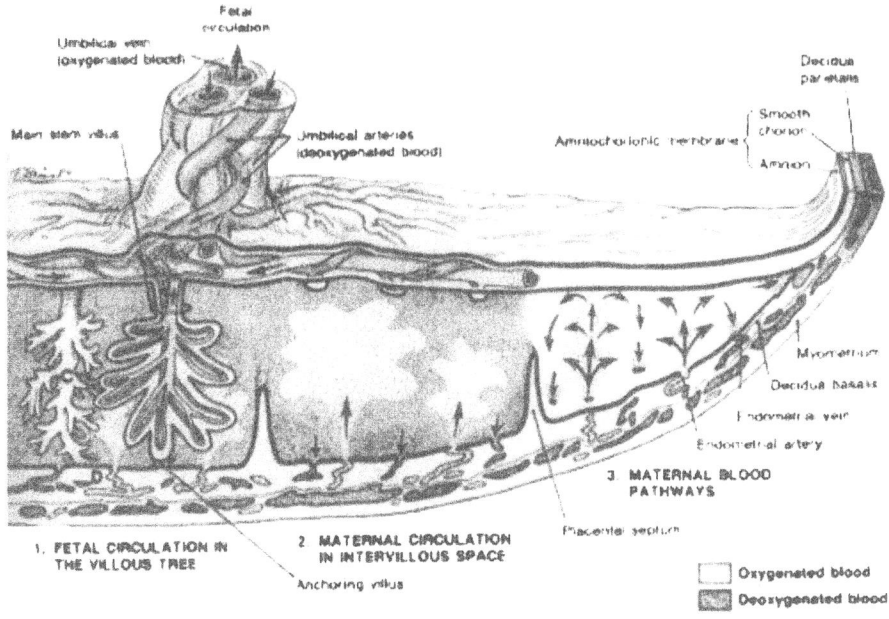

Figure 1. Anatomy and circulation of the term human placenta (with permission: William's Obstetrics, 1994).

3.   PLACENTAL OXYGEN TRANSPORT UPON ACUTE HIGH-ALTITUDE EXPOSURE

Upon acute high-altitude exposure, the pregnant woman undergoes a series of physiological responses that are altitude- and time-dependent. These responses act together to preserve oxygen delivery to the fetus. Initial, immediate responses are maternal cardiorespiratory compensations: an increase in minute ventilation (largely due to an increase in tidal volume), increased cardiac output (primarily through increased heart rate secondary to sympathetic activation), and increased systolic blood pressure. Thus, increased uterine artery and placental blood flow partially offset the fall in oxygen content. Intermediate-term acclimatization begins within hours of exposure to high altitude and develops over days to weeks. These intermediate responses include an increase in intra-erythrocyte 2,3-diphosphoglycerate (2,3-DPG) levels as soon as 3 hours after exposure, that shifts the hemoglobin-oxygen dissociation curve to the right (15), increasing oxygen availability for placental transfer. Erythropoietin elevation also becomes detectable 6-12 hours after altitude exposure; active erythropoiesis enhances the oxygen transport capacity of blood over days to weeks.

In fully acclimatized pregnant women above 4000 m, arterial oxygen tension is higher and pCO_2 lower than in acclimatized nonpregnant women at the same altitudes (11, 27,28).

Table 1. Hyperventilation decreases pCO_2 and increases pO_2 in fully acclimatized pregnant women as compared to non-pregnant women above 4000 m.

Altitude	Pregnant Women	Non-pregnant Women
	pO_2 pCO_2	pO_2 pCO_2
4400 meters	59 mm Hg 23 mm Hg	51 mm Hg 28 mm Hg
4300 meters		48 mm Hg 32 mm Hg
4200 meters	61 mm Hg 25 mm Hg	

At an altitude of approximately 4000 m, maternal arterial pO_2 is in the range of 55-60 mm Hg, uterine vein pO_2 35 mm Hg and umbilical vein pO_2 20 mm Hg (21). The decrease in fetal pO_2 is less than would be expected from the relative maternal hypoxemia at high altitude. While maternal pO_2 falls from 91 mm Hg at 150 m to 61 mm Hg at 4200 m, fetal scalp values have been documented to change only 3 mm Hg, from 22 mm Hg to 19 mm Hg over the same altitude range (27, 28).

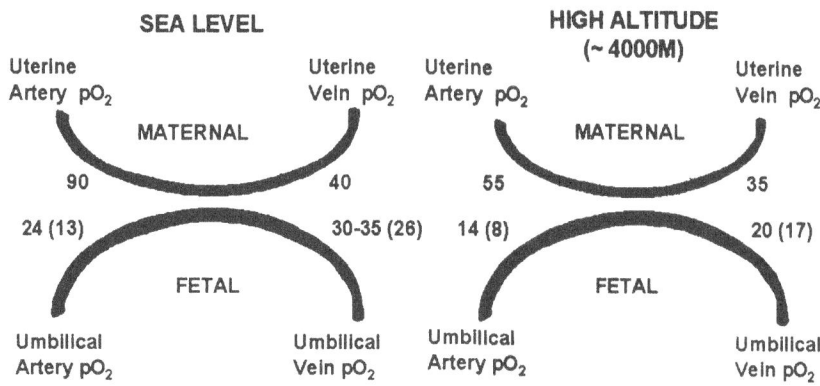

Figure 2. Figure 2. Maternal and fetal oxygenation at sea level and approximately 4000 m

To understand the time course and the periods of vulnerability during these maternal adjustments to high altitude, it is necessary to turn to animal models. The experimental model of the chronically instrumented pregnant sheep provides the most detailed information on fetal oxygen delivery with acute exposure to high altitude. Cotter and associates (7) studied catheterized pregnant ewes (uterine vein, femoral vein and artery, umbilical vein and artery catheters) in an altitude chamber at 5,000, 10,000, and 15,000 feet

(1524, 3048, and 4572 m). Ascent was at a rate of 1000 feet per minute (approximately 300m/min). Samples for blood gases, pH, hematocrit, and hemoglobin were obtained after 30 minutes at a given altitude. Values in 3 animals at 3048 m showed a fall in maternal arterial oxygen saturation (97 to 77%), with uterine vein saturations showing only a slight decline (68.6 to 64.5 %). Upon acute exposure, there was no noted increase in oxygen capacity of maternal or fetal blood. Oxygen saturations in the umbilical vein fell from 63 to 50 %, but with an estimated pO_2 change of only 29.3 to 23.6 mm Hg. Stability of the fetal oxygen tension resulted, in part, from the steep slope of the fetal oxygen dissociation curve in the range of 50% saturation. Increased uterine blood flow also contributed to preserved fetal oxygenation, as evidenced by a decrease in the maternal arteriovenous oxygen difference (1.61 to 0.68 mM/l) and in the coefficient of oxygen utilization (30.8 to 16.4%).

Studies by Makowski et al. in Colorado (19) extended these observations over a longer time period. They examined 6 ewes, chronically catheterized in the femoral artery, uterine vein, and fetal umbilical vein and artery, that were transported from Denver (1610 m) to Mount Evans (4346 m). Blood samples were drawn at the two altitudes and analyzed for oxygen content, oxygen combining capacity, pO_2, and [H+]. Samples were drawn every other day at altitude, until the catheters ceased functioning (7-18 days).

Maternal arterial and uterine venous pO_2 were acutely lower at 2-4 days post altitude exposure. Oxygen content in the uterine vein fell in all animals; however, after one week at high altitude, the uterine vein oxygen content returned to about 75% of the control value. The oxygen content in the umbilical vein showed an initial fall, then a return toward pre-altitude levels, with 2 of 5 fetuses showing a complete return to control values by days 10 and 16. Saturations in the umbilical vein paralled this pattern. Oxygen capacity rose in 4 ewes upon altitude exposure. Fetal oxygen capacity rose through the first week, to a value about 20% higher than in Denver (2 fetuses). Fetal oxygen supply was preserved, and the observations suggested that an increase in uterine blood flow initially was the important factor. With prolonged exposure to altitude, oxygen content rose in the umbilical circulation, due to a combination of increased oxygen saturation and hemoglobin content.

The pregnant visitor to high altitude will initially rely on additional hyperventilation and further increase in cardiac output and placental blood flow to maintain fetal oxygen delivery. Intermediate acclimatization, with changes in 2,3-DPG and hemoglobin, occurs after days to weeks.

Studies of acute maternal hypoxia, achieved by administration of hypoxic gas mixtures, have further defined fetal responses to limited oxygen supply. Early studies examined the use of hypoxic gas mixtures in pregnant women as a possible screen for detecting placental insufficiency (6, 16, 29). Using 8-15% oxygen, the observed patterns of FHR response were classified as normal (mild tachycardia, bradycardia or no change in heart rate), or abnormal (mild tachycardia or bradycardia with poststimulation tachycardia; profound bradycardia).

Studies in chronically instrumented sheep (24,25) demonstrated an increase in FHR variability (oscillation amplitude and frequency) which accompanied an overall 18% decrease in fetal heart rate over relatively brief hypoxia (26 minutes). This response was interpreted as adequate fetal compensation, that included redistribution of fetal blood flow to the brain and myocardium, decreased oxygen consumption, and development of metabolic acidosis reflecting anaerobic metabolism. These mechanisms resulted in conservation of oxygen and its preferential supply to vital organs (25). Fetal oxygen consumption decreased 39% in short-term studies (25) and up to 50% with hypoxia sustained for up to 47 minutes (24). The observed increase in FHR variability was ascribed to a generalized increase in α-adrenergic activity. The known association of decreased FHR variability with asphyxia likely represents a phase of fetal distress or decompensationn.

More recent human data on simultaneous maternal and fetal responses to acute high-altitude exposure come from observations performed in aircraft and altitude-chamber studies.

Ten pregnant women, with gestations ranging from 32 to 38 weeks, were studied on 20 domestic European scheduled flights (13). Battery-powered monitors recorded heart rate, blood pressure, and transcutaneous pO_2 and pCO_2 in the mothers, beat-to-beat cardiotocogram in the fetuses, and the cabin pressure. Cabin pressure at maximal altitude corresponded to altitudes of 1900 to 2635 m. Initial responses included a decrease in maternal pO_2, with a significant increase in heart rate and slight increase in blood pressure. There were no changes in pCO_2 or respiratory rate throughout the flight. Fetal heart rate monitoring showed no variations outside the normal range. There were no systematic fetal responses to key phases of flight, suggesting that the fetuses were largely "unaware" of flying.

A case report involving a gliding enthusiast provides data on chamber-simulated altitudes up to 3500 m under resting conditions. The fetal heart rate showed no changes or features of note (4).

A final group of observations came from in-flight monitoring of pregnant women during emergency obstetric transports (9). A feasibility study of in-flight FHR monitoring in 53 emergency obstetric transports found an 83% success rate for electronic monitoring. With cruising altitudes from 2900 to 7000 m and cabin altitudes from 340 to 2130 m, three cases showed mild variable decelerations in labor; no late decelerations (signs of fetal hypoxemia) were observed.

The available animal and human data suggest that acute and intermediate acclimatization responses maintain adequate oxygenation in healthy pregnancies for acute exposure to approximately 4000 m. Direct fetal monitoring has given no evidence of fetal effects at cabin altitudes encountered during commercial air travel.

4.   MATERNAL EXERCISE PERFORMANCE AND FETAL RESPONSE TO MATERNAL EXERCISE AT HIGH ALTITUDE

Exercise at high altitude introduces competition for blood supply between skeletal muscles and the placenta (17, 18). In 1985 Baumann et al. studied 12 sedentary women with uncomplicated pregnancies between 30 and 39 weeks gestation during short-term altitude exposure in the Swiss mountains (2). Subjects traveled from Zurich by car to the cable car station at 1080 m. After a rest phase, subjects ascended to the mountain station at 2228 m in a cable car, with an elevation gain of 1050 m in 10 minutes. Subjects rested for 5 minutes before exercising at 25 W for 3 minutes on a bicycle ergometer. After a 5-minute rest period, they descended by cable car to the valley station, where the 3-minute exercise at 25 W was repeated. Continuous documented transcutaneous pO_2 and pCO_2, respiratory rate, heart rate, uterine contractions, and fetal heart rate. Blood pressure was monitored intermittently.

The mean transcutaneous pO_2 fell from 71 mm Hg at the valley station to 58 mm Hg at the mountain station. pCO_2 did not change significantly with ascent or exercise. Maternal heart rate, respiratory rate and blood pressure increased during exercise. Six subjects experienced regular mild contractions during the cable car ascent; these did not increase during or after exercise. Mean FHR increased slightly from 138 to 142 beats/min during the cable car ascent. All FHR traces except one were normal in terms of baseline, variability, accelerations, and absence of late decelerations. The one notable trace was normal before exercise at the mountain station. Exercise was followed by mild bradycardia, then by reduced short-term variability. During descent, variability began to return and was normal upon arrival at the valley station. Of note, the mother – a 29 y.o. in week 38 of pregnancy - was a smoker who had smoked while at altitude.

Because of the one case of observed fetal bradycardia and loss of variability, subsequent studies were performed in proximity to the obstetric hospital in a low pressure chamber with simulation of altitudes of 1100 m and 2200 m (3). A similar protocol including exercise at 50 W was utilized in 6 women, ranging from 31 to 39 weeks gestation. Maternal responses followed the same pattern as in the mountain study, with slightly higher respiratory and heart rate increases during exercise. Five of the 6 FHR traces were normal; however, a 2-minute bradycardia occurred in one fetus after exercise at 50 W at 2200 m. Again, the mother (a 33 y.o. woman at week 39 of gestation) had smoked throughout pregnancy.

Artal and colleagues (1) examined the maternal and fetal responses to exercise at 50 m and 1800 m. Seven sedentary women at a mean gestational age of 34 weeks without medical or obstetrical risk factors completed a symptom-limited maximal exercise test and a submaximal cardiac output exercise test at workloads of 25 and 50 W. The pre-exercise examination included initiation of a continuous electrocardiogram, blood pressure assessment, and 30 minutes of fetal monitoring. Baseline metabolic and respiratory data were collected, then subjects pedaled at 50 rev/min for 5 minutes at 25, 50, and 75 W, followed by 2-minute periods at workloads increasing by 25 W increments until volitional fatigue. Post-exercise monitoring included electrocardiogram, blood pressure, fetal heart rate and uterine activity (minimum of 30 minutes).

Of the 10 subjects enrolled, data were obtained on only 7; 2 subjects dropped out for personal reasons, and one subject experienced persistent and frequent uterine activity after the first exercise test which precluded additional testing. This subject delivered 10 days later at 37 weeks gestation. Maximal levels of work on a bicycle ergometer were lower at altitude, as expressed in l/min (13% decrease) and ml/kg/min. Subjects did not meet the general criteria (heart rate and lactate concentration) for VO_2max in nonpregnant individuals; thus, the term peak VO_2 is used. Maximal heart rates and ventilation were similar at sea level and altitude; however, the work level during peak exercise at altitude was significantly lower. There were no significant altitude-induced differences in ventilation at rest; however, ventilation at 75W was significantly higher at altitude. Resting cardiac outputs were significantly higher at altitude than at sea level, as was resting stroke volume. The changes in stroke volume with exercise were smaller at altitude, reflecting a smaller reserve in stroke volume.

Fetal heart rate monitoring documented a few, random variable decelerations. One episode of fetal bradycardia to 105 beats/minute for 2 minutes occurred after exercise at high altitude in one subject. Another subject at 32 weeks' gestation had persistent, frequent uterine activity after exercise at altitude and was hospitalized for observation in labor and delivery for 72 hours. The subject went on to deliver at 39 weeks gestation.

Because the effects of altitude and exercise may be synergistic rather than additive, recommendations defining the safe upper limits of the two stresses are difficult to determine (14). Thus far, studies have focused on resident populations, or maximal altitude at rest and maximal exercise at moderate altitude. Published studies also focus on very acute altitude exposure, and fail to acknowledge underlying medical and obstetrical conditions and mediating environmental factors, which can produce serious pregnancy complications.

Epidemiological studies of pregnancy complications secondary to acute high-altitude exposure are absent in the literature. A Delphi survey of 12 Colorado obstetrical care providers in mountain communities and Denver referral centers focused on observed pregnancy complications and risk factors for pregnant women visiting high altitude. The most frequently reported pregnancy complications are listed in Table 2.

Table 2. Pregnancy complications in high altitude visitors, as reported by Colorado obstetrical care providers

Pregnancy Complication	Weeks of Gestation
Preterm Labor	26 – 36 weeks
Premature Rupture of Membranes	20 – 36 weeks
Placental Abruption	> 24 weeks
Spontaneous Abortion	6 – 12 weeks
Intrauterine Fetal Demise	> 24 weeks

Physicians who serve mountain communities reported acute mountain sickness at approximately the same, or slightly decreased frequency in pregnant visitors as in the general population. Dehydration and vigorous exercise were the most frequently cited factors increasing the risk of altitude-related complications among pregnant visitors. The baseline hyperventilation of pregnancy, which may be further accentuated by ascent, can lead to large insensible water losses and dehydration, especially in the dry environment of high altitude. Dehydration in pregnant women has been linked to uterine contractions; this effect may be mediated by anti-diuretic hormone, which is very similar in chemical structure to oxytocin. While exercise itself has not been linked to preterm labor in normal pregnancies, exercise at high altitude may serve to unmask previously undiagnosed problems of placental insufficiency or placental anatomic abnormalities.

Practitioners also cited the practical factors of changes in body mass and the center of gravity, which can result in problems with balance and coordination. Hormonal effects cause changes in ligaments, producing joint laxity. These alterations can predispose to accidents and trauma that may cause placental disruption (placental hematomas, placental abruption). Though emergency evacuation and medical attention are widely available in recreational areas, specialized services are focused on neurologic and orthopedic trauma, not diagnosis and management of preterm labor or potentially life-threatening placental complications.

Other medical and obstetrical conditions cited as risk factors are summarized in Table 3.

Table 3. Medical and obstetrical risk factors for pregnancy complications at high altitude

Chronic Hypertension
Pregnancy-induced Hypertension
Maternal Heart/Lung Disease (including smoking)
Intrauterine Growth Retardation
Impaired Placental Gas Exchange
Advanced Maternal Age
Sea Level Residence

While the placental oxygen transport system has abundant reserves under normal conditions; maternal problems, which interfere with oxygen, transport at the level of the lung or heart may diminish these reserves. Direct or indirect evidence of impaired placental function – such as diagnosis of a partial placental abruption, placenta previa, intervillous clots, fetal growth retardation, or oligohydramnios – also suggest a limited capacity to compensate for the hypoxia of high altitude (23).

5.   RECOMMENDATIONS FOR PREGNANT VISITORS TO HIGH ALTITUDE

Colorado obstetrical care providers were also questioned about their advice to pregnant women planning visits to high altitude regarding mode of travel, general precautions, and exercise. Air travel was generally preferred to travel by car because it minimized the amount of time spent sitting. During any form of travel, hourly breaks to walk and stretch for a few minutes were recommended to avoid excessive venous pooling of blood.

Once at altitude, all obstetrical care providers emphasized the importance of adequate hydration. All physicians recommended waiting at least 3 to 4 days for partial acclimatization to occur before beginning any exercise. Others recommended acclimatization periods of 2 to 6 weeks before strenuous exercise. Most counseled short-term visitors to not exceed or even to reduce slightly their usual level of exertion. Some advised avoiding exercise above 3000 m without full acclimatization. Most physicians reiterated cautions against activities, which might lead to falls, and many specifically cautioned against skiing.

The pregnant visitor to high altitude responds to the relative hypoxia with acute and intermediate changes of acclimatization. These serve to preserve oxygen delivery to the fetus at a level very similar to that during pregnancy at sea level. In addition, the fetus utilizes short-term compensatory strategies of reduced oxygen consumption, redistribution of blood flow to vital organs, and anaerobic metabolism during brief hypoxic exposures. Exercise at high altitude imposes a further stress by competing with placental blood supply. With intact maternal and placental oxygen transport, the limited data on exercise at high altitude suggest that sufficient placental reserves exist to permit vigorous exercise at moderately high altitude. However, underlying medical and obstetrical conditions, which impair oxygen transport at any level, may limit these reserves; in such circumstances, exercise may produce signs of fetal hypoxia or trigger preterm labor. Physical factors in the high-altitude environment increase the risk of dehydration and trauma, both of which can result in pregnancy complications. With respect for the process of acclimatization, most pregnant visitors to high altitude can meet the physiologic needs of their fetus and enjoy the mountains.

REFERENCES

1. Artal, R., V. Fortunato, A. Welton et al. A comparison of cardiopulmonary adaptations to exercise in pregnancy at sea level and altitude. *Am J Obstet Gynecol* 172:1170-1180, 1995.
2. Baumann, H., P. Bung, F. Fallenstein, et al: Reaktion von Mutter und Fet auf die körperlicher Belastung in der Höhe. *Geburtshilfe Frauenheilkd* 45:869-876, 1985.
3. Baumann, H., R. Huch. Höhenexposition und Höhenaufenthalt in der Schwangerschaft: *Auswirkungen auf Mutter und Fet. Zentralbl Gynäkol* 108:889-899, 1986.
4. Bung, P. Köperliche Belastung und Sport in der Schwangerschaft-Möglichkeiten und Gefahren unter besonderer Berückischtigung der klinischen Wertigkeit. *Habilitationsschrift Med. Fakultät Universität* Bonn, 1992.
5. Carter, A. M. Factors affecting gas transfer across the placenta and the oxygen supply to the fetus. *J Devel Physiol* 1989; 12:305-322.
6. Copher, D. E., C. P. Huber. Heart rate response of the human fetus to induced maternal hypoxia. *Am J Obstet Gynecol* 98:320-335, 1967.
7. Cotter, J. R., J. N. Blechner, H. Prystowsky. Observations on pregnancy at altitude. I. The respiratory gases in maternal arterial and uterine venous blood. *Am J Obstet Gynecol* 99:1-8, 1967.
8. de Swiet, M. Cardiovascular problems in pregnancy. In *Turnbull's Obstetrics* (2nd Ed) Ed. Geoffrey Chamberlain. Edinburgh: Churchill Livingstone, 1995, pp. 369, 370.
9. Elliott, J. P., R. N. Trujillo. Fetal monitoring during emergency obstetric transport. *Am J Obstet Gynecol* 157:245-247, 1987.
10. Fox, H. The placenta, membranes and umbilical cord. In *Turnbull's Obstetrics* (2nd Ed) Ed. Geoffrey Chamberlain. Edinburgh: Churchill Livingstone, 1995, pp. 45-60.
11. Hellegers, A., J. Metcalfe, W. E. Huckabee, et al. Alveolar pCO_2 and pO_2 in pregnant and nonpregnant women at high altitude. *Am J Obstet Gynecol* 82:241-245, 1961.
12. Huch, R. Maternal hyperventilation and the fetus. *J Perinat Med* 13:1-15, 1985.
13. Huch, R., H. Baumann, F. Fallenstein, et al. Physiologic changes in pregnant women and their fetuses during jet air travel. *Am J Obstet Gynecol* 154:996-1000, 1986.
14. Huch, R. Pregnancy and altitude: physical activity at high altitude, In Artal Mittelmark R., R. A. Wiswell, B. L. Drinkwater (eds): *Exercise in Pregnancy*. Baltimore, MD, Williams & Wilkins, 1991, pp. 247-260.

15. Huch, R. Physical activity at altitude in pregnancy. *Seminars in Perinatology* 20:303-314, 1996.

16. John, A. H. The effect of maternal hypoxia on the heart rate of the foetus in utero. *Brit J Anaesth* 37:515-519, 1965.

17. Koos, B. J., G. G. Power, L. D. Longo. Placental oxygen transfer with considerations for maternal exercise. In *Exercise in Pregnancy*, Artal R. and R. A. Wiswell (eds). Baltimore: Williams and Wilkins, 1986, pp. 155-180.

18. Longo, L. L. Respiratory gas exchange in the placenta. Handbook of Physiology. Section 3: *The Respiratory System*, Vol. 4. Bethesda, MD: American Physiological Society, 1987, pp. 351-401.

19. Makowski, E. L., F. C. Battaglia, G. Meschia, R. E. Behrman, J. Schruefer, et al. Effect of maternal exposure to high altitude upon fetal oxygenation. *Am J Obstet Gynecol* 100: 852-861, 1968.

20. Meschia, G. Supply of oxygen to the fetus. *J Reprod Med* 23:160-165, 1979.

21. Moore, L. G. Altitude, effects on humans. *Encyclopedia of Reproduction* 1:107-112, 1999.

22. Morton, M. J., M. S. Paul, G. R. Campos, M. V. Hart, J. Metcalfe. Exercise dynamics in late gestation: effects of physical training. *Am J Obstet Gynecol* 152:91-97, 1985.

23. Parer, J. Effects of hypoxia on the mother and fetus with emphasis on maternal air transport. *Am J Obstet Gynecol* 142:957-961, 1982.

24. Parer, J. T. The effect of acute maternal hypoxia on fetal oxygenation and the umbilical circulation in the sheep. *Europ J Obstet Gynecol Reprod Biol* 10:125-136, 1980.

25. Parer, J. T., H. R. Dijkstra, P. P. M. Vredebregt, J. L. Harris, T. R. Krueger, M. L. Reuss. Increased fetal heart rate variability with acute hypoxia in chronically instrumented sheep. *Europ J Obstet Gynecol Reprod Biol* 10:393-399, 1980.

26. Ramsey, E. M. Circulation of the placenta. Birth Defects, Original Articles Series 1:5-12, 1965.

27. Sobrevilla, L. A., M. T. Cassinelli, A. Carcelen, J. M. Malaga. Human fetal and maternal oxygen tension and acid-base status during delivery at high altitude. *Am J Obstet Gynecol* 111:1111-1118, 1971.

28. Sorenson, S., J. Severinghaus. Respiratory sensitivity to acute hypoxia in man born at sea level living at high altitude. *J Appl Physiol* 25:211-216, 1968.

29. Wood, C., J. Hammond, J. Lumley, W. Newman. Effect of maternal inhalation of 10% oxygen upon the human fetus. *Aust NZ J Obstet Gynecol* 11:85-90, 1971.

Chapter 6

High Altitude Pulmonary Edema
Introduction

Peter Bärtsch
Department of Sports Medicine, Rupprecht Karls University, Heidelberg, Germany

Key words: pulmonary circulation, alveolar fluid clearance, transepithelial sodium
clearance, pulmonary hypertension, pulmonary artery pressure

The aim of this section is to present the latest results on HAPE research
and to discuss their implications for understanding the pathophysiology of
HAPE. Although high pulmonary artery pressure appears to be a condition
'sine qua non' it is not clear what causes the exaggerated pressure response
and how it accounts for the leak. Animal models and findings in
bronchoalveolar lavage fluid indicate a role for increased permeability due to
inflammation. Furthermore, data obtained in cell cultures suggest that
hypoxia may reduce fluid clearance from the alveoli. Simon Gibbs will
review the data on pulmonary circulation in HAPE-susceptible subjects and
discuss hemodynamic concepts. Urs Scherrer will evaluate a possible role of
transepithelial sodium transport on edema formation and present data
obtained in vivo supporting the hypothesis of decreased alveolar fluid
clearance in HAPE.

Hypoxia: Into the Next Millennium,
Edited by R. C. Roach, *et al.* Kluwer Academic/Plenum Publishing, New York, 1999.

Chapter 7

Pulmonary Hemodynamics: Implications for High Altitude Pulmonary Edema (HAPE)
A Review

J. Simon R. Gibbs
National Heart & Lung Institute at Imperial College of Science, Technology and Medicine, London, UK

Key words: High altitude, pulmonary edema, hemodynamics, hypoxia

Abstract: The role of pulmonary hemodynamics is central to the pathogenesis of high altitude pulmonary edema (HAPE). High pulmonary artery pressure is a marker of HAPE susceptibility in hypoxia and to a lesser extent in normoxia. Compared to non-susceptible subjects high pulmonary artery pressure is present not only at rest, but also during exercise and sleep. The reasons for elevated pulmonary artery pressure in HAPE susceptible subjects include increased vasomotor tone, severe hypoxic vasoconstriction and diminished capacity of the pulmonary circulation. Overperfusion of some parts of the capillary bed and wave reflections in the pulmonary circulation may result in pressure transients in the peripheral circulation which are considerably greater than the pressure in the main arteries.

The mechanism by which pulmonary hypertension causes the pulmonary circulation to leak involves hydraulic stress. Patchy vasoconstriction may expose parts of the capillary bed to high pressure resulting in stress failure of the capillary wall. The development of an inflammatory process may then occur after the initiation of the leak.

1.   INTRODUCTION

In health and disease the pulmonary circulation exhibits great diversity in its structure and behaviour. There are variations not only between species

Hypoxia: Into the Next Millennium,
Edited by R. C. Roach, *et al.* Kluwer Academic/Plenum Publishing, New York, 1999.

but also between individuals within a species. These are marked in man and may affect pulmonary hemodynamics.

The pulmonary circulation is a compromise. While requiring a thin barrier for gas exchange, it must also be strong enough to support the hydraulic stress of the entire cardiac output during exercise.

High altitude pulmonary edema (HAPE) is one of a number of causes of non-cardiogenic pulmonary edema which may share a similar pathophysiology. HAPE occurs in otherwise healthy subjects who ascend to high altitude and, usually in association with vigorous exercise and cold, develops after the first day. The edema fluid contains large proteins and red cells as well as inflammatory markers (38). Individuals who have had one attack are at risk of further episodes on future ascents. If pulmonary edema does not develop by 5 days it is very unlikely to occur.

Pulmonary hemodynamics play a crucial role in the pathogenesis of HAPE. Subjects susceptible to HAPE have excessively high pulmonary artery pressure preceding and during pulmonary edema compared to subjects who are not prone to this condition. Furthermore HAPE is precipitated in susceptible subjects by activities which raise pulmonary artery pressure.

2.   PULMONARY HEMODYNAMICS

At high altitude, pulmonary artery pressure rises as a consequence of hypoxic vasoconstriction which occurs in the muscularized distal circulation and causes an increase in pulmonary vascular resistance. The pulmonary artery pressure has been shown to mirror vascular resistance.

Vasoconstriction is determined mainly by the oxygen tension in alveolar air (3)and occurs within seconds of the onset of hypoxia (22). This is seen from about 2100 m altitude. The major site of vasoconstriction is the small muscular pulmonary arteries between 30 and 200 microns diameter. The pulmonary veins also vasoconstrict during prolonged hypoxia (43).

At sea level hypoxic pulmonary vasoconstriction serves a useful purpose: as a homeostatic mechanism intrinsic to the lung it diverts blood away from poorly ventilated lung to well ventilated alveoli. This is especially important in the fetus but its role in adults to ensure ventilation perfusion matching and thus maximal arterial oxygenation may be less important.

Pulmonary hypertension causes an interaction between right and left ventricles which may result in a reduced cardiac output. In patients with pulmonary hypertension high right ventricular pressure causes significant displacement of the interventricular septum towards the left ventricle (26). Prolonged decrease in right ventricular tension results in prolongation of right ventricular systole into left ventricular diastole. The consequence is that right ventricular pressure is high at the instant of mitral valve opening (4) and thus left ventricular filling is impaired.

Hydraulic stress in the pulmonary capillaries may be amplified by wave reflections. These occur in the branching structure of the pulmonary circulation. Since forward waves generated by the right ventricle, backward waves reflected from the peripheral vessels and forward re-reflected waves may be additive, pressure transients up to twice as high as the pressure measured in the central pulmonary arteries may occur.

2.1 Sea Level

Pulmonary artery pressure is elevated at sea level in subjects who develop HAPE compared to those who do not develop HAPE. This has been observed in single measurements made at rest by pulmonary artery catheterization (7,18,23). That this finding is applicable during normal daily activities, exercise and at night has been confirmed by continuous ambulatory pulmonary artery pressure monitoring (11). Pulmonary artery pressure during the day in control subjects (in mm Hg) was 19/7 and in HAPE prone subjects was 23/9 (P<0.001). This difference was greater at night: in control subjects 24/10 and in HAPE prone subjects 31/14 (P<0.001).

The rise in pulmonary artery pressure in response to exercise in HAPE prone subjects is up to about twice that of control subjects (23). While pulmonary capillary wedge pressure is normal at rest, one study has shown a greater rise in wedge pressure in HAPE prone subjects compared to controls during heavy bicycle exercise (6). In this exercise study HAPE prone subjects had a higher pulmonary artery pressure for a given cardiac index.

2.2 High Altitude

Pulmonary artery pressure measured by cardiac catheterization during untreated HAPE has been reported in 21 cases at altitudes between 2935 m and 3750 m (1,19,24,33,36). The mean pulmonary artery pressure varied between 15 and 117 mm Hg with a normal or low pulmonary capillary wedge pressure.

Pulmonary artery pressure rises on ascent to high altitude in the absence of pulmonary edema to a greater extent in subjects prone to HAPE than controls, further exaggerating the difference observed at sea level. This has been shown by cardiac catheterization in high altitude laboratories and barochambers (11,18). An exaggerated pulmonary artery pressure response to exercise has been shown (6,18) without an excessive rise in pulmonary capillary wedge pressure.

Ambulatory pulmonary artery pressure monitoring has shown that the highest pulmonary artery pressures are observed at night and on exercise (Gibbs 1997}. During the day at 4000 m pulmonary artery pressure (in mm Hg) was 31/14 in control subjects and 47/23 in HAPE prone subjects (P<0.001), at night this rose to 40/19 in controls and 60/29 in HAPE prone subjects (P<0.001). None had pulmonary edema. Lying flat in bed is the main explanation for the nocturnal pressure rise. Pulmonary artery pressure is lowest standing upright because the assumption of orthostasis is associated with a fall in intrathoracic blood volume of about one third (39).

The significance of pulmonary hypertension at high altitude is that it has been shown to precede the formation of pulmonary edema (2). Lowering pulmonary artery pressure prevents or attenuates the development of pulmonary edema. It has been shown that administration of vasodilators reduces pulmonary artery pressure with associated improvement in symptoms (2) and gas exchange (14,37). This was shown in a randomized controlled trial of nifedipine. Nifedipine is also successful in preventing pulmonary edema (2).

At 4559 m nitric oxide abolished the excessive pulmonary hypertensive response in HAPE susceptible individuals, reducing pressure to the same level as control subjects and suggesting an endothelial defect in HAPE susceptible subjects (37). Nitric oxide is known to be important in the maintenance of low pulmonary vascular resistance in the normal pulmonary circulation (10).

Phentolamine also reduces pulmonary artery pressure and vascular resistance in HAPE susceptible subjects (14) suggesting a role for the sympathetic nervous system. This is activated at high altitude (28) as evidenced by increased sympathetic peroneal nerve traffic recorded during microneuronography (37).

Oxygen lowers pulmonary artery pressure in the first 24 h after arrival at high altitude but has started to lose its vasodilator effect by 2 days (12). This may be explained by vascular remodelling which involves increased amounts of smooth muscle and extracellular matrix in the pulmonary arterial wall (29). This smooth muscle growth may protect against capillary overperfusion (see below) and explain why pulmonary edema does not develop after the first 5 days at high altitude (44).

3.   EXAGGERATED RESPONSE OF PULMONARY ARTERY PRESSURE IN HAPE

HAPE prone subjects appear to have greater pulmonary vascular reactivity than control subjects as evidenced by their response to hypoxia

(7,18,33,47) and exercise (6,18,23). Kawashima et al showed a greater response to hypoxia at sea level in HAPE susceptible subjects compared to control subjects matched for pulmonary function (23). Pulmonary vascular resistance index increased 3 to 5 times more than controls with a concomitant increase in pulmonary artery pressure 3 to 4 times more than controls. The pressure drop across the pulmonary vascular bed was greater in HAPE susceptible subjects. Not all studies have confirmed this enhanced hypoxic response (42). These discrepancies might be explained by differences in measurement techniques and reproducibility of HAPE in susceptible subjects.

These differences in pulmonary hemodynamics might be consistent with the hypothesis that subjects prone to HAPE have a reduced cross-sectional area of their pulmonary circulation (6). An increased propensity to develop HAPE at <3000 m altitude caused by the reduced capacity of the pulmonary circulation in patients with congenital absence (13,35), hypoplasia (8) or acquired occlusion (40) of the right pulmonary artery could be explained by reduced capacity of the pulmonary circulation.

Table 1. Pulmonary function reported in published studies of high altitude pulmonary edema. The column labelled Difference indicates the difference between HAPE and control groups for a given test in litres. Where a difference was recorded the volume was always greater in the control group.

Author	HAPE subjects	Control subjects	Difference	P
Viswanathan	44	51	FVC 0.86	0.01
1969			TLC 0.98	0.01
Hultgren 1971	5	0	(VC 107%)	
Viswanathan	57	44	FVC	NS
1978			FEV1 0.40	0.05
Kawashima	5	5	FVC, FEV1	NS
1989			TLC	NS
Matsuzawa	10	8	FVC, FEV1	NS
1989			TLC	NS
Selland 1993	4	4	FVC	NS
			FEV1 0.44	0.05
Eldridge 1996	7	9	FVC 0.9	0.045
			FEV1	NS

Smaller lung volumes have also been cited as evidence for reduced pulmonary circulatory capacity but Table 1 shows that such a finding is not universal. Where lung volumes differ between HAPE susceptible and control subjects, the control subjects have larger than normal volumes and the HAPE susceptible subjects have volumes within the normal range. Whether the difference in lung volumes is sufficient to explain the hemodynamic differences is not clear. It is likely that smaller lung volumes will predispose to lower arterial oxygen saturation at high altitude and this would be exacerbated by the reduced hypoxic ventilatory response documented in these HAPE subjects (15,16,27).

A more likely explanation for the exaggerated pulmonary vascular response is raised pulmonary vascular tone in HAPE susceptible subjects. This might be related to enhanced sympathetic activity and reduced nitric oxide synthesis in the endothelium. A gene polymorphism affecting iNOS may be implicated.

4.   MECHANISMS OF PULMONARY EDEMA IN ACUTE PULMONARY HYPERTENSION

Two hypotheses to explain hydraulic stress induced pulmonary vascular leak have been proposed. The law of Laplace predicts that circumferential wall tension is related to pressure and radius. Lamé's equation states that circumferential wall stress is related to pressure and radius, and inversely related to wall thickness.

4.1   Large Capacitance Vessel Leak

Whayne and Severinghaus performed experimental arteriolar embolisation in rats using polystyrene beads 12 – 35 microns in diameter (46). This simulated uniform hypoxic vasoconstriction. A static pressure of 100 mm Hg was then applied to the pulmonary artery for 10 min. Perivascular edema was demonstrated in the lungs consistent with rupture of the wall of large capacitance vessels. This site of leak was confirmed in a further study (21) but further work has not been pursued.

4.2   Capillary Leak

Hultgren first proposed that pulmonary vasoconstriction might be uneven throughout the vascular bed (17). Evidence for this came from animal studies (9,25) and the chest radiographic appearance of patchy non-uniform edema at high altitude. On the basis of further animal studies he proposed the concept of overperfusion (Figure 1) (20). There is wide variation in the amount of pulmonary vasoconstriction in man and this may be determined by the amount of muscle in the distal arteries (34). An example of the variation in the amount of muscle in small arteries is shown in Figure 2.

High pressure in a thin walled capillary may lead to high levels of wall stress and the pressures described above are adequate to cause wall disruption. This paved the way for West's description of capillary stress failure, evidence for which has been provided by electron micrographs showing endothelial disruption, and endothelial, epithelial and basement membrane disruption in isolated rabbit lung preparations (5,45). West proposed that mechanical stress caused by elevated intravascular pressure could lead to stress failure of the thin capillary wall and that this was primarily determined by the tensile strength of the basement membrane. While cardiogenic, low protein edema occurred through an intact capillary wall, further mechanical stress resulted first in stretching of the endothelium with leak of red cells and fluid into the interstitium, and then tearing of the alveolar epithelium and rupture of basement membrane (45). This passive process could thus cause complete mechanical disruption of the wall with accompanying leak of red cells and large proteins into the alveoli. Interestingly, the chronically elevated pulmonary artery pressure in HAPE susceptible subjects does not appear sufficient to cause the protective structural changes in capillaries which are seen in chronic heart failure (41).

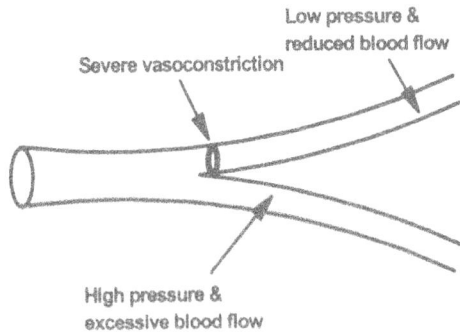

Figure 1. The concept of pulmonary capillary overperfusion proposed by Hultgren. Vasoconstriction in some vessels diverts blood flow to vessels which do not vasoconstrict thus causing overperfusion.

Recently, new data have suggested that the endothelial leak may occur not only between endothelial cells but also through transcellular openings. These openings have been demonstrated in frog mesentery on serial ultrathin electronmicrographs which are reconstructed in three dimensions (31). Hydraulic stress is a stimulus to their formation and there is rapid reversal of permeability when the pressure in the lumen drops (30). Cooling of these

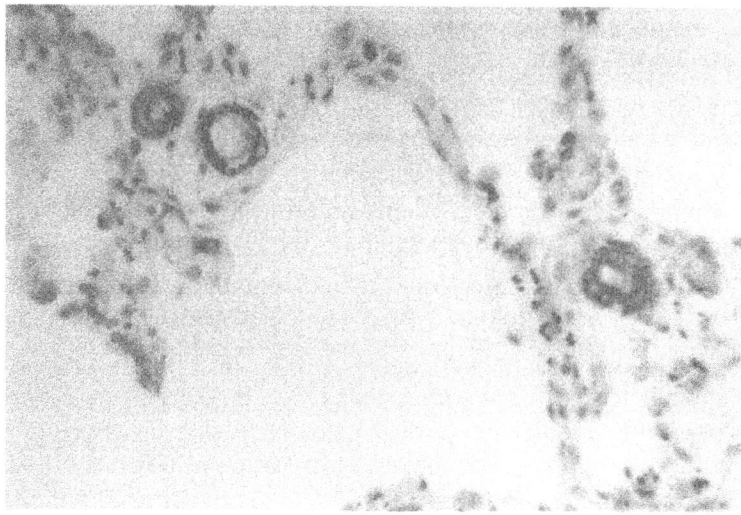

Figure 2. Variation in muscularisation of pulmonary arterioles in the human lung. Smooth muscle actin antibody stain. While two vessels have concentric muscle, the vessel in the middle has less muscle and exhibits a break in its muscle coat. Other arterioles may have no muscle. Courtesy Dr Mary Shepherd, Royal Brompton Hospital, London UK.

vessels increases the pressure at which they rupture (30) suggesting that the fragility of the capillaries may be affected by the endothelium. Evidence from isolated rat lungs suggests that microvascular filtration may be an active process and not simply the result of passive stretch (32).

5.   CONCLUSIONS

Any explanation for the difference between HAPE susceptible and control subjects must take account of the differences observed at sea level, at high altitude and during pulmonary edema. The single unifying feature appears to be the pulmonary vascular endothelium, which may combine differences in vasomotor tone and fragility with a propensity to leak under hydraulic stress and recover rapidly.

REFERENCES

1. Antezana, G., G. Leguia, G. Morales, J. Coudert, and H. Spielvogel. Hemodynamic study of high altitude pulmonary edema (12,200 ft). In: *High Altitude Physiology and Medicine*, edited by W. Brendel and R.A. Zink. New York, NY: Springer-Verlag, 1982, p. 232-241.
2. Bartsch, P., M. Maggiorini, M. Ritter, C. Noti, P. Vock, and O. Oelz. Prevention of high-altitude pulmonary edema by nifedipine. *NEJM* 325: 1284-1289, 1991.

3. Bergofsky, E.H. and S. Holtzman. A study of the mechanisms involved in the pulmonary arterial pressor response to hypoxia. *Circ. Res.* 20: 506-519, 1967.

4. Brecker, S.J., J.S. Gibbs, K.M. Fox, M.H. Yacoub, and D.G. Gibson. Comparison of Doppler derived hemodynamic variables and simultaneous high fidelity pressure measurements in severe pulmonary hypertension. *Br. Heart J.* 72: 384-389, 1994.

5. Costello, M.L., O. Mathieu-Costello, and J.B. West. Stress failure of alveolar epithelial cells studied by scanning electron microscopy. *Am Rev Respir Dis* 145: 1446-1455, 1992.

6. Eldridge, M.W., A. Podolsky, R.S. Richardson, D.H. Johnson, D.R. Knight, E.C. Johnson, S.R. Hopkins, H. Michimata, B. Grassi, J. Feiner, S.S. Kurdak, P.E. Bickler, P.D. Wagner, and J.W. Severinghaus. Pulmonary hemodynamic response to exercise in subjects with prior high-altitude pulmonary edema. *J. Appl. Physiol.* 81: 911-921, 1996.

7. Fasules, J.W., J.W. Wiggins, and R.R. Wolfe. Increased lung vasoreactivity in children from Leadville, Colorado, after recovery from high-altitude pulmonary edema. *Circulation* 72: 957-962, 1985.

8. Fiorenzano, G., V. Rastelli, V. Greco, A. Di Stefano, and M. Dottorini. Unilateral high-altitude pulmonary edema in a subject with right artery hypoplasia. *Respiration* 61: 51-54, 1994.

9. Fowler, K.T. and J. Read. Effect of alveolar hypoxia on zonal distribution of pulmonary blood flow. *J. Appl. Physiol.* 18: 244-250, 1963.

10. Gaston, B., J.M. Drazen, J. Loscalzo, and J.S. Stamler. The biology of nitrogen oxides in the airways. *Am. J. Respir. Crit. Care Med* 149: 538-551, 1994.

11. Gibbs, J.S.R., C. Schirlo, V. Pavlicek, P. Bartsch, E. Koller, U. Scherrer, and O. Oelz. High altitude pulmonary edema: differences in pulmonary artery pressure between susceptible and non-susceptible subjects in normoxia and hypoxia. *Circulation* 96 (Suppl): I426-I427, 1997.

12. Groves, B.M., J.T. Reeves, J.R. Sutton, P.D. Wagner, A. Cymerman, M.K. Malconian, P.B. Rock, P.M. Young, and C.S. Houston. Operation Everest II: Elevated high altitude pulmonary resistance unresponsive to oxygen. *J. Appl. Physiol.* 63: 521-530, 1987.

13. Hackett, P.H., C.E. Creagh, R.F. Grover, B. Honigman, C.S. Houston, J.T. Reeves, A.M. Sophocles, and H.M. Van. High-altitude pulmonary edema in persons without the right pulmonary artery. *NEJM* 302: 1070-1073, 1980.

14. Hackett, P.H., R.C. Roach, G.S. Hartig, E.R. Greene, and B.D. Levine. The effect of vasodilators on pulmonary hemodynamics in high altitude pulmonary edema: a comparison. *Int. J. Sports Med.* 13 Suppl 1: S68-S711992.

15. Hackett, P.H., R.C. Roach, R.B. Schoene, G.L. Harrison, and W.J. Mills. Abnormal control of ventilation in high-altitude pulmonary edema. *J. Appl. Physiol.* 64: 1268-1272, 1988.

16. Hohenhaus, E., A. Paul, R.E. McCullough, H. Kucherer, and P. Bartsch. Ventilatory and pulmonary vascular response to hypoxia and susceptibility to high altitude pulmonary oedema. *Eur. Respir. J.* 8: 1825-1833, 1995.

17. Hultgren, H.N. High altitude pulmonary edema. In: *Lung Water and Solute Exchange*, edited by N.C. Staub. New York, NY: Dekker, 1978, p. 437-469.

18. Hultgren, H.N., R.F. Grover, and L.H. Hartley. Abnormal circulatory responses to high altitude in subjects with a previous history of high-altitude pulmonary edema. *Circulation* 44: 759-770, 1971.

19. Hultgren, H.N., C.E. Lopez, E. Lundberg, and H. Miller. Physiologic studies of pulmonary edema at high altitude. *Circulation* 29: 393-408, 1964.

20. Hultgren, H.N. and E.A. Marticorena. High altitude pulmonary edema. Epidemiologic observations in Peru. *Chest* 74: 372-376, 1978.

21. Illiff, L.D. Extra-alveolar vessels and edema development in excised dog lungs. *Circ. Res.* 28: 524-532, 1971.

22. Jensen, K.S., A.J. Micco, J. Czartolomna, L. Latham, and N.F. Voelkel. Rapid onset of hypoxic vasoconstriction in isolated lungs. *J. Appl. Physiol.* 72: 2018-2023, 1992.

23. Kawashima, A., K. Kubo, T. Kobayashi, and M. Sekiguchi. Hemodynamic responses to acute hypoxia, hypobaria, and exercise in subjects susceptible to high-altitude pulmonary edema. *J. Appl. Physiol.* 67: 1982-1989, 1989.

24. Kobayashi, T., K. Kubo, M. Fukushima, K. Yoshimura, T. Shibamoto, K. Fujimoto, K. Hirai, A. Kawashima, S. Koyama, H. Yagi.Pulmonary hemodynamics in patients with high altitude pulmonary edema. *Nippon Kyobu Shikkan Gakkai Zasshi.* 25: 1284-1289, 1987.

25. Lehr, D., M. Triller, L. Fisher et al. Induced changes in the pattern of pulmonary blood flow in the rabbit. *Circ. Res.* 13: 119-131, 1963.

26. Louie, E.K., S. Rich, S. Levitsky, and B.H. Brundage. Doppler echocardiographic demonstration of the differential effects of right ventricular pressure and volume overload on left ventricular geometry and filling. *J. Am. Coll. Cardiol.* 19: 84-90, 1992.

27. Matsuzawa, Y., K. Fujimoto, T. Kobayashi, N.R. Namushi, K. Harada, H. Kohno, M. Fukushima, and S. Kusama. Blunted hypoxic ventilatory drive in subjects susceptible to high-altitude pulmonary edema. *J. Appl. Physiol.* 66: 1152-1157, 1989.

28. Mazzeo, R.S., G.A. Brooks, G.E. Butterfield, D.A. Podolin, E.E. Wolfel, and J.T. Reeves. Acclimatization to high altitude increases muscle sympathetic activity both at rest and during exercise. *Am. J. Physiol.* 269: R201-R207, 1995.

29. Meyrick, B. and L. Reid. Hypoxia-induced structural changes in the media and adventitia of the rat hilar pulmonary artery and their regression. *Am J Pathol* 100: 151-178, 1980.

30. Neal, C.R. and C.C. Michel. Openings in frog microvascular endothelium induced by high intravascular pressures. *J. Physiol. Lond.* 492: 39-52, 1996.

31. Neal, C.R. and C.C. Michel. Transcellular openings through frog microvascular endothelium. *Exp. Physiol.* 82: 419-422, 1997.

32. Parker, J.C., C.L. Ivey, and J.A. Tucker. Gadolinium prevents high airway pressure-induced permeability increases in isolated rat lungs. *J. Appl. Physiol.* 84: 1113-1118, 1998.

33. Penaloza, D. and F. Sime. Circulatory dynamics during high altitude pulmonary edema. *Am. J. Cardiol.* 23: 369-378, 1969.

34. Reid, L. The pulmonary circulation: remodelling in growth and disease. *Am. Rev. Respir. Dis.* 119: 531-546, 1979.

35. Rios, B., D.J. Driscoll, and D.G. McNamara. High-altitude pulmonary edema with absent right pulmonary artery. *Pediatrics* 75: 314-317, 1985.

36. Roy, S.B., J.S. Guleria, P.K. Khanna, S.C. Manchanda, J.N. Pande, and P.S. Subba. Haemodynamic studies in high altitude pulmonary oedema. *Br. Heart J.* 31: 52-58, 1969.

37. Scherrer, U., L. Vollenweider, A. Delabays, M. Savcic, U. Eichenberger, G.R. Kleger, A. Fikrle, P.E. Ballmer, P. Nicod, and P. Bartsch. Inhaled nitric oxide for high-altitude pulmonary edema. *NEJM* 334: 624-629, 1996.

38. Schoene, R.B., P.H. Hackett, W.R. Henderson, E.H. Sage, M. Chou, R.C. Roach, J. Mills, and T.R. Martin. High altitude pulmonary edema. Characteristics of lung lavage fluid. *JAMA* 256: 63-69, 1986.

39. Sjostrand, T. Volume and distribution of blood and their significance in regulating the circulation. *Physiol Rev* 33: 202-208, 1953.

40. Torrington, K.G. Recurrent high-altitude illness associated with right pulmonary artery occlusion from granulomatous mediastinitis. *Chest* 96: 1422-1423, 1989.

41. Townsley, M.I., Z. Fu, O. Mathieu-Costello, and J.B. West. Pulmonary microvascular permeability. Responses to high vascular pressure after induction of pacing-induced heart failure in dogs. *Circ. Res.* 77: 317-325, 1995.

42. Viswanathan, R., S.K. Jain, S. Subramanian, T.A. Subramanian, G.L. Dua, and J. Giri. Pulmonary edema of high altitude II. Clinical, aerohemodynamic, and biochemical studies in a group with history of pulmonary edema of high altitude. *Am Rev Respir Dis* 100: 334-341, 1969.

43. Welling, K.K., R. Sanchez, J.B. Ravn, B. Larsen, and O. Amtorp. Effect of prolonged alveolar hypoxia on pulmonary arterial pressure and segmental vascular resistance. *J. Appl. Physiol.* 75: 1194-1200, 1993.

44. West, J.B. and O. Mathieu-Costello. Vulnerability of pulmonary capillaries in heart disease. *Circulation* 92: 622-631, 1995.

45. West, J.B., K. Tsukimoto, O. Mathieu-Costello, and R. Prediletto. Stress failure in pulmonary capillaries. *J Appl Physiol* 70: 1731-1742, 1991.

46. Whayne, T.F. and J.W. Severinghaus. Experimental hypoxic pulmonary edema in the rat. *J. Appl. Physiol.* 25: 729-732, 1968.

47. Yagi, H., H. Yamada, T. Kobayashi, and M. Sekiguchi. Doppler assessment of pulmonary hypertension induced by hypoxic breathing in subjects susceptible to high altitude pulmonary edema. *Am. Rev. Respir. Dis.* 142: 796-801, 1990.

Chapter 8

High-Altitude Pulmonary Edema: From Exaggerated Pulmonary Hypertension to a Defect in Transepithelial Sodium Transport

Urs Scherrer, Claudio Sartori, Mattia Lepori, Yves Allemann, Hervé Duplain, Lionel Trueb, Pascal Nicod

Department of Internal Medicine, Centre Hospitalier Universitaire Vaudois, Lausanne (U.S., C.S., M.L., H.D., P.N.); the Department of Cardiology (Y.A.), University Hospital, Berne; and the Institute of Physiology (L.T.), University of Lausanne, Lausanne, Switzerland

Key words: high-altitude pulmonary edema, pulmonary hypertension, nitric oxide, endothelin, sympathetic nervous system, alveolar transepithelial sodium transport

Abstract: High-altitude pulmonary edema (HAPE) is a form of lung edema which occurs in otherwise healthy subjects, thereby allowing the study of underlying mechanisms of pulmonary edema in the absence of confounding factors. Exaggerated pulmonary hypertension is a hallmark of HAPE and is thought to play an important part in its pathogenesis. Pulmonary vascular endothelial dysfunction and augmented hypoxia-induced sympathetic activation may be underlying mechanisms contributing to exaggerated pulmonary vasoconstriction in HAPE. Recent observations by our group suggest, however, that pulmonary hypertension itself may not be sufficient to trigger HAPE. Based on studies in rats, indicating that perinatal exposure to hypoxia predisposes to exaggerated hypoxic pulmonary vasoconstriction in adulthood, we examined effects of high-altitude exposure on pulmonary-artery pressure in a group of young adults who had suffered from transient perinatal pulmonary hypertension. We found that these young adults had exaggerated pulmonary vasoconstriction of similar magnitude to that observed in HAPE-susceptible subjects. Surprisingly, however, none of the subjects developed lung edema. These findings strongly suggest that additional mechanisms are needed to trigger pulmonary edema at high-altitude. Observations in vitro, and in vivo suggest that a defect of the alveolar transepithelial sodium transport could act as a sensitizer to pulmonary edema. The aim of this article is to review very recent experimental evidence consistent with this concept. We will discuss data gathered in mice with targeted disruption of the gene of the α subunit of the amiloride-sensitive epithelial sodium channel (αENaC), and present preliminary data on measurements of transepithelial sodium transport in vivo in HAPE-susceptible and HAPE-resistant mountaineers.

1.   INTRODUCTION

Pulmonary edema is a problem of major clinical importance and results from a persistent imbalance between forces that drive water into the extravascular space and the biologic mechanisms for its removal. HAPE is a form of lung edema that occurs in otherwise healthy subjects. It thereby allows the study of underlying mechanisms of pulmonary edema in the absence of confounding factors such as coexisting cardiovascular or pulmonary disease, and drug therapy. The additional observation that there exist HAPE-resistant and HAPE-prone subjects suggests the possibility of a genetic and/or acquired predisposition (36, 39).

Exaggerated pulmonary hypertension is a hallmark of HAPE, and by leading to capillary leakage either by overperfusion (21) or stress failure (47), is thought to play an important part in alveolar fluid flooding at high altitude (16, 20, 36, 39, 40, 43). However, the mechanism(s) underlying the exaggerated hypoxic pulmonary vasoconstriction in HAPE-prone subjects is still unknown.

2.   MECHANISMS OF EXAGGERATED PULMONARY VASOCONSTRICTOR RESPONSIVENESS TO HIGH-ALTITUDE EXPOSURE IN HAPE-SUSCEPTIBLE SUBJECTS

2.1   Role of the pulmonary vascular endothelium

Recent studies from our group indicate that the endothelium may play an important part, and that both impaired release of relaxing factors and augmented release of vasoconstrictor factors contribute to exaggerated hypoxic pulmonary vasoconstriction and HAPE. The evidence is as follows. When administered by inhalation, nitric oxide (NO), an endothelium-derived relaxing factor which is synthesized locally by the endothelium from the amino acid L-arginine, attenuates the pulmonary vasoconstriction evoked by short-term hypoxia (13, 14). In a recent study, we examined effects of NO inhalation on pulmonary-artery pressure (and arterial oxygenation) in a group of HAPE-prone mountaineers, and in a group of subjects resistant to this condition (39). As expected, HAPE-prone subjects had more pronounced pulmonary vasoconstriction than those resistant to such edema. During NO inhalation, however, the pulmonary-artery pressure was similar in both groups, because the NO-induced decrease in pulmonary-artery pressure was much larger in HAPE-prone subjects (Figure 1). This observation is consistent with the hypothesis that a defect in NO-mediated pulmonary vasodilation - a mechanism that may act as a brake on pulmonary vasoconstriction (9) - contributes to HAPE-susceptibility.

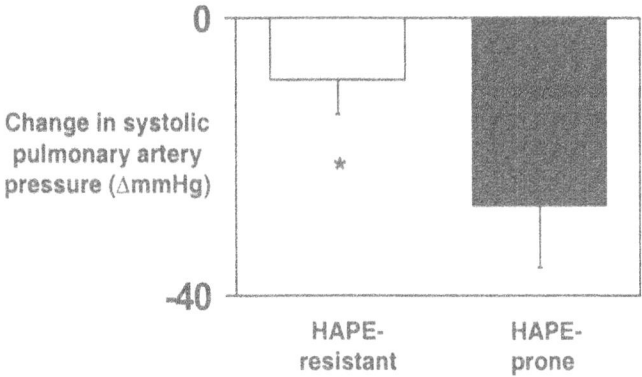

Figure 1. Effects of nitric oxide inhalation (40ppm for 20 min.) at high-altitude (4559 m) on systolic pulmonary artery pressure. Data are means±SE *for* 17 HAPE-resistant and 18 HAPE-prone subjects. * p<0.001 vs. HAPE-prone subjects. (Adapted from Scherrer et al. (39))

Consistent with this hypothesis, inhibition of nitric oxide synthesis by L-NMMA (a stereospecific inhibitor of the NO-synthase) infusion potentiates the pulmonary vasoconstrictor response to short-term hypoxic breathing in humans (2). Moreover, we and others have recently shown that endothelial NOS dysfunction predisposes to augmented pulmonary vasoconstrictor responsiveness to hypoxia in mice (10, 12, 45). For example, we have measured pulmonary-artery pressure (as estimated from systolic right ventricular pressure) in heterozygous eNOS (+/-) mice and wild type littermates (10). We found that under normoxic conditions pulmonary-artery pressure was comparable in both groups. In contrast, both short-term hypoxic breathing (F_IO_2 0.15 for 15 minutes), and more prolonged hypoxic exposure (F_IO_2 0.08 for 72 hours), evoked a roughly 50 percent larger increase in pulmonary-artery pressure in eNOS deficient than in wild type mice. Taken together these observations demonstrate that NO plays a key role in the regulation of the pulmonary vascular tone during hypoxic stress.

The findings are consistent with the hypothesis that in HAPE-prone subjects a defect in NO synthesis may be one of the factors contributing to exaggerated pulmonary vasoconstrictor responses at high-altitude.

In addition to relaxing factors, the endothelium also synthesizes vasoconstrictor factors. Endothelin-1 (ET-1) is the most potent among them (48), and plays a role in the regulation of pulmonary vascular tone during hypoxic stress. In rats and humans, endothelin receptor blockade attenuates the pulmonary vasoconstrictor response to hypoxia (6, 8). High-altitude exposure augments ET-1 plasma concentration in healthy subjects (15). To examine whether ET-1 may contribute to exaggerated pulmonary vasoconstriction in HAPE-prone subjects, in a recent study, we measured ET-1 plasma levels and pulmonary-artery pressure at low (580 m) and high altitude (4559 m), in HAPE-prone and HAPE-resistant mountaineers (37). We found that, at high altitude, ET-1 plasma levels were roughly 33 percent higher in mountaineers prone to pulmonary edema than in those resistant to edema (Figure 2). Moreover, there was a direct relationship between the changes, from low to high altitude, in ET-1 plasma levels and systolic pulmonary-artery pressure, and, between ET-1 plasma levels and pulmonary-artery pressure measured at high-altitude.

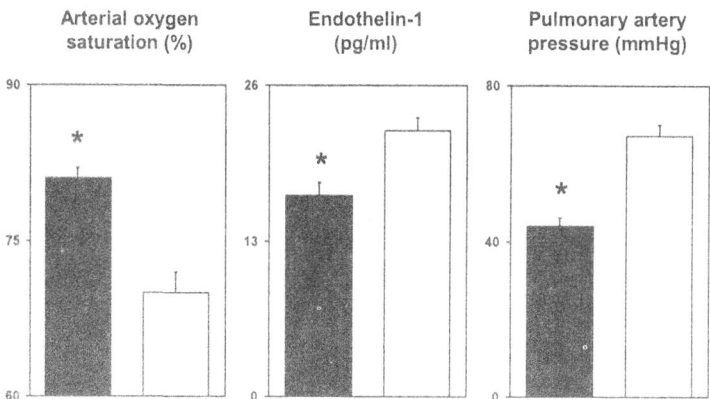

Figure 2. Bar graphs showing mean±SE values at high altitude (4559 m), for arterial oxygen saturation (SaO$_2$), *venous* endothelin-1 plasma concentration, and systolic pulmonary artery pressure in 16 HAPE-prone (open bars) and 16 HAPE-resistant subjects (filled bars). *P<0.05 patients vs. control subjects (From Sartori et al. (37)).

These findings are consistent with the hypothesis that an augmented release of the potent pulmonary vasoconstrictor peptide ET-1, and/or its reduced pulmonary clearance, could represent one of the mechanisms contributing to exaggerated pulmonary hypertension at high-altitude. Finally, and most interestingly, in human endothelial cells, NO inhibits the hypoxia-induced stimulation of ET-1 gene expression and synthesis (26). suggesting that the defect in NO-synthesis and augmented ET-1 synthesis could be causally related.

In summary, it is now clear that the endothelium plays a key role in the regulation of the pulmonary vascular responsiveness to hypoxic stress. In HAPE-prone mountaineers, recent studies have provided evidence consistent with the hypothesis that impaired endothelial synthesis of vasorelaxing factors and augmented synthesis of contracting factors could be involved in the pathogenesis of exaggerated altitude-induced pulmonary hypertension.

2.2   Role of the sympathetic nervous system

Cardiovascular adjustments to hypoxia are mediated, at least in part, by the sympathetic nervous system, and sympathetic activation promotes pulmonary vasoconstriction and alveolar fluid flooding in experimental animals (7, 27). Thus, it is possible that the sympathetic nervous system may contribute to exaggerated pulmonary hypertension in HAPE-susceptible subjects. To test this hypothesis, we measured, in HAPE-prone and -resistant mountaineers, sympathetic-nerve activity (using intraneural microelectrodes) targeted at the skeletal vasculature, and pulmonary-artery pressure during short-term hypoxic breathing at low altitude, and during high-altitude exposure at the high-altitude research laboratory Capanna Regina Margherita (4559 m) (11). We found that in subjects prone to pulmonary edema, short-term hypoxic breathing at low altitude evoked comparable hypoxemia, but a more than two times larger increase in the rate of the sympathetic-nerve firing than in subjects resistant to edema (Figure 3). Similarly, at high altitude, the sympathetic-firing rate in subjects prone to edema was markedly augmented, and the sympathetic overactivation preceded the development of lung edema. We also observed a direct relationship between sympathetic-nerve activity and pulmonary-artery pressure measured at low and high-altitude in the two groups.

These data provide the first evidence for an exaggerated sympathetic activation in HAPE-prone subjects, both during short-term hypoxic breathing at low altitude, and during actual high-altitude exposure. They suggest that sympathetic overactivation may contribute to high-altitude induced exaggerated pulmonary hypertension in HAPE-susceptible subjects. Consistent with this hypothesis, in subjects suffering from HAPE, infusion of the alpha-adrenergic blocking agent phentolamine evokes markedly larger decreases in pulmonary-artery pressure than other, non-specific vasodilators (17).

What we have seen so far, is that there exist HAPE-prone and HAPE-resistant subjects. The former are characterized by exaggerated pulmonary hypertension which may be related to endothelial dysfunction and sympathetic overactivation. The factors predisposing individual subjects to such augmented altitude-induced pulmonary vasoconstriction are not known.

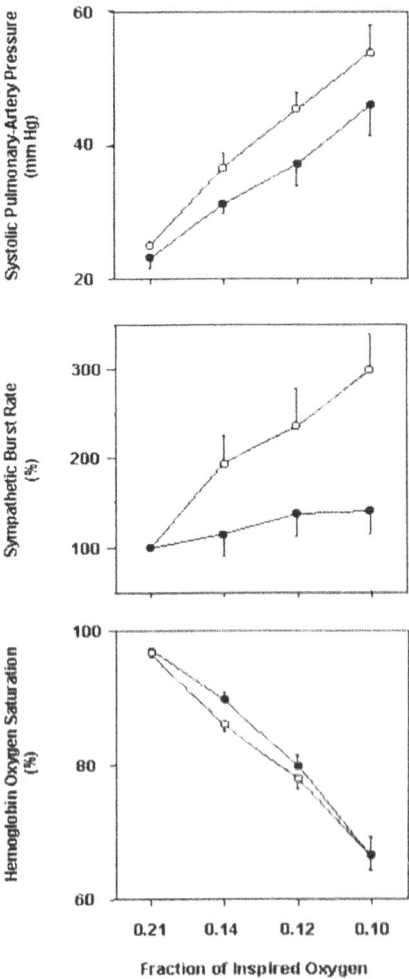

Figure 3. Effects (mean±SE) of short term hypoxic breathing at low altitude on arterial oxygen saturation, muscle sympathetic-nerve activity (MSNA), and systolic pulmonary artery pressure in 8 *HAPE*-prone (open circles) and 7 HAPE-resistant (*filled* circles) mountaineers. The subjects were sequentially breathing each of the hypoxic gas mixtures for 20 minutes. Measurements were performed during the last 4 minutes of each step. The hypoxia-induce sympathetic and pressor effects were augmented in HAPE-prone subjects (P<0.001 for the comparison between HAPE-prone and HAPE-resistant subjects) (From Duplain et al. (11)).

3.   EXAGGERATED PULMONARY HYPERTENSION *PER SE*, IS NOT SUFFICIENT TO TRIGGER HAPE

Epidemiological studies suggest that adverse events in utero are associated with cardiovascular and metabolic disease in adulthood (1). During the perinatal period the pulmonary circulation undergoes important structural and functional changes to allow the sudden transition from gas exchange by the placenta to gas exchange by the lungs (30). These changes allow a dramatic, roughly ten-fold increase in pulmonary blood flow and a corresponding decrease in pulmonary vascular resistance. During the perinatal period the pulmonary circulation is particularly vulnerable to noxious stimuli such as hypoxia (18, 30). Studies in rats have suggested that transitory exposure to hypoxia during the first few days of life, which induces transient pulmonary hypertension (18), predisposes to augmented pulmonary vasoconstrictor responses to hypoxia in adult life (5, 18, 32). This augmented responsiveness may be related, at least in part, to endothelial dysfunction (41).

To test for the existence of such a predisposition in man, we measured pulmonary vasoconstrictor responses to high-altitude exposure (4559 m) in a group of young healthy adults who were born at or near term ($\geq$34 weeks of gestation), and who had suffered from transient hypoxic pulmonary hypertension during their perinatal period, and compared these responses with those observed in young adults who had not suffered from any complication during the perinatal period (34). We found that in young adults who during their perinatal period had suffered from transient pulmonary hypertension, the altitude-induced increase in pulmonary artery pressure was more than 50 percent larger than in control subjects (Figure 4). This augmented pulmonary vasoconstrictor response could not be attributed to more severe oxygen desaturation in the circulating blood, because the degree of the altitude-induced hypoxemia was comparable in both groups (34).

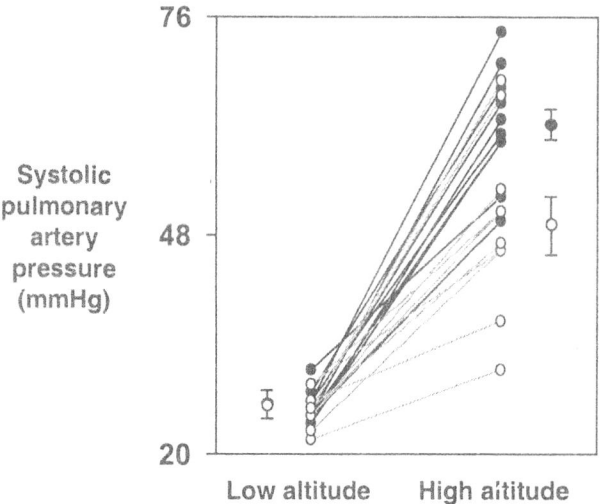

Figure 4. Effects of high-altitude exposure (4559 m) and nitric oxide inhalation at high-altitude on mean±SE systolic pulmonary-artery pressure in 10 healthy young adults with a history of transient perinatal pulmonary hypertension [filled circles] and in 10 control subjects [open circles]. The high-altitude induced increase in pulmonary-artery pressure was significantly (P=0.01) larger in patients than in control subjects (From Sartori et al. (34)).

The underlying mechanism causing the exaggerated pulmonary vasoconstrictor responsiveness is not known. Structural and functional defects need to be considered. Infants dying from neonatal pulmonary hypertension exhibit thickening of the pulmonary vascular wall, due to vascular smooth muscle cell hypertrophy (19, 44). It is not known whether in infants who survive, these structural anomalies of the vascular wall persist, but if so, they could predispose to exaggerated vasoconstrictor responses. Alternatively, one may speculate that the perinatal defect of nitric oxide synthesis (19) observed in neonates with pulmonary hypertension persists into adult life, and predisposes to exaggerated altitude-induced pulmonary vasoconstriction in these subjects. In line with this speculation, in rats exposed to transitory hypoxia during their first few days of life, the augmented hypoxia-induced pulmonary vasoconstriction in adult life is associated with impaired nitric-oxide synthase mRNA expression in the lungs (41).

The exaggerated pulmonary vasoconstriction in these young adults was of similar magnitude as observed previously in HAPE-prone mountaineers studied under the same conditions (39). Surprisingly, however none of the subjects had clinical, radiographic, or laboratory (widening of the alveolar-arterial oxygen difference) evidence of alveolar fluid flooding (Figure 5).

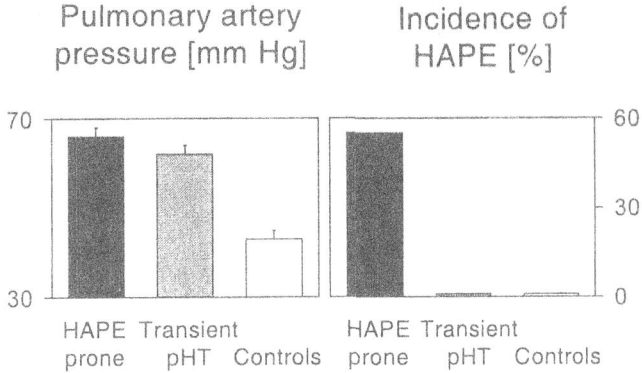

Figure 5. Effects of high-altitude exposure (4559 m) on pulmonary artery pressure and incidence of HAPE in 18 HAPE prone subjects, 10 healthy young adults with a history of transient *perinatal* pulmonary *hypertension*, and 17 HAPE-resistant control subjects (Adapted from Scherrer et al. (39) and Sartori et al. (34)).

This finding contrasts with the roughly 60 percent incidence of pulmonary edema which has consistently been found in HAPE-prone subjects studied under the same conditions (36, 39). This very important observation suggests that exaggerated pulmonary hypertension per se may not always be sufficient to trigger HAPE, and that additional mechanisms play a role. A defect in transepithelial alveolar sodium transport may represent such a candidate mechanism.

4. DOES A DEFECT OF ALVEOLAR TRANSEPITHELIAL SODIUM TRANSPORT ACT AS A SENSITIZER TO PULMONARY EDEMA?

Pulmonary edema results from an imbalance between the leak of fluid into the airspace, and its removal (42). While for many years, it was believed that Starling forces and lymphatic drainage entirely account for the removal of excess intraalveolar fluid, it is now clear that both active and facilitated transepithelial sodium transport play an important part. Sodium is taken up by the alveolar cells at the apical surface, primarily through the amiloride-sensitive sodium channel (ENaC). Once taken up, the sodium is then pumped out of the cell by the Na-K-ATPase located at the basolateral membrane (29, 38) (Figure 6).

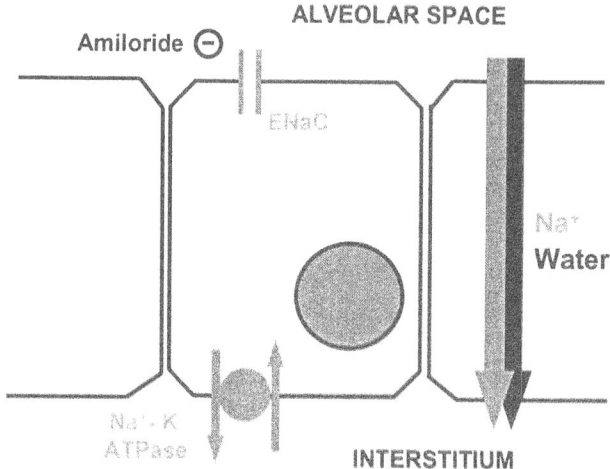

Figure 6. Mechanisms involved in the alveolar transepithelial sodium (and water) transport. Sodium is taken up by the alveolar cell at the apical surface, primarily through the amiloride-sensitive sodium channel (ENaC). Once taken up, the sodium is then pumped out of the cell into the lung interstitium by the Na-K-ATPase located at the basolateral membrane.

The amiloride sensitive sodium channel, ENaC, is a heteromultimeric protein made up of three homologous subunits (α, β, and γ) (3, 4). *In vitro*, assembly and expression of active sodium channels is strictly dependent on αENaC, the β and γ subunits by themselves are unable to induce an amiloride-sensitive sodium current (4). ENaC is thought to be the limiting step of transepithelial sodium transport. In isolated animal lungs, in *ex vivo* resected human lungs, and in intact animals (29), the amiloride-sensitive sodium transport accounts for approximately 40-60 percent of the alveolar fluid clearance. The key role of this transport, in keeping the airspace free of fluid, has recently been further, and rather dramatically, demonstrated by transgenic mice deficient for the α-subunit of the ENaC which develop respiratory distress and die shortly after birth from failure to clear their lungs of liquid (22). This raises the question, whether under conditions of augmented alveolar fluid flooding, ENaC dysfunction could lead to pulmonary edema. Interestingly, in the context of HAPE, hypoxia and cold temperature (two conditions universally associated with high-altitude exposure) impair the sodium transport *in vitro* by inhibiting the ENaC (31, 33, 46). If also present in vivo, such an impairment, possibly in conjunction with preexistent infraclinical ENaC dysfunction, could favor lung edema.

Transgenic expression of αENaC driven by a CMV promoter in αENaC(-/-) knockout mice [αENaC(-/-)Tg], rescues the perinatal lethal pulmonary phenotype (23). Surviving adult [αENaC(-/-)Tg] mice, have normal or near normal lung water content, but the amiloride-sensitive sodium transport in the lung is lower than in littermate control mice, demonstrating infraclinical ENaC dysfunction. To study the effects of such dysfunction on susceptibility to lung edema, we measured wet/dry (W/D) lung weight ratio (an indicator of lung water content) after hypoxic exposure (F_1O_2 0.08 for 72 hours) in such mice and their wild type littermates. We found that at normoxia, the W/D lung weight ratio was similar in both groups. In contrast, during hypoxia, the W/D lung weight ratio was markedly augmented in transgenic as compared with wild type mice (28).

These preliminary findings provide the first evidence *in vivo* that infraclinical ENaC dysfunction, which under normal conditions (normoxia) had no detectable effect on fluid content of the lungs, leads to pulmonary water accumulation during hypoxic stress, and may therefore act as a sensitizer to lung edema. It is important to note here that the difference in alveolar fluid accumulation between [αENaC(-/-)Tg] mutant mice and wild type littermates appears to be related specifically to ENaC dysfunction, because the hypoxia-induced pulmonary vasoconstrictor responses are comparable in the two groups (Duplain et al., unpublished observations).

We wondered whether a similar mechanism could be operational in humans, and if so, may contribute to HAPE-susceptibility. We measured, at low altitude, nasal potential difference (a marker of the sodium transport across the respiratory epithelium of the lower respiratory tract (24, 25), in HAPE-prone and HAPE-resistant mountaineers (35). To assess specifically the contribution of the ENaC, we also measured the effects of amiloride superfusion on the nasal potential difference. We found that in HAPE-prone subjects, the nasal PD was roughly 30 percent lower than in mountaineers resistant to edema. This impairment appears to be related, at least in part, to a defect in ENaC function, because amiloride superfusion induced a significantly smaller decrease in the nasal potential difference in HAPE-prone than in HAPE-resistant subjects. These exciting preliminary findings provide the first evidence for an impairment of the respiratory transepithelial sodium and water transport in a human form of pulmonary edema.

5. CONCLUSION

Based on our results, we suggest the following new concept for the pathogenesis of HAPE (Figure 7). Pulmonary edema results from a persistent imbalance between the forces that drive water into the airspace, and the biologic mechanisms for its removal. In HAPE-prone subjects, alveolar fluid flooding is augmented, because of exaggerated pulmonary hypertension which appears to be related, at least in part, to endothelial dysfunction and sympathetic overactivation. Exaggerated pulmonary hypertension per se, however, is not sufficient to trigger HAPE, as evidenced by studies in young adults with transient perinatal pulmonary hypertension, and additional mechanisms appear to play a role. Our findings suggest that HAPE-prone subjects are characterized by a, possibly genetic, defect of the transepithelial sodium (and water) transport which during high-altitude exposure may be further impaired by environmental factors such as hypoxia and cold temperature. The conjunction of these pulmonary vascular endothelial and alveolar epithelial defects ultimately leads to high-altitude pulmonary edema.

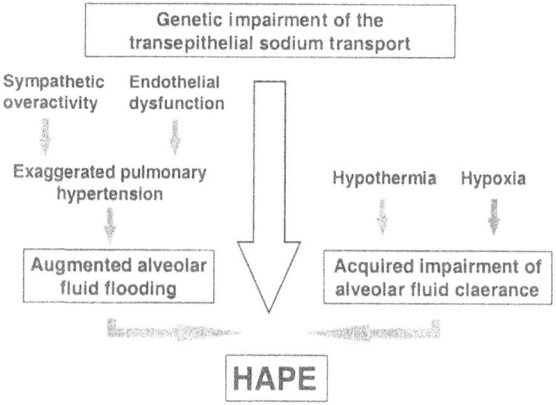

Figure 7. Mechanisms involved in the pathogenesis of HAPE.

ACKNOWLEDGMENTS

The authors' research was supported by grants from the Swiss National Science Foundation, the International Olympic Committee, the Fondazione Dottor PierLuigi Crivelli, and the Placide Nicod Foundation.

We would like to thank Franziska Keller, Edith Hummler, PhD, Laurent Vollenweider, MD, Denis Randin, MD, Alain Delabays, MD, Milos Savcic MD, and Bernd-Michael Löffler, MD, for their invaluable contributions to the authors' studies; and Peter Bärtsch, MD, Marco Maggiorini, MD, Bernard Rossier, MD, and Peter E. Ballmer, MD, for many stimulating discussions. We are indebted to our subjects; to the Sezione Varallo del Club Alpino Italiano for providing the locations in the Capanna Regina Margherita; to our mountain guides Andrea Enzio and Osvaldo Antonietti for leading our subjects safely to the high altitude research laboratory; to the Hewlett-Packard Corporation for providing the echocardiographic equipment; and the Swiss Army for providing the radiographic equipment and transporting part of the material.

REFERENCES

1. Barker, D. J. P. *Mothers, babies, and disease in later life.* London: BMJ Books, 1994.
2. Blitzer, M. L., E. Loh, M. A. Roddy, J. S. Stamler, and M. A. Creager. Endothelium-derived nitric oxide regulates systemic and pulmonary vascular resistance during acute hypoxia in humans. *J Am Coll Cardiol* 28: 591-6, 1996.
3. Canessa, C. M., J. D. Horisberger, and B. C. Rossier. Epithelial sodium channel related to proteins involved in neurodegeneration. *Nature* 361: 467-70, 1993.
4. Canessa, C. M., L. Schild, G. Buell, B. Thorens, I. Gautschi, J. D. Horisberger, and B. C. Rossier. Amiloride-sensitive epithelial Na+ channel is made of three homologous subunits. *Nature* 367: 463-7, 1994.
5. Caslin, A., D. Heath, and P. Smith. Influence of hypobaric hypoxia in infancy on the subsequent development of vasoconstrictive pulmonary vascular disease in the Wistar albino rat. *J Pathol* 163: 133-111, 1991.
6. Chen, S.-J., Y.-F. Chen, Q. C. Meng, and S. Oparil. The endothelin receptor antagonist Bosentan prevents short term hypoxia induced pulmonary hypertension in the rats (Abstract). *Circulation* 90: I-151, 1994.
7. Dauber, I. M., and J. V. Weil. Lung injury edema in dogs. Influence of sympathetic ablation. *J Clin Invest* 72: 1977-86, 1983.
8. DiCarlo, V. S., S. J. Chen, Q. C. Meng, J. Durand, M. Yano, Y. F. Chen, and S. Oparil. ETA-receptor antagonist prevents and reverses chronic hypoxia-induced pulmonary hypertension in rat. *Am J Physiol* 269: L690-7, 1995.
9. Dinh-Xuan, A. T., T. W. Higenbottam, C. A. Clelland, J. Pepke-Zaba, G. Cremona, A. Y. Butt, S. R. Large, F. C. Wells, and J. Wallwork. Impairment of endothelium-dependent pulmonary-artery relaxation in chronic obstructive lung disease. *N Engl J Med* 324: 1539-47, 1991.
10. Duplain, H., K. L. Peterson, M. Lepori, C. Sartori, E. Hummler, P. Nicod, and U. Scherrer. Augmented hypoxic pulmonary vasoconstriction and increased susceptibility to lung edema in heterozygous endothelial nitric oxide synthase (eNOS) deficient mice (Abstract). *Am J Respir Crit Care Med* 159: A355, 1999.
11. Duplain, H., L. Vollenweider, A. Delabays, P. Nicod, P. Bartsch, and U. Scherrer. Augmented sympathetic activation during short-term hypoxia and high-altitude exposure in subjects susceptible to high-altitude pulmonary edema. *Circulation* 99: 1713-8, 1999.
12. Fagan, K. A., B. W. Fouty, R. C. Tyler, K. G. Morris, Jr., L. K. Hepler, K. Sato, T. D. LeCras, S. H. Abman, H. D. Weinberger, P. L. Huang, I. F. McMurtry, and D. M. Rodman. The pulmonary circulation of homozygous or heterozygous eNOS-null mice is hyperresponsive to mild hypoxia. *J Clin Invest* 103: 291-9, 1999.
13. Frostell, C., M.-D. Fratacci, J. C. Wain, R. Jones, and W. M. Zapol. Inhaled nitric oxide. A selected pulmonary vasodilatator reversing hypoxic pulmonary vasoconstriction. *Circulation* 83: 2038-2047, 1991.
14. Frostell, C. G., H. Blomqvist, G. Hedenstierna, J. Lundberg, and W. M. Zapol. Inhaled nitric oxide selectively reverses human hypoxic pulmonary vasoconstriction without causing systemic vasodilation. *Anesthesiology* 78: 427-35, 1993.

15. Goerre, S., M. Wenk, P. Bärtsch, T. F. Luescher, F. Niroomand, E. Hohenhaus, O. Oelz, and W. H. Reinhart. Endothelin-1 in pulmonary hypertension associated with high-altitude exposure. *Circulation* 90: 359-364, 1995.

16. Hackett, P. H., and R. C. Roach. High altitude pulmonary edema. *J Wilderness Med* 1: 3-26, 1990.

17. Hackett, P. H., R. C. Roach, G. S. Hartig, E. R. Greene, and B. D. Levine. The effect of vasodilators on pulmonary hemodynamics in high altitude pulmonary edema: a comparison. *Int J Sports Med* 13: S68-71, 1992.

18. Hampl, V., and J. Herget. Perinatal hypoxia increases hypoxic pulmonary vasoconstriction in adult rats recovering from chronic exposure to hypoxia. *Am Rev Respir Dis* 142: 619-24, 1990.

19. Haworth, S. G. Pulmonary vascular remodeling in neonatal pulmonary hypertension. State of the art. *Chest* 93: 133S-138S, 1988.

20. Hultgren, H. N. High altitude pulmonary edema. In: *Lung Water and Solute Exchange*, edited by N. C. Staub. New York, NY: Dekker, 1978, p. 437-469.

21. Hultgren, H. N. High-altitude pulmonary edema: current concepts. *Annu Rev Med* 47: 267-84, 1996.

22. Hummler, E., P. Barker, J. Gatzy, F. Beermann, C. Verdumo, A. Schmidt, R. Boucher, and B. C. Rossier. Early death due to defective neonatal lung liquid clearance in alpha-ENaC-deficient mice. *Nat Genet* 12: 325-8, 1996.

23. Hummler, E., P. Barker, C. Talbot, Q. Wang, C. Verdumo, B. Grubb, J. Gatzy, M. Burnier, J. D. Horisberger, F. Beermann, R. Boucher, and B. C. Rossier. A mouse model for the renal salt-wasting syndrome pseudohypoaldosteronism. *Proc Natl Acad Sci U S A* 94: 11710-5, 1997.

24. Knowles, M. R., W. H. Buntin, P. A. Bromberg, J. T. Gatzy, and R. C. Boucher. Measurements of transepithelial electric potential differences in the trachea and bronchi of human subjects in vivo. *Am Rev Respir Dis* 126: 108-12, 1982.

25. Knowles, M. R., J. L. Carson, A. M. Collier, J. T. Gatzy, and R. C. Boucher. Measurements of nasal transepithelial electric potential differences in normal human subjects in vivo. *Am Rev Respir Dis* 124: 484-90, 1981.

26. Kourembanas, S., L. P. McQuillan, G. K. Leung, and D. V. Faller. Nitric oxide regulates the expression of vasoconstrictors and growth factors by vascular endothelium under both normoxia and hypoxia. *J Clin Invest* 92: 99-104, 1993.

27. Krasney, J. A. A neurogenic basis for acute altitude illness. *Med Sci Sports Exerc* 26: 195-208, 1994.

28. Lepori, M., E. Hummler, F. Feihl, C. Sartori, P. Nicod, B. Rossier, and U. Scherrer. Amiloride sensitive sodium transport dysfunction augments susceptibility to hypoxia-induced lung edema (Abstract). *FASEB J* 12: A328, 1998.

29. Matthay, M. A., H. G. Folkesson, and A. S. Verkman. Salt and water transport across alveolar and distal airway epithelia in the adult lung. *Am J Physiol* 270: L487-503, 1996.

30. Morin, F. C., 3rd, and K. R. Stenmark. Persistent pulmonary hypertension of the newborn. *Am J Respir Crit Care Med* 151: 2010-32, 1995.

31. Planes, C., B. Escoubet, M. Blot-Chabaud, G. Friedlander, N. Farman, and C. Clerici. Hypoxia downregulates expression and activity of epithelial sodium channels in rat alveolar epithelial cells. *Am J Respir Cell Mol Biol* 17: 508-18, 1997.

32. Rabinovitch, M., W. J. Gamble, O. S. Miettenen, and L. Reid. Age and sex influence on pulmonary hypertension of chronic hypoxia and on recovery. *Am J Physiol* 240: H62-H72, 1981.

33. Sakuma, T., G. Okaniwa, T. Nakada, T. Nishimura, S. Fujimura, and M. A. Matthay. Alveolar fluid clearance in the resected human lung. *Am J Respir Crit Care Med* 150: 305-10, 1994.

34. Sartori, C., Y. Allemann, L. Trueb, A. Delabays, P. Nicod, and U. Scherrer. A perinatal vascular insult predisposes to augmented vasoreactivity in adult life (In Press). *Lancet* , 1999.

35. Sartori, C., M. Lepori, M. Maggiorini, Y. Allemann, P. Nicod, and U. Scherrer. Impairment of amiloride-sensitive sodium transport in individuals susceptible to high altitude pulmonary edema (Abstract). *FASEB J* 12: A231, 1998.

36. Sartori, C., L. Trueb, and U. Scherrer. High-altitude pulmonary edema. Mechanisms and management. *Cardiologia* 42: 559-67, 1997.

37. Sartori, C., L. Vollenweider, B. M. Loffler, A. Delabays, P. Nicod, P. Bartsch, and U. Scherrer. Exaggerated endothelin release in high-altitude pulmonary edema. *Circulation* 99: 2665-8, 1999.

38. Saumon, G., and G. Basset. Electrolyte and fluid transport across the mature alveolar epithelium. *J Appl Physiol* 74: 1-15, 1993.

39. Scherrer, U., L. Vollenweider, A. Delabays, M. Savcic, U. Eichenberger, G. R. Kleger, A. Fikrle, P. E. Ballmer, P. Nicod, and P. Bartsch. Inhaled nitric oxide for high-altitude pulmonary edema. *N Engl J Med* 334: 624-629, 1996.

40. Schoene, R. B. Pulmonary edema at high altitude: Review, pathophysiology and update. *Clin Chest Med* 6: 491-507, 1985.

41. Smith, A. P. L., C. J. Emery, and T. W. Higenbottam. Perinatal chronic hypoxia decreases endothelial nitric oxide synthase (NOS III) and increases preproendothelin-1 (ppET-1) mRNA levels in rat (Abstract). *Eur Respir J* 10: 433s, 1997.

42. Staub, N. C. Pulmonary edema. *Physiol Rev* 54: 678-811, 1974.

43. Staub, N. C. Pulmonary edema--hypoxia and overperfusion (Editorial). *N.Engl.J.Med.* 302: 1085-1086, 1980.

44. Stenmark, K. R., E. C. Orton, J. T. Reeves, N. F. Voelkel, E. C. Crouch, W. C. Parks, and R. P. Mecham. Vascular remodeling in neonatal pulmonary hypertension. Role of the smooth muscle cell. *Chest* 93: 127S-133S, 1988.

45. Steudel, W., M. Scherrer-Crosbie, K. D. Bloch, J. Weimann, P. L. Huang, R. C. Jones, M. H. Picard, and W. M. Zapol. Sustained pulmonary hypertension and right ventricular hypertrophy after chronic hypoxia in mice with congenital deficiency of nitric oxide synthase 3. *J Clin Invest* 101: 2468-77, 1998.

46. Suzuki, S., Y. Hoshikawa, S. Ono, T. Sakuma, K. Koike, T. Tanita, and S. Fujimura. [Effects of subacute hypoxia on alveolar epithelial ion transport in rats]. *Nihon Kyobu Shikkan Gakkai Zasshi* 34: 52-6, 1996.

47. West, J. B., and O. Mathieu Costello. High altitude pulmonary edema is caused by stress failure of pulmonary capillaries. *Int J Sports Med* 13: S54-8, 1992.

48. Yanagisawa, M., H. Kurihara, S. Kimura, Y. Tomobe, M. Kobayashi, Y. Mitsui, Y. Yazaki, K. Goto, and T. Masaki. A novel potent vasoconstrictor peptide produced by vascular endothelial cells. *Nature* 332: 411-5, 1988.

Chapter 9

Frontiers in Neuroscience
Hypoxia and the Blood-Brain Barrier: Introduction

John A. Krasney

Department of Physiology and Biophysics, University at Buffalo, School of Medicine and Biomedical Sciences, 124 Sherman Hall, Buffalo, NY 14214, USA

Key words: high-altitude cerebral edema, vasogenic edema, cytotoxic edema, cerebral vascular pressures, cerebral blood flow, cerebral energetics

It is now generally accepted that acute mountain sickness (AMS) is caused by a mild form of high-altitude cerebral edema (HACE). In susceptible individuals AMS may progress to a lethal form of HACE and/or high-altitude pulmonary edema (3). Two hypotheses have been promulgated to account for HACE: the vasogenic edema hypothesis and the cytotoxic edema hypothesis (3,4). Since cerebral energetics are unchanged during AMS-HACE in an experimental sheep model (7), evidence favors the view that HACE is vasogenic in nature, although cytotoxic edema has not been ruled out specifically.

It has been suggested that vasogenic edema in hypoxia is similar to the "autoregulatory breakthrough" postulated to occur in hypertensive encephalopathy (1,3). While systemic hypertension in excess of 160 mm Hg reproducibly causes reversible opening of the blood-brain barrier (1,5), it is questionable whether capillary or venous hydrostatic pressures rise high enough to elicit autoregulatory breakthrough in HACE. Experimental hypertension causes pial venous pressures to increase in excess of 24 mm Hg (5) whereas in experimental AMS-HACE cerebral venous pressures only rise transiently to ~ 10 mm Hg (7). Moreover, sustained cerebral vasodilation elicited either by systemic hypercapnia or by infusions of nitroglycerin fails to elicit brain responses or clinical signs of AMS-HACE (4).

In the absence of evidence supporting vascular hydrostatic gradients large enough to open the blood-brain barrier, it seems reasonable to focus on the question of whether sustained hypoxia elicits one or more dysfunctional changes in the blood-brain barrier itself. Hypoxia has been shown to increase the susceptibility to oxidant stress and to increase the permeability of brain capillary endothelial cells in culture (6). There is evidence that histamine and cyclic nucleotides may play a role at the blood-brain barrier in edema associated with brain hypoxia (2). Lastly, Xu and Severinghaus have postulated an important role for vascular endothelial growth factor (VEGF) in HACE (8). Accordingly, the present section has been organized to provide an Overview of the Blood-brain Barrier by Dr Lester Drewes and a presentation of the Role of Mediators in the Etiology of Cerebral Edema by Dr Lothar Schilling. These important presentations will provide the background and theoretical framework for exploring the extent and nature of the potential pivotal role of the blood-brain barrier in acute altitude illness.

REFERENCES

1. Johannsson, B.B. Hypertension and the blood-brain barrier. In: *Implications of the blood-brain barrier and its manipulation.* Edited by E.A Neuwelt. New York: Saunders, 1989, 389-410.
2. Joo, F. Brain microvascular cyclic nucleotides and protein phosphorylation. In: *The Blood-Brain Barrier*, Edited by W.M Pardridge, New York: Raven Press, 1993, Chap 13, p 267-302.
3. Krasney, J.A. A neurogenic basis for acute altitude illness. *Med Sci. Sports Exercise.* 26:195-208, 1994.
4. Krasney, J.A. Cerebral hemodynamics and high altitude cerebral edema. In. *Hypoxia: Women at Altitude, Edited by* C.S Houston , G Coates. Burlington, Vt: Queen City Printers, Chap 30: 1997, p254-267.
5. Mayhan, W.G. and D.D. Heistad, Role of veins and cerebral venous pressure in disruption of the blood-brain barrier. *Circ Res.* 59:216-220, 1986.
6. Plateel, M. , M-P. Dehouck, , G. Torpier,., R. Cecchelli, and E. Tessier. Hypoxia increases the susceptibility to oxidant stress and the permeability of the blood-brain barrier endothelial cell monolayer. *J. Neurochem.* 65:2138-2145, 1995.
7. Yang, S-P., G.W. Bergo, E. Krasney and J.A. Krasney. Cerebral pressure-flow and metabolic responses to sustained hypoxia: Effect of CO_2. *J. Appl. Physiol.* 76:303-313,1994.
8. Xu, F., and J.W. Severinghaus. Rat brain VEGF expression in alveolar hypoxia: possible role in high-altitude cerebral edema. *J. Appl. Physiol.* 85:53-57, 1998.

Chapter 10

What is the Blood-Brain Barrier? A Molecular Perspective
Cerebral Vascular Biology

Lester R. Drewes

Department of Biochemistry & Molecular Biology, School of Medicine, University of Minnesota, Duluth, MN 55812, USA

Key words: brain, transporter, monocarboxylic acid, endothelial cell, vascular biology, transcellular transport, adhesion molecules, leukocyte, multidrug resistance, amino acid, tight junction, asymmetric, P-glycoprotein, luminal membrane, abluminal membrane

Abstract: The term "blood-brain barrier" was coined over one hundred years ago as a result of the observation that vital dyes introduced into the circulation quickly penetrated and stained nearly all organs and tissues of the mammalian body except the brain which retained its pale creamy appearance. Advances in microscopy revealed that, in contrast to other vascular beds, the brain endothelial cells lining the vascular wall are tightly linked with junctional complexes that eliminate gaps or spaces between cells and prevent any free diffusion of blood-borne substances into the brain parenchymal space. The endothelial cells, situated at the interface between blood and brain, therefore, play a critical role in performing essential biological functions including transport of micro- and macronutrients, receptor-mediated signaling, leukocyte trafficking, and osmoregulation. A number of molecular components responsible for some of these unique properties have now been identified and are being characterized under physiological and disease conditions. These include the proteins involved in formation and assembly of tight junctions; the plasma membrane-embedded proteins that are responsible for transport of brain energy substrates and nutrients (glucose, monocarboxylic acids, nucleosides, amino acids, others); the multi-drug transporter protein, p-glycoprotein, and other drug-rejecting proteins that protect the brain from foreign, potentially disruptive chemicals. These and other recent findings, taken as a whole, reveal the brain endothelium as a complex and dynamic biological system, in contrast to the simple, inert and rigid barrier initially perceived.

1.   INTRODUCTION

The functioning brain is one of the most energy-dependent tissues of mammalian organisms. Although the human brain weighs approximately 1.4 kg or about 2% of the adult body weight, this organ uses about one quarter of all oxygen and glucose consumed by the whole body under resting conditions. The fuels and nutrients to maintain this high metabolic state are delivered to the brain via the arterial blood supply and the extensive cerebral vasculature. This complex vascular network is highly branched with, for the most part, an irregular and extensive pattern projecting from major arterial vessels that descend into the parenchyma from the cortical surface. Capillary density in brain tissue is high, and it is estimated from morphometric studies that in one gram of brain tissue the total length of all vessels is 425 m and the total capillary surface area is 240 cm^2 (2).

The vascular system of the brain was recognized by natural scientists such as Paul Ehrlich roughly a century ago to be unique compared to those of other organ systems. Ehrlich observed that organic dyes infused into the mammalian circulation quickly penetrated and stained nearly all tissues within a few minutes. However, even after several hours the brain at autopsy remained its pale, creamy color. These observations led Goldman later to coin the term "blood-brain barrier" (7).

The anatomic basis for the blood-brain barrier was a disputed subject for many years, until the debate was resolved by application of electron microscopy. This technique permitted the observation that endothelial cells that line the brain capillaries form close junctional contacts and eliminate any gaps or spaces between cells for diffusion or bulk flow of plasma components (1)(Fig. 1). Thus, paracellular transport is greatly retarded or eliminated by these tight junctions. Additionally, the plasma cell membrane, consisting of a lipid bilayer and its hydrophilic core, is a major deterrent to passage of ionized molecules and hydrophilic molecules. Thus, substances entering the brain must traverse two plasma membranes of the capillary endothelial cell, one on the luminal side facing the blood, and the second on the abluminal side facing the extracellular space and neuropil.

A layer of cells with extensively formed and developed tight junctions is a poor conductor of ionized species and exhibits a high electrical resistance. The brain endothelium is among the tightest monolayer of cells and its transendothelial electrical resistance is estimated to be between 1000 and 3000 ohm·cm^2 (3). Other cells with extensive tight junction formation and high electrical resistance include the intestinal epithelium, kidney epithelia and the pigment epithelium of the retina.

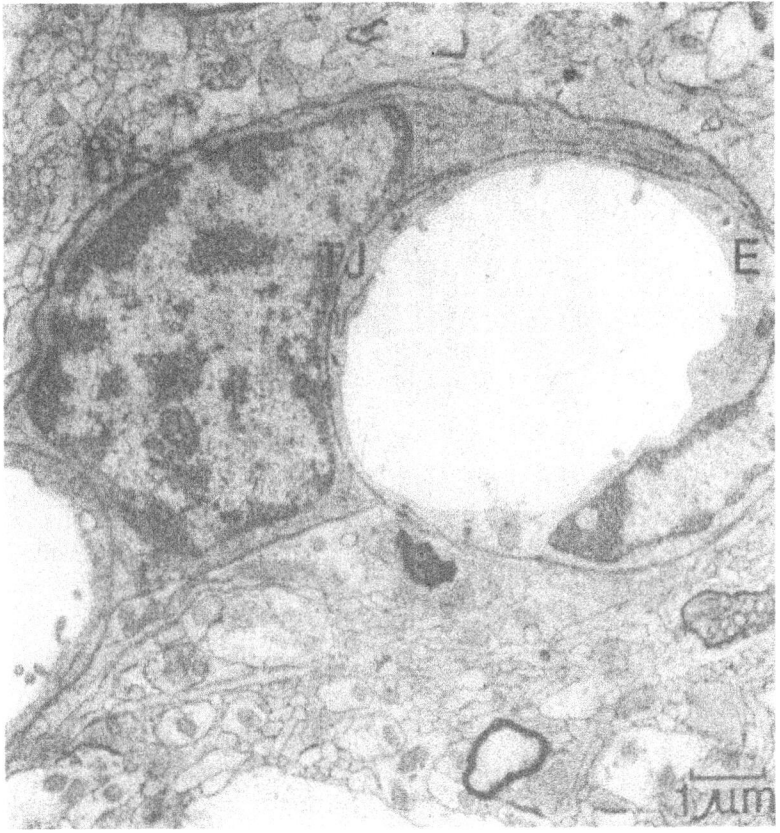

Figure 1. Electron micrograph of a brain capillary. An endothelial cell (E) of canine cerebral cortex is shown with a tight junction (tj). Astrocytic endfeet surround the vessel and are separated from the endothelial cell by a basement membrane.

Tight junctions are composed of multiple components assembled in complex structures at the plasma membranes between two homologous cells. Two membrane proteins that appear to be major components of these junctional complexes are occludin and claudin (Fig. 2). Occludin-1 was the first to be discovered and is a polypeptide of 504 amino acids with four putative transmembrane segments, and its short amino terminal and larger carboxyl terminal end in the cytoplasm (4). The two major extracellular

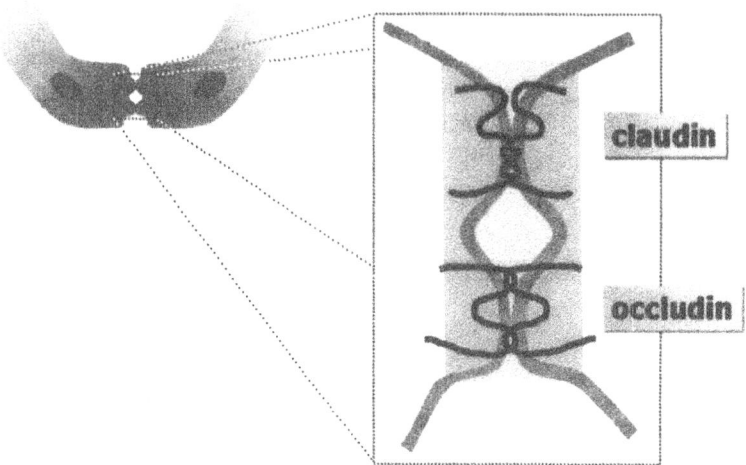

Figure 2. Tight-junction proteins of brain endothelium. Junctional contacts between endothelial cells involve complex structures. Occludin-1 and claudin-1 are two major proteins that are components of endothelial tight junctions. Each contains four membrane-spanning segments.

loops are speculated to interact with similar loops on adjacent cells, thus providing noncovalent binding and a form of adhesion between cells. Other soluble proteins that concentrate at tight junctions such as ZO-1, ZO-2, ZO-3 (*zonula occludens* proteins) and cingulin may strongly associate with the carboxyl domain of occludin, and play important roles in complex assembly and in linkage to the cellular cytoskeleton. Claudin-1, a 211-amino acid membrane protein, has no sequence similarity to occludin, but also has four putative transmembrane domains and two substantive extracellular loops (5). As with occludin, the extracellular loops may be important in chemical contact with neighboring cells. Recent discoveries that occludin-1 and claudin-1 are each members of two larger families of proteins with tissue-specific expression patterns, suggest that the molecular anatomy of tight junctions may be heterogeneous. Although transcripts for occludin-1 and claudin-1 are present in brain, the identity of the proteins in brain endothelial tight junctions is not know with certainty.

2.   TRANSPORTERS

Transcellular transport (transport across both the luminal and abluminal membranes) is the major pathway for entry (and exit) of fuels and nutrients of the brain. This occurs by membrane proteins, synthesized and embedded by the brain endothelial cell, that recognize substrates and deliver them to the opposite side of the membrane. This process is believed to involve substrate-specific recognition, association at the binding site, protein conformational change, and dissociation from the binding site on the opposite membrane surface. The first cloned and most studied transporter, the glucose transporter (GLUT1), is a 492 amino acid protein with 12 putative membrane-spanning segments, a glycosylation site on an extracellular loop, and the amino and carboxyl terminal ends located on the cytoplasmic surface (10). Although neither the three dimensional structure nor the mechanistic detail of glucose transport is known, GLUT1 is a facilitative carrier, exhibits Michaelis-Menten-like kinetics, carries glucose down its concentration gradient, and operates reversibly to carry glucose in either direction across the membrane. GLUT1 is equally distributed between the luminal and abluminal membranes of canine brain endothelial cells (6), but is asymmetrically distributed in other species such as the rat.

Transport systems for several other major brain substrates have been detected and localized to the luminal and abluminal membranes of brain endothelium, by functional analysis or molecular probes (Fig. 3). These

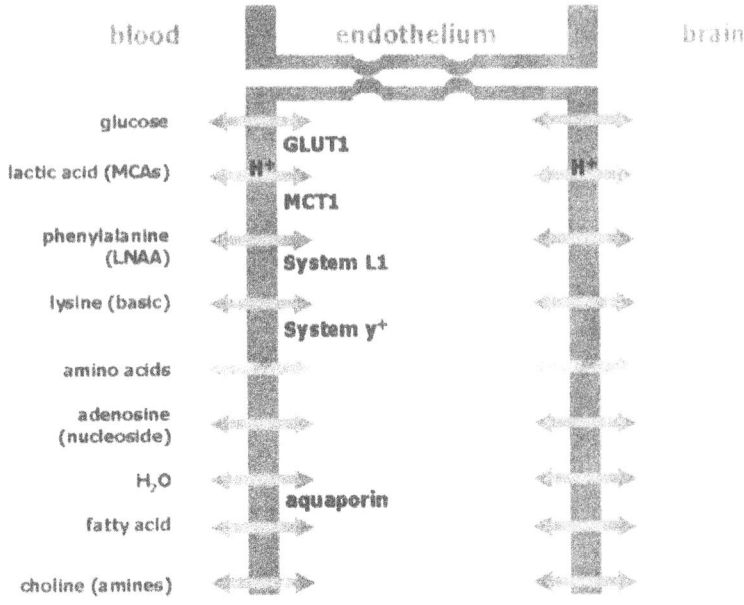

Figure 3. Facilitative transport systems of brain endothelial cells. Several carrier-mediated transport systems for energy substrates and metabolites are present in the luminal and abluminal membranes of brain endothelial cells. See text for details.

include the monocarboxylic acid transporter, large neutral amino acid (system L1) transporter, basic amino acid (system y+) transporter, and nucleoside transporter (equilibrative). Additional carriers for fatty acids, choline, other amino acids, water channels (aquaporin), various vitamins, and cofactors also probably are present, but at low abundance.

3.   CELL MEMBRANE ASYMMETRY

Several proteins involved in blood-brain transport are asymmetrically distributed between the luminal and abluminal surfaces of the endothelial cell (Fig. 4). In general, these transporters or channels are involved in primary active (ATP required) or secondary active (electrochemical gradient energy required) transport. Among the most interesting and potentially

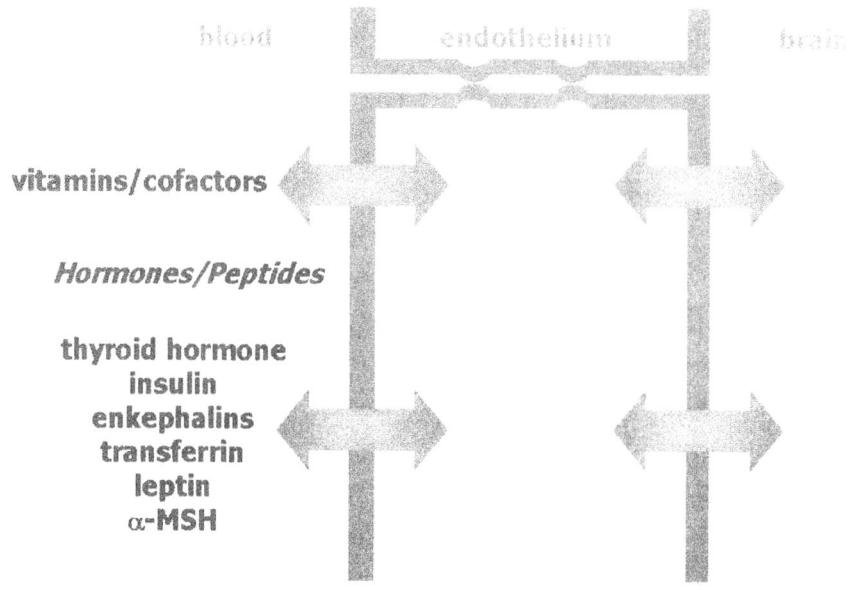

Figure 4. Blood-brain transport of vitamins, hormones and proteins. Various low capacity, but highly specific mechanisms for transport of vitamins, hormones and proteins are present in brain endothelial cells. The molecular components and mechanistic details of these systems remain to be elucidated.

medically relevant of these are the proteins that give cells the attribute of excluding lipophilic drugs. First discovered in cancer cells, the multidrug resistance gene product, P-glycoprotein, is able to expel against a concentration gradient potentially harmful agents, by an ATP-dependent pumping mechanism. P-glycoprotein is a member of a large family of ABC (ATP binding cassette) transporters that includes the CFTR protein (chloride transporter) of cystic fibrosis. These proteins have 12 membrane-spanning domains, one or two ATP-binding domains, large intracellular loops and long terminal-end domains. Mice lacking the P-glycoprotein (mdr -/-) have the identical phenotype as the wild type, until they are challenged with a toxic agent such as ivermectin or the anticancer drug vincristine (11). Then, they exhibit symptoms of severe neurotoxicity. Subsequent studies have shown that the P-glycoprotein is highly expressed in the luminal membrane of the brain endothelial cell, and presumably protects the neurons and glia from xenobiotics by active extrusion at the blood-brain interface. Not only does the endothelium facilitate the entry of essential fuels and nutrients, it also actively guards against the entry of potentially neurotoxic substances.

Ion transport by the brain endothelial cell is important for maintaining the ionic composition of interstitial fluid, for volume regulation, and for contributing to the formation of cerebral spinal fluid (8). These transport systems include on the luminal membrane a Na^+/H^+ exchanger, an amelioride-sensitive Na^+ channel, and a $Na^+/K^+/Cl^-$ system (Fig. 5). On the abluminal side, the transport into the endothelial cell of small, neutral amino acids against their concentration gradient is facilitated by co-transport with Na^+, and is driven by sodium's electrochemical gradient. The Na^+/K^+ ATPase pump located predominantly on the abluminal membrane serves to restore and maintain the physiological distribution of these ions across the plasma membranes.

The evidence suggests that entry of protein hormones or peptide signaling molecules occurs by receptor-mediated mechanisms. Binding of the blood-borne peptide is specific, saturable, and inhibited by structural analogs. However, the receptor-bound peptide undergoes endocytosis and subsequent release at the abluminal-interstitial fluid interface (Fig. 5). Cell biological details of this process are not well understood.

4. ENZYMATIC BARRIER

The cerebral vascular endothelium serves as an enzymatic barrier because of chemical modifications that are made to various substrates by enzymes that are attributed to the endothelial cell. The best example of this involves the action of monoamine oxidase (MAO) on catecholamine

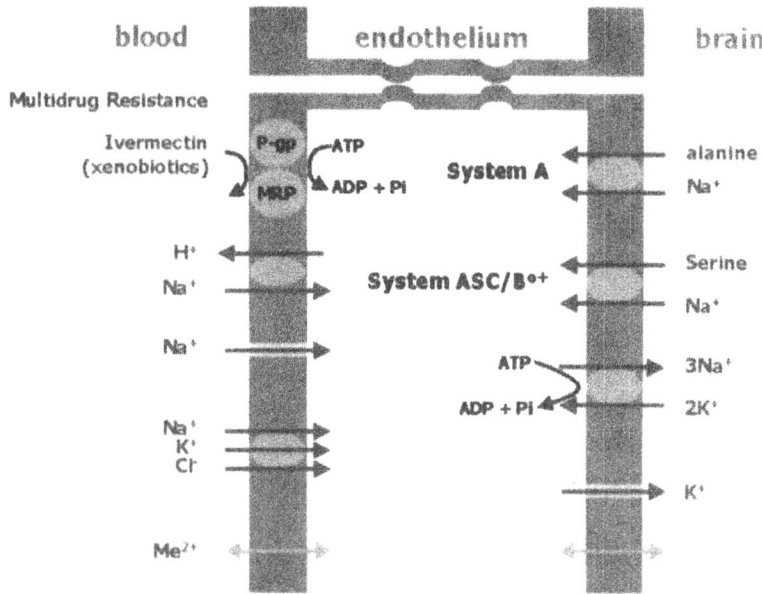

Figure 5. Primary and secondary active transport systems of brain endothelium. ATP-dependent systems include the P-glycoprotein and Na+/K+ATPase that appear to be asymmetrically distributed between the luminal and abluminal sides of the endothelial cell. Other specific carriers for various mono- and divalent ions have also been demonstrated.

neurotransmitters synthesized in the brain, released from neurons, and transported by diffusion to the vicinity of the capillaries (Fig. 6). Dopamine is readily transported into the endothelial cell via abluminal amino acid transporters (system L1, system A, etc.). However, high intracellular MAO activity converts the neurotransmitter to its pharmacologically inactive metabolite, dihydroxyphenyl acetic acid (DOPAC), which readily effluxes to the circulating plasma where it produces minimal systemic effects and is mostly excreted.

Another example of the brain endothelium serving as an enzymatic barrier is carbonic anhydrase isozyme IV, located on the extracellular side of the luminal membrane (Fig. 6). Based on this enzyme's location in other tissues and vascular beds, carbonic anhydrase IV is believed to increase the CO_2 gradient from its source to its site of removal by rapidly converting CO_2 to bicarbonate and hydrogen ion. In brain vasculature, carbonic anhydrase IV may be important in increasing CO_2 efflux from highly respiring, activated neurons by acting, in a sense, as a sink for CO_2 and increasing the neuronal to plasma CO_2 ratio. Such a process would be enhanced by the

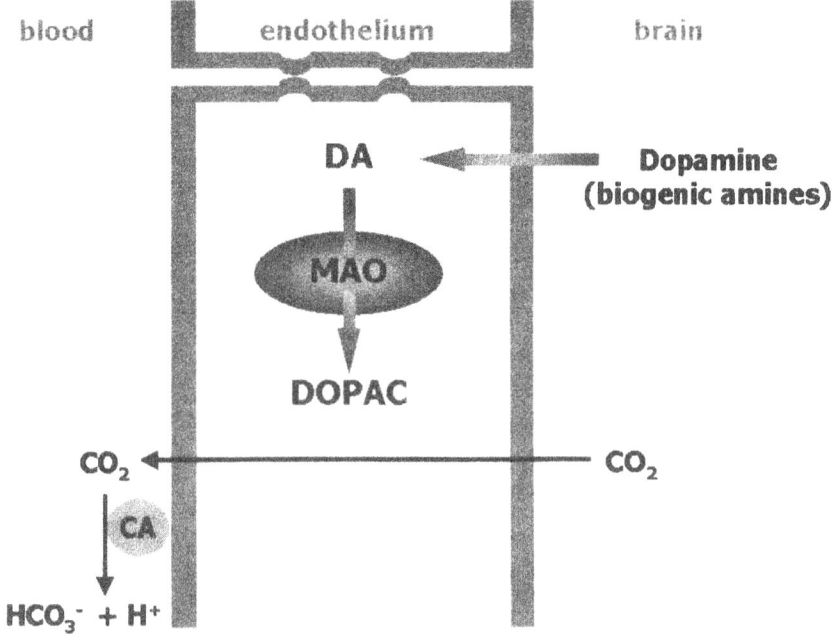

Figure 6. Brain endothelial cells as an enzymatic barrier. Enzymes for catecholamine metabolism such as monoamine oxidase (MAO) are enriched in endothelial cells and inactivate neurotransmitters by forming metabolites during transit through he endothelium. An isoform of carbonic anhydrase (CA-IV) is located on the luminal endothelial membrane.

presence of water channels (aquaporin). These channels significantly enhance CO_2 diffusion and are expressed by astrocytes and enriched in their endfeet surrounding capillaries.

In the absence of a lymphatic system and other components for immune surveillance, the brain under physiological conditions does not have as strong an immune response as other organs. However, it is now recognized that lymphocytes readily traverse the brain vascular wall, and this activity is greatly stimulated under neuroinflammatory conditions, such as during multiple sclerosis and following stroke. Trafficking of cells through the endothelium involves the concerted action of several cell adhesion molecules and their receptors on the membrane surfaces of endothelial cells and lymphocytes. Prominent among them are ICAM-1, VCAM-1, and the E- and P-selectins. In a poorly understood process the lymphocytes make initial contact with the endothelial wall and minimal adhesion occurs. This allows more and varied adhesion molecules on the lymphocytes and endothelial cells to form greater contacts and stronger adhesion. Activation of these receptors signals further intracellular events and eventually the endothelial luminal and abluminal membranes contact, fuse and form a passageway for the lymphocyte to transmigrate to the abluminal side of the endothelium. Activation of extracellular enzymes presumably allows for penetration through the surrounding basement membrane.

5.   FUTURE DIRECTIONS

Advances in molecular and cell biology have expanded greatly our knowledge and understanding of the original observation of the blood-brain barrier. During the next years rapid and major advancements are predicted. Among the many possible fruitful areas, speculation on three is presented here. First is the area of selective induction and expression of desirable transporters by brain endothelial cells. This will require greater knowledge about the transcriptional factors and mechanisms of gene expression. However, with the further completion of various genome projects and development of related technologies, the nucleic acid sequences critical for specific genes or families of genes will become targets for pharmacological agents. It will become possible to activate, for example, an amino acid transporter, vitamin transporter or other transporter for which the activity or function is considered beneficial. Second is the area of transporter accessory proteins (Fig. 7). Several groups have recently reported that functional

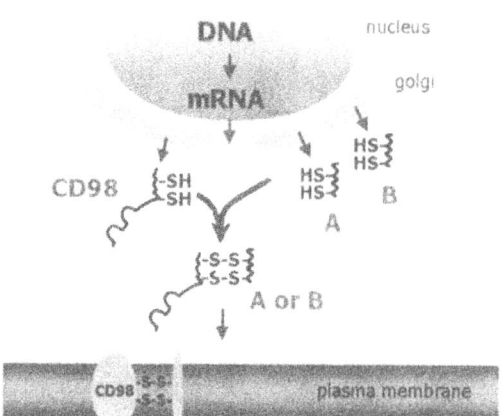

Figure 7. Transport systems and the role of accessory proteins. The activity of membrane transporters may be regulated by either covalent or noncovalent interactions with accessory proteins. The accessory proteins may be essential for transporter function and activity.

amino acid transporters in the plasma membranes are covalently linked to a second protein forming a heterodimer (9,12). Neither of these proteins is capable independently of transporting amino acids. The light chains have the prototypic 12 transmembrane segment structure, while the heavy chain has hydrophobic character, but with 1 to 4 transmembrane segments. It has been speculated that the heavy chain plays a role in intracellular trafficking of the light chain from the Golgi to the destination membrane. Thus, the heavy chain serves as an accessory or chaperone-like function, while the light chain provides the transporter specificity and function.

Finally, the endothelial cell is juxtaposed at the interface between the brain and the circulating blood, and therefore is perfectly suited for genetic manipulation, modification, and replacement. For example, cells with an endothelial lineage might be obtained from a patient's muscle or other tissue and cultured in vitro. By genetic manipulation the genotype of the cells will be altered to express new and beneficial traits. The cells then are returned to the patient by intra-venous or intra-arterial infusion. This grafting of new endothelial cells, possessing new genetic or functional properties may be useful for correcting genetic abnormalities or for improving drug delivery to the central nervous system.

ACKNOWLEDGMENTS

The skill and efforts of Dave Gerhart, Rick Leino, Roman Duelli, Mary Sneve, and Brad Enerson are gratefully acknowledged. These studies were supported by the National Institute of Neurological Diseases and Stroke (NS-37764), American Heart Association, Minnesota Medical Foundation and the Duluth Clinic Education and Research Foundation.

REFERENCES

1. Brightman, M.W., and T.S. Reese. Junctions between intimately apposed cell membranes in the vertebrate brain. *J. Cell Biol.* 40: 648-677, 1969.
2. Crone, C. The permeability of capillaries in various organs as determined by use of the "indicator diffusion" method. *Acta Physiol. Scand.* 58: 292-305, 1963.
3. Crone, C., and S.-P. Olesen. Electrical resistance of brain microvascular endothelium. *Brain Res.* 241: 49-55, 1982.
4. Furuse, M., T. Hirase, M. Itoh, A. Nagafuchi, S. Yonemura, S. Tsukita, and S. Tsukita. Occludin: a novel integral membrane protein localizing at tight junctions. *J. Cell Biol.* 123: 1777-1788, 1993.
5. Furuse, M., K. Fujita, T. Hiiragi, K. Fujimoto, and S. Tsukita. Claudin-1 and –2: novel integral membrane proteins localizing at tight junctions with no sequence similarity to occludin. *J. Cell Biol.* 141: 1539-1550, 1998.
6. Gerhart, D.Z., R.J. LeVasseur, M.A. Broderius, and L.R. Drewes. Glucose transporter localization in brain using light and electron immunocytochemistry. *J. Neurosci. Res.* 22: 464-472, 1989.
7. Goldmann, E.E., *Vitalfarbung am Zentralnervensystem*. Berlin. 1913.

8. Keep, R.F., S.R. Ennis, and L. Betz. *Introduction to the Blood-Brain Barrier.* Edited by W.M. Pardridge. Cambridge. Cambridge University Press. 1998: 207-213.

9. Mannion, B.A., T.V. Kolesnikova, S. Hwa Lin, S. Wang, N.L. Thompson, and M.E. Hemler. The light chain of CD98 is identified as E16/TA1 protein. *J. Biol.Chem.* 273: 33127-33129, 1998.

10. Mueckler, M., C. Caruso, S.A. Baldwin, M. Panico, I. Blench, H.R. Morris, W.I. Allard, G.E. Lienhard, H.F. Lodish. Sequence and structure of a human glucose transporter. *Science.* 229: 941-945, 1985.

11. Schinkel, A.H., J.J. Smit, O. van Tellingen, J.H. Beijnen, E. Wagenaar, L. van Deemter, C.A. Mol, M.A. van der Valk, E.C. Robanus-Maandag, H.P. te Riele, et al. Disruption of the mouse mdr1a P-glycoprotein gene leads to a deficiency in the blood-brain barrier and to increased sensitivity to drugs. *Cell.* 77:491-502, 1994.

12. Torrents, D., R. Esteves, M. Pineda, E. Fernandez, J. Lloberas, Y. Shi, A. Zorzano, and M. Palacin. Identification and characterization of a membrane protein (y^+L amino acid transporter-1) that associates with 4F2hc to encode the amino acid transporter activity y^+L. *J. Biol. Chem.* 273: 32437-32445, 1998.

Chapter 11

Mediators of Cerebral Edema

Lothar Schilling and Michael Wahl*

*Dept. Neurosurg., Div. Neurosurg. Res., Fac. Clin. Med., Mannheim, Univ. Heidelberg, Theodor Kutzer-Ufer 1-3, D-68135 Mannheim, Germany and *Dept. Physiol., Univ. Munich, Pettenkoferstr. 12, D-8 D-80336 Munich, Germany*

Key words: blood brain barrier, histamine, bradykinin, arachidonic acid, free radicals

Abstract: The blood-brain barrier (BBB) which is located in the continuous endothelial lining of cerebral blood vessels rigidly controls exchange of water soluble compounds under physiological conditions. Under pathological conditions such as trauma or ischemia, BBB permeability may increase thus allowing plasma constituents to escape into brain tissue. This "opening" of the BBB may, at least in part, be mediated by massive release of autacoids resulting in vasogenic brain edema. Five criteria have to be fulfilled by an individual autacoid to be considered a mediator candidate of cerebral edema: i) a permeability-enhancing action under physiological conditions, ii) a vasodilatory action, iii) the ability to induce vasogenic brain edema, iv) an increase of concentration in the tissue or interstitial fluid under pathological conditions, and v) a decrease of brain edema by specific interference with the release or action of a given autacoid. Among the mediator candidates considered, bradykinin is the only one to meet all criteria. Histamine, arachidonic acid and free radicals including nitric oxide may also be considered mediators of brain edema, but for each of these compounds evidence is less clear than for bradykinin. Although the concept of mediators inducing brain edema is well established by experimental studies, only a bradykinin receptor antagonist has so far gained entrance into clinical evaluation.

Hypoxia: Into the Next Millennium,
Edited by R. C. Roach, *et al.* Kluwer Academic/Plenum Publishing, New York, 1999.

1.   INTRODUCTION

In the brain two types of edema may be distinguished according to the location of water accumulating in the tissue: i) a cytotoxic type of edema which is characterized by an increase of intracellular water content, and ii) a vasogenic type of edema which is accompanied by an accumulation of water in the interstitial space. The vasogenic type of brain edema is characterized by the entrance of plasma constitutents and water into the brain interstitial space due to a disturbance of the blood-brain barrier (BBB). Although the cerebral vasculature is largely endowed with a BBB, it is absent in a few areas, the so-called circumventricular organs and the choroid plexus. The circumventricular organs being neurosecretion control centers and chemosensitive areas are involved in the maintenance of body homeostasis such as regulation of cardiovascular function, of extracellular sodium content, of fluid osmolality and body fluid turnover (37). In the choroid plexus the cerebrospinal fluid contained in the ventricular system is secreted (94).

2.   THE BLOOD-BRAIN BARRIER (BBB): MORPHOLOGICAL CHARACTERISTICS AND FUNCTIONAL IMPLICATIONS

Under physiological conditions the entrance of hydrophilic plasma constituents into the brain is strictly controlled by the BBB the morphological substrate of which is the continuous endothelial lining of the cerebral blood vessels (12,77). The chemical mediators and mechanisms which may be involved in alterations of BBB function resulting in development of brain edema will be described in detail below thereby updating previous reviews on this topic (87,112,114)

The BBB closely resembles a tight epithelial layer by a number of ultrastructural and functional features:

2.1   Expression of complex interendothelial junctions.

The complexity of junctions has been shown in the vessels in situ, in freshly isolated brain microvessels, and in cultured endothelial cells (77,123). However, the complexity of tight junction appears to be lower in cultured endothelial cells than in vivo (123). Studies using electron-dense compounds of different molecular weight such as La^{3+} ions, microperoxidase, and horseradish peroxidase have shown the presence of these tracers in the interendothelial junctions but not beyond them (12,13,77,97) indicating the tightness of these complex junctions.

2.2 Lack of considerable vesicular transport.

Approximately 4 transport vesicles were found per μm^2 in cerebral endothelial cells under physiological conditions (26,97). However, most of these structures may represent pits instead of free transport vesicles (11,20).

2.3 High density of mitochondria.

Using stereological methods Oldendorf and coworkers (66) have compared the amount of endothelial cell volume covered by mitochondria in blood vessels from different organs. They found up to 11% of the endothelial cytoplasmic volume occupied by mitochondria in cerebral vessel endothelial cells but only 2 - 5% in peripheral blood vessels. This figure emphasizes the large apparent working capacity of BBB-forming endothelial cells.

2.4 Specific transport systems and ion channels.

In BBB-forming cells a couple of highly specific transport systems are distributed symmetrically or asymmetrically in the cell membrane. Glucose supply of brain tissue is provided by specific transporters of the GLUT1 subtype (19,75). This transporter displays a higher density on the abluminal side of the BBB (18). A marked increase in GLUT1 expression was found in recovery after hypoxic-ischemic brain damage consistent with a higher glucose transport and utilisation under these conditions (107). Supply of amino acids is provided by a couple of Na^+-dependent and Na^+-independent transport systems present in the luminal and abluminal membrane of cerebral endothelial cells (84,99). Exchange of electrolytes is accomplished by ion channels, ion exchange mechanisms, and the Na^+/K^+-ATPase the latter one originally detected on the abluminal side of BBB-forming cells (6) but later on found in the luminal membrane as well (62,83). In addition, p-glycoprotein expression has recently been demonstrated in brain microvessel endothelium from different species including man (43,55,101).

2.5 Marked enzyme activity.

In addition to the above mentioned Na^+/K^+-ATPase and the p-glycoprotein a variety of enzymes have been identified in BBB-forming endothelial cells by methods of cytochemistry, biochemistry, immunohistochemistry, and molecular biology. The enzymes present include ecto-nucleotidase, alkaline phosphatase, gamma-GTP, and the monoamine oxidase (45,83,108).

2.6   High transendothelial potential and resistance.

In brain surface (so-called pial) vessels of the rat there is a potential difference of approximately -4 mV between the intra- and extraluminal compartment with the lumen being negative (79). The transendothelial resistance as measured in frog and rat pial vessels is approximately 1500 - 2000 Ω cm^2, in arteries usually higher than in veins (1,14,21,68). In comparison, the transendothelial resistance in peripheral vessels located in the striated muscle or the mesentery is by a factor of 100 or even more lower than in brain vessels (1). In cultured cerebral endothelial cells, however, the transendothelial resistance is substantially lower than in vivo despite the presence of tight junctions (8,49), and it suffers dramatic decrease during periods of ischemia/hypoxia (49).

2.7   High reflection coefficient and low hydraulic conductivity.

The reflection coefficient for polar compounds such as sucrose is at least one order of magnitude higher than in non-brain vessels, and the difference is even more marked for the hydraulic conductivity as summarized elsewhere (1,67).

Due to its unique morphological construction, i.e. the virtually impermeable paracellular pathway along with highly delicate and efficient systems of transporters, channels and enzymes the BBB takes responsibility for the homeostasis in brain tissue. The special composition of the central nervous system interstitial fluid compartment is the prerequisite for adequate neuronal function.

3.   THE MEDIATOR CONCEPT OF CEREBRAL EDEMA

Under pathological conditions, such as trauma or ischemia the permeability of the cerebral blood vessels may increase allowing plasma constituents to gain access to the brain interstitial fluid compartment ("opening" of the BBB). Entrance of low and high molecular weight plasma components results in net water influx and development of vasogenic brain edema. The compliance of the brain is limited since it is encapsulated in the rigid skull bone. Therefore, an increase of BBB permeability will eventually lead to an increase of intracranial pressure which is a life-threatening complication in many patients suffering from severe brain damage. Release of autacoids from injured brain tissue appears to play a major role in the pathophysiological sequelae leading to vasogenic cerebral edema. In order to be considered a potential mediator a number of criteria has to be fulfilled by an individual autacoid as outlined previously (114). The criteria defined in the mediator concept of cerebral edema are: i) a direct effect on BBB permeability. Application of a test compound should increase permeability under physiological conditions, ii) the vasomotor action upon cerebral blood vessels. Although arterial (and venous) dilatation will usually not by itself induce opening of the BBB it will augment extravasation by increasing vessel surface area and the driving force for transmural bulk flow once the permeability is enhanced, iii) the capability of inducing cerebral edema. When applied under physiological conditions a presumed mediator should result in development of cerbral edema, iv) expression in damaged brain tissue. Clearly, under pathological conditions a mediator compound must be present in the brain tissue or in the interstitial space, and v) therapeutic efficacy. A decrease or inhibition of edema formation should result from specific interference with the synthesis, release or action of a given autacoid. The above given criteria will be discussed for a number of autacoids considered mediator candidates.

3.1   BRADYKININ (BK)

3.1.1   Effect on BBB permeability.

Using intravital fluorescence microscopy the BBB permeability-increasing action of BK has been demonstrated. Intracarotid infusion as well as cortical superfusion of BK resulted in a leakage of the low molecular weight tracer Na^+-fluorescein from cat pial vessels (104,113). However, neither fluorescein isothiocyanate (FITC)-coupled albumin (MW, 67,000) nor FITC-dextran (MW, 19,400 - 62,000) was found to pass the BBB during challenge with BK (104,113). Therefore, a "selective" increase of BBB permeability induced by BK was postulated supposing generation of small functional pores (upper limit of pore diameter, $> 1.1 < 6$ nm since Na^+ fluorescein with a Stokes' radius of 5.5 Å could leak but FITC-dextran 19,000 with a Stokes' radius of 30 Å could not). The concept of "selective" opening of the BBB by BK is in agreement with studies showing an immediate increase of ion permeability over the BBB in frogs and rats by intra- and extravascularly applied BK (14,68) but exclusion of ink- and Evans blue-coupled albumin from the brain during challenge with BK (34,86). However, extravasation of horseradish peroxidase (MW, 44,000) following intracarotid injection of BK in rats has been observed in one study (76).

Leakage of tracer induced by BK is apparently mediated by activation of B_2 receptors. This conclusion is based on studies in which the increase of BBB-permeability induced by BK or a BK receptor agonist was not affected by B_1 receptor antagonists but reduced by B_2 receptor antagonists (30,104). The B_2 receptors appear to be present on the luminal and abluminal side of the endothelial cells because intra- as well as extravascularly applied BK stimulated leakage of Na^+-fluorescein (104).

The route of extravasation induced by BK is still controversial. The rapid decrease of transendothelial resistance during cortical superfusion with BK (14,68) appears to argue for activation of a paracellular pathway. This assumption is supported by a recent electron microscopic study showing penetration of La^{3+} ions into and even through the tight junctions after intravenous application of the BK analogue RMP-7 (85). However, stimulation of vesicular transport has also been suggested (76).

In view of its BBB permeability-enhancing action, BK has recently been employed for unlocking BBB in order to increase substrate delivery (e.g. cytostatic agents) to tumor-bearing brain tissue. A selective increase of blood-tumor barrier for small and high molecular weight tracers was described by Nakano and coworkers (63), while Elliott et al. (30) found an increase of carboplatin entrance into the tumor and, although to a lower degree, into the peritumoral tissue. Whether or not this approach will also be useful in humans remains to be determined.

3.1.2   Vasomotor actions.

Bradykinin exerts potent relaxation of cerebral arteries in vitro and in vivo (36,116) which is mediated by activation of a B_2 recepotor subtype (32,121). This receptor appears to be located on the abluminal membrane since in vivo cerebroarterial dilatation and increase of cerebral blood flow occurred only when BK was applied from the extravascular side (32,50,51,116) The BK-induced dilatation is endothelium-dependent, and several transduction molecules have been identified, first of all nitric oxide (36,56,69). However, depending on the species and the location of the artery studied release of prostanoids (50,125), free radicals (51,81,93), or leukotrienes (121) may also be involved.

3.1.3   Induction of cerebral edema.

Intracerebral infusion of BK (either via the ventriculo-cisternal route or into the forebrain white matter) resulted in development of brain edema

(102,122). This observation is in good agreement with the BBB permeability-enhancing and dilatory actions of BK.

3.1.4   Local concentration of BK.

Brain tissue may synthesize and release BK becaue it contains all components of a kallikrein-kinin system as reviewed elsewhere (110,111,115). While under physiological conditions virtually no BK is present in the brain, activation of the cerebral kallikrein-kinase system occurs under pathological conditions. Thus, an increase in brain tissue content of BK has been found following cold lesion (53) and concussive brain trauma (31), and also in ischemia-reperfusion and traumatic spinal cord injury (47,124). Synthesis of BK may even be enhanced by kininogen uptake from the plasma (53).

3.1.5   Therapeutic studies.

In animal experiments brain swelling after cold lesion and ischemia-reperfusion injury could be significantly diminished by treatment with aprotinin to inhibit kallikrein activity (47,103). In addition, application of the recently developed B_2-kininergic receptor antagonist CP-0127 proved to be effective in reducing edema development in the rat cold lesion model as described in a recent review by Wahl et al.(115). In rats subjected to an ischemia-reperfusion damage treatment with a newly developed potent B_2 receptor antagonist, CP-0597 yielded evidence for a significant decrease of brain swelling and a marked neuroprotective effect of this compound (78). Moreover, the fairly specific B_2 receptor antagonist, CP-0127, has only recently been tested in a small number of patients suffering from traumatic brain injury of mild to moderate degree. Continuous subdural infusion of the antagonist resulted in a lower peak increase of intracranial pressure and a marked decrease of the therapy intensity level (64). Although these results are very promising, further studies with larger number of patients are necessary to confirm these preliminary results. In conclusion, BK meets all criteria of a mediator candidate of cerebral edema.

3.2   HISTAMINE (HA)

3.2.1   Effect on BBB permeability.

Cortical superfusion with HA resulted in a decrease of transendothelial pial vascular resistance (14,15) and extravasation of Na^+-fluorescein and FITC-dextran 62,000 and 145,000 (Stokes' radius, 87 Å) (90). Similarly, local application of HA to individual pial venules enhanced permeability for Lucifer yellow (MW, 457) (28). Thus "unspecific" opening of the BBB by HA allows escape of low and high molecular weight tracer compounds. During cortical superfusion extravasation of Na^+-fluorescein started at concentrations as low as 1 nM HA in the superfusate when no dilatation of pial arteries was observed (90). This clearly indicates that the permeability-enhancing and the diameter-increasing actions of a given compound may occur independent of each other. Intravascular application of HA also resulted in an increase of BBB permeability for differently sized tracers (24,33,39,40). The BBB opening action of HA is well established although it could not be confirmed in a small number of studies (34,68,86,117). These negative results may be explained by species-related features or technical reasons.

Widening of the tight junctions due to endothelial contraction has been suggested to be the route of HA-induced extravasation. This mechanism could well explain the rapid fall of transendothelial resistance observed in rats during topical application of HA (14,15). On the other hand, stimulation of vesicular transport by HA has been consistently found in electron microscopic studies (26,39). The conclusion of vesicular transport stimulated by HA appears to receive further support from the observation of a "reverse pinocytosis" induced by intraventricularly applied HA without signs of brain edema (25).

3.2.2   Vasomotor actions.

The main vasomotor effect exerted by HA is relaxation/dilatation of cerebral blood vessels in vitro and in vivo and an increase of cerebral blood flow, although in rabbit cerebral arteries HA induces constriction as reviewed extensively elsewhere (89). The dilatory effect of HA is predominantly due to activation of H_2 receptors (38,109) which are located on the smooth muscle cells. However, activation of H_1 receptors located on endothelial cells and coupled to release of nitric oxide may also contribute substantially to cerebroarterial relaxation induced by HA (100) (for review see Schilling and Wahl (89)).

3.2.3   Induction of cerebral edema.

In accord with its permeability enhancing and dilatory action, intracarotid application of HA has been found to induce cerebral edema as reflected by an increased tissue water content and swelling of perivascular glial endfeet (26,39).

3.2.4   Local concentration of HA.

In the brain mast cells are the main source of HA (41,71,95). However, HA is also present in cells of the vessel wall itself, in perivascular nerve terminals (96) and in neurons (35,95,118). A significant increase of tissue HA content was found after induction of cold lesion and stab injury (60,70), spinal cord contusion (61) and ischemia or ischemia-reperfusion injury (2,98).

3.2.5   Therapeutic studies.

A couple of different histaminergic receptor antagonists has been used in animal experiments to decrease development of brain edema. Application of the H_2 receptor antagonists metiamide, ranitidine and cimetidine were shown to decrease brain edema following induction of pneumothorax, brain radiation and stab injury (22,27,44,60). However, no decrease of ischemia- and cold lesion-induced brain edema by treatment with cimetidine, zolantidine or mepyramine was observed in rats (52,88). Similarly, application of a newly developed antagonist at the intracellular HA affinity site, N,N-diethyl-2-[4-phenylmethyl)phenoxy]ethanamine, did not decrease albumin extravasation into brin tissue following transient ischemia (65).

3.3   ARACHIDONIC ACID (AA)

3.3.1   Effect on BBB permeability.

A decrease of transendothelial resistance in frogs (68) and extravasation of differently sized tracers in cats were observed during cortical superfusion with AA (106,113,120). Similarly, tracer extravasation also occurred after intracerebral injection of AA (9,16,73). Whether or not the BBB permeability-enhancing effect is brought about by AA itself as suggested by Unterberg and coworkers (106) or by metabolites such as leukotrienes or free radicals (9,73,120) is not yet clear. However, a leukotactic action may be involved since polymorphonuclear leukocytes sticking to and even migrating through the endothelial cells of cerebral blood vessels were found in electron micrographs following cortical superfusion with AA (106).

3.3.2   Vasomotor actions.

Descriptions of the vasomotor action of AA are not uniform. During topical application of AA pial arteries have been found to exert weak constriction (82,106) or marked dilatation (51). Thus, it is questionable whether the vasomotor effects of AA would enhance tracer extravasation significantly.

3.3.3   Induction of cerebral edema.

Using the intraparenchymal injection technique AA was found to induce cerebral edema in rats (9,16,73).

3.3.4   Local concentration of AA.

In pathological states such as ischemia and experimental head injury, an increase of AA tissue content was found (3,7). A concentration of up to 2 x 10^{-4} M AA in the interstitial space was estimated after cold lesion (3) which is a concentration range where tracer extravasation was observed during cortical superfusion with AA (106).

3.3.5   Therapeutic studies.

Inhibition of phospholipase A_2 has yielded controversial results with respect to inhibition of edema.Thus, glucocorticoids proved efficient in decreasing brain edema following ischemia with or without hypoxia (4,46) but failed to do so after experimental brain trauma (23,91). Possibly the negative results reflect insufficient pharmacological inhibition of AA release under these conditions. In agreement with these pharmacologic studies, a smaller degree of post-ischemic edema occurs in mice lacking the cytosolic phospholipase A_2 (10).

3.4   NITRIC OXIDE (NO) AND OXYGEN-DERIVED FREE RADICALS

3.4.1   Effect on BBB permeability.

Application of a free radical generating system has been found to result in a moderate extravasation of Na^+-fluorescein (105) and Evans blue-tagged albumin (17) and a decrease of transendothelial resistance in vivo (68) or in cultured cerebral microvascular endothelial cells (42). Indirect evidence in support of a BBB-permeability enhancing action of free radicals is provided by studies in which superoxide dismutase and/or catalase was found to result in a decrease of tracer extravasation (28,120). Furthermore, there is some evidence suggesting a BBB-opening action of NO. Thus, leakage of Na^+-fluorescein, sucrose and Evans blue-tagged albumin was found after intracarotid infusion of exogenous NO donors (92). In addition, leakage of

FITC-dextran (MW, 10,000) induced by topically applied glutamate was slightly enhanced by cortical superfusion with an exogenous NO donor, and a decrease of tracer extravasation induced by arterial hypertension or topical application of glutamate or histamine, respectively, by a NO synthase inhibitor has been reported (57-59).

3.4.2   Vasomotor actions.

Oxygen-derived free radicals have been claimed to induce dilatation of cerebral arteries (80,119), but discrepant results have also been reported (105). In contrast, the vasodilatory action of NO is well established and its role in cerebrovascular regulation has been reviewed extensively (29).

3.4.3   Induction of cerebral edema.

Whether or not intravascular or intracerebral application of NO results in induction of brain edema has not yet been studied. In contrast, intraparenchymal infusion of a mixture containing hypoxanthine/xanthin oxidase to generate oxygen-derived free radicals has been shown to induce cerebral edema (17).

3.4.4   Local concentration of free radicals.

Brain tissue content of oxygen-derived free radicals or associated lipid peroxides have been shown to be increased after ischemia-reperfusion injury and contusion trauma (48). Furthermore, in a rat model of ischemia-reperfusion injury a rapid and transient increase of the NO concentration in the brain interstitial fluid was measured after induction of carotid artery occlusion and again immediately after allowing reperfusion (54).

3.4.5   Therapeutic studies.

With regard to the therapeutic efficacy of blocking release of NO, a decrease of brain edema development has been found after application of a NO synthase inhibitor in the rat cold lesion-model of brain trauma (72). In ischemia-reperfusion injury, however, discrepant results have been obtained, possibly due to differences in experimental design as discussed by Pelligrino (74). One important factor may be whether or not gene expression of the type II NO synthase (the so-called inducible NO synthase) will occur. Once inducible NO synthase becomes active, large amounts of NO will be continuously released possibly leading to formation of peroxynitrites and lipid peroxidation (5). Insufficient inhibition of NO release under these conditions may explain failure of NO synthase inhibitor application to reduce brain edema. Thus further studies appear necessary for establishing a mediator role of NO.

4.   CONCLUSION

In conclusion, the BBB which consists of a continuous endothelium with tight junctions and specific transendothelial transport systems may be disrupted under pathological conditions. The resulting vasogenic edema appears to be mediated by several mediators. All criteria favor BK as a mediator of brain edema. Much evidence also supports a mediator role of HA, AA, and free radicals including NO.

REFERENCES

1. Abbott, N. J., and P. A. Revest. Control of brain endothelial permeability. *Cerebrovasc. Brain Metab. Rev.* 3: 39-72, 1991.
2. Adachi, N., Y. Itoh, R. Oishi, and K. Saeki. Direct evidence for increased continuous histamine release in the striatum of conscious freely moving rats produced by middle cerebral artery occlusion. *J. Cereb. Blood Flow Metab.* 12: 477-483, 1992.
3. Baethmann, A., K. Maier-Hauff, L. Schürer, M. Lange, C. Guggenbichler, W. Vogt, K. Jacob, and O. Kempski. Release of glutamate and of free fatty acids in vasogenic brain edema. *J. Neurosurg.* 70: 578-591, 1989.
4. Barbosa-Coutinho, L. M., A. Hartmann, K.-A. Hossmann, and T. Rommel. Effect of dexamethasone on serum protein extravasation in experimental brain infarcts of monkey: an immunohistochemical study. *Acta Neuropathol.* 65: 255-260, 1985.
5. Beckman, J. S. The double-edged role of nitric oxide in brain function and superoxide-mediated injury. *J. Develop. Physiol.* 15: 53-59, 1991.
6. Betz, A. L., J. A. Firth, and G. W. Goldstein. Polarity of the blood-brain barrier: distribution of enzymes between the luminal and antiluminal membranes of brain capillary endothelial cells. *Brain Res.* 192: 17-28, 1980.
7. Bhakoo, K. K., H. A. Crockard, and P. T. Lascelles. Regional studies of changes in brain fatty acids following experimental ischaemia and reperfusion in the gerbil. *J. Neurochem.* 43: 1025-1031, 1984.
8. Biegel, D., D. D. Spencer, and J. S. Pachter. Isolation and culture of human brain microvessel endothelial cells for the study of blood-brain barrier properties in vitro. *Brain Res.* 692: 183-189, 1995.
9. Black, K. L., and J. T. Hoff. Leukotrienes increase blood-brain barrier permeability following intraparenchymal injections in rats. *Ann. Neurol.* 18: 349-351, 1985.
10. Bonventre, J. V., Z. Huang, M. R. Taheri, E. O'Leary, E. Li, M. A. Moskowitz, and A. Sapirstein. Reduced fertility and postischaemic brain injury in mice deficient in cytosolic phospholipase A_2. *Nature* 390: 622-625, 1997.

11. Brightman, M. W. The anatomic basis of the blood-brain barrier. In: *Implications of the blood-brain barrier and its manipulation*, edited by E. A. Neuwelt. New York: Plenum, 1989, p. 53-83.

12. Brightman, M. W., T. S. Reese, and N. Feder. Assessment with the electromicroscope of the permeability to peroxidase of cerebral endothelium and epithelium in mice and sharks. In: *Capillary permeability*, edited by C. Crone and N. A. Lassen. Copenhagen: Munksgaard, 1970, p. 468-476.

13. Bundgaard, M. Ultrastructure of frog cerebral and pial microvessels and their impermeability to lanthanum ions. *Brain Res.* 241: 57-65, 1982.

14. Butt, A. M. Effect of inflammatory agents on electrical resistance across the blood-brain barrier in pial microvessels of anaesthetised rats. *Brain Res.* 696: 145-150, 1995.

15. Butt, A. M., and H. C. Jones. Effect of histamine and antagonists on electrical resistance across the blood-brain barrier in rat brain-surface microvessels. *Brain Res.* 569: 100-105, 1992.

16. Chan, P. H., R. A. Fishman, J. Caronna, J. W. Schmidley, G. Prioleau, and J. Lee. Induction of brain edema following intracerebral injection of arachidonic acid. *Ann. Neurol.* 13: 625-632, 1983.

17. Chan, P. H., J. W. Schmidley, R. A. Fishman, and S. M. Longar. Brain injury, edema, and vascular permeability changes induced by oxygen-derived free radicals. *Neurology* 34: 315-20, 1984.

18. Cornford, E. M., S. Hyman, and W. M. Pardridge. An electron microscopic immunogold analysis of developmental up-regulation of the blood-brain barrier GLUT1 glucose transporter. *J. Cereb. Blood Flow Metab.* 13: 841-854, 1993.

19. Cornford, E. M., S. Hyman, and B. E. Swartz. The human brain GLUT1 glucose transporter: ultrastructural localization to the blood-brain barrier endothelia. *J. Cereb. Blood Flow Metab.* 14: 106-112, 1994.

20. Crone, C. Modulation of solute permeability in microvascular endothelium. *Federation Proc.* 45: 77-83, 1986.

21. Crone, C., and S. P. Olesen. Electrical resistance of brain microvascular endothelium. *Brain Res.* 241: 49-55, 1982.

22. Csanda, E. Radiation brain edema. In: *Brain Edema*, edited by J. Cervos-Navarro and R. Ferszt. New York: Raven Press, 1980, p. 125-146.

23. Dick, A. R., M. E. McCallum, J. A. Maxwell, and S. R. Nelson. Effect of dexamethasone on experimental brain edema in cats. *J. Neurosurg.* 45: 141-147, 1976.

24. Domer, F. R., S. B. Boertje, E. G. Bing, and I. Reddix. Histamine- and acetylcholine-induced changes in the permeability of the blood-brain barrier of normotensive and spontaneously hypertensive rats. *Neuropharmacology* 22: 615-619, 1983.

25. Dux, E., T. Doczi, F. Joó, P. Szerdahelyi, and L. Siklos. Reverse pinocytosis induced in cerebral endothelial cells by injection of histamine into the cerebral ventricle. *Acta Neuropathol.* 76: 484-488, 1988.

26. Dux, E., and F. Joó. Effects of histamine on brain capillaries. Fine structural and and immunohistochemical studies after intracarotid infusion. *Exp. Brain Res.* 47: 252-258, 1982.

27. Dux, E., P. Temesvari, P. Szerdahelyi, A. Nagy, J. Kovacs, and F. Joó. Protective effects of antihistamines on cerebral oedema induced by experimental pneumothorax in newborn piglets. *Neuroscience* 22: 317-321, 1987.

28. Easton, A. S., M. H. Sarker, and P. A. Fraser. Two components of blood-brain barrier disruption in the rat. *J. Physiol.* 503: 613-623, 1997.

29. Ehrenreich, H., and L. Schilling. New developments in understanding cerebral vasoregulation and vasospasm. The endothelin-nitric oxide network. *Cleveland Clin. J. Med.* 62: 105-116, 1995.

30. Elliott, P. J., N. J. Hayward, M. R. Huff, T. L. Nagle, K. L. Black, and R. T. Bartus. Unlocking the blood-brain barrier: a role of RMP-7 in brain tumor therapy. *Exp. Neurol.* 141: 214-224, 1996.

31. Ellis, E. F., J. Chao, and M. L. Heizer. Brain kininogen following experimental brain injury: evidence for a secondary event. *J. Neurosurg.* 71: 437-442, 1989.

32. Ellis, E. F., M. L. Heizer, G. S. Hambrecht, S. A. Holt, J. M. Stewart, and R. J. Vavrek. Inhibition of bradykinin- and kallikrein-induced cerebral arteriolar dilation by a specific bradykinin antagonist. *Stroke* 18: 792-795, 1987.

33. Földes, I., and B. Kelentei. Studies on the haemato-encephalic barrier II. The effects of histamine with special reference to the passage of antibiotics. *Acta Physiol. Acad. Sci. Hung.* 5: 149-161, 1954.

34. Gabbiani, G., M. C. Badonnel, and G. Majno. Intra-arterial injections of histamine, serotonin, or bradykinin: a topograhic study of vascular leakage. *Proc. Soc. Exp. Biol. Med.* 135: 447-452, 1970.

35. Garbarg, M., G. Barbin, J. Feger, and J.-C. Schwartz. Histaminergic pathway in rat brain evidenced by lesions of the medial forebrain bundle. *Science* 186: 833-835, 1974.

36. Görlach, C., and M. Wahl. Bradykinin dilates rat middle cerebral artery and its large branches via endothelial B_2 receptors and release of nitric oxide. *Peptides* 17: 1373-1378, 1996.

37. Gross, P. M. *Circumventricular organs and body fluids.* Boca Raton: CRC Press, 1987.

38. Gross, P. M., A. M. Harper, and G. M. Teasdale. Cerebral circulation and histamine: 2. responses of pial veins and arterioles to receptor agonists. *J. Cereb. Blood Flow Metab.* 1: 219-225, 1981.

39. Gross, P. M., G. M. Teasdale, D. I. Graham, W. J. Angerson, and A. M. Harper. Intra-arterial histamine increases blood-brain transport in rats. *Amer. J. Physiol.* 243: H307-H317, 1982.

40. Hurst, E. W., and O. L. Davies. Studies on the blood-brain barrier. II. Attempts to influence the passage of substances into the brain. *Brit. J. Pharmacol.* 5: 147-164, 1950.

41. Ibrahim, M. Z. M. The mast cells of the mammalian central nervous system. Part I. Morphology, distribution and histochemistry. *J. Neurol. Sci.* 21: 431-478, 1974.

42. Imaizumi, S., T. Kondo, M. A. Deli, G. Gobbel, F. Joó, C. J. Epstein, T. Yoshimoto, and P. H. Chan. The influence of oxygen free radicals on the permeability of the monolayer of cultured brain endothelial cells. *Neurochem. Int.* 29: 205-211, 1996.

43. Jetté, L., J.-F. Pouliot, G. F. Murphy, and R. Béliveau. Isoform I (mdr3) is the major form of P-glycoprotein expressed in mouse brain capillaries. *Biochem. J.* 305: 761-766, 1995.

44. Joó, F., A. Szücs, and E. Csanda. Metiamide-treatment of brain oedema in animals exposed to ^{90}yttrium irradiation. *J. Pharm. Pharmacol.* 28: 162-163, 1976.

45. Kalaria, R. N., and S. I. Harik. Blood-brain barrier monoamine oxidase: enzyme characterization in cerebral microvessels and other tissues from six mammalian species, including human. *J. Neurochem.* 49: 856-864, 1987.

46. Kalayci, Ö., S. Cataltepe, and O. Cataltepe. The effect of bolus methylprednisolone in prevention of brain edema in hypoxic ischemic brain injury: an experimental study in 7-day-old rat pups. *Brain Res.* 569: 112-116, 1992.

47. Kamiya, T., Y. Katayama, F. Kashiwagi, and A. Terashi. The role of bradykinin in mediating ischemic brain edema in rats. *Stroke* 24: 571-576, 1993.

48. Kawauchi, N., S., M. Yunoki, Y. Noguchi, M. Kawauchi, S. Asari, and T. Ohmoto. Detection of lipid peroxidation and hydroxyl radicals in brain contusion of rats. *Acta Neurochir. Suppl.* 70: 84-86, 1997.

49. Kondo, T., H. Kinouchi, M. Kawase, and T. Yoshimoto. Astroglial cells inhibit the increasing permeability of brain endothelial cell monolayer following hypoxia/reoxygenation. *Neurosci. Lett.* 208: 101-104, 1996.

50. Kontos, H. A., E. P. Wei, R. C. Kukreja, E. F. Ellis, and M. L. Hess. Differences in endothelium-dependent cerebral dilation by bradykinin and acetylcholine. *Amer. J. Physiol.* 258: H1261-H1266, 1990.

51. Kontos, H. A., E. P. Wei, J. T. Povlishock, and C. W. Christman. Oxygen radicals mediate the cerebral arteriolar dilation from arachidonate and bradykinin in cats. *Circ. Res.* 55: 295-303, 1984.

52. Leistra, H. P. J. M., and H. H. Dietrich. Effect of the histamine antagonist cimetidine on infarct size in the rat. *J. Neurotrauma* 10: 83-89, 1993.

53. Maier-Hauff, K., A. J. Baethmann, M. Lange, L. Schürer, and A. Unterberg. The kallikrein-kinin system as a mediator in vasogenic brain edema. Part 2: Studies on kinin formation in focal and perifocal brain tissue. *J. Neurosurg.* 61: 97-106, 1984.

54. Malinski, T., F. Bailey, Z. G. Zhang, and M. Chopp. Nitric oxide measured by a porphyrinic microsensor in rat brain after transient middle cerebral artery occlusion. *J. Cereb. Blood Flow Metab.* 13: 355-358, 1993.

55. Mándi, Y., I. Ocsovszki, D. Szabo, Z. Nagy, J. Nelson, and J. Molnar. Nitric oxide production and MDR expression by human brain endothelial cells. *Anticanc. Res.* 18: 3049-3052, 1998.

56. Mayhan, W. G. Impairment of endothelium-dependent dilatation of basilar artery during chronic hypertension. *Amer. J. Physiol.* 259: H1455-H1462, 1990.

57. Mayhan, W. G. Role of nitric oxide in disruption of the blood-brain barrier during acute hypertension. *Brain Res.* 686: 99-103, 1995.

58. Mayhan, W. G. Role of nitric oxide in histamine-induced increases in permeability of the blood-brain barrier. *Brain Res.* 743: 70-76, 1996.

59. Mayhan, W. G., and S. P. Didion. Glutamate-induced disruption of the blood-brain barrier in rats. Role of nitric oxide. *Stroke* 27: 965-970, 1996.

60. Mohanty, S., P. K. Dey, H. S. Sharma, S. Singh, J. P. N. Chansouria, and Y. Olsson. Role of histamine in traumatic brain edema. An experimental study in the rat. *J. Neurol. Sci.* 90: 87-98, 1989.

61. Naftchi, N. E., M. Demeny, V. DeCrescito, J. J. Tomasula, E. S. Flamm, and J. B. Campbell. Biogenic amine concentrations in traumatized spinal cords of cats. Effect of drug therapy. *J. Neurosurg.* 40: 52-57, 1974.

62. Nag, S. Ultracytochemical localization of Na+,K+-ATPase in cerebral endothelium in acute hypertension. *Acta Neuropathol.* 80: 7-11, 1990.

63. Nakano, S., K. Matsukado, and K. L. Black. Increased brain tumor microvessel permeability after intracarotid bradykinin infusion is mediated by nitric oxide. *Cancer Res.* 56: 4027-4031, 1996.

64. Narotam, P. K., T. C. Rodell, S. S. Nadvi, K. D. Bhoola, J. M. Troha, R. Parbhoosingh, and J. R. van Dellen. Traumatic brain contusions: a clinical role for the kinin antagonist CP-0127. *Acta Neurochir.* 141: 793-803, 1998.

65. Németh, L., M. A. Deli, A. Falus, C. Szabó, and C. S. Ábraham. Cerebral ischemia reperfusion-induced vasogenic brain edema formation in rats: effect of an intracellular histamine receptor antagonist. *Eur. J. Pediatr. Surg.* 8: 216-219, 1998.

66. Oldendorf, W. H., E. M. Cornford, and W. J. Brown. The large apparent work capability of the blood-brain barrier: a study of the mitochondrial content of capillary endothelial cells in brain and other tissue of the rat. *Ann. Neurol.* 1: 409-417, 1977.

67. Olesen, S.-P. An electrophysiological study of microvascular permeability and its modulation by chemical mediators. *Acta Physiol. Scand.* 136 (Suppl 579): 7-28, 1989.

68. Olesen, S.-P., and C. Crone. Substances that rapidly augment ionic conductance of endothelium in cerebral venules. *Acta Physiol. Scand.* 127: 233-241, 1986.

69. Onoue, H., N. Kaito, M. Tomii, S. Tokudome, M. Nakajima, and T. Abe. Human basilar and middle cerebral arteries exhibit endothelium-dependent responses to peptides. *Amer. J. Physiol.* 267: H880-H886, 1994.

70. Orr, E. L. Cryogenic lesions induce a mast cell-dependent increase in cerebral cortical histamine levels in the mouse. *Neurochem. Pathol.* 8: 43-51, 1988.

71. Orr, E. L., and K. R. Pace. The significance of mast cells as a source of histamine in the mouse brain. *J. Neurochem.* 42: 727-732, 1984.

72. Oury, T. D., C. A. Piantadosi, and J. D. Crapo. Cold-induced brain edema in mice. Involvement of extracellular superoxide dismutase and nitric oxide. *J. Biol. Chem.* 268: 15394-15398, 1993.

73. Papadopoulos, S. M., K. L. Black, and J. T. Hoff. Cerebral edema induced by arachidonic acid: role of leukocytes and 5-lipoxygenase products. *Neurosurgery* 25: 369-372, 1989.

74. Pelligrino, D. A. Saying NO to cerebral ischemia. *J. Neurosurg. Anesthesiol.* 5: 221-231, 1993.

75. Rahner-Welsch, S., J. Vogel, and W. Kuschinsky. Regional congruence and divergence of glucose transporters (GLUT1) and capillaries in rat brains. *J. Cereb. Blood Flow Metab.* 15: 681-686, 1995.

76. Raymond, J. J., D. M. Robertson, and H. B. Dinsdale. Pharmacological modification of bradykinin induced breakdown of the blood-brain barrier. *Can. J. Neurol. Sci.* 13: 214-220, 1986.

77. Reese, T. S., and M. J. Karnovsky. Fine structural localization of a blood-brain barrier to exogenous peroxidase. *J. Cell Biol.* 34: 207-217, 1967.

78. Relton, J. K., V. E. Beckey, W. L. Hanson, and E. T. Whalley. CP-0597, a selective bradykinin B_2 receptor antagonist, inhibits brain injury in a rat model of reversible middle cerebral artery occlusion. *Stroke* 28: 1430-1436, 1997.

79. Revest, P. A., H. C. Jones, and N. J. Abbott. Transendothelial electrical potential across pial vessels in anaesthetised rats: a study of ion permeability and transport at the blood-brain barrier. *Brain Res.* 652: 76-82, 1994.

80. Rosenblum, W. I. Effects of free radical generation on mouse pial arterioles: probable role of hydroxyl radicals. *Amer. J. Physiol.* 245: H139-H142, 1983.

81. Rosenblum, W. I. Hydroxyl radical mediates the endothelium-dependent relaxation produced by bradykinin in mouse cerebral arterioles. *Circ. Res.* 61: 601-603, 1987.

82. Rosenblum, W. I., and G. H. Nelson. Endothelium-dependent constriction demonstrated in vivo in mouse cerebral arterioles. *Circ. Res.* 63: 837-843, 1988.

83. Sánchez del Pino, M. M., R. A. Hawkins, and D. R. Peterson. Biochemical discrimination between luminal and abluminal enzyme and transport activities of the blood-brain barrier. *J. Biol. Chem.* 270: 14907-14912, 1995.

84. Sánchez del Pino, M. M., D. R. Peterson, and R. A. Hawkins. Neutral amino acid transport characterization of isolated luminal and abluminal membranes of the blood-brain barrier. *J. Biol. Chem.* 270: 14913-14918, 1995.

85. Sanovich, E., R. T. Bartus, P. M. Friden, R. L. Dean, H. Q. Le, and M. W. Brightman. Pathway across blood-brain barrier opened by the bradykinin agonist, RMP-7. *Brain Res.* 705: 125-135, 1995.

86. Saria, A., J. M. Lundberg, G. Skofitsch, and F. Lembeck. Vascular protein leakage in various tissues induced by substance P, capsaicin, bradykinin, serotonin, histamine and by antigen challenge. *Naunyn-Schmiedeberg's Arch. Pharmacol.* 324: 212-218, 1983.
87. Schilling, L., and M. Wahl. Brain edema: pathogenesis and therapy. *Kidney Int.* 51, Suppl. 59: S69-S75, 1997.
88. Schilling, L., and M. Wahl. Effects of antihistaminics on experimental brain edema. *Acta Neurochir.* 60 (Suppl): 79-82, 1994.
89. Schilling, L., and M. Wahl. Histaminergic effects on cerebral hemodynamics. In: *The regulation of cerebral blood flow*, edited by J. W. Phillis. Boca Raton: CRC Press, 1993, p. 114-128.
90. Schilling, L., and M. Wahl. Opening of the blood-brain barrier during cortical superfusion with histamine. *Brain Res.* 653: 289-296, 1994.
91. Shapira, Y., E. Davidson, Y. Weidenfeld, S. Cotev, and E. Shohami. Dexamethasone and indomethacin do not affect brain edema following head injury in rats. *J. Cereb. Blood Flow Metab.* 8: 395-402, 1988.
92. Shukla, A., M. Dikshit, and R. C. Srimal. Nitric oxide-dependent blood-brain barrier permeability alterations in the rat brain. *Experientia* 52: 136-140, 1996.
93. Sobey, C. G., D. D. Heistad, and F. M. Faraci. Mechanisms of bradykinin-induced cerebral vasodilatation in rats. Evidence that reactive oxygen species activate K+ channels. *Stroke* 28: 2290-2295, 1997.
94. Spector, R., and C. E. Johanson. The mammalian choroid plexus. *Sci. Amer.* 261: 68-74, 1989.
95. Steinbusch, H. W. M., and A. H. Mulder. Immunohistochemical localization of histamine in neurons and mast cells in the rat brain. In: *Handbook of Chemical Neuronanatomy. Vol.3: Classical Transmitters and Transmitter Receptors in the CNS. Part II*, edited by A. Björklund, T. Hökfelt and M. J. Kuhar. Amsterdam: Elsevier, 1984, p. 126-140.
96. Steinbusch, H. W. M., and A. A. J. Verhofstad. Immunocytochemical demonstration of noradrenaline, serotonin and histamine and some observations on the innervation of the intracerebral blood vessels. In: *Neural Regulation of Brain Circulation*, edited by C. Owman and J. E. Hardebo. Amsterdam: Elsevier, 1986, p. 181-194.
97. Stewart, P. A., and E. M. Hayakawa. Interendothelial junctional changes underlie the developmental 'tightening' of the blood-brain barrier. *Develop. Brain Res.* 32: 271-281, 1987.
98. Subramanian, N., D. Theodore, and J. Abraham. Experimental cerebral infarction in primates: Regional changes in brain histamine content. *J. Neural Transm.* 50: 225-232, 1981.
99. Tayarani, I., J. M. LeFauconnier, F. Roux, and J. M. Bourre. Evidence for an alanine, serine, and cysteine system of transport in isolated brain capillaries. *J. Cereb. Blood Flow Metab.* 7: 585-591, 1987.
100. Toda, N. Mechanism underlying responses to histamine of isolated monkey and human cerebral arteries. *Amer. J. Physiol.* 258: H311-H317, 1990.
101. Tsuji, A., T. Terasaki, Y. Takabatake, Y. Tenda, I. Tamai, T. Yamashima, S. Moritani, T. Tsuruo, and J. Yamashita. P-glycoprotein as the drug efflux pump in primary cultured bovine brain capillary endothelial cells. *Life Sci.* 51: 1427-1437, 1992.
102. Unterberg, A., and A. J. Baethmann. The kallikrein-kinin system as mediator in vasogenic brain edema. Part 1: Cerebral exposure to bradykinin and plasma. *J. Neurosurg.* 61: 87-96, 1984.
103. Unterberg, A., C. Dautermann, A. Baethmann, and W. Müller-Esterl. The kallikrein-kinin system as mediator in vasogenic brain edema. Part 3: Inhibition of the kallikrein-kinin system in traumatic brain swelling. *J. Neurosurg.* 64: 269-276, 1986.

104. Unterberg, A., M. Wahl, and A. Baethmann. Effects of bradykinin on permeability and diameter of pial vessels in vivo. *J. Cereb. Blood Flow Metab.* 4: 574-585, 1984.

105. Unterberg, A., M. Wahl, and A. Baethmann. Effects of free radicals on permeability and vasomotor response of cerebral vessels. *Acta Neuropathol.* 76: 238-244, 1988.

106. Unterberg, A., M. Wahl, F. Hammersen, and A. Baethmann. Permeability and vasomotor responses of cerebral vessels during exposure to arachidonic acid. *Acta Neuropathol.* 73: 209-219, 1987.

107. Vannucci, S. J., L. B. Seaman, and R. C. Vannucci. Effects of hypoxia-ischemia on GLUT1 and GLUT3 glucose transporters in immature rat brain. *J. Cereb. Blood Flow Metab.* 16: 77-81, 1996.

108. Vorbrodt, A. W., A. S. Lossinsky, and H. M. Wisniewski. Enzyme cytochemistry of blood-brain barrier (BBB) disturbance. *Acta Neuropathol.* Suppl. VIII: 43-57, 1983.

109. Wahl, M., and W. Kuschinsky. The dilating effect of histamine on pial arteries of cats and its mediation by H_2 receptors. *Circ. Res.* 44: 161-165, 1979.

110. Wahl, M., and L. Schilling. Effects of bradykinin in the cerebral microcirculation. In: *The regulation of cerebral blood flow*, edited by J. W. Phillis. Boca Raton: CRC Press, 1993, p. 315-328.

111. Wahl, M., L. Schilling, A. Unterberg, and A. Baethmann. Autacoids as mediators of vasogenic brain oedema. In: *New concepts of a blood-brain barrier*, edited by J. Greenwood, D. J. Begley and M. B. Segal. New York: Plenum Press, 1995, p. 147-157.

112. Wahl, M., L. Schilling, A. Unterberg, and A. Baethmann. Mediators of vascular and parenchymal mechanisms in secondary brain damage. *Acta Neurochir.* 57 (Suppl): 64-72, 1993.

113. Wahl, M., A. Unterberg, and A. Baethmann. Intravital fluorescence microscopy for the study of blood-brain-barrier function. *Int. J. Microcirc. Clin. Exp.* 4: 3-18, 1985.

114. Wahl, M., A. Unterberg, A. Baethmann, and L. Schilling. Mediators of blood-brain barrier dysfunction and formation of vasogenic brain edema. *J. Cereb. Blood Flow Metab.* 8: 621-634, 1988.

115. Wahl, M., E. T. Whalley, A. Unterberg, L. Schilling, A. A. Parsons, A. Baethmann, and A. R. Young. Vasomotor and permeability effects of bradykinin in the cerebral microcirculation. *Immunopharmacology* 33: 257-263, 1996.

116. Wahl, M., A. R. Young, L. Edvinsson, and F. Wagner. Effects of bradykinin on pial arteries and arterioles in vitro and in situ. *J. Cereb. Blood Flow Metab.* 3: 231-237, 1983.

117. Watanabe, M., and W. I. Rosenblum. In vivo studies of pial vascular permeability to sodium fluorescein: absence of alterations by bradykinin, histamine, serotonin, or arachidonic acid. *Stroke* 18: 1157-1159, 1987.

118. Watanabe, T., Y. Taguchi, H. Hayashi, J. Tanaka, S. Shiosaka, M. Tohyama, H. Kubota, Y. Terano, and H. Wada. Evidence for the presence of a histaminergic neuron system in the rat brain: an immunohistochemical analysis. *Neurosci. Lett.* 39: 249-254, 1983.

119. Wei, E. P., C. W. Christman, H. A. Kontos, and P. J.T. Effects of oxygen radicals on cerebral arterioles. *Amer. J. Physiol*. 248: H157-H162, 1985.

120. Wei, E. P., M. D. Ellison, H. A. Kontos, and J. T. Povlishock. O2 radicals in arachidonate-induced increased blood-brain barrier permeability to proteins. *Amer. J. Physiol.* 251: H693-H699, 1986.

121. Whalley, E. T., Y. O. Amure, and R. H. Lye. Analysis of the mechanism of action of bradykinin on human basilar artery in vitro. *Naunyn-Schmiedeberg's Arch. Pharmacol.* 335: 433-437, 1987.

122. Whittle, I. R., I. R. Piper, and J. D. Miller. The role of bradykinin in the etiology of vasogenic brain edema and perilesional brain dysfunction. Acta Neurochir. 115: 53-59, 1992.

123. Wolburg, H., J. Neuhaus, U. Kniesel, B. Krauß, E.-M. Schmid, M. Öcalan, C. Farrell, and W. Risau. Modulation of tight junction structure in blood-brain barrier endothelial cells. Effects of tissue culture, second messengers and cocultured astrocytes. J. Cell Sci. 107: 1347-1357, 1994.

124. Xu, J., C. Y. Hsu, H. Junker, S. Chao, E. L. Hogan, and J. Chao. Kininogen and kinin in experimental spinal cord injury. J. Neurochem. 57: 975-980, 1991.

125. Yang, S.-T., W. G. Mayhan, and D. D. Heistad. Endothelium-dependent responses of cerebral blood vessels during chronic hypertension. Hypertension 17: 612-618, 1991.

Chapter 12

The Hypoxic Brain
Introduction

Thomas F. Hornbein

Departments of Anesthesiology and Phsiology and Biopyhsics, University of Washington, Seattle, Washington, USA

Key words: brain, hypoxia, acute mountain sickness, high altitude cerebral edema, brain injury, brain imaging

The brain thrives on oxygen. High altitude poses a tax upon the oxygen supply. In spite of adaptations to a low partial pressure of oxygen, notably a resetting of cerebral blood flow, the paucity of oxygen in high places can make a lasting impression on our most precious organ. Among the physiological questions are: How does real-time hypoxia affect judgement and performance at high altitude? How might the hypoxia of high altitude cause long-lasting injury to the brain? How does hypoxia cause AMS, particularly its most common symptom, headache, and is AMS just early HACE? What tools can we apply to studying the human brain to begin to obtain answers to questions such as those above? In this section, we will explore three pieces of these various puzzles: 1) how brain cells get injured (Hossman); 2) what causes headache (Moskowitz); and 3) how we might better probe the mysteries of what's going on inside the human brain at high altitude (Raichle).

Hypoxia: Into the Next Millennium.
Edited by R. C. Roach, *et al.* Kluwer Academic/Plenum Publishing, New York, 1999.   143

Chapter 13

High Altitude Headache
Lessons from Headaches at Sea Level

Margarita Sanchez del Rio and Michael A. Moskowitz
Stroke & Neurovascular Regulation Laboratory, Massachusetts General Hospital, Harvard Medical School, Boston, MA 02129, USA

Key words: pain, headache, hypoxia, high altitude

Abstract: There is little known about high altitude headache, except that it is an important and serious problem that often heralds the onset of acute mountain sickness. We do know that the brain itself is an insensate organ except for its meninges which contain sensory axons projecting from the trigeminal nerve. These nerve fibers travel in proximity to meningeal blood vessels and constitute an important component of the trigeminovascular system. Signals generated at high altitude which may activate the trigeminovascular system can arise from brain, blood or the blood vessel wall, include protons, neurotransmitters and other potential noxious agents which can discharge or sensitize small unmyelinated fibers. Brain edema and raised intracranial pressure may cause headache by compressing brain structures leading to displacement and stretching of the pain-sensitive intracranial structures. Small hemorrhage may irritate and discharge these fibers chemically. Furthermore, high altitude seems capable of decreasing the threshold of response to sensory stimulation. Therefore, headache can be attributed to activation of a common pathway, the trigeminovascular system by both chemical or mechanical stimulation.

1.   INTRODUCTION

There is little information known about the pathogenesis of headache at normal altitude, and even less so under conditions of high altitude. We do know, however, that the brain itself is an insensate organ with only its coverings, or meninges containing sensory nerve fibers projecting from the largest of the 12 cranial nerves, the trigeminal nerve.

These nerve cells reside at the base of the brain and send their axonal projections to invest predominantly meningeal blood vessels including the thick covering, or dura mater, and blood vessels which lay on the surface of the brain. These axons contain vasoactive neuropeptides which can promote leakage of plasma protein. They also contain receptors and ion channels which can sense the presence of protons, and high concentrations of nociceptive or pain generating chemicals like potassium, histamine, serotonin, bradykinin and metabolites of arachidonic acids, such as prostaglandins.

Under conditions of real or threatened tissue injury, these axons discharge and transmit information centrally to promote the perception of headache. In addition, discharging axons promote (particularly in the dura mater) an inflammatory response with degranulation of mast cells. Trigeminal axons are ideally positioned to sample and detect the existence of an abnormal perivascular environment either generated from the brain proper or from the blood or blood vessel wall. These axons also discharge during raised intracranial pressure, or mechanical stimulation. Hence, the genesis of headache may arise from each of these three tissues. Signals generated at high altitude which may participate in the activation of the trigeminovascular system and generate headache include protons, neurotransmitter release and other potential noxious agents from sequestered compartments, brain edema and raised intracranial pressure, or shift in the threshold for depolarization and activation in individuals susceptible to headache.

This chapter is intended to provide a framework for understanding the origins and pathogenesis of headache. The consequences of related changes in brain and blood vessel function will help clarify the relevance of this framework to the pathogenesis of high altitude headache.

2.   ANATOMICAL SUBSTRATES OF CEPHALIC
PAIN

The meninges (pia mater, arachnoid and dura mater) and attendant blood vessels are pain-sensitive and the most likely source of headache (25,33). Distension, stretching or stroking of meningeal vessels causes pain during surgical exposure in awake patients whereas constriction does not. Rhythmical vessel distension produces throbbing pain and nausea as does insufflation of an intraluminal balloon catheter. The thick dura mater is also capable of generating pain particularly when stimulated in proximity to arteries, veins and venous sinuses. These extraordinary findings, performed in the 1940s laid the foundation for research in headache for decades thereafter.

The pia mater, dura mater and arachnoid receive axonal projections from ophthalmic division of the trigeminal nerve and upper cervical dorsal root ganglia. This network of sensory fibers originates in large part from bipolar neurons whose cell bodies lie within the trigeminal ganglia and defines the trigeminovascular system, an important substrate and final common pathway for the transmission of pain. Trigeminal fibers are predominantly small unmyelinated C fibers which distribute themselves to the anterior, middle, posterior cerebral arteries, and anterior and posterior communicators on the same side. Preserved laterality and extensive axonal branching explains the strictly unilateral distribution of many vascular headaches, the diffuse quality of pain, and the difficulties distinguishing between pain from each of the three vessels. A few trigeminal cells project bilaterally, particularly to midline blood vessels which accounts for the bilateral pain following stimulation of a single blood vessel. Some ganglion cells project divergent axon collaterals to innervate both the middle meningeal and middle cerebral arteries, which probably explains why the pain of pial and dural origin are indistinguishable.

Sensory fibers not only transmit nociceptive information to the trigeminal nucleus caudalis (TNC) within brain stem but also promote a sterile inflammatory response within target tissues by releasing vasodilating and permeability-promoting peptides from perivascular nerve endings. Lewis in 1937 suggested the term *nocifensor system* to recognize the role of neurogenic inflammation as a potent endogenous defense in the early phase of tissue damage. It has been well established that SP (an 11 amino acid-containing peptide), neurokinin A (a decapeptide), and CGRP (a 37 amino acid-containing peptide) released from peripheral sensory axons mediate some or all of neurogenic inflammation (28). All three peptides are vasoactive and dilate blood vessels. SP and neurokinin A but not CGRP promote the leakage of albumin from blood vessels, most likely by an action at the postcapillary venule. None of these peptides is capable of disrupting the blood-brain barrier and, because of their size and charge, penetrate the barrier poorly under normal circumstances.

Neurogenic vasodilatation provides a mechanism to explain the blood flow changes that sometimes develop during the headache phase and explain the occurrence of hyperalgesia. In the latter instance, sensory axons become sensitized to previously innocuous stimuli (e.g. vessel pulsations or venous pressure changes) (30). Most likely, sensitization develops as well within brain stem structures after repeated noxious stimulation.

It is important to emphasize that vascular headaches exhibit several features in common with visceral pains originating in other organs, such as bladder, heart, and bowel. For example, both are poorly localized and diffuse and are referred to superficial organs such as skin and muscle. Visceral pains and headaches are often accompanied by intense motor and autonomic responses, such as muscle spasms, sweating, and increased heart rate and blood pressure. Furthermore, visceral organs are relatively insensate except for the organ capsule, the meninges providing an equivalent of the brain's capsule.

Neurogenic inflammation has been observed in several tissues at portals of entry, including the skin (28), the respiratory tract (16,28), the genitourinary system (17,21), and parts of the gastrointestinal tract (8). Neurogenic inflammation occurs almost exclusively in those tissues possessing neuropeptide-containing fibers innervating blood vessels and can be attenuated by specific receptor blockers (e.g., SP) or by drugs that inhibit the release of neuropeptides from these fibers (32). Despite the evidence for its existence in numerous tissues, neurogenic inflammation has not yet been demonstrated within human meninges, perhaps because existing techniques are not sufficiently sensitive.

In summary, the perivascular primary sensory neuron and its axons within meninges may be viewed as a final common pathway, subject to activation or modulation by local factors within the vessel lumen and vessel wall.

3.   ACUTE MOUNTAIN SICKNESS AND HIGH ALTITUDE CEREBRAL EDEMA

Little is known about headache under high altitude conditions but it is estimated to affect between 25% to 50% of persons at 2000-5000m (18,20). The International Headache Society (IHS) classification committee considers headache as secondary to hypoxia when it occurs within 24 hours after sudden ascent to altitudes above 3000m (14). The headache can arise either due to worsening of a preexisting headache condition in individuals predisposed to headache, or by the development of a new one, possibly reflecting the early stages of acute mountain sickness. The quality of the pain may be described as migrainous, tension-type or cluster headache. Because so little descriptive or investigative information is available, it is important to develop an accurate classification of headache to avoid nonspecific diagnostic parameters as well as to compare groups between studies.

High altitude headache is the most common and persistent symptom in Acute mountain sickness (AMS), a condition which if left untreated, might progress to high altitude cerebral edema (HACE). In addition to severe headache, HACE includes vomiting, hallucinations, ataxia, seizures, focal neurological symptoms, papilledema and stupor or coma. Hypoxia has been implicated as a triggering factor but the pathogenesis of AMS and HACE is still not well understood. In normal individuals, high-altitude exposure increases ventilation, hypocapnia, respiratory alkalosis, and compensatory renal excretion of bicarbonate, resulting in blunting of the ventilatory response to hypoxia. Acetazolamide is used to treat AMS based partly on its capacity to augment ventilation (31). Inappropriate hypoventilation with impaired gas exchange leading to decreased arterial oxygen saturation has been found to be associated with an increased risk of AMS (SaO_2% of 81.5% or lower has a PPV of 0.81, NPV of 0.67)(10,26).

The pathogenesis of high altitude headache has been subject of debate. Magnetic resonance brain imaging of subjects with clinical evidence of HACE showed increased T2 signals along white matter tracts, with sparing of gray matter structures, a pattern consistent with edema of vasogenic origin (13). Although still unclear, vasogenic edema may develop from an increase in plasma hydrostatic pressure secondary to increased flow with compromised autoregulation and disruption of the BBB. Hypoxic cerebral vasodilatation on ascent to high altitude is well documented (15). Significant decreases in PaO_2 provides a strong stimulus for increased global cerebral blood flow. An increase in global blood flow of 36% was recently measured by PET during normobaric hypoxia; increases in flow within hypothalamus (32.8%) and thalamus (19%) were also detected (4).

Disruption of the blood-brain-barrier (BBB) may play an important role in the pathogenesis of cerebral edema. The BBB is influenced by neurotransmitters, nitric oxide, histamine, substance P, free oxygen radicals, 5-Hytroxytryptamine, cytokines and endothelial growth factors, some of which are known to be altered during hypoxia in animal models (1,11,24,34). Local hypoxia triggers a complex cascade of cellular responses resulting in an increase in lactate, altered redox state, capillary basement dissolution and rupture with plasma extravasation. Vascular endothelial growth factor (VEGF) may be the most potent identified agent which disrupts the basement membrane and promotes edema (34). VEGF has not only been shown to be upregulated by hypoxia in rats (34) but also in human plasma after physical exercise at high altitude (2) and potently causes leakage of plasma proteins and water from blood vessels.

Mazzone and colleagues investigated the regulation of substance P (SP) receptors in the rat brain stem by acute hypoxia using homogenate radioligand and quantitative autoradiography (19). In the rat spinal trigeminal tract (Sp5) a significant and persistent decrease of (^{125}I)-Bolton-Hunter-SP (BHSP) binding was observed, suggesting enhanced internalization and processing of receptor. Chemical or mechanical stimulation of peripheral nerves has been shown to release SP from the central terminals of primary afferent nociceptive C-fibers, leading to internalization of NK-1 receptors in laminae I-III in the spinal cord. Hypoxia is known to markedly increase the release of SP from the brain stem terminals of carotid body afferents. Mazzone and colleagues reported that hypoxia reduces the number of NK-1 receptors in various brain stem nuclei, including Sp5.

Relief of AMS by dexamethasone provides indirect evidence for the importance of cerebral edema and inflammation in the genesis of headache. Dexamethasone is known to suppress lipid peroxidation, block vascular endothelial growth factor and reduce permeability of endothelial cells in part by inhibiting deacylation of phospholipids. Arachidonic acid and its products (prostaglandins, leucotrienes and lipoxins) mediate inflammation and brain damage. Furthermore, aspirin which N-acetylates cycloxygenase reportedly decreases vascular headaches at high altitude when taken prophylactically (randomized, double blind, placebo controlled study) (5).

4.   POSSIBILITIES AND A FORMULATION

The etiology of high altitude headache is difficult to establish without objective studies (i.e., functional imaging), and will likely be multifactorial. There is certain to be a population at risk, just as there is for pulmonary edema. Various factors such as barometric pressure, photic stimulation, exercise and most of all, hypoxia may play a major role in sensitizing or priming the nervous system including those structures associated with the trigeminovascular system. Altered CNS function may contribute. Alterations in the threshold for sensory activation have been observed repeatedly. For example, there is a 25-40% decrease in threshold to smell, taste or touch, early-on at altitudes higher than 3000m (9,12,23). Noel-Jorand and colleagues also found that pain perception is altered during hypoxia (23). A 30% decrease in pain threshold is observed at high altitudes (1300-5600 m) compared to controls when determined in 6 volunteers by cutaneous electrical stimulation. The authors attribute this decrease in threshold to an adaptive mechanism, similar to the increased respiratory sensation found in lowlanders during the first stages of adaptation to altitude hypoxia (22).

Pending further studies, it is difficult to discern whether such threshold reductions develop as an adaptive response to adverse conditions or merely reflect the consequences of a noxious environment upon nervous system function. On the other hand, it is also difficult to establish whether altered thresholds develop from hypoxia alone or from the combined effects of low temperature, high intensity lighting conditions, hypobaric pressure, fatigue or sleep deprivation. What seems true is that high altitude renders the nervous system more sensitive, and possibly more susceptible to afferent inputs, possibly also from the trigeminovascular system, to generate headache.

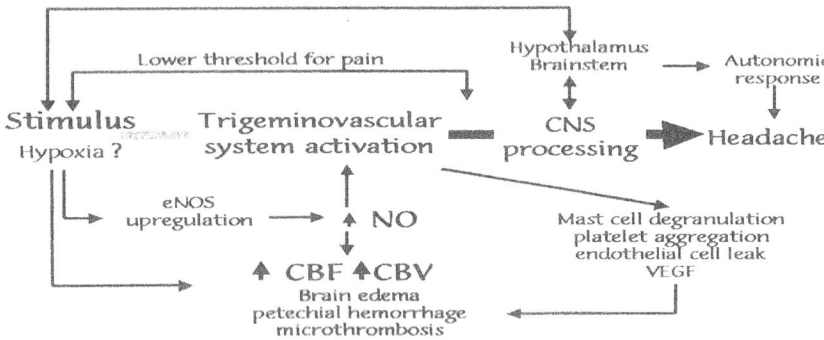

Figure 1. Summary of possible mechanisms involved in high altitude headache

We know from studies at sea level that the trigeminovascular system, as other surveillance systems, detects real or threatened tissue injury within the vicinity of the meningeal blood vessel, and can respond to locally generated (vessel wall/brain) stimuli or to molecules carried from afar and generated under high altitude conditions. Triggering factors associated with high altitude hypoxia include release substances (e.g. nitric oxide) that activate or sensitize trigeminovascular fibers, which reside in the outer layer of arteries and venous sinuses. One hypothesis suggests that protons or hydrogen ions, potassium, arachidonic metabolites, serotonin, histamine and nitric oxide, substances which discharge or sensitize small unmyelinated fibers conveying pain in most tissues, accumulate in proximity to trigeminovascular fibers to possibly provide the cause of headache. On the other hand, the increased cerebral blood flow and volume can be due to hypoxia but also to substances such as nitric oxide that will not only directly stimulate c-fibers but also generate vasodilation. We speculate that the increase in cerebral blood flow plus the action of peptides such as VEGF that disrupt the blood brain barrier, contribute to cerebral edema. With severe edema, brain structures are compressed leading to displacement and stretching of the pain-sensitive intracranial structures. Therefore at this stage, headache can be attributed to chemical and mechanical stimulation of a common pain pathway: the trigeminovascular system (see Figure 1).

5.   REFERENCES

1. Arregui, A., Barer, G.R., and Emson, P.C. Neurochemical studies in the hypoxic brain: substance P, met-enkephalin, GABA and angiotensin converting enzyme. *Life Sci.* 28:2925-9,1981.
2. Asano, M., Kaneoka, K., Nomura, T., Asano, K., Sone, H., Tsurumaru, K., Yamashita, K., Matsuo, K., Suzuki, H., and Okuda, Y. Increase in serum vascular endothelial growth factor levels during altitude training. *Acta Physiol Scand.* 162:455-459, 1998.
3. Bonnon, M., Noel-Jorand, MC., and Therme, P. Psychological changes during altitude hypoxia. *Aviat Space Environ Med.* 66:330-5, 1995.
4. Buck, A., Schirlo, C., Jasinsky, V., Weber, B., Burger, C., von Schulthess, G.K., Koller, E.A., and Pavlicek, V. Changes of cerebral blood flow during short-term exposure to normobaric hypoxia. *J Cereb Blood Flow Metab.*18:906-10, 1998.
5. Burtscher, M., Likar, R., Nachbauer, W., and Philadelphy, M. Aspirin for prophylaxis against headache at high altitudes: randomised, double blind, placebo controlled trial. *BMJ.* 316:1057-8, 1998.
6. Dimitriadou, V., Buzzi, M.G., Moskowitz, M.A., and Theoharides, T.C. Trigeminal sensory fiber stimulation induces morphological changes in rat dura mater mast cells. *Neuroscience.* 44:97-112, 1991.
7. Dimitriadou, V., Buzzi, M.G., Theoharides,T., and Moskowitz, M.A. Ultrastructural evidence for neurogenically mediated changes in blood vessels of the rat dura mater and tongue following antidromic trigeminal stimulation. *Neuroscience.* 48:187-203, 1992.
8. Figini, M., Emanueli, C., Grady, E.F., Kirkwood, K., Payan, D.G., Ansel, J., Gerard, C., Geppetti, P., and Bunnett, N. Substance P and bradykinin stimulate plasma protein extravasation in the mouse gastrointestinal tract and pancreas. *Am J Physiol.* 272:785-793,1997.
9. Fleisch, A., and Von Muralt, A. *Klimaphysiologische untersuchungen in der Schweiz.* Part II. 1948. Bemo Schwabe, Basel.
10. Forwand, S.A., Landowne, M., Follansbee, J.N., and Hansen, J.E. Effect of acetazolamide on acute mountain sickness. *NEJM.* 279:839-845, 1968.
11. Gotoh, K., Kikuchi, H., Kataoka, H., Nagata, I., Nozaki, K., Takahashi, J.C., and Hazama, F. Nitric oxide synthase immunoreactivity related to cold-induced brain edema. *Neurol Res.* 20:637-42, 1998.
12. Grandjean, E. Physiologie du climat de montagne. *J Physiol.* 40:1-96,1948.
13. Hackett, P.H., Yarnell, P.R., Hill, R., Reynard, K., Heit, J., and McCormick, J. High-altitude cerebral edema evaluated with magnetic resonance imaging: clinical correlation and pathophysiology *JAMA.* 280:1920-5, 1998.
14. Headache Classification Committee of the International Headache society. Classification and diagnostic criteria for headache disorders, cranial neuralgias and facial pain. *Cephalalgia.* 8 (Suppl 7), 1988.

15. Jensen, J.B., Sperling, B., Severinghaus, J.W., and Lassen, N.A. Augmented hypoxic cerebral vasodilation in men during 5 days at 3,810 m altitude. *J Appl Physiol*.4:1214-8, 1996.

16. Lundberg, J.M., Brodin, E., and Hua, X., and Saria, A. Vascular permeability changes and smooth muscle contraction in relation to capsaicin-sensitive substance P afferents in guinea pig. *Acta Physiol Scand*. 120:217-227, 1984.

17. Maggi CA. the dual function of capsaicin-sensitive sensory nerves in the bladder and urethra. *Ciba Found Symp*.151:77-83, 1990.

18. Maggiorini, M., Buhler, B., Walter, M., and Oelz, O. Prevalence of acute mountain sickness in the Swiss Alps. *BMJ*. 301:853-5, 1990.

19. Mazzone, S.B., Hinrichsen, C.F., and Geraghty, D.P. Substance P receptors in brain stem respiratory centers of the rat: regulation of NK1 receptors by hypoxia. *J Pharmacol Exp Ther*. 282:1547-56,1997.

20. Montgomery, A.B., Mills, J., and Luce, J.M. Incidence of acute mountain sickness at intermediate altitude. *JAMA*.261:732-4, 1989.

21. Nimmo, A.J., Whitaker, E.M., Castairs, J.R., and Morrison, J.F. The autoradiographic localization of calcitonin gene-related peptide and substance P receptors in human fallopian tube. *Q J Exp Physiol*. 74:955-958, 1989.

22. Noel-Jorand, M.C., and Burnet, H. Changes in human respiratory sensation induced by acute high altitude hypoxia. *Neuroreport*. 5:1561-6, 1994.

23. Noel-Jorand, M.C., Bragard, D., and Plaghki, L. Pain perception under chronic high-altitude hypoxia. *Eur J Neurosci*. 8:2075-9,1996.

24. Rapoport S. Brain edema and the blood-brain barrier. In: *Primer on cerebrovascular diseases*. Ed: Welch et al. Academic Press. 1997; 25-28.

25. Ray, B.S., and Wolff, H.G. Experimental studies on headache pain: pain sensitive structures of the head and their significance in headache. *Arch Surg*. 41:813-856,1940.

26. Roach, R.C., Greene, E.R., Schoene, R.B., and Hackett, P.H. Arterial oxygen saturation for prediction of acute mountain sickness. *Aviat Space Environ Med*.12:1182-5. 1998.

27. Rosenberg, M.E., and Pollard, A.J. Altitude-dependent changes of directional hearing in mountaineers. *Br J Sports Med*.26:161-5, 1992

28. Saria, A.L., Lundberg, J., Skofitsch, G., and Lembeck, F. Vascular leakage in various tissues induced by substance P, capsaicin, bradykinin, serotonin, histamine and antigen challenge. *Naunyn Schmiedebergs Arch Pharmacol*.324.1983

29. Schilling, L., and Wahl, M. Brain edema: pathogenesis and therapy. *Kidney Int Suppl*. 59:S69-75, 1997.

30. Strassman, A.M., Raymond, S.A., and Burstein, R. Sensitization of meningeal sensory neurons and the origin of headaches. *Nature*. 12;384:560-4, 1996

31. Wagenaar, M., Teppema, L., Berkenbosch, A., Olievier, C., and Folgering, H. Effect of low-dose acetazolamide on the ventilatory CO_2 response during hypoxia in the anaesthetized cat. *Eur Respir J*.12:1271-7, 1998.

32. Williamson, D.J., Hargreaves, R.J., Hill, R.G., and Shepheard, S.L. Intravital microscope studies on the effects of neurokinin agonists and calcitonin gene-related peptide on dural vessel diameter in the anaesthetized rat. *Cephalalgia*. 17:518-524,1997

33. Wolff, H.G. *Headache and other head pain*. New York: Oxford University Press 1972.

34. Xu, F., Severinghaus, J.W. Rat brain VEGF expression in alveolar hypoxia: possible role in high-altitude cerebral edema. *J Appl Physiol*.85:53-7, 1998.

Chapter 14

The Hypoxic Brain
Insights from Ischemia Research

Konstantin-A. Hossmann
Max-Planck-Institute for Neurological Research, Department of Experimental Neurology, Cologne, Germany

Key words: ischemia, threshold concept, penumbra, delayed neuronal death, selective vulnerability, endoplasmic reticulum, protein synthesis

Abstract: The high energy requirements compared to the low energy reserves render the brain particularly vulnerable to hypoxic conditions. To protect the brain against hypoxia, powerful cerebrovascular regulatory systems assure an increase of blood flow to compensate for the reduced arterial oxygen content. This system is so efficient that during respiratory hypoxia brain metabolism is little disturbed as long as cardiac function does not fail. Only with declining blood pressure cerebral blood flow also declines, and brain energy metabolism rapidly collapses.

Under experimental conditions, oxygen delivery to the brain is therefore more readily impaired by reducing blood flow in the first place, e.g. by occluding a supplying brain artery. With declining flow values metabolic and electrophysiological functions stepwise disappear according to the threshold concept of brain ischemia: first the most complex functions such as protein synthesis or the spontaneous electrical activity are suppressed, followed at much lower flow values by the breakdown of energy state and the depolarisation of cell membranes. The tissue supplied at a flow range between functional impairment and the suppression of vital functions has been called penumbra to characterize its potential revivability, provided oxygen supply is resumed.

Besides its immediate effects, hypoxia causes delayed functional and metabolic disturbances which may even progress to cell death. The brain regions most sensitive to this type of injury are parts of the hippocampus, the dorsolateral caudate nucleus and the reticular nucleus of thalamus. Mechanisms contributing to delayed injury include coupling disturbances

Hypoxia: Into the Next Millennium.
Edited by R. C. Roach, *et al.* Kluwer Academic/Plenum Publishing, New York, 1999.

155

between brain function and blood flow, glutamate-propagated functional disturbances such as spreading depression, free radical mediated changes, disturbances of signal transduction pathways and complex abnormalities in the genomic expression patterns leading, in the worst case, to programmed cell death. A key mechanism in this complex stress response is the disturbed calcium homoeostasis of the endoplasmic reticulum which, among others, leads to the inhibition of protein synthesis at the translational level. Modulations of these pathological interactions are a major area of current ischemia research.

1.   INTRODUCTION

The healthy brain covers its energy requirements almost exclusively by oxidative metabolism of glucose. With adequate oxygen supply, combustion of 1 mol glucose produces almost 38 mol ATP which is used in equal parts for supporting the brain's electrical activity and its vital functions. Under conditions of reduced oxygen availability, part of glucose can be metabolized anaerobically but the energy yield per mol glucose is only 2 mol ATP which is too low to maintain normal brain function even when glycolytic rate is increased. Moreover, the end-product of anaerobic glycolysis, lactate acid, accumulates in brain tissue and results in acidosis and osmotically induced brain edema. The brain is protected against this potentially adverse situation by powerful regulatory systems which compensate any reductions in arterial oxygen supply by increasing the rate of cerebral circulation (22). Under experimental conditions respiratory hypoxia down to an arterial pO_2 of 35 Torr which corresponds to an altitude of about 9000 meter reduces oxygen saturation of hemoglobin to 65% but increases blood flow by about 100%, resulting even in overcompensation of oxygen delivery to the brain. However, if heart function is impaired at low ambient oxygen pressure, cerebral blood flow precipitously declines, leading to sharp reduction of oxygen supply and oxidative glucose metabolism. From an experimental point of view, it is therefore difficult to maintain the brain in a steady state of graded hypoxia by manipulating respiratory pO_2. This is different when oxygen supply to the brain is lowered by reducing blood flow. Occlusion of a major brain artery such as the middle cerebral artery, results in a gradient of reduced flow declining steadily from the peripheral to the central parts of the vascular supplying territory. Oxygen delivery declines accordingly, and the effect of various levels of hypoxia can be studied without interference of disturbed cardiac function by correlating regional cerebral blood flow with regional functional and/or metabolic disturbances. One of the most important lessons learned from ischemia research was the finding that irrespective of its immediate effects on brain energy metabolism, hypoxia may produce delayed neuronal injury. These delayed effects are mediated by complex molecular disturbances and are presumably of similar importance for other kinds of brain hypoxia including that induced at high altitude. In the following, the immediate and late effects of ischemia will be described separately.

2. IMMEDIATE EFFECTS OF ISCHEMIA

Graded brain hypoxia as induced by cerebrovascular occlusion affects the energy consuming processes of the brain in a sequential way: first, the functional activity is impaired followed, at a more severe degree of hypoxia, by the suppression of the metabolic activity required to maintain structural integrity. As demonstrated by the German physiologists Opitz and Schneider already 50 years ago, EEG reversibly flattens as soon as the oxygen pressure of cerebrovenous blood falls to below 19 Torr but when it further declines to below 12 Torr, EEG suppression becomes irreversible and structural damage evolves.

The concept of the two thresholds of hypoxia was later refined by Symon and his coworkers (83) who used a model of acute focal ischemia in the baboon to identify the respective rates of blood flow. The experiments were carried out by combining local blood flow measurements with recordings of the EEG, sensory evoked potentials and extracellular potassium activity, respectively. By placing electrodes at different parts of the cortical territory of the occluded artery, they noted that the amplitude of evoked potentials and of spontaneous EEG activity collapsed at flow values below 0.15 ml/g/min or 30% of control whereas extracellular potassium activity remained undisturbed unless blood flow further declined below 0.10 ml/g/min or 20% of control (4). At this threshold extracellular potassium sharply rose, due to the sudden depolarization of cell membranes. In the normothermic mammalian brain, maintenance of transmembrane ion gradients is an active energy-consuming process and, therefore, a sign of cell viability. The demonstration of two flow thresholds, a higher one leading to "electrical failure" and a substantially lower one associated with "membrane failure" suggests that in the flow range between these two thresholds cerebral cortex is functionally silent but structurally intact. In focal ischemia this flow range corresponds to a coronal region intercalated between the necrotic infarct core and the normally perfused brain tissue. It has been termed "penumbra" in analogy to the partly illuminated area around the complete shadow of the moon in full eclipse to characterize its intermediate state between life and death (5).

More recent studies expanded the concept of functional thresholds to that of metabolic disturbances (29). Here again complex biochemical functions such as protein synthesis are affected at much higher flow levels than basic metabolic pathways as the energy producing metabolism. In rats, protein synthesis declines by 50% at about 0.55 ml/g/min, and it is completely suppressed below 0.35 ml/g/min. These values are clearly above the threshold of mRNA synthesis which begins to decline below 0.25 - 0.35 ml/g/min (42). At this level also changes of glucose utilization are present: in small rodents glycolysis transiently increases at a flow rate below 0.35 ml/g/min before it sharply declines below 0.25 ml/g/min (73). The upper level of glucose activation corresponds to the stimulation of anaerobic glycolysis, as reflected by the beginning acidosis and the beginning accumulation of lactate (2, 28, 46, 67, 69). At flow rates below 0.26 ml/g/min tissue acidosis becomes very pronounced (2) and both PCr and ATP begin to decline (2, 28, 46, 63, 67, 69, 73). Naritomi et al. (67) reported a slightly higher threshold for the depletion of PCr (0.18 - 0.23 ml/g/min) than that for ATP (0.13 - 0.14 ml/g/min) which is in line with the faster PCr decline under conditions of complete ischemia (44).

Anoxic depolarization has been assessed by recording extracellular potassium activity (4, 9, 23, 64) or by measuring the tissue contents of sodium and potassium (36, 76). The sodium/potassium ratio of brain tissue increases at flow values below 0.10-0.15 ml/g/min (36), and the extracellular potassium rises between 0.06 and 0.15 ml/g/min (4, 9, 23, 64). At the same threshold extracellular calcium declines due to the opening of calcium channels (23, 24). The metabolic and ionic disturbances in the periphery of focal ischemia thus proceed in the following order: initially protein synthesis is inhibited (at a threshold of about 0.55 ml/g/min), followed by the suppression of mRNA synthesis and a stimulation of anaerobic glycolysis (below 0.35 ml/g/min), the breakdown of energy state (at about 0.20 ml/g/min) and anoxic depolarization of the cell membranes (below 0.15 ml/g/min).

As far as the electrophysiological functions are concerned, the first change is the slowing of EEG activity, followed by amplitude reduction of EEG and evoked potentials. Complete suppression of EEG activity occurs between 0.15 and 0.23 ml/g/min (5, 64, 67, 77); evoked potentials disappear between 0.15 and 0.25 ml/g/min (3, 10, 64, 78) and spontaneous unit activity at a mean value of 0.18 ml/100g/min (26, 27). Neurological studies suggest that reversible hemiparalysis appears in monkeys at about 0.23 ml/g/min, followed by irreversible paralysis below 0.17-0.18 (40, 64). All these values are distinctly below the threshold of the suppression of protein synthesis and even below that of the beginning activation of anaerobic glycolysis but they fall into the range of the beginning energy crisis, indicating that functional suppression is, in the first place, the result of energy failure. This is also true for the release of neurotransmitters into the extracellular compartment, as measured by interstitial dialysis techniques. In cats and rats both inhibitory and excitatory neurotransmitters are released at about 0.2 ml/g/min with a possibly slightly higher threshold for glycine, adenosine and GABA than for glutamate (53, 58, 78, 79, 84, 85). Dopamine and serotonin release has been measured in a graded global ischemia model of rat and was found to increase transiently at flow values below 21-48% of control before it permanently increased at a flow rate below 14% (48). The release of neurotransmitters is probably unspecific because other intracellular metabolites are co-released (21, 57).

A direct consequence of the metabolic disturbances associated with focal ischemia is the rise of cell osmolality which causes a shift of water from the extra- into the intracellular compartment (60). The resulting decline in the fluid volume of the extracellular space can be detected by measurements of electrical impedance (36, 59, 76) or by diffusion-weighted NMR imaging (6, 8, 11, 28, 46, 65). Two hours after vascular occlusion the thresholds for the beginning rise of electrical impedance or the rise of signal intensity in diffusion-weighted imaging range between 0.3 and 0.4 ml/g/min (46, 59). These thresholds are distinctly higher than the threshold of brain edema - defined as the volumetric increase of water content - which is close to 0.1 ml/g/min (36). This difference explains why T_2-weighted NMR imaging which detects alterations of tissue water content, is less sensitive to ischemic changes than diffusion-weighted imaging (65).

In contrast to the biochemical and functional changes which appear shortly after vascular occlusion, histological lesions require some time before they become visible. The threshold of histological changes, therefore, depends both on the density and the duration of the flow reduction. Under conditions of permanent focal ischemia, the threshold of pan-necrosis is between 0.17 and 0.24 ml/g/min (40, 86). At flow values below 0.80 ml/g/min, i.e. far above the threshold of pan-necrosis, selective neuronal loss may occur (61). Interestingly, this loss is not threshold-dependent: the flow rate correlates linearly with the number of surviving neurons which suggests a coupled decrease in parallel to the reduced metabolic requirements of the tissue. This interpretation is in line with the hypothesis that the peri-infarct brain tissue suffers pathological changes which are not necessarily caused by a critical reduction of blood flow (see below).

Obviously, brain tissue viability is immediately endangered when blood flow declines below the threshold of energy depletion. The duration of energy depletion the brain is able to survive (survival time), has been a matter of controversy and depends not only on the severity of ischemia but also on the quality of post-ischemic reperfusion (30). Under clinical conditions global energy failure as induced by cardiac arrest is tolerated only for a few minutes because conventional cardiac resuscitation methods are complicated by a no-reflow phenomenon. However, recovery of brain function was observed after up to 1 h normothermic circulatory arrest when post-ischemic blood recirculation was carefully controlled (35). A further prolongation of the brain revival time can be achieved by pre-ischemic protective interventions such as deep hypothermia (87) but these interventions are of clinical relevance only for induced cerebrocirculatory arrest as for aneurysma surgery. If blood flow remains above the threshold of energy depletion, i.e. in the penumbra range, cellular viability is initially preserved. The original concept of the ischemic penumbra predicted that this state could be survived indefinitely (5) but later findings revealed that metabolic disturbances progress, leading to neuronal death within a few hours (51). Similarly, tissue that has been successfully reperfused after severe ischemia, may undergo delayed neuronal injury despite the initial restoration of energy state (43). These observations have led to the concept that ischemia may initiate molecular disturbances which „maturate" despite the reversal of the initial hemodynamic/metabolic injury and which lead to delayed neuronal death by other mechanisms than energy failure (45). In the following, some of the putative mechanisms of this type of injury will be discussed.

3.   LATE EFFECTS OF CEREBRAL ISCHEMIA

3.1   Late injury in the ischemic penumbra

In the peripheral parts of the supplying territory of an acutely occluded brain vessel, blood flow may be reduced to a flow range which is above the threshold of energy failure but below the threshold of other functional or metabolic disturbances, notably the suppression of protein synthesis. This penumbral region can be visualized by multiparametric imaging and has been submitted to pixel analysis for the evaluation of the dynamics of metabolic thresholds. Such measurements revealed that with ongoing ischemia time, the threshold of ATP depletion but not that of inhibition of protein synthesis steadily rises, leading to the gradual expansion of the infarct core into the peri-infarct penumbra (63). The volume expansion can be followed by diffusion-weighted MR imaging because the signal intensity of this imaging mode reflects the cellular uptake of fluid from the extracellular compartment after anoxic depolarization of cell membranes (34). According to these studies, infarct core reaches its largest expansion within about 6 hours after vascular occlusion, indicating that during this interval penumbral injury becomes irreversible (28). Various mechanisms have been proposed to explain this adverse transformation. The most widely cited mechanism is the calcium/excitotoxicity hypothesis of neuronal injury (14). According to this hypothesis the release from ischemic neurons of the excitatory neurotransmitter glutamate opens glutamate-operated calcium channels, resulting in cytosolic calcium flooding. This process is further enhanced by depletion of intracellular calcium stores via signaling pathways initiated by the activation of metabotropic glutamate receptors, and by the opening of voltage operated calcium channels subsequent to glutamate-mediated depolarization of cell membranes (12). Cytosolic calcium flooding, in turn, evokes multiple adverse cellular reactions which are thought to lead to gradual deterioration of cellular viability (50). Although the toxicity of glutamate-mediated effects has been amply documented in cell cultures, its relevance for ischemic injury *in vivo* has been questioned (31). Glutamate rises to high levels in the infarct core (where the tissue necroses due to energy failure) but not in the penumbra where excitotoxic mechanisms are thought to prevail (70). Even if a critical threshold of glutamate would be reached, the calcium-conducting NMDA receptor-operated ion channel does not open because penumbral neurons - by definition - do not suffer cell depolarization. This, however, is a requirement to release the magnesium block from this channel (39). Further, the penumbral activation of anaerobic glycolysis causes tissue acidosis which is known to alleviate glutamate toxicity *in vitro* (41). Other arguments against glutamate toxicity are the different effect of ischemia and glutamate exposure on protein synthesis (16), the simultaneous release from ischemic neurons of inhibitory neurotransmitters (78) and the different dynamics of neuronal injury. In fact, glutamate-induced cell death maturates over 24 h (13) whereas the penumbra rarely survives more than 6 hours (28). On the other hand, a strong argument for glutamate-mediated cell injury is the dramatic reduction by glutamate antagonists of infarct volume (74). However, this effect is not necessarily related to the alleviation of glutamate neurotoxicity. In fact, glutamate is involved in the propagation of spreading depression-like depolarizations which are evoked by the ischemic release of intracellular potassium (33). These depolarizations pose substantial metabolic stress on the hypoperfused penumbra, leading to the fatal aggravation of the mismatch between oxygen supply and oxygen needs of the tissue (7). Suppression of the propagation of spreading depressions by glutamate antagonists alleviates this additional workload and, therefore, provides a plausible explanation for the observed protective effect (62). Another molecular mechanism of penumbral injury which has received considerable attention over the past years, is programmed cell death or apoptosis (55). Strong arguments in favor of apoptosis are the expression of various apoptosis-associated genes such as p53, bax, c-myc or gadd45 (52, 66), the demonstration of DNA fragments of characteristic length („DNA laddering") (54) or the reduction of infarct volume by drugs that inhibit the activity of the „executioner" of apoptosis, caspase 3 (20). On the other hand, imaging of DNA fragmentation by TUNEL revealed appearance of such changes only in the infarct core following ATP depletion but not in the penumbra where they would be expected to occur if they contribute to infarct expansion. The role of apoptosis for infarct expansion is, therefore, less obvious than widely assumed.

3.2   Late injury after transient ischemia

Reperfusion of brain tissue after transient ischemia results in rapid restoration of energy metabolism, provided the survival time of the tissue has not elapsed (see above). However, despite this initial metabolic recovery a delayed type of injury may evolve depending on the kind of ischemia and the anatomical site of injury. Following *transient focal ischemia*, full restoration of energy state is possible after vascular occlusion of one hour or longer (Hata et al., in preparation) but with ongoing recirculation time, a secondary energy depletion may occur, starting in the central part of the previously ischemic territory and gradually expanding to the volume of the initial injury. The delay of this secondary injury depends on the duration of the initial ischemia. After 30 min MCA occlusion, development of secondary infarction may take as long as 2 weeks (18); after 1 h MCA occlusion, this latency declines to 1 day, and after 2 h occlusion to 6 hours (Hata et al., in preparation). Also for this type of delayed neuronal injury, various molecular mechanisms have been proposed most of which have been inferred from the effects of pharmacological interventions. Particular attention has been addressed to free radical mediated peroxidative alterations of phospholipid membranes. At the plasma membrane these changes result in the release of biologically active fatty acids, such as arachidonic acid, which in turn leads to multiple adverse tissue reactions (1). At the mitochondrial membrane the opening of a permeability transition pore causes delayed cell death either by stimulating pro-apoptitic genomic responses or by impairing mitochondrial oxidative phosphorylation (80). In a recent study from our laboratory, evidence was provided that both DNA fragmentation and the manifestation of secondary energy depletion were preceded by severe inhibition of protein synthesis. Since similar disturbances precede also other types of delayed ischemic cell death, a causal role should be considered (see below).After *transient global ischemia*, as induced by cardiac arrest, the dominating pathophysiology is delayed neuronal death in the selectively vulnerable areas (75). Although brain energy metabolism may recover after complete cerebrocirculatory arrest of as long as one hour, delayed neuronal death occurs in anatomically defined brain regions after brief ischemia times of 5-10 min (43). These selectively vulnerable areas include the CA1 sector of hippocampus, the dorsolateral part of striate nucleus, the reticular nucleus of thalamus, layers 2 and 5 of paramedian cortex and the cerebellar Purkinje cells. Similar to transient focal ischemia, this type of injury is manifested the later, the shorter the duration of the initial ischemia (maturation phenomenon, (38)), and it is also preceded by persisting inhibition of protein synthesis (88). The mechanisms of cell damage are therefore probably similar to those observed after transient focal ischemia, however with the important difference that in the selectively vulnerable areas the ischemia time required for the initiation of injury is much shorter. Therapeutic interventions suggest that multiple pathophysiological pathways may contribute to selective vulnerability. Mild hypothermia, free radical scavengers, glutamate antagonists, calcium blockers, inhibition of apoptosis-promoting pathways, inhibition of corticosteroid receptors - to name only a few - are all effective in reducing cell injury under threshold conditions, i.e. after brief periods of circulatory arrest (19). However, the efficacy of the intervention declines when ischemia time is prolonged, suggesting that the affected pathways are modulators rather than initiators of delayed neuronal death. In this context the pathophysiological role of post-ischemic disturbance of the coupling between brain function and blood flow should be recalled. This disturbance leads to post-ischemic hypoperfusion and may cause delayed hypoxic episodes in regions with increased functional and/or metabolic activity (30). In hippocampal subfield CA1 the vascular resistance of the supplying arteries is higher (81) and the number of capillaries is smaller (37) than in the more resistant parts of the brain. Since hippocampal functional activity increases after recovery from global ischemia (82) this mismatch may contribute to the observed delayed injury in this region.

4. IMPLICATIONS OF BRAIN ISCHEMIA RESEARCH FOR HIGH ALTITUDE HYPOXIA

One of the main differences between ischemic hypoxia and high altitude induced hypoxia is the fact that ischemia - but not high altitude - impairs clearance of metabolic waste products from the brain. This results in differences of tissue pCO_2, tissue lactate, extracellular concentrations of neurotransmitters and many other flow-dependent variables. However, hypoxia of any origin produces a stereotyped metabolic disturbance preceding anoxic cell death, i.e. an inhibition of global protein synthesis (32). Morphological and biochemical studies revealed that the inhibition is caused by selective impairment of polypeptide chain initiation whereas the elongation and termination steps remain undisturbed (49). Obviously, sustained reduction of protein synthesis deprives cells of enzymes or trophic factors essential for their survival but there may be also more immediate effects such as the disinhibition of feedback controlled mRNA synthesis, leading to the superinduction of short-lived gene products (47).The activity of polypeptide chain initiation factors responsible for the control of protein synthesis is regulated by the endoplasmic reticulum (17). A decline of endoplasmic reticulum calcium activity stimulates protein kinase R (PKR) which, in turn, inactivates polypeptide chain initiation by phosphorylating the eukaryotic initiation factor eIF2α (15). Paschen (71) hypothesized that it is the decrease of calcium in the endoplasmic reticulum rather than the increase of calcium in the cytosol that accounts for the cellular stress response observed under ischemic and post-ischemic conditions. An important mechanism for calcium mobilization from endoplasmic reticulum is the phosphoinosite signaling pathway (89). Another mechanism could be denaturation and/or misfolding of proteins which leads to the expression of molecular chaperones such as heat stress protein hsp72 (56). The comparison of hsp expression with the inhibition of protein synthesis revealed a remarkable coincidence in neurons destined to die, irrespective of the underlying ischemic condition: in the peri-infarct penumbra during permanent focal ischemia (25), in the central parts of the ischemic territory after transient focal ischemia (Hata, in preparation) or in the selectively vulnerable neurons after global ischemia (68). Under various cellular stress conditions both, expression of hsp72 and the inhibition of protein synthesis, are mediated by hsp40, a regulatory protein associated with endoplasmic reticular dysfunction. Since hsp40 mRNA markedly rises after ischemia (72) these findings further add to the hypothesis that delayed ischemic cell death is caused by dysfunction of the endoplasmic reticulum. Obviously, these molecular changes are of relevance to high altitude hypoxia only under the condition that the reduced arterial oxygen partial pressure is not compensated by an increase of cerebral blood flow. However, the combination of low oxygen pressure with cardiac or cerebrovascular insufficiency will result in a pathophysiological situation that is very similar to the ischemia experiments described in this article. Similarly, neuroprotective interventions that succeeded in ameliorating ischemic injury may also improve cerebral dysfunction at high altitude. Experimental investigations into this interesting field of research are, therefore, strongly recommended.

REFERENCES

1. Abe K, Yoshidomi M , Kogure K. Arachidonic acid metabolism in ischemic neuronal damage. *Ann NY Acad Sci* 559:259-268, 1989.
2. Allen KL, Busza AL, Proctor E, King MD, Williams SR, Crockard HA , Gadian DG. Controllable graded cerebral ischaemia in the gerbil - Studies of cerebral blood flow and energy metabolism by hydrogen clearance and ^{31}P NMR spectroscopy. *NMR Biomed* 6:181-186, 1993.
3. Astrup J, Symon L, Branston NM , Lassen NA. Cortical evoked potential and extracellular K^+ and H^+ at critical levels of brain ischemia. *Stroke* 8:51-57, 1977.
4. Astrup J, Symon L, Branston NM , Lassen NA. Cortical evoked potential and extracellular K^+ and H^+ at critical levels of brain ischemia. *Stroke* 8:51-57, 1977.
5. Astrup J, Symon L , Siesjö BK. Thresholds in cerebral ischemia - The ischemic penumbra. *Stroke* 12:723-725, 1981.
6. Back T, Hoehn-Berlage M, Kohno K , Hossmann K-A. Diffusion nuclear magnetic resonance imaging in experimental stroke. Correlation with cerebral metabolites. *Stroke* 25:494-500, 1994.
7. Back T, Kohno K , Hossmann K-A. Cortical negative DC deflections following middle cerebral artery occlusion and KCl-induced spreading depression - Effect on blood flow, tissue oxygenation, and electroencephalogram. *J Cereb Blood Flow Metab* 14:12-19, 1994.
8. Benveniste H, Hedlund LW , Johnson GA. Mechanism of detection of acute cerebral ischemia in rats by diffusion-weighted magnetic-resonance microscopy. *Stroke* 23:746-754, 1992.
9. Branston NM, Strong AJ , Symon L. Extracellular potassium activity, evoked potential and tissue blood flow. Relationships during progressive ischaemia in baboon cerebral cortex. *J Neurol Sci* 32:305-321, 1977.
10. Branston NM, Symon L, Crockard HA , Pasztor E. Relationship between the cortical evoked potential and local cortical blood flow following acute middle cerebral artery occlusion in the baboon. *Exp Neurol* 45:195-208, 1974.
11. Busza AL, Allen KL, King MD, van den Bruggen N, Williams SR , Gadian DG. Can diffusion-weighted magnetic-resonance-imaging detect critical cerebral blood-flow thresholds and energy failure during cerebral-ischemia? *Eur J Neurosci* 1992:242, 1992.
12. Choi DW. *Glutamate receptors and the induction of excitotoxic neuronal death*, Elsevier Science Publ B V, Amsterdam, 1994.
13. Choi DW. Glutamate neurotoxicity in cortical cell culture is calcium dependent. *Neurosci Lett* 58:293-297, 1985.
14. Choi DW , Rothman SM. The role of glutamate neurotoxicity in hypoxic-ischemic neuronal death. *Annu. Rev. Neurosci.* 13:171-182, 1990.
15. Degracia DJ, Neumar RW, White BC , Krause GS. Global brain ischemia and reperfusion: Modifications in eukaryotic initiation factors associated with inhibition of translation initiation. *J Neurochem* 67:2005-2012, 1996.
16. Djuricic B, Röhn G, Paschen W , Hossmann K-A. Protein synthesis in the hippocampal slice: Transient inhibition by glutamate and lasting inhibition by ischemia. *Metab Brain Dis* 9:235-247, 1994.
17. Doutheil J, Gissel C, Oschlies U, Hossmann K-A , Paschen W. Relation of neuronal endoplasmic reticulum calcium homeostasis to ribosomal aggregation and protein synthesis - implications for stress-induced suppression of protein synthesis. *Brain Res* 775:43-51, 1997.

18. Du C, Hu R, Csernansky CA, Hsu CY , Choi DW. Very delayed infarction after mild focal cerebral ischemia: A role for apoptosis? *J Cereb Blood Flow Metab* 16:195-201, 1996.

19. Ferger D , Krieglstein J. Cerebral ischemia: Pharmacological bases of drug therapy. *Dementia* 7:161-168, 1996.

20. Fink K, Zhu J, Namura S, Shimizu-Sasamata M, Endres M, Ma J, Dalkara T, Yuan J , Moskowitz MA. Prolonged therapeutic window for ischemic brain damage caused by delayed caspase activation. *J Cereb Blood Flow Metab* 18:1071-1076, 1998.

21. Hagberg H, Andersson P, Lacarewicz J, Jacobson I, Butcher S , Sandberg M. Extracellular adenosine, inosine, hypoxanthine, and xanthine in relation to tissue nucleotides and purines in rat striatum during transient ischemia. *J Neurochem* 49:227-231, 1987.

22. Harper AM. Regulation of cerebral circulation. Sci Basis Med Ann Rev 60-81, 1969.

23. Harris RJ , Symon L. Extracellular pH, potassium, and calcium activities in progressive ischaemia of rat cortex. *J Cereb Blood Flow Metab* 4:178-186, 1984.

24. Harris RJ, Symon L, Branston NM , Bayhan M. Changes in extracellular calcium activity in cerebral ischaemia. *J Cereb Blood Flow Metab* 1:203-209, 1981.

25. Hata R, Mies G, Wiessner C , Hossmann KA. Differential expression of c-fos and hsp72 mRNA in focal cerebral ischemia of mice. *Neuroreport* 9:27-32, 1998.

26. Heiss W-D, Hayakawa T , Waltz AG. Cortical neuronal function during ischemia. Effects of occlusion of one middle cerebral artery on single-unit activity in cats. *Arch Neurol* 33:813-820, 1976.

27. Heiss W-D , Rosner G. Functional recovery of cortical neurons as related to degree and duration of ischemia. *Ann Neurol* 14:294-301, 1983.

28. Hoehn-Berlage M, Norris DG, Kohno K, Mies G, Leibfritz D , Hossmann K-A. Evolution of regional changes in apparent diffusion coefficient during focal ischemia of rat brain: The relationship of quantitative diffusion NMR imaging to reduction in cerebral blood flow and metabolic disturbances. *J Cereb Blood Flow Metab* 15:1002-1011, 1995.

29. Hossmann K-A. Viability thresholds and the penumbra of focal ischemia. *Ann Neurol* 36:557-565, 1994.

30. Hossmann K-A. Reperfusion of the brain after global ischemia - hemodynamic disturbances. *Shock* 8:95-101, 1997.

31. Hossmann K-A. Glutamate-mediated injury in focal cerebral ischemia - The excitotoxin hypothesis revised. *Brain Pathol* 4:23-36, 1994.

32. Hossmann K-A. Disturbances of cerebral protein synthesis and ischemic cell death. Progr. Brain Res. 96:161-177, 1993.

33. Hossmann K-A. Periinfarct depolarizations. *Cerebrovasc Brain Metab Rev* 8:195-208, 1996.

34. Hossmann K-A , Hoehn-Berlage M. Diffusion and perfusion MR imaging of cerebral ischemia. *Cerebrovasc Brain Metab Rev* 7:187-217, 1995.

35. Hossmann K-A, Schmidt-Kastner R , Grosse Ophoff B. Recovery of integrative central nervous function after one hour global cerebro- circulatory arrest in normothermic cat. *J Neurology Sci*. 77:305-320, 1987.

36. Hossmann K-A , Schuier FJ. Experimental brain infarcts in cats. I. Pathophysiological observations. *Stroke* 11:583-592, 1980.

37. Imdahl A , Hossmann K-A. Morphometric evaluation of post-ischemic capillary perfusion in selectively vulnerable areas of gerbil brain. *Acta Neuropathol* 69:267-271, 1986.

38. Ito U, Kirino T, Kuroiwa T , Klatzo I. *Maturation phenomenon in cerebral ischemia*, Springer, Berlin, 1992.

39. Johnson JW , Ascher P. Voltage-dependent block by intracellular Mg^{2+} of N-methyl-D-aspartate-activated channels. *Biophys J* 57:1085-1090, 1990.

40. Jones TH, Morawetz RB, Crowell RM, Marcoux FW, FitzGibbon SJ, DeGirolami U , Ojemann RG. Thresholds of focal cerebral ischemia in awake monkeys. *J Neurosurg* 54:773-782, 1981.
41. Kaku DA, Giffard RG , Choi DW. Neuroprotective effects of glutamate antagonists and extracellular acidity. *Science* 260:1516-1518, 1993.
42. Kamiya T, Jacewicz M, Pulsinelli WA , Nowak TSJ. CBF thresholds for mRNA and protein synthesis after focal ischemia and the effect of MK-801. *J Cereb Blood Flow Metab* 15, Supplement 1:1, 1995.
43. Kirino T. Delayed neuronal death in the gerbil hippocampus following ischemia. *Brain Res* 239:57-69, 1982.
44. Kloiber O, Miyazawa T, Hoehn-Berlage M , Hossmann K-A. Simultaneous ^{31}P NMR-spectroscopy and laser-Doppler flowmetry of rat brain during global-ischemia and reperfusion. *NMR Biomed* 6:144-152, 1993.
45. Kogure K, Hossmann K-A, Siesjö BK , Welsh FA. *Molecular mechanisms of ischemic brain damage*, Elsevier, Amsterdam, 1985.
46. Kohno K, Hoehn-Berlage M, Mies G, Back T , Hossmann K-A. Relationship between diffusion-weighted magnetic resonance MR images, cerebral blood flow and energy state in experimental brain infarction. *Magn Reson Imaging* 13:73-80, 1995.
47. Koistinaho J , Hokfelt T. Altered gene expression in brain ischemia (review). *Neuroreport* 8:R:1-R 8, 1997.
48. Kondoh T, Korosue K, Lee SH, Heros RC , Low WC. Evaluation of monoaminergic neurotransmitters in the rat striatum during varied global cerebral ischemia. *Neurosurgery* 35:278-285, 1994.
49. Krause GS , Tiffany BR. Suppression of protein synthesis in the reperfused brain. *Stroke* 24:747-755, 1993.
50. Kristian T , Siesjö BK. Calcium-related damage in ischemia. Life Sci 59:357-367, 1996.
51. Lassen NA, Fieschi C, Lenzi GL. Ischemic penumbra and neuronal death: comments on the therapeutic window in acute stroke with particular reference to thrombolytic therapy. *Cerebrovasc Dis* 1,Suppl.1:32-35, 1991.
52. Li Y, Chopp M, Powers C , Jiang N. Apoptosis and protein expression after focal cerebral ischemia in rat. *Brain Res* 765:301-312, 1997.
53. Mackay KB, Galbraith S, Patel TR , McCulloch J. Kappa receptor agonist (Ci-977) inhibits glutamate release in the focal ischaemic penumbra. *J Cereb Blood Flow Metab* 15, Suppl. 1:143, 1995.
54. MacManus JP, Hill IE, Huang ZG, Rasquinha I, Xue D , Buchan AM. DNA damage consistent with apoptosis in transient focal ischaemic neocortex. *NeuroReport* 5:493-496, 1994.
55. MacManus JP , Linnik MD. Gene expression induced by cerebral ischemia - an apoptotic perspective (review). *J Cereb Blood Flow Metab* 17:815-832, 1997.
56. Massa SM, Swanson RA , Sharp FR. The stress gene response in brain. *Cerebrovasc Brain Metab Rev* 8:95-158, 1996.
57. Matsumoto K, Graf R, Rosner G, Shimada N , Heiss W-D. Flow thresholds for extracellular purine catabolite elevation in cat focal ischemia. *Brain Res* 579:309-314, 1992.
58. Matsumoto K, Graf R, Rosner G, Taguchi J , Heiss W-D. Elevation of neuroactive substances in the cortex of cats during prolonged focal ischemia. *J Cereb Blood Flow Metab* 13:586-594, 1993.
59. Matsuoka Y , Hossmann K-A. Cortical impedance and extracellular volume changes following middle cerebral artery occlusion in cats. *J Cereb Blood Flow Metab* 2:466-474, 1982.

60. Matsuoka Y , Hossmann K-A. Brain tissue osmolality after middle cerebral artery occlusion in cats. *Exp Neurol* 77:599-611, 1982.

61. Mies G, Auer LM, Ebhardt G, Traupe H , Heiss W-D. Flow and neuronal density in tissue surrounding chronic infarction. *Stroke* 14:22-27, 1983.

62. Mies G, Iijima T , Hossmann K-A. Correlation between periinfarct dc shifts and ischemic neuronal damage in rat. *NeuroReport* 4:709-711, 1993.

63. Mies G, Ishimaru S, Xie Y, Seo K , Hossmann K-A. Ischemic thresholds of cerebral protein synthesis and energy state following middle cerebral artery occlusion in rat. *J Cereb Blood Flow Metab* 11:753-761, 1991.

64. Morawetz RB, Crowell RH, DeGirolami U, Marcoux FW, Jones TH , Halsey JH. Regional cerebral blood flow thresholds during cerebral ischemia. Fed Proc 38:2493-2494, 1979.

65. Moseley ME, Cohen Y, Mintorovitch J, Chileuitt L, Shimizu H, Kucharczyk J, Wendland MF , Weinstein PR. Early detection of regional cerebral ischemia in cats: comparison of diffusion- and T2-weighted MRI and spectroscopy. *Magn Reson Med* 14:330-346, 1990.

66. Nakagomi T, Asai A, Kanemitsu H, Narita K, Kuchino Y, Tamura A , Kirino T. Up-regulation of c-myc gene expression following focal ischemia in the rat brain. *Neurol Res* 18:559-563, 1996.

67. Naritomi H, Sasaki M, Kanashiro M, Kitani M , Sawada T. Flow thresholds for cerebral energy disturbance and Na^+ pump failure as studied by in vivo ^{31}P and ^{23}Na nuclear magnetic resonance spectroscopy. *J Cereb Blood Flow Metab* 8:16-23, 1988.

68. Nowak TS, Zhou Q, Valentine WJ, Harrub JB , Abe H. Regulation of heat shock genes by ischemia. *Stress Proteins* 136:173-199, 1999.

69. Obrenovitch TP, Garofalo O, Harris RJ, Bordi L, Ono M, Momma F, Bachelard HS , Syomon L. Brain tissue concentrations of ATP, phosphocreatine, lactate, and tissue pH in relation to reduced cerebral blood flow following experimental acute middle cerebral artery occlusion. *J Cereb Blood Flow Metab* 8:866-874, 1988.

70. Obrenovitch TP, Urenjak J, Richards DA, Ueda Y, Curzon G , Symon L. Extracellular neuroactive amino-acids in the rat striatum during ischemia - comparison between penumbral conditions and ischemia with sustained anoxic depolarization. *J Neurochem* 61:178-186, 1993.

71. Paschen W. Disturbances of calcium homeostasis within the endoplasmic reticulum may contribute to the development of ischemic cell damage. Med Hypotheses 47:283-288, 1996.

72. Paschen W, Linden T , Doutheil J. Effects of transient cerebral ischemia on hsp40 mRNA levels in rat brain. *Mol Brain Res* 55:341-344, 1998.

73. Paschen W, Mies G , Hossman K-A. Threshold relationship between cerebral blood-flow, glucose-utilization, and energy metabolites during development of stroke in gerbils. *Exp Neurol* 117:325-333, 1992.

74. Prass K , Dirnagl U. Glutamate antagonists in therapy of stroke (review). *Restorative Neurology & Neuroscience* 13:3-10, 1998.

75. Pulsinelli WA, Brierley JB , Plum F. Temporal profile of neuronal damage in a model of transient forebrain ischemia. *Ann Neurol* 11:491-498, 1982.

76. Schuier FJ , Hossmann K-A. Experimental brain infarcts in cats. II. Ischemic brain edema. *Stroke* 11:593-601, 1980.

77. Sharbrough FW, Messick JM , Sundt TM. Correlation of continuous electroencephalograms with cerebral blood flow measurements during carotid endarterectomy. *Stroke* 4:674-683, 1973.

78. Shimada N, Graf R, Rosner G , Heiss W-D. Differences in ischemia-induced accumulation of amino acids in the cat cortex. *Stroke* 21:1445-1451, 1990.

79. Shimada N, Graf R, Rosner G, Wakayama A, George CP , Heiss W-D. Ischemic flow threshold for extracellular glutamate increase in cat cortex. *J Cereb Blood Flow Metab* 9:603-606, 1989.

80. Siesjö BK , Siesjö P. Mechanisms of secondary brain injury. Europ. J. of Anaesthesiol. 13:247-268, 1996.

81. Spielmeyer W. Zur Pathogenese örtlich elektiver Gehirnveränderungen. *Z. ges. Neurol. und Psych.* 99:756-776, 1925.

82. Suzuki R, Yamaguchi T, Li C-L , Klatzo I. The effects of 5-minute ischemia in mongolian gerbils: II. Changes of spontaneous neuronal activity in cerebral cortex and CA1 sector of hippocampus. *Acta Neuropathol* 60:217-222, 1984.

83. Symon L, Branston NM, Strong AJ , Hope TD. The concepts of thresholds of ischaemia in relation to brain structure and function. *J Clin Path* 30, Suppl.11:149-154, 1977.

84. Takagi K, Ginsberg MD, Globus MYT, Dietrich WD, Martinez E, Kraydieh S , Busto R. Changes in amino acid neurotransmitters and cerebral blood flow in the ischemic penumbral region following middle cerebral artery occlusion in the rat - correlation with histopathology. *J Cereb Blood Flow Metab* 13:575-585, 1993.

85. Takagi K, Ginsberg MD, Globus MYT, Martinez E , Busto R. Effect of hyperthermia on glutamate release in ischemic penumbra after middle cerebral artery occlusion in rats. *American Journal of Physiology - Heart and Circulatory Physiology* 36:H1770-H1776, 1994.

86. Tamura A, Graham DI, McCulloch J , Teasdale GM. Focal cerebral ischaemia in the rat: 2. Regional cerebral blood flow determined by (^{14}C)iodoantipyrine autoradiography following middle cerebral artery occlusion. *J Cereb Blood Flow Metab* 1:61-69, 1981.

87. White RJ, Austin PE, Austin JC, Taslitz N , Takoaka Y. Recovery of the subhuman primate after deep cerebral hypothermia and prolonged ischaemia. *Resuscitation* 2:117-122, 1973.

88. Widmann R, Kuroiwa T, Bonnekoh P , Hossmann K-A. (14C)leucine incorporation into brain proteins in gerbils after transient ischemia: relationship to selective vulnerability of hippocampus. *J Neurochem* 56:789-796, 1991.

89. Zhang SX, Zhang JP, Fletcher DL, Zoeller RT , Sun GY. In situ hybridization of mRNA expression for IP3 receptor and IP3-3-kinase in rat brain after transient focal cerebral ischemia. *Mol Brain Res* 32:252-260, 1995.

Chapter 15

Food for Thought: Altitude versus Normal Brain Function

Marcus E. Raichle

Washington University School of Medicine, 4525 Scott Avenue, St Louis, Missouri 63110, USA

Key words: brain blood flow, brain metabolism, brain imaging, cognition

Abstract: This paper presents a general overview of the implementation of cognitive skills in the normal human brain as viewed from a modern functional brain imaging perspective. It is hoped that information of this type will assist eventually in developing a more informed neurobiological basis for the understanding of the cognitive impairments that occur all too frequently during sojourns to extreme altitude.

1.   INTRODUCTION

Popular as well as scientific accounts of human cognitive function at extreme altitude have repeatedly documented decrements in performance. In recent years data have accumulated suggesting that permanent residual cognitive deficits can accrue also (15). At the moment our understanding of the pathophysiology of both the transient and permanent deficits is meager.

On the other hand, our understanding of the relationship between normal brain function and metabolism is rapidly growing as the result of a revolution in functional brain imaging with positron emission tomography (PET) and functional magnetic resonance imaging (fMRI). These tools combined with the developing of the field of cognitive neuroscience, in which they are extensively used, could eventually provide a rational basis for studying the neurobiology of hypoxia-induced cognitive deficits.

Over the past 10 years the field of cognitive neuroscience has emerged as a very important growth area in neuroscience. Cognitive neuroscience

Hypoxia: Into the Next Millennium,
Edited by R. C. Roach, *et al.* Kluwer Academic/Plenum Publishing, New York, 1999.

combines the experimental strategies of cognitive psychology with various techniques to actually examine how brain function supports mental activities. Leading this research in normal humans are the new techniques of functional brain imaging: PET and MRI along with event related potentials (ERP's) obtained from electroencephalography (EEG) or magneto-encephalography (MEG).

Emerging from work in cognitive neuroscience is a new appreciation of the complex, distributed nature of brain areas involved in such activities as language, attention and memory. In addition, our concept of the metabolic and circulatory activities supporting such functions is being rapidly revised to include an important role for aerobic glycolysis in astrocytes and an intimate metabolic "working" relationship between astrocytes, neurons and blood vessels (27). Understanding how hypoxia, sleep deprivation, fatigue and inadequate nutrition can upset such relationships is the challenge facing those interested in understanding better cognitive performance deficits during and after a sojourn to extreme altitude.

This chapter reviews how functional brain imaging with PET and MRI is used in cognitive neuroscience to understand human brain function. The strategies presently employed in normal subjects at sea level are applicable to the study of human cognition under the stress of hypoxia. To date no such studies have been performed. In addition, this chapter also reviews new knowledge about the relationship between brain metabolism and blood flow and brain function.

2.   FUNCTIONAL IMAGING IN COGNITIVE NEUROSCIENCE

The signal used in functional brain imaging to measure brain function is based on the fact that changes in the cellular activity of the brain of normal, awake humans and unanesthetized laboratory animals are invariably accompanied by changes in local blood flow (for a review see (28)). Soon after its introduction in the early 1970's, it was realized that highly accurate measurements of brain blood flow could be measured in humans with PET (14, 30). While brain function could be assessed with either measurements of blood flow or metabolism (28), blood flow became the favored technique because it could be measured quickly (<1 min) using an easily produced radiopharmaceutical ($H_2^{15}O$) with a short half life (123 sec) which allowed many repeat measurements in the same subject.

The study of human cognition with PET was aided greatly by the involvement of cognitive psychologists in the 1980's whose experimental designs for dissecting human behaviors using information-processing theory fit extremely well with the emerging functional brain imaging strategies (25). It may well have been the combination of cognitive science and systems neuroscience with brain imaging that lifted this work from a state of indifference and obscurity in the neuroscience community in the 1970's to its current role of prominence in cognitive neuroscience.

As a result of collaboration among neuroscientists, imaging scientists and cognitive psychologists, a distinct behavioral strategy for the functional mapping of neuronal activity emerged. This strategy was based on a concept introduced by the Dutch physiologist Franciscus C. Donders in 1868 (reprinted in (9)). Donders proposed a general method to measure thought processes based on a simple logic. He subtracted the time needed to respond to a light (say, by pressing a key) from the time needed to respond to a particular color of light. He found that discriminating color required about 50 msec. In this way, Donders isolated and measured a mental process for the first time by subtracting a control state (i.e., responding to a light) from a task state (i.e., discriminating the color of the light). An example of the manner in which this strategy has been adopted for functional imaging is illustrated in Figure 1.

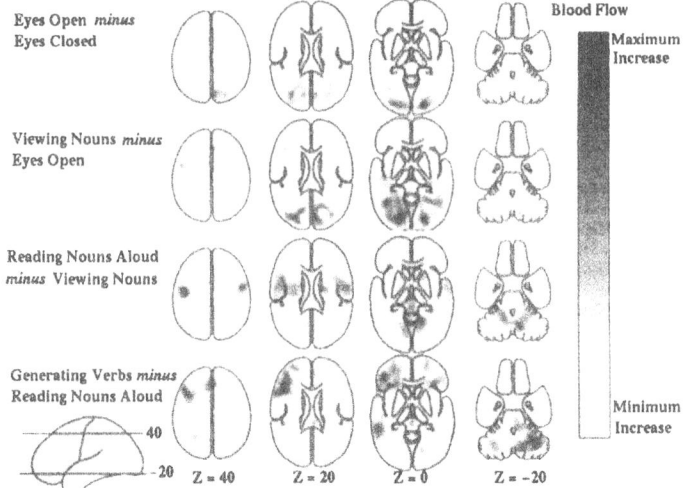

Figure 1. Four different hierarchically organized conditions are represented in these mean blood flow difference images obtained with PET. All of the changes shown in these images represent increases over the control state for each task. A group of normal subjects performed these tasks involving common English nouns (23, 24, 29) to demonstrate the spatially distributed nature of the processing by task elements going on in the normal human brain during a simple language task. Task complexity was increased from simply opening the eyes (row 1) through passive viewing of nouns on a television monitor (row 2); reading aloud the nouns as they appear on the screen (row 3); and saying aloud an appropriate verb for each noun as it appeared on the screen (row 4). These horizontal images are oriented with the front of the brain on top and the left side to the reader's left. The markings "Z = 40" indicate millimeters above and below a horizontal plane through the brain marked "Z = 0".

One criticism of this approach has been that the time necessary to press a key after a decision to do so has been made is affected by the nature of the decision process itself. By implication, the nature of the processes underlying key press, in this example, may have been altered. Although this issue (known in cognitive science jargon as the assumption of pure insertion) has been the subject of continuing discussion in cognitive psychology, it finds its resolution in functional brain imaging, where changes in any process are directly signaled by changes in observable brain states. Events occurring in the brain are not hidden from the investigator as in the purely cognitive experiments. Careful analysis of the changes in the functional images reveals whether processes (e.g., specific cognitive decisions) can be added or removed without affecting ongoing processes (e.g., motor processes). Processing areas of the brain that become inactive during the

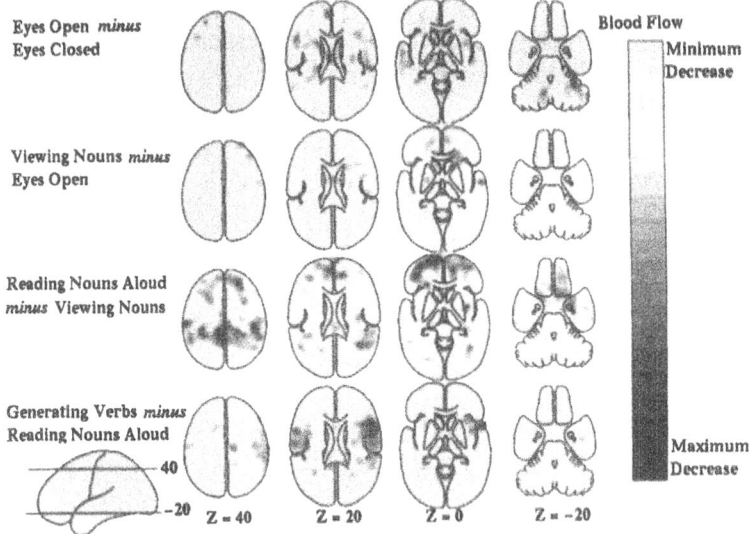

Figure 2. Hierarchically organized subtractions involving the same task conditions as shown in Figure 1 with the difference being that these images represent areas of decreased activity in the task condition as compared to the control condition. Note that the major decreases occurred when subjects read the visually presented nouns aloud as compared to viewing them passively as they appeared on the television monitor (row 3); and, when they said aloud an appropriate verb for each noun as it appeared on the television monitor as compared to reading the noun aloud (row 4). Combining the information available in Figures 1 and 2 provides a fairly complete picture of the interactions between tasks and brain systems in hierarchically organized cognitive tasks when studied with functional brain imaging.

course of a particular cognitive paradigm are illustrated in Figure 2. By examining the images in Figures 1 and 2 together, a more complete picture emerges of the changes taking place in the cognitive paradigm illustrated together in these two figures. Clearly, some areas of the brain active at one stage in a hierarchically designed paradigm can become inactive as task complexity is increased. While changes of this sort are hidden from the view of the cognitive scientist they become obvious when brain imaging is employed.

A final caveat with regard to certain cognitive paradigms is that the brain systems involved do not necessarily remain constant through many repetitions of the task. While simple habituation might be suspected when a task is tedious, this is not the issue referred to here. Rather, when a task is novel and, more importantly, conflicts with a more habitual response to the presented stimulus major changes can occur in the systems allocated to the task. A good example relates to the task shown in Figures 1 and 2 (row 4) where subjects are asked to generate an appropriate verb for visually presented nouns rather than simply read the noun aloud as they had been doing (29). In this task, regions uniquely active when the task is first performed (Figure 1, row 4 and Figure 3, row 1) are replaced by regions active when the task has become well practiced (Figure 3, row 2). Such

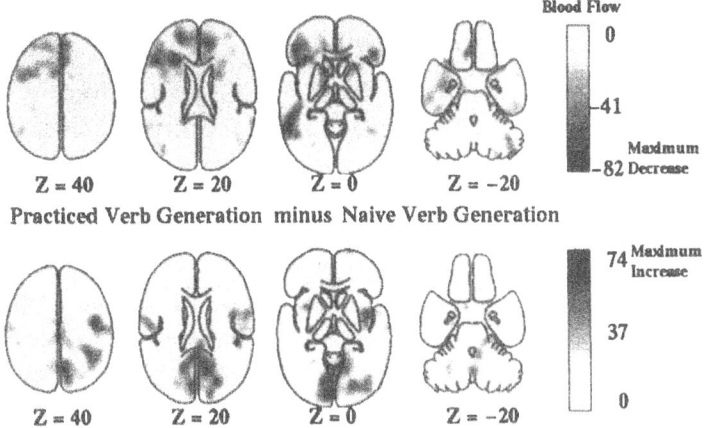

Figure 3. Practice-induced changes in brain systems involve both the disappearance of activity in systems initially supporting task performance (row 1) and the appearance of activity in other systems concerned with practiced performance (row 2). In this example, generating verbs aloud for a visually presented nouns (see also row 4 of Figures 1 and 2 for changes during the naïve performance of the task) subjects acquired proficiency on the task after 10 minutes of practice. This improved performance was associated with a disappearance of activity in areas of frontal and temporal cortex and the right cerebellum (row 1) and the appearance of activity in Sylvian-insular and occipital cortex (row 2). These images were created by subtracting the naïve performance of verb generation from the practiced performance of the task. More details on these changes can be obtained from Raichle et al (29).

changes have both practical and theoretical implications when it comes to the design and interpretation of cognitive activation experiments. Functional brain imaging obviously provides a unique perspective that is unavailable in the purely cognitive experiment.

Finally, another technology emerged contemporaneously with PET and CT. This was magnetic resonance imaging (MRI). MRI is based upon yet another set of physical principles that have to do with the behavior of hydrogen atoms or protons in a magnetic field. These principles were discovered independently by Felix Block (4) and Edward Purcell and his colleagues in 1946 (26) and expanded to imaging by Paul Lauterbur in 1973 (18). Initially MRI provided superb anatomical information but inherent in the data also was important metabolic and physiological information. An opening for MRI in the area of functional brain imaging emerged when it was discovered that during changes in neuronal activity there are local changes in the amount of oxygen in the tissue (10, 11). By combining this observation with a much earlier observation by Pauling and Coryell (22) that changing the amount of oxygen carried by hemoglobin changes the degree to which hemoglobin disturbs a magnetic field, Ogawa and colleagues (20) were able to demonstrate that in vivo changes in blood oxygenation could be detected with MRI. The MRI signal (technically known as T2* or "tee-two-star") arising from this unique combination of brain physiology (10) and nuclear magnetic resonance physics (22) (34) became known as the blood oxygen level dependent or BOLD signal (20). There quickly followed several demonstrations of BOLD signal changes in normal humans during functional brain activation (2, 17, 21) giving birth to the rapidly developing field of functional MRI or fMRI.

In the discussion to follow it is important to keep in mind that when a BOLD signal is detected blood flow to a region of brain has changed out of proportion to the change in oxygen consumption (16). When blood flow changes more than oxygen consumption, in either direction, there is a reciprocal change in the amount of deoxyhemoglobin present locally in the tissue changing the local magnetic field properties. As is frequently observed, both increases and decreases occur in the BOLD signal in the normal human brain.

3.   METABOLIC REQUIREMENTS OF COGNITION

While many had assumed that behaviorally induced increases in local blood flow would be reflected in local increases in the oxidative metabolism of glucose (32), evidence from brain imaging studies with PET (10, 11) and fMRI (16) have indicated otherwise. Fox and his colleagues (10, 11) demonstrated that in normal, awake adult humans, stimulation of the visual or somatosensory cortex results in dramatic increases in blood flow but minimal increases in oxygen consumption. Increases in glucose utilization occur in parallel with blood flow (11) (5), an observation fully anticipated by the work of others (33, 38). However, changes in blood flow and glucose utilization were much in excess of the changes in oxygen consumption, an observation contrary to most popularly held notions of brain energy metabolism (32). These results suggested that the additional metabolic requirements associated with increased neuronal activity might be supplied largely through glycolysis alone.

Another element of the relationship between brain circulation and brain function which was not appreciated prior to the advent of functional brain imaging was that regional blood flow and the fMRI BOLD signal not only increase in some areas of the brain appropriate to task performance but also decrease from a resting baseline in other areas (31) as shown in Figure 2.

Physiologists have long recognized that individual neurons in the cerebral cortex can both increase or decrease their activities from a resting, baseline firing pattern depending upon task conditions. Examples abound in the neurophysiological literature (12). A parsimonious view of these decreases in neuronal activity is that they reflect the activity of inhibitory interneurons acting within local neuronal circuits of the cerebral cortex. Because inhibition is energy requiring (1) it is impossible to distinguish inhibitory from excitatory cellular activity on the basis of changes in either blood flow or metabolism. Thus, on this view a local increase in inhibitory activity would be as likely to increase blood flow and the fMRI BOLD signal as would a local increase in excitatory activity. How, then, might decreases in blood flow or the fMRI BOLD signal arise?

To understand the possible significance of the decreases in blood flow in functional imaging studies it is important to distinguish two separate conditions in which they might arise. The less interesting and more usually referred to circumstance arises when two images are compared in which one contains a regional increase in blood flow due to some type of task activity (e.g., let us consider hand movement which produces increases in contralateral motor cortex blood flow) and a control image that does not (i.e., in this example, no hand movement). In our example, subtracting the image associated with no hand movement from the image associated with hand movement reveals the expected increase in blood flow in motor cortex. Simply reversing the subtraction produces an image with a decrease in the same area. While this example may seem trivial and obvious, such subtraction reversals are often presented in the analysis of very complex tasks and in such a manner as to be quite confusing even to those working the field.

The second circumstance in which decreases in blood flow and the fMRI BOLD signal appear is not due to the above type of data manipulations (i.e., an active task image subtracted from a passive state image). Rather, blood flow and the fMRI BOLD signal actually decrease from the passive baseline state (i.e., the activity in a region of brain has not been first elevated by a task). The usual baseline conditions from which this occurs consist of lying quietly but fully awake in an MRI or PET scanner with eyes closed or passively viewing a television monitor and its contents, be it a fixation point or even a more complex stimulus (Fig. 2, row 3). In the examples discussed by Shulman and colleagues (31) areas of the medial orbital frontal cortex, the posterior cingulate cortex and precuneus consistently showed decreased blood flow when subjects actively processed a wide variety of visual stimuli as compared to a passive baseline condition (compare with the example shown in Fig. 2).

The hypothesis one is led to consider, regarding these rather large area reductions in blood flow, is that a large number of neurons reduce their activity together (for one of the few neurophysiological references to such a phenomenon see (7)). Such group reductions could not be mediated by a local increase in the activity of inhibitory interneurons as this would be seen as an increase in activity by PET and fMRI. Rather, such reductions are likely mediated through the action of diffuse projecting systems like dopamine, norepinephrine and serotonin or a reduction in thalamic inputs to the cortex. The recognition of such changes probably represents an important contribution of functional brain imaging to our understanding of cortical function and should stimulate increased interest in the manner in which brain resources are allocated on a large systems level during task performance.

The metabolic accompaniments of these functionally induced decreases in blood flow from a passive baseline condition were not initially explored and it was tacitly assumed that such reductions would probably be accompanied by coupled reductions in oxygen consumption. Therefore, it came as a surprise that the fMRI BOLD signal, based on tissue oxygen availability, detected both increases and decreases during functional activation. Decreases in the BOLD signal during a task state as compared to a passive, resting state have been widely appreciated by investigators using fMRI although, surprisingly, no formal publications on the subject have yet to appear.

Taken together the data we have at hand suggest that blood flow changes more than oxygen consumption in the face of increases as well as decreases in local neuronal activity. Glucose utilization also changes more than oxygen consumption during increases in brain activity (we presently have no data on decreases in glucose utilization) and may equal the changes in blood flow in both magnitude and spatial extent (5, 11).

Interpretations of these blood flow-metabolism relationships during changes in functional brain activity are presently controversial. Several schools of thought have emerged. Pierre Magistretti most eloquently articulates one hypothesis, which addresses the role of glycolysis in brain functional activation based on their work with cultured astrocytes (3, 35). On this theory increases in neuronal activity stimulated by the excitatory amino acid transmitter glutamate result in relatively large increases in glycolytic metabolism in astrocytes. The energy supplied through glycolysis in the astrocyte is used to metabolize glutamate to glutamine before being recycled to neurons. Coupled with estimates that increased firing rates of neurons require little additional energy over and above that required for the normal maintenance of ionic gradients (8) leads to the hypothesis that the primary metabolic change associated with changes (at least increases) in neuronal activity are glycolytic and occur in astrocytes.

Not surprisingly the above hypothesis has been challenged and alternatives offered to explain the observed discrepancy between changes in blood flow and glucose utilization, which appear to change in parallel, and oxygen consumption, which changes much less than either. Probably the most popular alternative hypothesis is based on optical imaging work on physiologically stimulated visual cortex by Grinvald and his associates (19). In their work they measure changes in reflected light from the surface of visual cortex in anesthetized cats. Using wavelengths of light sensitive to deoxyhemoglobin and oxyhemoglobin they note an almost immediate increase in deoxyhemoglobin concentration followed, after a brief interval, by an increase in oxyhemoglobin which, while centered at the same location as the change in deoxyhemoglobin, is greater in magnitude and extends over a much larger area of the cortex than do the changes in deoxyhemoglobin (19). They interpret these results to mean that increases in neuronal activity are associated with highly localized increases in oxygen consumption which stimulate a vascular response, delayed by several seconds, that is large in relation to both the magnitude of the increase in oxygen consumption and the area of cerebral cortex that is active. In other words, by their theory increases in neuronal activity in the cerebral cortex are associated with increased oxidative metabolism of glucose. Because the blood flow response to the change in neuronal activity is relatively slow, oxygen reserves in the area of activation are temporarily depleted. When the blood flow response does occur, after a delay of 1-3 seconds, it exceeds the needs of the tissue, delivering to the active area of cortex and its surroundings oxygen in excess of metabolic needs.

Support for the hypothesis of Malonek and Grinvald (19) comes from theoretical work by Buxton and Frank (6). In their modeling work they show that in an idealized capillary tissue cylinder in the brain, an increase in blood flow in excess of the increased oxygen metabolic demands of the tissue is needed in order to maintain proper oxygenation of the tissue. This results from the poor diffusivity and solubility of oxygen in brain tissue. On this theory, blood flow remains coupled to oxidative metabolism but in a non-linear fashion designed to overcome the diffusion and solubility limitations of oxygen in brain tissue in order to maintain adequate tissue oxygenation.

While the hypothesis that reactive hyperemia is a normal and necessary consequence of increased neuronal activity merits careful consideration, several observations remain unexplained. First, it does not account for the increased glucose utilization that parallels the change in blood flow observed in normal humans (5, 11) and laboratory animals (13, 36, 37). Second, it does not agree with the observations of Woolsey and his associates (37) as well as others (13) who have demonstrated a remarkably tight spatial relationship between changes in neuronal activity within a single, rat whisker barrel and the response of the vascular supply as well as glucose metabolism to that barrel. There is little evidence in these studies for spatially diffuse reactive hyperemia surrounding the stimulated area of cortex. Third, in the paper by Malonek and Grinvald (19) the initial rise in deoxyhemoglobin seen with activation is not accompanied by a fall in oxyhemoglobin as would be expected with a sudden rise in local oxygen consumption which precedes the onset of increased oxygen delivery to the tissue. In the presence of somewhat conflicting evidence on capillary recruitment in brain (80-82) which could explain this observation, we should exercise caution in accepting uncritically the data of Malonek and Grinvald (19) until an explanation for this particular discrepancy is found and better concordance is achieved with other experiments. Clearly, more information is needed on the exact nature of the microvascular events surrounding functional brain activation. Finally, we are left without an explanation for the observation that when blood flow decreases below a resting baseline during changes in the functional activity of a region of the brain (Fig. 2), a negative BOLD signal arises due to the fact that blood flow decreases more than the oxygen consumption.

So what are we to conclude at this point in time? Any theory designed to explain functional brain imaging signals must accommodate three observations. First, local increases and decreases in brain activity are reliably accompanied by changes in blood flow. Second, these blood flow changes exceed any accompanying change in the oxygen consumption. If this were not the case, fMRI based on the BOLD signal changes could not exist. Third, while paired data on glucose metabolism and blood flow are limited they suggest that blood flow changes are accompanied by changes in glucose metabolism of approximately equal magnitude and spatial extent.

ACKNOWLEDGEMENTS

I would like to acknowledge many years of generous support from NINDS, NHLBI, The McDonnell Center For Studies of Higher Brain Function at Washington University as well as The John D. and Katherine T. MacArthur Foundation and The Charles A. Dana Foundation.

REFERENCES

1. Ackerman, R. F., D. M. Finch, T. L. Babb, and J. Engel, Jr. Increased glucose metabolism during long-duration recurrent inhibition of hippocampal cells. *Journal of Neuroscience* 4: 251-264, 1984.
2. Bandettini, P. A., E. C. Wong, R. S. Hinks, R. S. Tikofsky, and J. S. Hyde. Time course EPI of human brain function during task activation. *Magnetic Resonance in Medicine* 25: 390-397, 1992.
3. Bittar, P. G., Y. Charnay, L. Pellerin, C. Bouras, and P. Magistretti. Selective distribution of lactate dehydrogenase isoenzymes in neurons and astrocytes of human brain. *Journal of Cerebral Blood Flow and Metabolism* 16: 1079-1089, 1996.
4. Block, F. Nuclear introduction. Physiology Review 70: 460-474, 1946.
5. Blomqvist, G., R. J. Seitz, I. Sjogren, C. Halldin, S. Stone-Elander, L. Widen, O. Solin, and M. Haaparanta. Regional cerebral oxidative and total glucose consumption during rest and activation studied with positron emission tomography. *Acta Physiologica Scandinavica* 151: 29-43, 1994.
6. Buxton, R. B., and L. R. Frank. A model for the coupling between cerebral blood flow and oxygen metabolism during neural stimulation. *Journal of Cerebral Blood Flow and Metabolism* 17: 64-72, 1997.
7. Creutzfeldt, O., G. Ojemann, and E. Lettich. Neuronal activity in the human temporal lobe. *Experimental Brain Research* 77: 451-475, 1989.
8. Crutzfeldt, O. D. Neurophysiological correlates of different functional states of the brain. In: *Brain Work: The Coupling of Function, Metabolism and Blood Flow in the Brain*, edited by D. H. Ingvar and N. A. Lassen. Copenhagen: Munksgaard, 1975, p. 21-46.
9. Donders, F. C. On the speed of mental processes. *Acta Psychologia* 30: 412-431, 1969.
10. Fox, P. T., and M. E. Raichle. Focal physiological uncoupling of cerebral blood flow and oxidative metabolism during somatosensory stimulation in human subjects. *PNAS* 83: 1140-1144, 1986.
11. Fox, P. T., M. E. Raichle, M. A. Mintun, and C. Dence. Nonoxidative glucose consumption during focal physiologic neural activity. *Science* 241: 462-464, 1988.
12. Georgopoulos, A. P., J. F. Kalaska, R. Caminiti, and J. T. Massey. On the relations between the direction of two-dimensional arm movements and cell discharge in primate motor cortex. *Journal of Neuroscience* 2: 1527-1537, 1982.
13. Greenberg, J. H., N. W. Sohn, and P. J. Hand. Vibrissae-deafferentation produces plasticity in cerebral blood flow in response to somatosensory activation. *Journal of Cerebral Blood Flow and Metabolism* 17: S561, 1997.
14. Herscovitch, P., J. Markham, and M. E. Raichle. Brain blood flow measured with intravenous H2(15)O. I. Theory and error analysis. Journal of Nuclear Medicine 24: 782-9, 1983.

15. Hornbein, T. F., B. D. Townes, R. B. Schoene, J. R. Sutton, and C. S. Houston. The cost to the central nervous system of climbing to extremely high altitude. *N Engl J Med* 321: 1714-1719, 1989.

16. Kim, S. G., and K. Ugurbil. Comparison of blood oxygenation and cerebral blood flow effects in fMRI: estimation of relative oxygen comsumption change. *Magnetic Resonance Medicine* 38: 59-65, 1997.

17. Kwong, K. K., J. W. Belliveau, D. A. Chesler, I. E. Goldberg, R. M. Weiskoff, B. P. Poncelet, D. N. Kennedy, B. E. Hoppel, M. S. Cohen, R. Turner, H. M. Cheng, T. J. Brady, and B. R. Rosen. Dynamic magnetic resonance imaging of human brain activity during primary sensory stimulation. *PNAS* 89: 5675-5679, 1992.

18. Lauterbur, P. Image formation by induced local interactions: examples employing nuclear magnetic resonance. *Nature* 242: 190-191, 1973.

19. Malonek, D., and A. Grinvald. Interactions between electrical activity and cortical microcirculation revealed by imaging spectroscopy: Implications for functional brain mapping. *Science* 272: 551-554, 1996.

20. Ogawa, S., T. M. Lee, A. R. Kay, and D. W. Tank. Brain magnetic resonance imaging with contrast depedent on blood oxygenation *PNAS* 87: 9868-9872, 1990.

21. Ogawa, S., D. W. Tank, R. Menon, J. M. Ellermann, S.-G. Kim, H. Merkle, and K. Ugurbil. Intrinsic signal changes accompanying sensory stimulation: Functional brain mapping with magnetic resonance imaging. *PNAS* 89: 5951-5955, 1992.

22. Pauling, L., and C. D. Coryell. The magnetic properties and structure of hemoglobin, oxyghemoglobin and caronmonoxyhemoglobin. *PNAS* 22: 210-216, 1936.

23. Petersen, S. E., P. T. Fox, M. I. Posner, M. Mintum, and M. E. Raichle. Positron emission tomographic studies of the cortical anatomy of single-word processing. *Nature* 331: 585-589, 1988.

24. Petersen, S. E., P. T. Fox, M. I. Posner, M. A. Mintun, and M. E. Raichle. Positron emission tomographic studies of the processing of single words. *Journal of Cognitive Neuroscience* 1: 153-170, 1989.

25. Posner, M. I., and M. E. Raichle. *Images of Mind.* New York: W.H. Freeman & Company, 1994.

26. Purcell, E. M., H. C. Torry, and R. V. Pound. Resonance absorption by nuclear magnetic moments in a solid. *Physiological Review* 69: 37, 1946.

27. Raichle, M. E. Behind the scenes of function brain imaging: A historical and physiological perspective. *PNAS* 95: 765-772, 1998.

28. Raichle, M. E. Circulatory and metabolic correlates of brain function in normal humans. In: *Handbook of Physiology: The Nervous System V. Higher Functions of the Brain*, edited by F. Plum. Bethesda: American Physiological Society, 1987, p. 643-674.

29. Raichle, M. E., J. A. Fiez, T. O. Videen, A. M. MacLeod, J. V. Pardo, P. T. Fox, and S. E. Petersen. Practice-related changes in human brain functional anatomy during nonmotor learning. *Cerebral Cortex* 4: 8-26, 1994.

30. Raichle, M. E., W. R. W. Martin, P. Herscovitch, M. A. Mintun, and J. Markham. Brain blood flow measured with intravenous H215O. II. Implementation and validation. *Journal of Nuclear Medicine* 24: 790-798, 1983.

31. Shulman, G. L., J. A. Fiez, M. Corbetta, R. L. Buckner, F. M. Miezin, M. E. Raichle, and S. E. Petersen. Common blood flow changes across visual tasks: II. Decreases in cerebral cortex. *Journal of Cognitive Neurosciences* in press, 1997b.

32. Siesjo, B. K. *Brain Energy Metabolism.* New York: John Wiley & Sons, 1978.

33. Sokoloff, L., M. Reivich, C. Kennedy, M. H. Des Rosiers, C. S. Patlak, K. D. Pettigrew, O. Sakurada, and M. Shinohara. The [14C]deoxyglucose method for the measurement of

local glucose utilization: theory, procedure and normal values in the conscious and anesthetized albino rat. *Journal of Neurochemistry* 28: 897-916, 1977.

34. Thulborn, K. R., J. C. Waterton, P. M. Matthews, and G. K. Radda. Oxygenation dependence of the transverse relaxation time of water protons in whole blood at high field. *Biochimica et Biophysica* Acta 714: 265-270, 1982.

35. Tsacopoulos, M., and P. J. Magistretti. Metabolic coupling between glia and neurons. *Journal of Neuroscience* 16: 877-885, 1996.

36. Ueki, M., F. Linn, and K.-A. Hossmann. Functional activation of cerebral blood flow and metabolism before and after global ischemia of rat brain. *Journal of Cerebral Blood Flow and Metabolism* 8: 486-494, 1988.

37. Woolsey, T. A., C. M. Rovainen, S. B. Cox, M. H. Henegar, G. E. Liang, D. Liu, Y. E. Moskalenko, J. Sui, and L. Wei. Neuronal units linked to microvascular modules in cerebral cortex: response elements for imaging the brain. *Cerebral Cortex* 6, 1996.

38. Yarowsky, P., M. Kadekaro, and L. Sokoloff. Frequency-dependent activation of glucose utilization in the superior cervical ganglion by electrical stimulation of cervical sympathetic trunk. *PNAS* 80: 4179-4183, 1983.

Chapter 16

Are Arterial, Muscle and Working Limb Lactate Exchange Data Obtained on Men at Altitude Consistent with the Hypothesis of an Intracellular Lactate Shuttle?

George A. Brooks

Exercise Physiology Laboratory, Department of Integrative Biology, University of California, Berkeley, CA 94720 USA

Key words: mitochondria, LDH, MCT1, hypoxia, cell redox, exercise, exertion

Abstract: The "Lactate Shuttle" Hypothesis posits that lactate removal requires exchange among producing and consuming cells. The "Intra-cellular Lactate Shuttle" hypothesis posits that lactate exchange occurs among compartments within cells, and that mitochondria are the major sites of cellular lactate disposal. Thus, cells with high mitochondrial densities (cardiocytes, myocytes, hepatocytes) are those which participate in lactate clearance. The model of an Intracellular Lactate Shuttle recognizes that the K_{eq} for LDH is 3.6×10^4 M^{-1}; thus, glycolysis results in cytosolic lactate production regardless of the intracellular PO_2. The model also requires presence of a mitochondrial monocarboxylate transporter (MCT) that allows uptake of lactate as well as pyruvate, and intra-mitochondrial LDH whose function is linked to the ETC, and which permits lactate→pyruvate conversion and oxidation. Recently, we have shown that liver, heart and muscle mitochondria readily oxidize lactate and contain LDH and MCT1. Accordingly, we have concluded that lactate is the predominant monocarboxylate oxidized by mitochondria *in vivo*. The model of an "Intra-cellular Lactate Shuttle" is consistent with many of the observations on men at sea level and altitude. The observations include: oxidation is the primary fate of lactate disposal during rest and exercise; lactate production and oxidation occur simultaneously within resting and working muscle; increasing $[lactate]_a$ increases muscle lactate extraction, and that by increasing SaO_2 acclimatization reduces blood [lactate].

1.   INTRODUCTION

Since the initial observations of Edwards (18), blood lactate responses to exercise at altitude have been observed to demonstrate several unexplained features. Not only has the term "lactate paradox" been used, but investigators have used different definitions for the "paradox" (24, 27, 34). However, since the initial observations and subsequent articulation of terms, our understanding of carbohydrate metabolism at altitude has grown immensely (5-9, 12, 27, 36, 37). Rather than dwell on any specific term whose utility may have passed, in this report the effort will be to use new knowledge in an attempt to explain blood metabolite responses to altitude.

Commencing with brief reviews and presentation of data necessary to illustrate presence of the "Cell-Cell" and "Intra-cellular Lactate Shuttles," an attempt will be made to evaluate whether those concepts are of use in understanding apparently disparate data observed on men at altitude.

2.   PHENOMENA TO EXPLAIN:

- Why is arterial [lactate] elevated during exercise at a given power output at altitude compared to sea level?
- Is the elevation in arterial [lactate] at altitude attributable to increased production and appearance in the blood (Ra), or are lactate disposal (Rd) and clearance rates (MCR) inhibited at altitude?
- How can working human muscle display a "Stainsby Effect" at altitude wherein the start of contractions results in muscle net lactate release. Thereafter, net lactate release follows the fall of lactate [v-a] with net release declining to zero even as arterial [lactate] is elevated and constant?
- If there is a "Stainsby Effect" at altitude, what explains the elevation in arterial [lactate]?
- How can working muscle simultaneously release, consume and oxidize lactate at altitude?

3.   WHAT IS THE CELL-CELL LACTATE SHUTTLE?

The original "Cell-Cell" lactate shuttle posited that shuttling of lactate through the interstitium and vasculature provides a significant carbon source for oxidation and gluconeogenesis during rest and exercise (4, 5). In Figure 1, Type IIB (fast-glycolytic) fibers are indicated to be lactate producing

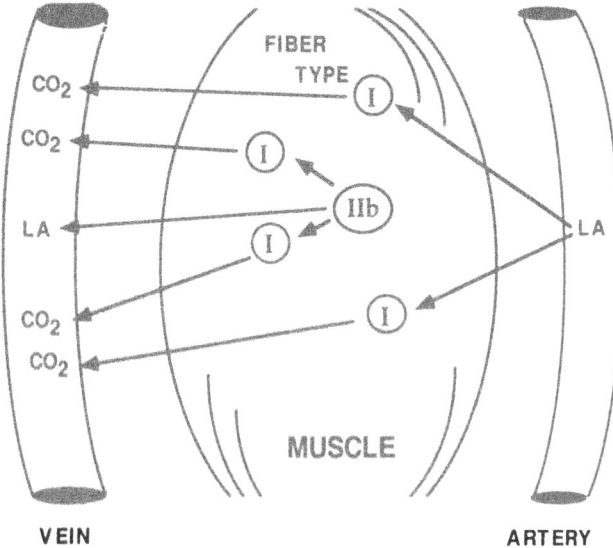

Figure 1. Model of the "Cell-Cell" Lactate Shuttle. Lactate is formed in fast-twitch white (type IIb) skeletal muscle fibers, or transiently in populations of red fibers at the start of exercise. Lactate released into the interstitium from cellular sites of production can be taken up and oxidized by adjacent lactate consuming (type I) muscle fibers. Alternatively, during exercise some lactate released into the circulation reperfuses the active muscle bed within a fraction of a minute, where uptake and oxidation in red, highly oxidative fibers occurs. Some of the lactate released from an active muscle bed can be taken up by the heart and oxidized, or taken up by the liver and kidneys where lactate serves as a gluconeogenic precursor. Redrawn from (4).

cells, whereas Type I fibers are indicated as sites of lactate oxidation. This hypothesis was developed at a time when fiber heterogeneity in skeletal muscle was recognized (1, 3). Further, the hypothesis was based on results of rats and dogs made to exercise and infused with radioactive glucose and lactate tracers (10, 11, 16, 17). On those species it was shown that during exercise lactate turnover and oxidation exceed glucose turnover and oxidation. Subsequently, the same phenomena of lactate flux and oxidation were demonstrated in humans (30, 43). Data in Figure 2 shows the direct relationships between lactate turnover and metabolic rate and between lactate oxidation and metabolic rate (30). Lactate turnover is high at rest and increases as a direct function of exercise intensity and metabolic power output. Further, lactate disposal through oxidation (approximately 50% at rest), increases both absolutely and relatively during exercise such that oxidation accounts for 75% of lactate disposal during exercise.

While systemic lactate flux and whole-body oxidation data supported the concept of a lactate shuttle, the technology could not be used to demonstrate tissue lactate exchange. Therefore, studies were conducted to determine the lactate concentration differences across active (leg) and inactive (arm)

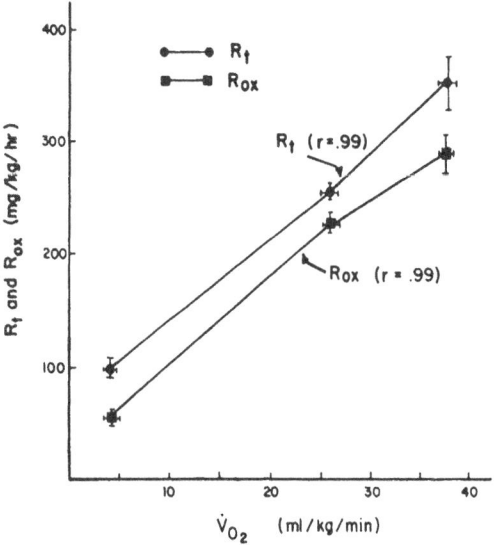

Figure 2. Lactate turnover determined with [1-^{13}C]lactate tracer in men at sea level during rest, exercise at 50% VO$_2$max, and exercise at 75% VO$_2$max. Data from Mazzeo et al. (30).

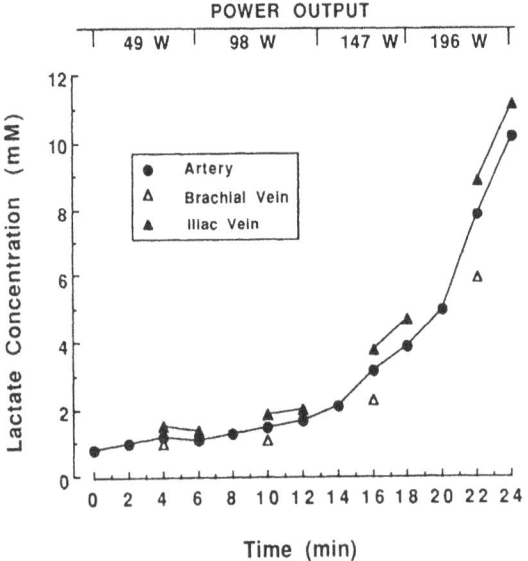

Figure 3. [Lactate] in blood sampled simultaneously from the radial artery, brachial vein, and iliac vein in men during continual, progressive exercise protocol. The results illustrate tissue lactate exchange through the blood during exercise. From Stanley et al. (42).

muscle beds during progressive leg cycling exercise. The results (42) (Figure 3) demonstrate lactate release from active (leg) muscle beds, transit through the vasculature, and uptake by inactive muscle (arm) beds. In the same set of studies, measurements of arterial-coronary sinus concentration differences and coronary blood flow indicated that exogenous lactate becomes the major fuel for the heart during exercise (22). Further, in those studies the appearance of ^{13}C and ^{14}C in blood glucose following tracer-lactate infusion indicated participation of the Cori Cycle in lactate removal (41, 43). Thus, skeletal as well as cardiac muscle and liver participate in lactate exchange and metabolism during exercise.

With regard to the issue of oxygen insufficiency as the cause of lactate production in muscle, the results obtained on resting, as well as contracting muscle indicate that lactate production occurs in well perfused and fully oxygenated tissues (47). Not only is lactate always present in resting muscle, but lactate release and oxidation occur simultaneously (6) while cardiac output and limb blood flow rise so that oxygen transport meets demand, and significant O_2 remains in femoral venous blood. Data on intact functioning humans as well as animal muscle preparations indicate that lactate production occurs under fully aerobic conditions (14, 15, 25).

4.   WHAT IS THE INTRACELLULAR LACTATE SHUTTLE?

To resolve the dilemma of tissue lactate production under fully aerobic conditions, the "Intracellular Lactate Shuttle" was posited. While there was good evidence to support activity of the "Cell-Cell Lactate Shuttle" during exercise, at rest recruitment of Type IIB fibers could not be invoked. A better model that allowed for lactate production in all fiber types during rest and exercise was necessary (6). The "Intracellular" Shuttle (Figure 4) allows that glycolysis in the cytosol results in lactate production, and lactate shuttles to mitochondria within the cell of production for oxidative removal (7).

That glycolysis inevitably results in cytosolic lactate production relates to the energetics of the terminal enzyme, lactate dehydrogenase (LDH). The K_{eq} for LDH is $3.6 \times 10^4 \, M^{-1}$, and the free energy change ($\Delta G^{o\prime}$) approximates -6 kcal/mol. This means that glycolysis inevitably proceeds to lactate production, and that its reversal in the cytosol is unlikely *in vivo*. How then is lactate oxidized?

To evaluate the role of mitochondria in balancing lactate production and oxidation as part of an "Intra-cellular Lactate Shuttle," isolated rat cardiac, skeletal muscle and liver mitochondria were respired with lactate and pyruvate in presence or absence of known inhibitors of metabolism. As well, efforts were made to detect the presence of LDH isoforms in mitochondria by electrophoresis and electron microscopy. Results support the conclusion of a mitochondrial role in cellular lactate oxidation (6, 7), and provide an explanation for the high correlation between lactate clearance during exercise and muscle mitochondrial respiratory capacity (2, 31).

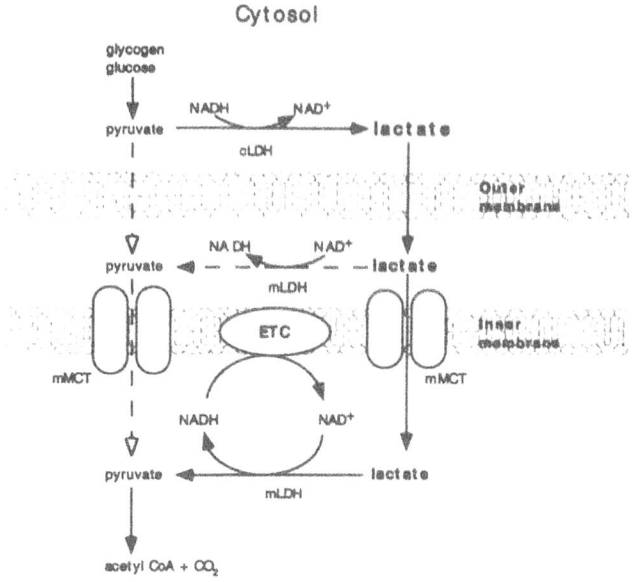

Matrix

Figure 4. Depiction of the functional relationship between mLDH and mMCT in operation of the "Intra-cellular Lactate Shuttle." The predominant monocarboxylate entering the mitochondrial inter-membrane space is lactate. Entry of lactate and pyruvate into the mitochondrial matrix is facilitated by mMCT. Thus, lactate enters mitochondria; lactate is oxidized to pyruvate via mLDH when mitochondrial Redox decreases, and pyruvate is oxidized via the TCA Cycle and ETC. From Brooks et al. (7).

In one experiment, mitochondria were isolated and respired with pyruvate-malate and lactate-malate as substrates. Respiration was stimulated by the presence of ADP. Figure 5 shows that maximal, ADP-stimulated respiration rates were obtained with both lactate and pyruvate as substrates (7). Further, the figure shows that addition of the known LDH inhibitor oxamate, blocks mitochondrial lactate oxidation. Thus, LDH is necessary for mitochondrial lactate oxidation.

To determine if LDH existed in mitochondria, organelles from rat liver, heart and skeletal muscle were isolated. Agarose gel electrophoresis of LDH isoenzyme patterns in cytosolic fractions of different tissues (Figure 6) are consistent with results of previous investigations showing tissue specificity (e.g., 29). However, mitochondrial fractions also revealed presence of LDH isoenzymes. Further, LDH isoenzyme patterns differed among tissues, and between mitochondria and the surrounding cytosol in each tissue. Heart and muscle mitochondria were noted by prevalence of both LDH-1 (H4) and LDH-5 (M4), while liver mitochondria were distinguished by presence of LDH-5 (M4) (7).

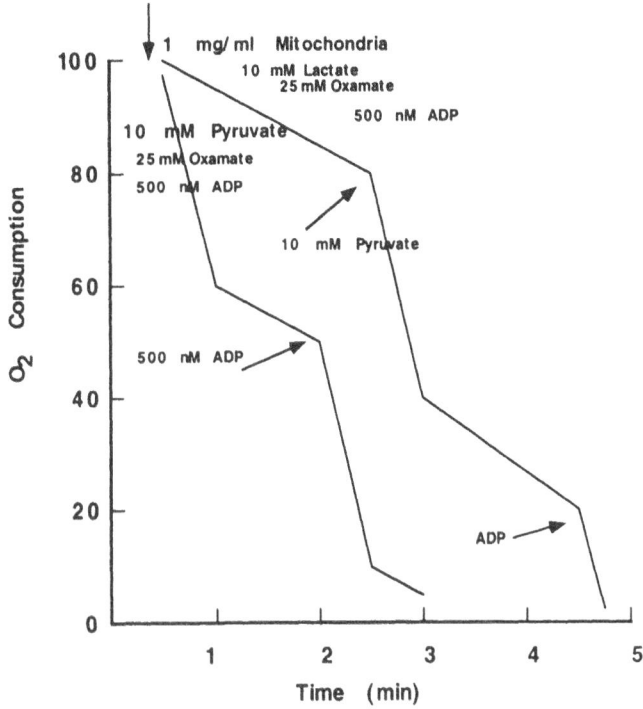

Figure 5. Depiction of a Clarke-O_2 electrode tracing showing that oxamate blocks lactate, but not pyruvate oxidation. Such experiments indicate that the ability of mitochondria isolated from muscle, liver and heart to oxidize lactate requires LDH for conversion to pyruvate within mitochondria. Data from Brooks et al. (7).

Even though studies with oxamate indicated functionality of mitochondrial LDH (Figure 5), and electrophoresis showed mitochondrial LDH (Figure 6), to further exclude the possibility of isolation artifacts, antibodies to LDH isoforms were used to detect presence of mitochondrial LDH, *in situ*. The electron micrograph in Figure 7 clearly shows a mitochondrial location of LDH (7).

The model of an "Intracellular Lactate Shuttle" (6, 7) depends heavily on presence of a mitochondrial lactate-pyruvate, or monocarboxylate transporter (MCT) (38, 39). To demonstrate the effects of inhibiting the mitochondrial lactate-pyruvate transporter, mitochondria were respired in the presence or absence of the known MCT inhibitor, cinnamate (CINN); results are shown in Figure 8. CINN blocked respiration of both substrates. However, in the presence of CINN, State 3 respiration was restored with

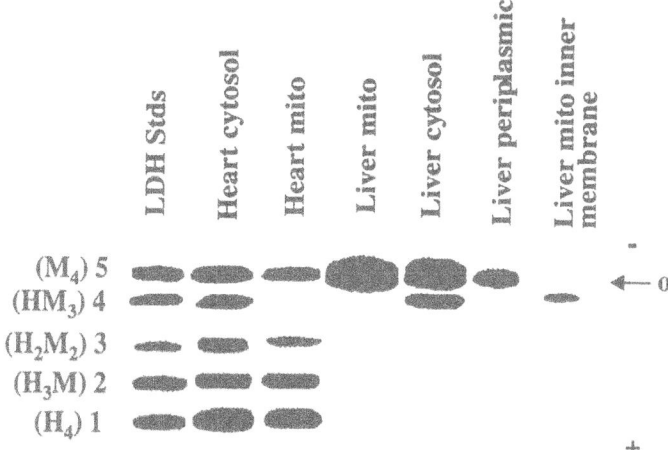

Figure 6. Agarose gel electrophoresis of LDH in mitochondria from rat liver and heart. LDH isoenzyme patterns differ between cytosol and mitochondria in both tissues. From Brooks et al. (7).

addition of either succinate or glutamate. Restoration of respiration with succinate or glutamate indicates that CINN does not block mitochondrial respiratory Complex I (glutamate, an NADH linked substrate), or Complex II (succinate, an $FADH_2$-linked substrate). Upstream inhibition of mitochondrial lactate and pyruvate oxidation, such as a transport limitation, by CINN is indicated. Thus, consistent with the concept of an "Intracellular Lactate Shuttle" (Figure 4), results as in Figures 5 and 8 show that mitochondrial lactate oxidation proceeds very rapidly requiring a transporter and LDH.

To date, preliminary studies have been conducted to identify the mitochondrial lactate-pyruvate transporter. Several possibilities exist. The cDNA of the first sarcolemmal lactate transporter from the hamster ovary cells was isolated by expression cloning (28). The protein was expressed in several tissues including heart, red skeletal muscle and erythrocytes (21). The cDNA was subsequently used for the screening of hamster liver cDNA library and resulted in isolation of the second transporter isoform which was expressed mainly in liver (20). These isoforms shared 60% identity with each other. The third MCT isoform was initially isolated as a protein exclusively expressed in the chicken retinal epithelium (32). All three isoforms stimulate proton-coupled lactate and pyruvate uptake when expressed in a heterologous system and show high affinities for propionate and ketone bodies (20, 21), and were named monocarboxylate transporters (MCT1, MCT2 and MCT3). More recently, four new mammalian monocarboxylate transporter (MCT) homologues were cloned and sequenced (33), and other candidates exist (Aivazachvili and Brooks, unpublished). Although scattered and partial homology exists among the

MCT isoforms, it is unlikely that all isoforms are lactate-pyruvate transporters. Most probably, MCT1 and MCT4 are the lactate transporters present in muscle (46).

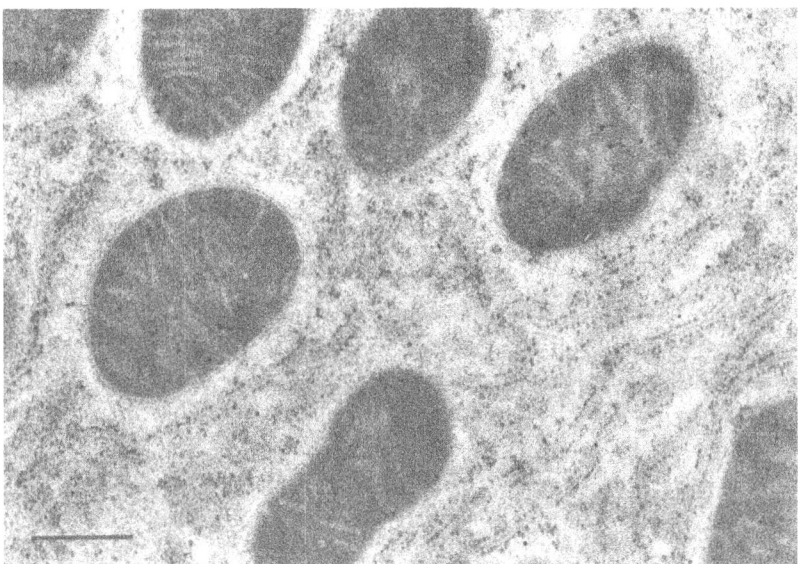

Figure 7. Electron micrograph of high pressure frozen rat liver showing mitochondria, rough ER, and cytosol. Immunolocalization of anti-LDH-5 (M4) antibodies is indicated by the 15 nm gold particles. Magnification = 54,100 X and scale bar = 400 nm. Note presence of LDH-5 in mitochondria and surrounding matrix and organelles. From Brooks et al. (7).

Figure 8. Cinnamate blocks oxidation of lactate and pyruvate. Because muscle, liver and heart mitochondria can respire both glutamate (donates electrons at Complex I) and succinate (donates electrons at Complex II), the blockage of cinnamate is upstream of PDH, GDH or SDH. The essential role of a mitochondrial MCT (lactate/pyruvate) transporter is illustrated. Data from Brooks et al. (7).

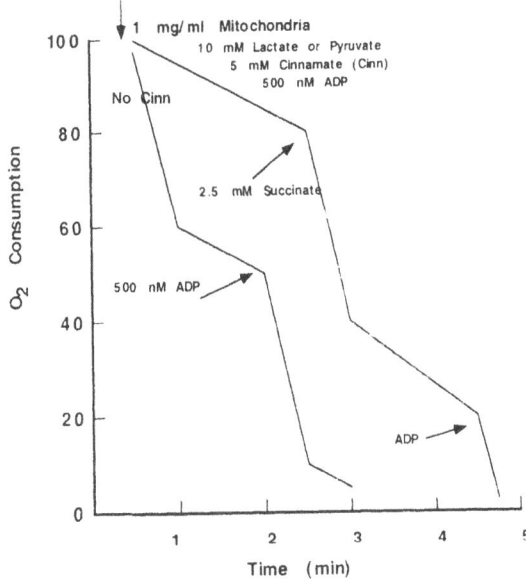

Because there was a good relationship between the oxidative capacity of muscle and the abundance of MCT1, we raised an antibody to the C-terminus of rat MCT1. Western blots of cardiac and skeletal muscle mitochondria prepared from rats show presence of MCT1 in striated muscle mitochondria. Further, electron microscopy and immunolocalization techniques show MCT1 on inner mitochondrial membranes (Brooks, et al., unpublished). Thus, MCT1 is a candidate mitochondrial lactate/pyruvate transporter.

5.   STUDIES ON MEN EXERCISING AT ALTITUDE

Having now introduced the Cell-Cell and Intracellular Lactate Shuttle Concepts, the pertinent data on men exercising at altitude will be reviewed and presented with an eye toward evaluating whether the concepts are of assistance in evaluating the data.

When men are acutely exposed to moderate altitude (e.g., 4,300 m on Pikes Peak), the circulating [lactate] is elevated during exercise compared to during the same, sub-maximal power output as at sea level. In each environmental condition portrayed (sea level, acute and chronic altitude exposure), the arterial [lactate] is elevated, and stable during exercise (Figure 9A). On acute altitude exposure, the greatest lactate concentration response is observed. With acclimatization, the circulating [lactate] declines even though whole body and working limb VO_2 are unchanged at altitude compared to sea level. Thus, there can be no possibility of a change in lactate production due to O_2 lack.

Figure 9B shows the sympathetic effect on circulating lactate level. β–adrenergic blockade with the non-specific β-antagonist propranolol decreases arterial [lactate] by approximately 60%, a result most obvious on acute altitude exposure. At altitude, β–blockade attenuates, but does not completely block the blood lactate response to exercise. What is the source of circulating lactate during exercise at altitude?

6.   LACTATE TURNOVER (PRODUCTION) AT
ALTITUDE

In the 1988 Pikes Peak study, fluxes of glucose and lactate were determined simultaneously using primed-continuous infusions of [6,6-

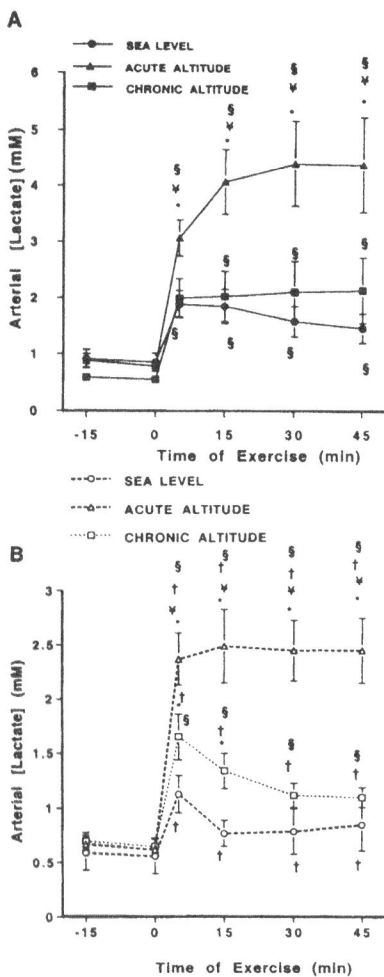

Figure 9. Arterial lactate concentrations (mean ± SEM) over time in: (A) control (n = 5), and (B) β-blocked subjects (n = 6) at sea level (SL), upon acute exposure and chronic (3-wk) exposure to 4,300 m altitude; symbols: * different from SL, ¥ different from A1, § different from rest, † different from control, p < 0.05. From Brooks et al. (6).

[2H]glucose and [3-13C]lactate. The results for sea level and acute exposure to 4,300 m are shown in Figure 10. During rest at sea level, glucose disposal (Rd) exceeds lactate appearance (Ra). Upon altitude exposure, glucose Rd rises significantly, but lactate Ra rises relatively more. During exercise at 50% VO2max at sea level, glucose flux rises compared to rest, and lactate flux rises to approximate glucose flux. Then, during exercise upon acute altitude exposure, lactate flux exceeds glucose flux. Thus, it is clear that altitude exposure causes a shift to carbohydrate metabolism, with both glucose and lactate fluxes exaggerated compared to sea level. Most importantly, blood lactate flux, a key measure of tissue lactate production, is increased significantly at altitude.

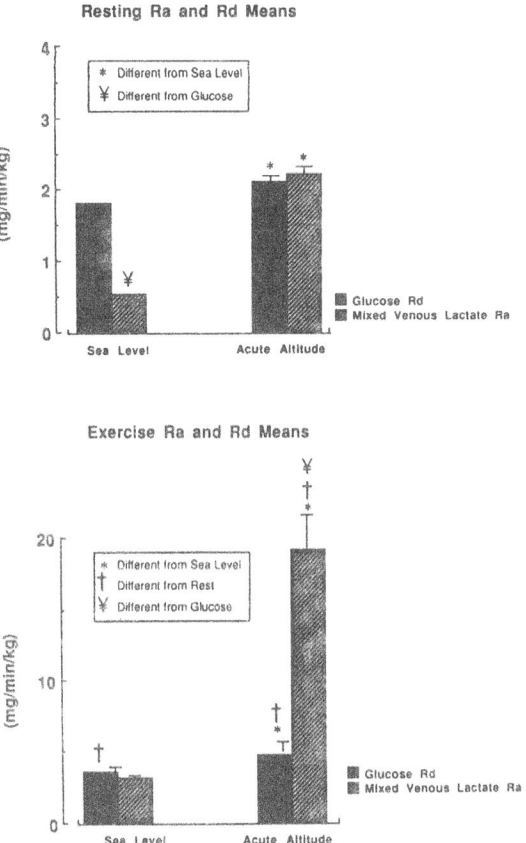

Figure 10. Blood glucose disposal rate (Rd), determined with [6,6-^{2}H]glucose, and lactate appearance rate (Ra), determined with [3-^{13}C]lactate, in men during rest (top) and exercise (bottom), at sea level (left) and acute exposure to 4,300 m altitude (right). During acute altitude exposure, lactate flux exceeds glucose flux during exercise. From Brooks et al. (13).

7.   ILLUSTRATION OF THE "STAINSBY EFFECT" BY WORKING HUMAN MUSCLE AT ALTITUDE

To evaluate the role of working muscle in contributing to the circulating lactate load during exercise at high altitude, femoral arterial and venous catheterizations were performed and limb blood flow rates as well as [v-a] lactate differences were determined. In this way, net lactate release rates ($\dot{L}$) were determined during rest and exercise under each environmental condition (12). That canine muscle preparations made to contract *in situ* release lactate on a net basis when exercise starts, and then switch to zero release or net consumption as contractions progress was first made by Stainsby and associates (40, 45). A similar 'Stainsby Effect' is observable in working human limbs (12) (Figure 11). Under all non-β-blocked conditions studied, resting limbs released lactate on a net basis. Then, when contractions started, there was a burst of lactate release, an occurrence most exaggerated upon acute altitude exposure (Figure 11A). However, even then, $\dot{L}$ declined to zero as exercise continued, all the while arterial [lactate] remained elevated and constant. Clearly, working muscle contributes to the circulating lactate load when exercise starts. However, the persistence of an elevation in circulating lactate (Figure 9), despite rapid turnover (Figure 10), must be attributable to tissue sites other than working muscle.

At present, the extra-muscular sites of lactate production and release during exercise at altitude are undetermined. In dogs made to exercise under normoxic (44) and hypoxic conditions (45), the liver is a site of net lactate release. However, similar data are not available on humans. Other possibilities include adipose and skin, both of which respond to adrenergic stimulation by increasing glycolysis and lactate release (19, 26).

At altitude, β-adrenergic blockade had some perplexing effects on muscle lactate exchange (Figure 11B). On acute exposure under β-blockade, there was a negative lactate [v-a], indicting uptake. This result was different from that observed under all blocked and unblocked conditions. The start of exercise upon acute exposure with β-blockade resulted in increased net lactate release, but release was blunted. Interestingly, net lactate release from the working limb was greatest after acclimatization, when the circulating [lactate] had returned almost to sea level values (Figure 9). As discussed previously (12), muscle and femoral venous lactate contents were minimally effected by β-blockade at altitude. Therefore, the lactate [v-a] was exaggerated due to the lesser circulatory lactate load.

8. LACTATE EXTRACTION AND OXIDATION DURING NET RELEASE:

Previously, Stanley et al. (42) demonstrated that working human muscle is capable of simultaneous lactate extraction and release with almost all of the extraction attributable to oxidation in working muscle. Leg extraction and oxidation can be calculated in two ways, which usually yield good agreement in the steady state. One method is to compare the amount of tracer lactate leaving the limb with that entering. The difference (i.e., the decrease in tracer mass leaving the leg) is quantitatively related to the increase in labeled CO_2 release. The alternative method is to compare the mass of tracer CO_2 entering and leaving the leg.

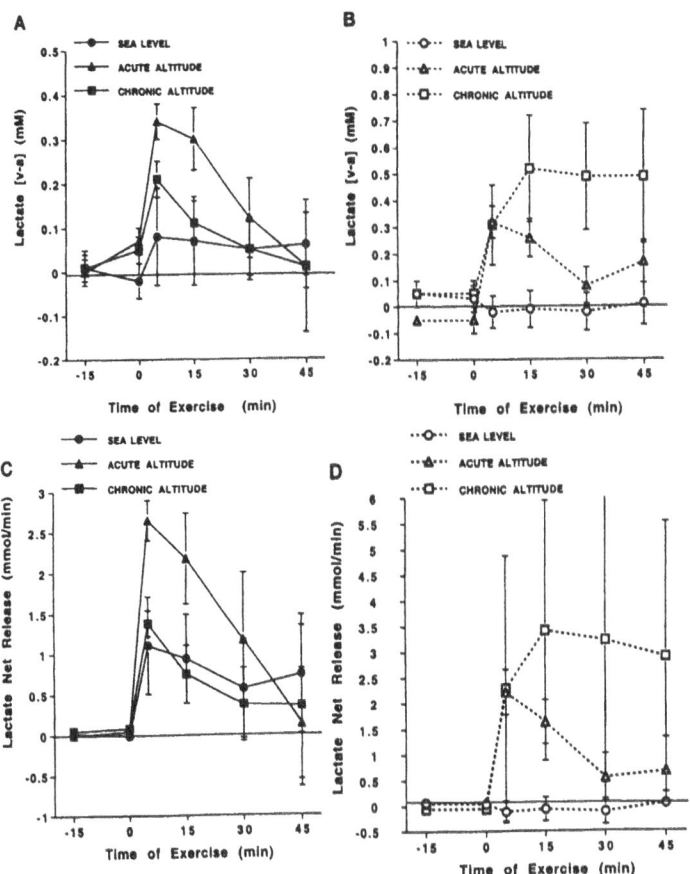

Figure 11. Mean (± SEM) leg net lactate venous-arterial concentration differences at rest and over time during exercise at sea level, upon acute exposure to 4,300 m altitude, and after a 3-wk acclimatization period: (A) control (n = 5), and (B) β-blocked subjects (n = 6). Corresponding mean (± SEM) net lactate release from the two legs over time during rest and exercise time in the same: (C) control, and (D) β -blocked subjects. From Brooks et al. (6).

Figure 12 portrays lactate extraction by leg muscles of men during rest and altitude at sea level, upon acute exposure to 4,300 m, and after a 3-week acclimatization period (9). The values were calculated from the decrease in tracer ([3-^{13}C]lactate) mass across limbs. Not shown is that during exercise extraction equaled oxidation (i.e., the rise in $^{13}CO_2$ equaled the decrease in ^{13}C-lactate). As shown in Figure 12, lactate extraction and oxidation are directly related to arterial lactate concentration. Thus, greatest lactate extraction and oxidation rates were observed upon acute altitude exposure when the arterial lactate concentration was highest.

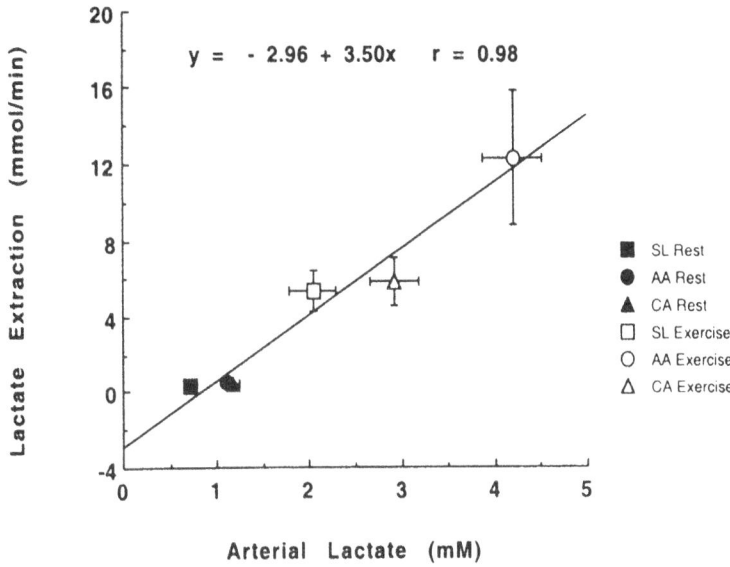

Figure 12. Leg blood lactate extraction as a function of arterial lactate concentration during rest (closed symbols) and leg cycling exercise (open symbols) at sea level (squares), upon acute exposure to 4,300 m altitude (circles), and after 3-wk acclimatization (triangles). Each point n = 6-7, mean ± SEM. Lactate extraction is highly correlated with arterial concentration. From Brooks et al. (13).

Although the results portrayed in Figure 12 are unique to men working at altitude, they are not unique in nature. With canine muscle preparations made to contract *in situ*, Gladden and associates (23) showed that by raising the arterial [lactate], working muscle switches from net release to uptake. Similarly, by adding arm to leg exercise (arm exercise raises the arterial [lactate]), Richter et al. (35) showed that leg muscle switches from net release to uptake. Thus, based on either chemical balance (Figures 3 and 9), or isotope tracers (Figure 12), muscle is capable of lactate exchange and oxidation.

9.   RESOLUTION OF QUESTIONS:

The Cell-Cell and Intramuscular Lactate Shuttle Concepts may be of assistance in understanding several phenomena observed in men exercising at altitude. Such phenomena of interest include: elevated arterial lactate levels, response of circulating lactate concentration to β-blockade, temporal variation in lactate [v-a] and net release, and simultaneous lactate release, extraction and oxidation by working muscle beds. The Lactate Shuttle Concepts accommodate all of these phenomena.

Arterial [lactate] is elevated at altitude because lactate Ra (production) is increased. However, it is clear working muscle is not the sole contributor to the circulating lactate load. Non-working muscle, skin, adipose and liver are all candidates as contributors to the circulating lactate load during exercise at altitude. Lactate production in non-contracting tissues appears to be under β-adrenergic control.

Lactate production is increased at altitude because glycolysis is stimulated. This stimulation occurs transiently in working muscle, but persists elsewhere in the body.

Working human muscle displays a "Stainsby Effect" during exercise at altitude. The start of contractions results in net lactate release followed the fall of lactate [v-a] and net release to zero. However, measurements of working limb (muscle) lactate concentration differences are inadequate to reveal active intramuscular production and oxidation.

Working skeletal muscle can consume and oxidize lactate at altitude. Further, working muscle lactate extraction and oxidation depend on the arterial lactate concentration. Because lactate extraction and oxidation are related to arterial [lactate], the greatest intramuscular lactate oxidation is observed during exercise upon acute altitude exposure.

It is now known that muscle possesses at least two MCT isoforms that facilitate sarcolemmal exchange of lactate; these are MCT1 and MCT4. The effects of chronic hypoxia on expression of these lactate transport proteins is unknown. However, the model (Figure 4) indicates a major role of sarcolemmal lactate transporters at altitude. Probably, MCT1 is present in mitochondria and sarcolemmal membranes whereas MCT4 is the constitutive muscle cell membrane isoform.

In addition to skeletal muscle, numerous other cells and tissues (erythrocytes, heart, liver, kidneys, brain, testes) express lactate transporter isoforms. Again, the effects of hypoxia are unknown.

Intra-myocyte, -hepatocyte, and -cardiocyte lactate oxidation depends on the presence of mitochondrial lactate-pyruvate transporter. When cytosolic [lactate] is high, lactate enters mitochondria where it is oxidized. Apparently, lactate oxidation in muscle is facilitated by high mitochondrial density and oxygen consumption rates.

Intra-myocyte, -hepatocyte, and -cardiocyte lactate oxidation depends on the presence of mitochondrial LDH. In mitochondria, LDH probably exists in the inter-membrane space as well as on the inner membrane. Mitochondrial LDH is essential for the oxidation of lactate.

10.   CONCLUSION

The Cell-Cell and Intramuscular Lactate Shuttle Concepts appear be of assistance in understanding several phenomena observed in men exercising at altitude. Further work is needed to evaluate the effects of hypoxia on expression of mitochondrial and extra-mitochondrial lactate transporters and lactate dehydrogenase isoforms.

ACKNOWLEDGEMENT

Supported by NIH grants DK19577 and AR 42906.

REFERENCES

1. Baldwin, K.M., P.J. Campbell, and D.A. Cooke. Glycogen, lactate and alanine changes in muscle during graded exercise. *J. Appl. Physiol.* 43:288-291, 1977.
2. Baldwin, K.M., A.M. Hooker, and R.E. Herrick. Lactate oxidative capacity in different types of muscle. *Biochem. Biophys. Res. Comm.* 83:151-157, 1978.
3. Barnard, R., V.R. Edgerton, T. Furukawa, and J.B. Peter. Histochemical, biochemical and contractile properties of red, white, and intermediate fibers. *Am. J. Physiol.* 220:410-414, 1971.
4. Brooks, G.A. Lactate: Glycolytic product and oxidative substrate during sustained exercise in mammals--the "lactate shuttle," In: *Comparative Physiology and Biochemistry* - Current Topics and Trends, Volume A, Respiration - Metabolism - Circulation, R. Gilles (Ed.), Berlin, Springer-Verlag, 1985, pp. 208-218.
5. Brooks, G.A. Current concepts in lactate exchange. *Med. Sci. Sports Exerc.* 23:895-906, 1991.
6. Brooks, G.A. Mammalian Fuel Utilization During Sustained Exercise. *Comp. Biochem. Physiol.* 120:89-107, 1998.
7. Brooks, G.A, H. Dubouchaud, M. Brown, J. P. Sicurello, and C.E. Butz. Role of mitochondrial lactic dehydrogenase and lactate oxidation in the 'intra-cellular lactate shuttle.' *Proc. Natl. Acad. Sci.* USA 96:1129-1134, 1999.
8. Brooks, G.A., G.E. Butterfield, R.R. Wolfe, B.M. Groves, R.S. Mazzeo, J.R. Sutton, E.E. Wolfel, and J.T. Reeves. Increased dependence on blood glucose after acclimatization to 4,300m. *J. Appl. Physiol.* 70:919-927, 1991.
9. Brooks, G.A., G.E. Butterfield, R.R. Wolfe, B.M. Groves, R.S. Mazzeo, J.R. Sutton, E.E. Wolfel, and J.T. Reeves. Decreased reliance on lactate during exercise after acclimatization to 4,300 m. *J .Appl .Physiol.* 71:333-341, 1991.
10. Brooks, G.A. and C.M. Donovan. Effect of training on glucose kinetics during exercise. *Am. J. Physiol.* 244 (Endocrinol. Metab. 7):E505-E512, 1983.
11. Brooks, G.A. and G.A. Gaesser. End points of lactate and glucose metabolism after exhausting exercise. *J. Appl. Physiol.* 49:1057-1069, 1980.
12. Brooks, G.A., E. E. Wolfel, G. E. Butterfield, A. Cymerman, A.C. Roberts, R.S. Mazzeo, and J.T. Reeves. Poor relationship between arterial [lactate] and leg net release during

steady-rate exercise at 4,300 m altitude. *Am. J. Physiol.* 275 (Regulatory Integrative and Comparative Physiol. 44): R1192-1201, 1998.

13. Brooks, G.A. E.E. Wolfel, B.M. Groves, P.R. Bender, G.E. Butterfield, A. Cymerman, R.S. Mazzeo, J.R. Sutton, R.R. Wolfe, and J.T. Reeves. Muscle accounts for glucose disposal but not blood lactate appearance during exercise after acclimatization to 4,300 m. *J. Appl .Physiol.* 72:2435-2445, 1992.

14. Connett, R.J., T.E.J. Gayeski, and C.R. Honig. Lactate accumulation in fully aerobic, working, dog gracilis muscle. *Am. J. Physiol.* 246:H120-H128, 1984.

15. Connett, R.J., C.R. Honig, T.E.J. Gayeski, and G.A. Brooks. Defining hypoxia: a systems view of VO2, glycolysis, energetics and intracellular PO2. *J. Appl. Physiol.* 68:833-842, 1990.

16. Depocas, F., Y. Minaire, and J. Chatonnet. Rates of formation and oxidation of lactic acid in dogs at rest and during moderate exercise. *Can. J. Physiol. Pharmacol.* 47:603-610, 1969.

17. Donovan, C.M. and G.A. Brooks. Endurance training affects lactate clearance, not lactate production. *Am. J. Physiol.* 244 (Endocrinol. Metab. 7) 244:E83-E92, 1983.

18. Edwards, H.T. Lactic acid at rest and work at high altitudes. *Am. J. Physiol.* 116:367-375, 1936.

19. Faintrenie, G. and A. Géloën. Alpha-1 adrenergic regulation of lactate production in white adipocytes. *J. Pharmacol. and Experimental Therapeutics.* 277:235-238, 1995.

20. Garcia, C. K., M.S. Brown, R.K. Pathak, and J.L. Goldstein. cDNA cloning of MCT2, a second monocarboxylate transporter expressed in different cells than MCT1. *J. Biol. Chem.* 270: 1843-1849, 1995.

21. Garcia, C. K., J.L. Goldstein, R.K. Pathak, R.G. Anderson, and M.S. Brown. Molecular characterization of a membrane transporter for lactate, pyruvate and other monocarboxylates: implications for the Cori cycle. *Cell* 76: 865-873, 1994.

22. Gertz, E.W., J.A. Wisneski, W.C. Stanley, and R.A. Neese. Myocardial substrate utilization during exercise in humans. Dual carbon-labeled carbohydrate isotope experiments. *J. Clin. Invest.* 82:2017-2025, 1988.

23. Gladden, L.B., R.E. Crawford, and M.J Webster. Effect of lactate concentration and metabolic rate on net lactate uptake by canine skeletal muscle. *Am. J. Physiol.* 266:R1095-101, 1994.

24. Hochachka, P.W. The lactate paradox: analysis of underlying mechanisms. *Ann. Sports Med.* 4:184-188, 1989.

25. Jöbsis F.F. and W. N. Stainsby. Oxidation of NADH during contractions of circulated skeletal muscle. *Resp. Physiol.* 4:292-300, 1968.

26. Johnson, J.A. and R.M. Fusaro. The role of skin in carbohydrate metabolism. *Adv. Metab. Disord.* 6:1-55, 1972.

27. Kayser, B. Lactate during exercise at high altitude. *Eur. J. Appl. Physiol.* 74: 195-205, 1996.

28. Kim, C.M., J.L. Goldstein, and M.S. Brown. cDNA cloning of MEV, a mutant protein that facilitates cellular uptake of mevalonate, and identification of the point mutation responsible for its gain of function. *J. Biol. Chem.* 267: 23113-23121, 1992.

29. Kopperschlager G. and Kirchberger J. Methods for the separation of lactate dehydrogenases and clinical significance of the enzyme. *J. Chromat. B, Biomed. App.* 684:25-49, 1996.

30. Mazzeo, R.S., G.A. Brooks, D.A. Schoeller and T.F. Budinger. Disposal of [1-13C]lactate during rest and exercise. *J. Appl. Physiol.* 60:232-241, 1986.

31. Molé, P.A., P.A. VanHandel, and W.R. Sandel. Extra O2 consumption attributable to NADH2 during maximum lactate oxidation in the heart. *Biochem. Biophys. Res. Comm.* 85:1143-1149, 1978.

32. Philp, N., P. Chu, T-C. Pan, R.Z. Zhng, M-L. Chu, K. Stark, D. Boettinger, H. Yoon, and T. Kieber-Emmons. Developmental expression and molecular cloning of REMP, a novel membrane protein. *Exp. Cell Res.* 219: 64-73, 1995.

33. Price, N. T., V.N. Jackson, and A.P. Halestrap. Cloning and sequencing of four new mammalian monocarboxylate transporter (MCT) homologues confirms the existence of transporter family with an ancient past. *Biochem. J.* 329: 321-328, 1998.

34. Reeves. J.T., E.E. Wolfel, H.J. Green, R.S. Mazzeo, A.J. Young, J.R. Sutton, and G.A. Brooks. Oxygen transport during exercise at high altitude and the lactate paradox: lessons from Operation Everest II and Pikes Peak. In: *Exercise and Sports Sciences Reviews.* K.B. Pandolf (Ed.), Vol. 20, Williams and Wikins, 1992, pp. 275-296.

35. Richter, E.A., B. Kiens, B. Saltin, N.J. Christensen, and G. Savard. Skeletal muscle glucose uptake during dynamic exercise in humans: role of muscle mass. *Am. J. Physiol.* 254:E555-E561, 1988.

36. Roberts, A.C., G.E. Butterfield, J.T. Reeves, A. Cymerman, E.E. Wolfel, and G.A. Brooks. Altitude and ß-blockade augment glucose utilization during submaximal exercise. *J. Appl. Physiol.* 80:606-615, 1996.

37. Roberts, A.C., G.E. Butterfield, A. Cymerman, J.T. Reeves, E.E. Wolfel, and G.A. Brooks. Acclimatization to 4,300 m altitude decreases reliance on fat as a substrate. *J. Appl. Physiol.* 81:1762-1771, 1996.

38. Roth, D.A. and G.A. Brooks. Lactate and pyruvate transport is dominated using a pH gradient-sensitive carrier in rat skeletal muscle sarcolemmal vesicles. *Arch. of Biochem. Biophys.* 279:386-394, 1990.

39. Roth, D.A. and G.A. Brooks. Lactate transport is mediated by a membrane-borne carrier in rat skeletal muscle sarcolemmal vesicles. *Arch. of Biochem. Biophys.* 279:377-385, 1990.

40. Stainsby, W.N. and G.A. Brooks. Control of lactic acid metabolism in contracting muscles and during exercise. In: *Exercise and Sport Sciences Reviews.* K.B. Pandolf and J.O. Holloszy (Eds.). Baltimore: Williams and Wilkins, 1990, pp. 29-63.

41. Stanley, W.C., E.W. Gertz, J.A. Wisneski, D.L. Morris, R. Neese, and G.A. Brooks. Systemic lactate turnover during graded exercise in man. *Am. J. Physiol.* (Endocrinol. Metab. 12). 249:E595-E602, 1985.

42. Stanley, W.C., E.W. Gertz, J.A. Wisneski, D.L. Morris, R. Neese, and G.A. Brooks. Lactate metabolism in exercising human skeletal muscle: Evidence for lactate extraction during net lactate release. *J. Appl. Physiol.* 60:1116-1120, 1986.

43. Stanley, W.C., J.A. Wisneski, E.W. Gertz, R.A. Neese, and G.A. Brooks. Glucose and lactate interrelations during moderate intensity exercise in man. Metabolism 37:850-858, 1988.

44. Wasserman, D.H., D.B. Lacey, D.R. Green, P.E. Williams, and A.D. Cherrington. Dynamics of hepatic lactate and glucose balances during prolonged exercise and recovery in the dog. *J. Appl. Physiol.* 63:2411-2417, 1987.

45. Welch, H.G. and W.N. Stainsby. Oxygen debt in contracting dog skeletal muscle in situ. *Resp. Physiol.* 3:229-242, 1967.

46. Wilson, M.C., V.N. Jackson, C. Heddle, N.T. Price, H. Pilegaard, C. Juel, A. Bonen, I. Montgomery, O.F. Hutter, and A.P. Halestrap. Lactic acid efflux from white skeletal muscle is catalyzed by the monocarboxylate transporter isoform MCT3. *J. Biol. Chem.* 273:15920-15926, 1998.

47. Wolfel, E.E., B.M. Groves, G.A. Brooks, G.E. Butterfield, R.S. Mazzeo, L.G. Moore, J.R. Sutton, P.R. Bender, T.E. Dahms, R.E. McCullough, R.G. McCullough, S.-Y. Huang, S.-F. Sun, R.F. Grover, H.N. Hultgren, and J.T. Reeves. Oxygen transport during steady-state submaximal exercise in chronic hypoxia. *J. Appl. Physiol.* 70:1129-1136, 1991.

48. Yoon, H., A. Fanelli, E. F. Grollman, and N. J. Philp. Identification of a unique monocarboxylate transporter (MCT3) in retinal pigment epithelium. *Biochem. Biophys. Res. Comm.* 234: 90-94, 1997.

49. Zinker, B.A., R.D. Wilson, and D.H. Wasserman. Interaction of decreased arterial PO_2 and exercise on carbohydrate metabolism in the dog. *Am. J. Physiol.* 269:E409-417, 1995.

Chapter 17

Role of Pyruvate Dehydrogenase in Lactate Production in Exercising Human Skeletal Muscle

George J.F. Heigenhauser and Michelle L. Parolin
Department of Medicine, McMaster University, Hamilton, Ontario L8N 3Z5, Canada

Key words: glycogen, glycogen phosphorylase, oxidative phosphorylation, phosphocreatine

Abstract: The mechanisms responsible for lactate production with increased intensity of muscle contraction are controversial. Some investigators suggest that the mitochondria are O_2-limited, whereas others suggest that lactate production occurs when O_2 to the mitochondria is adequate and that the increased lactate production is due to a "mass-action effect" when pyruvate production exceeds the rate of pyruvate oxidation. Pyruvate dehydrogenase is a rate-limiting enzyme for pyruvate entry into the tricarboxylic acid cycle; its catalytic activity influences both pyruvate oxidation and lactate production. Since lactate dehydrogenase is an equilibrium enzyme, increased lactate production will be due to a mass-action effect exerted by increases in pyruvate concentrations. Because the equilibrium constant of the lactate dehydrogenase reaction markedly favors lactate over pyruvate, small increases in pyruvate concentration will result in large increases in lactate concentration. At higher exercise intensities, which are more reliant on glycogen as substrate, the rate of pyruvate production exceeds the catalytic activity of pyruvate dehydrogenase, and lactate production occurs. Studies using dichloroacetate, induced acid-base changes, diet and short-term endurance training, indicate that lactate production is related to complex interactions of metabolic pathways and not related to inadequate O_2 supply. As pyruvate dehydrogenase plays a central role in the integration of carbohydrate and fat metabolism, and in the entry of pyruvate into the tricarboxylic acid cycle, this enzyme plays a key role in lactate production.

1.   INTRODUCTION

Classic studies (7) have shown that with increased intensity of exercise there is an increase in lactate production. The mechanism of lactate production with increasing exercise intensity is controversial. Some investigators suggest that the mitochondria are oxygen-limited, whereas others suggest that lactate production occurs when oxygen to the mitochondria is adequate.

Classically, lactate production during high intensity exercise has been attributed to an increased rate of glycolysis due to limited oxygen supply. The limitation of oxygen has been thought to result in substrate limitation at cytochrome oxidase, which in turn leads to an accumulation of NADH and ADP. In support of this concept is the measurement of whole cell NADH and NAD^+ (27,28), which suggests that the mitochondria become more reduced with increases in exercise intensity. Similarly, measurement of the pyruvate/lactate in both muscle and blood also suggest that the mitochondria become more reduced (5). However, the conclusions of these studies must be viewed with caution, since these methods estimate the redox state of the whole muscle, and do not reflect the mitochondrial redox state or availability of oxygen at the mitochondria. There is evidence that the K_m of oxygen of the mitochondria is extremely low (0.5 Torr), and that the mitochondrial oxygen availability remains above this critical level (3).

Recently, investigators have suggested that oxygen is not limiting during exercise in normoxia, and that lactate production is simply due to a reduced energy state of the exercising muscle. The mechanism for lactate production is simply due to a "mass-action effect" when the rate of pyruvate production is greater than its rate of oxidation. Studies using direct measurements of redox state of the mitochondria by surface fluorometry (19), indirect estimates of the mitochondrial redox state by the glutamate dehydrogenase reaction (10) and measurements of myoglobin saturation by cryospectrophotometry (4), suggest that mitochondrial oxygen is not limiting and that the mitochondria become more oxidized when lactate is produced in exercising muscle.

This controversy regarding whether the mitochondria is oxygen-limited cannot be presently resolved since the partial pressure of oxygen and the redox state cannot be measured or estimated reliably (14). It should be recognized that the mechanisms responsible for lactate production are complex and appear to be multifactorial. Although acute hypoxia has been shown to increase lactate production during exercise, studies using induced acid-base changes (13,19,20,30,31), diet (26), and short-term endurance training (2,11,12,23) all indicate that lactate production is the result of complex interactions between metabolic pathways and not related to inadequate oxygen supply alone.

In human skeletal muscle, the range of ATP turnover rates can vary 100-fold from rest to maximal exercise (38,39). Because the available ATP pool in muscle is small, the rate of ATP resynthesis must closely balance demand or ATP stores would be rapidly depleted. Tight coupling of metabolic pathways is required to allow ATP supply to respond to changes in ATP demand as exercise intensity increases. However, Newsholme (21) has pointed out that the large change in flux rates in a given metabolic pathway and the integration of flux rates between several metabolic pathways cannot be dependent upon mass-action regulated (equilibrium) enzymes. These conclusions were based on the observation that the small changes in substrates and products, such as ADP, inorganic phosphate (P_i), H^+, NADH, and NAD^+, cannot account for the large changes in ATP turnover rates, sustained by glycolysis and oxidative phosphorylation, as observed in human skeletal muscle. In addition, the changes in the glycolytic intermediates (25) and tricarboxylic acid cycle intermediates (9,29) increase by only 3-5 fold, compared with resting conditions, much less than implied by the large changes in ATP turnover rate.

Large changes in flux can be achieved by activation or deactivation of regulatory (or non-equilibrium) enzymes, whose catalytic rates are controlled allosterically. To control the overall rate and direction of the metabolic pathway, these enzymes must have the lowest catalytic rate in the metabolic pathway, and the reactions must be irreversible. Since these enzymes are always saturated with their substrates, large changes in pathway flux can occur with only small changes in substrate concentration.

Glycogen phosphorylase and pyruvate dehydrogenase are both flux-regulatory enzymes whose catalytic rates are important in lactate production (Fig. 1). Phosphorylase regulates the overall flux through glycolysis. Pyruvate dehydrogenase initiates and regulates the irreversible flux of pyruvate into the tricarboxylic acid cycle, not only regulating carbohydrate oxidation, but also determining the maximal rate of tricarboxylic acid cycle activity (1). Since pyruvate is also the substrate for the equilibrium enzyme lactate dehydrogenase, the activity of the pyruvate dehydrogenase complex determines the rate of lactate production when glycolytic flux exceeds the rate of pyruvate entering the tricarboxylic acid cycle (25).

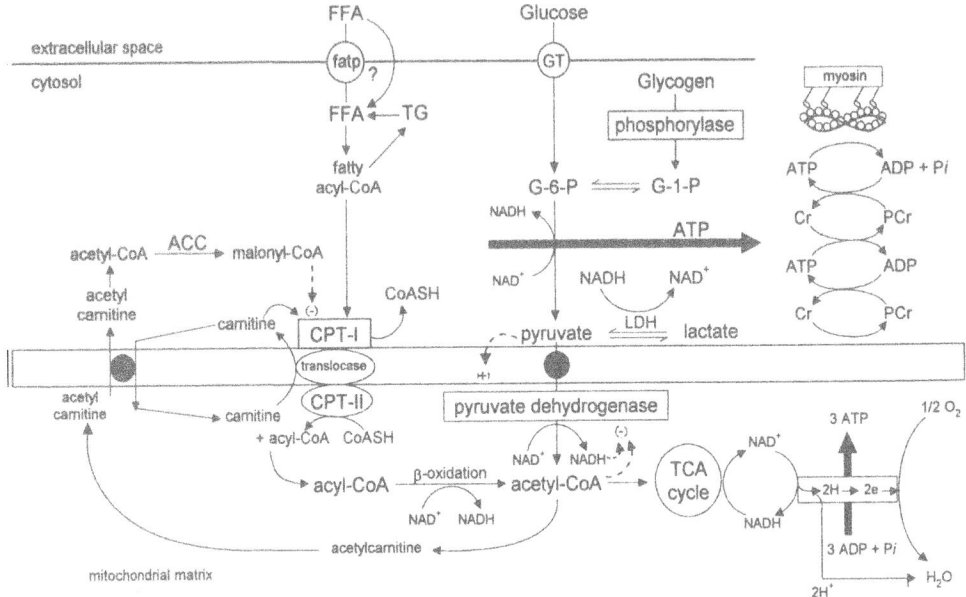

Figure 1. Schematic diagram of fat and carbohydrate metabolic pathways. Some intermediates have been eliminated for clarity. GT, glucose transporter; fatp, fatty acid transport protein; G-6-P, glucose-6-phosphate; G-1-P, glucose-1-phosphate; TCA cycle, tricarboxylic acid cycle; ACC, acteyl CoA carboxylase; CPT, carnitine palmitoyl transferase; TG, tiacylglycerol; ETC, electron transport chain.

Glycogen phosphorylase (Fig. 2) catalyzes the first step in the glycolytic pathway: $(Glycogen)_n + P_i^{2-} \rightarrow (Glycogen)_{n-1} + Glucose-1-Phosphate$

It exists as two interconvertible forms: an active **a** form and a less active **b** form. Phosphorylase **b** is allosterically activated by AMP and IMP, and inhibited by ATP and glucose-6-phosphate. In response to Ca^{2+} and epinephrine, phosphorylase **b** is phosphorylated to phosphorylase **a** by phosphorylase kinase as part of a cascade system initiated by 3'-5' cyclic AMP. Phosphorylase **a** is not dependent on AMP. Dephosphorylation, converting phosphorylase **a** to phosphorylase **b**, is catalyzed by phosphorylase phosphatase. Increases in the availability of substrates, P_i and glycogen increase the activity of phosphorylase **a** and phosphorylase **b**. AMP lowers the K_m of P_i for phosphorylase **a** (See (17) for review).

During exercise glycogen phosphorylase appears to be regulated by a two-step process. The initial step is the transformation of phosphorylase by Ca^{2+} from the less active **b** to its more active **a** form. This initial step appears to be a gross control mechanism which determines the upper limits of glycogenolytic flux. The second step finely tunes glycolytic flux to the ATP demands via regulators linked to the energy state of the cytoplasm. In this step post-transformational control of the active **a** form occurs by increased availability of its substrate, P_i, and by allosteric regulation of AMP.

Pyruvate dehydrogenase (Fig. 3) is a multi-enzyme complex located in the inner matrix of mitochondria; it catalyzes the non-reversible oxidative decarboxylation of pyruvate with conversion of coenzyme A (CoASH) to acetylCoA: Pyruvate + NAD^+ + CoASH → AcetylCoA + NADH + H^+ + CO_2

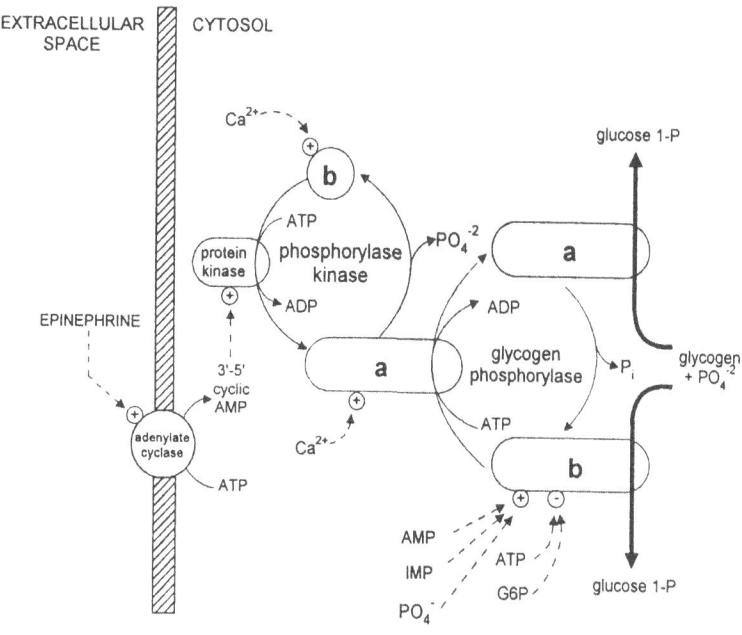

Figure 2. Schematic diagram of glycogen phosphorylase regulation.

The reaction is catalyzed sequentially by a complex of three enzymes: E1 (pyruvate dehydrogenase), E2 (lipoate acetyltransferase) and E3 (dihydrolipoyl dehydrogenase), and is regulated by both end-product inhibition (acetylCoA and NADH) and by reversible covalent modification (phosphorylation-dephosphorylation). The pyruvate dehydrogenase complex exists in two interconvertible forms, active dephosphorylated (**a** form) and inactive phosphorylated (**b** form). Phosphorylation with concomitant inactivation is catalyzed by an ATP-specific kinase tightly bound to the pyruvate dehydrogenase complex. Dephosphorylation with activation is catalyzed by a loosely bound phosphatase. Both kinase and phosphatase require Mg^{2+}. Kinase activity is stimulated by acetyl CoA, NADH and ATP, and inhibited by ADP, CoASH, NAD^+ and pyruvate. Phosphatase activity is stimulated by Ca^{2+} and insulin, and inhibited by NADH (see (6,8,32) for review).

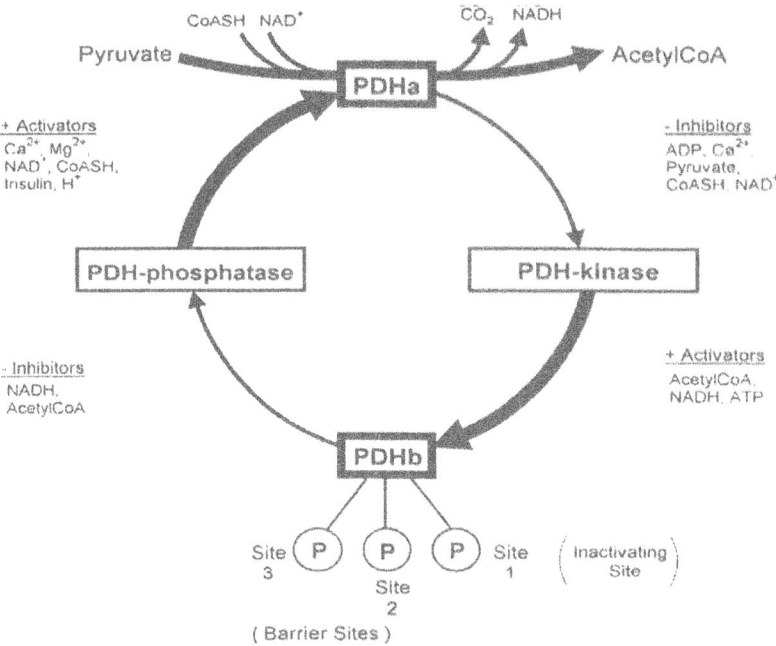

Figure 3. Schematic diagram of pyruvate dehydrogenase regulation.

When pyruvate dehydrogenase flux is estimated in exercising skeletal muscle, it corresponds closely with the catalytic rate of the active **a** form (26). However, the regulation of the transformation of pyruvate dehydrogenase to its active form is complex and not well understood in exercising skeletal muscle. Similar to glycogen phosphorylase, the transformation of pyruvate dehydrogenase to its active form is a two-step process. The initial step and primary stimulus for transformation appears to be release of Ca^{2+} at the onset of exercise. The remaining activation of pyruvate dehydrogenase during exercise appears to be related to the energy status (ATP/ADP), the redox state (NADH/NAD$^+$) and substrate availability (pyruvate). Although acetyl CoA/CoASH appears to play a regulatory role in resting skeletal muscle, its role in contracting skeletal muscle appears to be minor (26).

2.   ROLE OF PYRUVATE DEHYDROGENASE IN LACTATE PRODUCTION

Our laboratory (15,16,22,24) and others (14,33,35-37) have suggested that the rate of lactate production is determined by the balance between pyruvate production and pyruvate oxidation. Pyruvate dehydrogenase is the rate-limiting enzyme for pyruvate entry into the tricarboxylic acid cycle; therefore, its activity influences both pyruvate oxidation and lactate production. Since lactate dehydrogenase is an equilibrium enzyme, increased lactate production will be due to a mass action effect exerted by increases in the [pyruvate] and [NADH]. Because the equilibrium constant of the lactate dehydrogenase reaction markedly favors lactate over pyruvate, small increases in the [pyruvate] and [NADH] will result in large increases in [lactate]. At lower exercise (<40% maximum oxygen uptake) intensities, pyruvate production is equal to pyruvate oxidation, and NADH is transported into the mitochondria at the same rate as it is produced by the glycerol-3-phosphate dehydrogenase reaction;` thus [lactate] and [pyruvate] do not increase above resting values. At moderate exercise intensities (~60% maximum oxygen uptake), pyruvate production exceeds pyruvate oxidation even though pyruvate dehydrogenase is not fully activated, and all NADH appears to be transported into the mitochondria at the same rate it is produced; thus small increases in [pyruvate] will result in larger increases in lactate accumulation. At higher exercise intensities (>90% maximum oxygen uptake) there is a greater reliance on glycogen as substrate, pyruvate production exceeds its rate of oxidation and the rate of NADH production exceeds the rate that it is transported into the mitochondria. This results in an increase in NAD^+ and lactate production. The NAD^+ would then be utilized in the glycerol-3-phosphate dehydrogenase reaction to maintain glycolytic flux. Thus, as exercise intensities increase, the rate of pyruvate production exceeds its rate of oxidation, and both NADH and pyruvate accumulation result in increased lactate production.

The importance of pyruvate dehydrogenase in pyruvate oxidation or reduction is appreciated if the difference in ATP synthesis by glycolysis and oxidative phosphorylation is taken into account. At a similar pyruvate production, an increase in pyruvate dehydrogenase flux in which pyruvate is fully oxidized rather than being reduced to lactate, will result in a 12-fold increase in ATP resynthesis. A decrease in pyruvate dehydrogenase flux of 0.5 mmol kg^{-1}·min^{-1} (wet weight) will result in an increase in lactate production of 26 mmol kg^{-1}·min^{-1} (dry weight). Thus, at high rates of ATP turnover, as in exercise, a small mismatch in which glycolytic flux exceeds pyruvate oxidation (pyruvate dehydrogenase flux) will result in a small increase in [pyruvate] but a large increase in [lactate].

During muscle contraction it is important that oxidative phosphorylation is rapidly activated to provide oxidative ATP production. The overall reaction of oxidative phosphorylation is:

$$3\ ADP^{3-} + 3\ P_i^{2-} + NADH + \tfrac{1}{2}\ O_2 + H^+ \rightarrow 3\ ATP^{4-} + NAD^+ + H_2O$$

Oxidative phosphorylation is a near-equilibrium reaction; therefore, the provision of substrate ADP, P_i, NADH and oxygen will increase the rate of oxidative phosphorylation. Increases in [ADP] and [P_i] occur when there is a transient mismatch between the rates of ATP utilization and its rate of resynthesis. To maintain [ATP], ATP is resynthesized by the phosphocreatine kinase and the adenylate deaminase reactions resulting in increases in [ADP] and [P_i]. As the intensity of exercise increases, the greater the mismatch becomes, resulting in greater [ADP] and [P_i], and hence, oxidative phosphorylation. Increased NADH is provided mainly from the dehydrogenase reactions in the tricarboxylic acid cycle. Although pyruvate dehydrogenase is not a mitochondrial enzyme, it regulates the flux through the tricarboxylic acid cycle, by controlling pyruvate entry into the mitochondria, thus supplying not only acetyl CoA to the tricarboxylic acid cycle, but also NADH, which can be directly utilized by the electron transport chain. Since mitochondrial partial pressure of oxygen is also a determinant of oxidative phosphorylation, the delivery of oxygen to the working muscle is important. Although the critical partial pressure of oxygen to maintain the maximum rate of oxidative phosphorylation is extremely low, there is controversy as to whether the partial pressure of oxygen is ever limiting.

Recently, our laboratory (16) investigated the activation of glycogen phosphorylase and pyruvate dehydrogenase in human subjects at three power outputs, 35%, 65% and 90% of their maximum oxygen uptake. The amount of glycogen phosphorylase (Fig. 4A) in the active **a** form (approximately 25%) was similar at all power outputs; however, the transformation of pyruvate dehydrogenase to its active **a** form (Fig. 4B) increased as a function of power output. At 35% of their maximum oxygen uptake, muscle lactate production (Fig. 5), phosphocreatine hydrolysis (Fig. 6A), and free P_i (Fig. 6B), free ADP (Fig. 6C), and free AMP (Fig. 6D) accumulation were unchanged from rest, but rose significantly at 65% and 90%, with the accumulation being higher at 90% of their maximum oxygen uptake. From this data, it appears that the transformation of glycogen phosphorylase to its active **a** form is necessary to maintain glycogenolysis during exercise; but the transformation to the active **a** form does not relate to the catalytic rate. The transformation to the active **a** form, occurs at the onset of exercise, due to the stimulation of phosphorylase a kinase by Ca^{2+} released from the sarcoplasmic reticulum. However, a second stage of control regulates the catalytic rate of glycogen phosphorylase by increasing substrate (P_i) and allosteric regulation by increases in AMP. In contrast to

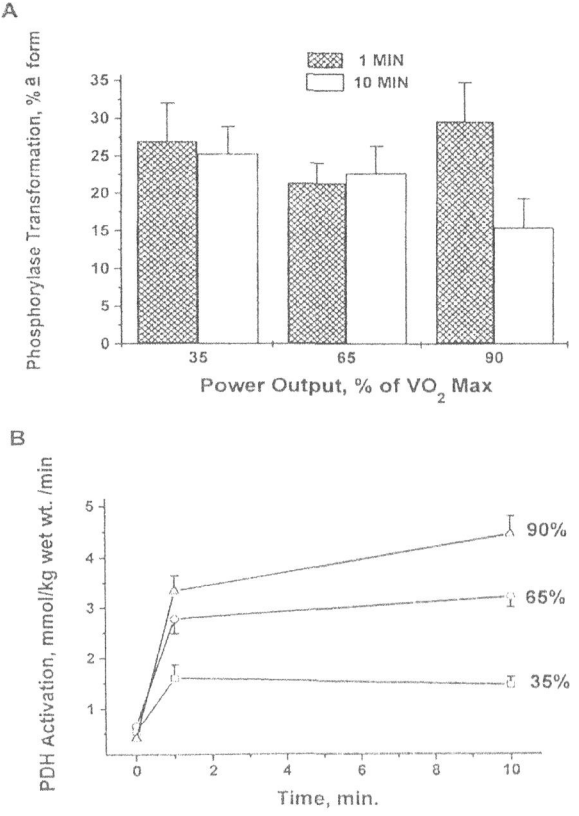

Figure 4. Glycogen phosphorylase (A) and pyruvate dehydrogenase (B) transformation during cycling at the various power outputs.

glycogen phosphorylase, the transformation of pyruvate dehydrogenase to its active **a** form increases as a function of exercise intensity, probably due to Ca^{2+} release from the sarcoplasmic reticulum and accumulation of [pyruvate], both of which are increasing with higher power outputs.

The increases in power output also require greater rates of ATP resynthesis from oxidative metabolism. As power output increases, a greater mismatch in ATP demand and supply occurs at the onset of exercise. At the lowest power output, only small changes occur in phosphocreatine hydrolysis. However, with increases in power output, there becomes a greater mismatch in ATP utilization and supply, resulting in greater phosphocreatine hydrolysis and accumulation of ADP, P_i and AMP. These changes not only initiate oxidative phosphorylation, but also activate glycogen phosphorylase and pyruvate dehydrogenase. The greater [ADP] and [P_i] will increase the flux through the active **a** form of glycogen phosphorylase, thus increasing glycogen breakdown and pyruvate production. The increase in [pyruvate] will increase the transformation of pyruvate dehydrogenase to its active *a* form, thus supplying acetyl CoA for the tricarboxylic acid cycle to maintain oxidative phosphorylation. Since lactate dehydrogenase is an equilibrium reaction, the increased [pyruvate] with increasing power output will result in a marked rise in lactate production. At 60% of maximum oxygen uptake, it is interesting to note, lactate production occurs despite the fact that pyruvate dehydrogenase is not fully transformed and could potentially support greater oxidation of pyruvate. At 90% maximum oxygen uptake, pyruvate dehydrogenase is fully activated and pyruvate production exceeds the rate of pyruvate oxidation, resulting in lactate production.

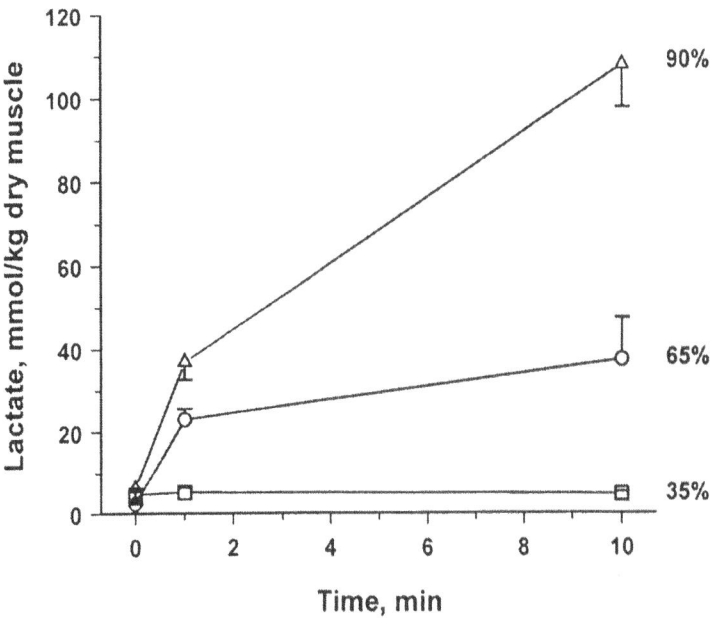

Figure 5. Muscle lactate content during cycling at various power outputs.

Timmons et al. (34,36,37) have suggested that the mismatch of ATP demand and ATP supply is not due to an oxygen limitation, but due to inadequate supply of substrate to the tricarboxylic acid cycle at the onset of exercise. A transient lag in pyruvate dehydrogenase transformation to the **a** form would limit substrate (acetyl CoA) to the tricarboxylic acid cycle and NADH to the electron transport chain. In a series of studies using an ischemic canine skeletal muscle model and an ischemic human leg model, these authors showed that activation of pyruvate dehydrogenase by

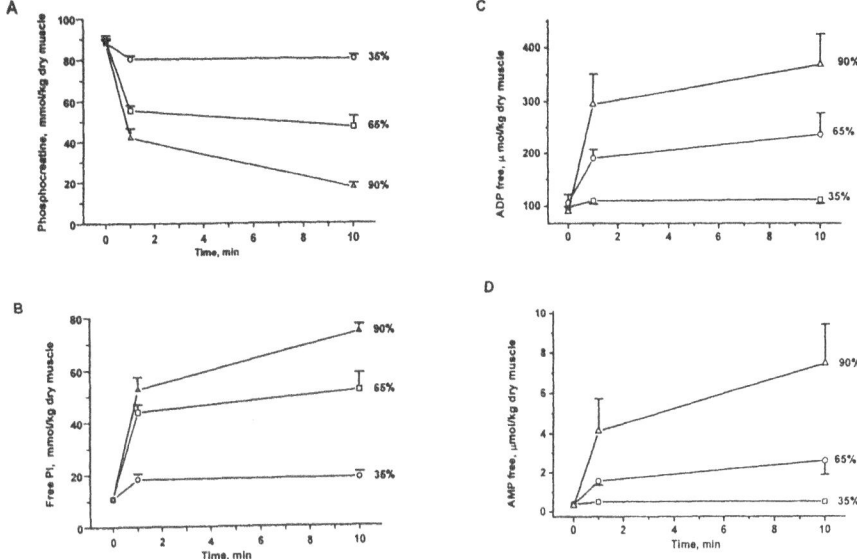

Figure 6. Muscle phosphocreatine (A), P_i (B), free ADP (C) and free AMP (D) contents during cycling at the various power outputs.

dichloroacetate prior to muscle contraction decreased phosphocreatine degradation, glycogen utilization and lactate production during muscle contraction. They concluded that even when oxygen delivery to contracting muscle is compromised, increased substrate delivery to the tricarboxylic acid cycle at the onset of muscle contraction decreases lactate production.

3. CONCLUSION

Until recently, the major cause of lactate production during exercise has been thought to be an oxygen limitation at the mitochondria. However, there has been a paradigm shift toward the mechanisms which integrate metabolic fuel utilization. Recent evidence suggests that the accumulation of lactate is primarily due to a "mass-action effect" and not due to an oxygen limitation. As glycogenolysis increases, pyruvate production exceeds its rate of oxidation by pyruvate dehydrogenase, and because of the near-equilibrium nature of lactate dehydrogenase, lactate is formed. Recent studies using dichloroacetate suggest that lactate production may be due to a limitation of oxidative substrate at the onset of exercise rather than an oxygen limitation at the mitochondria.

ACKNOWLEDGEMENTS

We would like to acknowledge the support of the operating grants to G.J.F Heigenhauser from the Medical Research Council and to L.L. Spriet from the Natural Sciences and Engineering Research Council of Canada. We would also like to acknowledge the contributions of N.L. Jones, L.L. Spriet, R.A. Howlett, C.T. Putman, and M.G. Hollidge-Horvat. M.L. Parolin was supported by a Natural Sciences and Engineering Research Council scholarship and by the Ontario Thoracic Society. G.J.F. Heigenhauser is a Career Investigator of the Heart and Stroke Foundation of Ontario.

REFERENCES

1. Balaban, R. S. Regulation of oxidative phosphorylation in the mammalian cell. *Am. J. Physiol.* 258: C377-C389, 1990.
2. Cadefau, J., H. J. Green, R. Cussó, M. Ball-Burnett, and G. Jamieson. Coupling of muscle phosphorylation potential to glycolysis during submaximal exercise of varying intensity after short-term training. *J. Appl. Physiol.* 76: 2586-2593, 1994.
3. Chance, B. and B. Quistorff. Study of tissue oxygen gradients by single and multiple indicators. *Adv. Exp. Med. Biol.* 94: 331-338, 1978.
4. Connett, R. J., T. E. J. Gayeski, and C. R. Honig. Lactate efflux is unrelated to intracellular PO_2 in a working red muscle in situ. *J. Appl. Physiol.* 61: 402-408, 1986.
5. Cooper, D. M., D. H. Wasserman, M. Vranic, and K. Wasserman. Glucose turnover in response to exercise during high- and low-FI_{O2} breathing in man. *Am. J. Physiol.* 251: E209-E214, 1986.
6. Denton, R. M., P. J. Randle, B. J. Bridges, R. H. Cooper, A. L. Kerbey, H. T. Pask, D. L. Severson, D. Stansbie, and S. Whitehouse. Regulation of mammalian pyruvate dehydrogenase. *Mol. Cell. Biochem.* 9: 27-53, 1975.
7. Dill, D. B. The economy of muscular exercise. *Physiol. Rev.* 16: 263-291, 1936.
8. Evans, O. B. Human muscle pyruvate dehydrogenase activity. *Neurology* 33: 51-56, 1983.
9. Gibala, M. J., D. A. MacLean, T. E. Graham, and B. Saltin. Tricarboxylic acid cycle intermediate pool size and estimated cycle flux in human muscle during exercise. *Am J Physiol* 275: E235-E242, 1998.
10. Graham, T. E. Mitochondrial redox state in skeletal muscle cannot be estimated with glutamate dehydrogenase system. *Am. J. Physiol.* 254: C588-C590, 1988.
11. Green, H., R. Helyar, M. Ball-Burnett, N. Kowalchuk, S. Symon, and B. Farrance. Metabolic adaptations to training precede changes in muscle mitochondrial capacity. *J. Appl. Physiol.* 72: 484-491, 1992.
12. Green, H. J., S. Jones, M. E. Ball-Burnett, D. Smith, J. Livesey, and B. W. Farrance. Early muscular and metabolic adaptations to prolonged exercise training in man. *J. Appl. Physiol.* 70: 2032-2038, 1991.
13. Heigenhauser, G. J. F. and N. L. Jones. Bicarbonate loading. In: *Ergogenics - Enhancement of Performance in Exercise and Sport*, edited by D. R. Lamb and M. H. Williams. Carmel,IN: W.C.B. Brown and Benchmark, 1991, p. 183-212.
14. Heinrich, R., S. Schuster, and H. G. Holzhutter. Mathematical analysis of enzymic reaction systems using optimization principles. *Eur. J. Biochem.* 201: 1-21, 1991.

15. Howlett, R. A., G. J. F. Heigenhauser, E. Hultman, M. G. Hollidge-Horvat, and L. L. Spriet. Effects of dichloroacetate infusion on human skeletal muscle metabolism at the onset of exercise. *Am J Physiol* 1998.

16. Howlett, R. A., L. M. Parolin, D. J. Dyck, E. Hultman, N. L. Jones, G. J. F. Heigenhauser, and L. L. Spriet. Regulation of skeletal muscle glycogen phosphorylase and pyruvate dehydrogenase at different exercise power outputs. *Am. J. Physiol.* 275: R418-R425, 1998.

17. Johnson, L. N. Glycogen phosphorylase: control by phosphorylation and allosteric effects. *FASEB J.* 6: 2274-2282, 1992.

18. Jöbsis, F. F. and W. N. Stainsby. Oxidation of NADH during contractions of circulated mammalian skeletal muscle. *Respir. Physiol.* 4: 292-300, 1968.

19. Jones, N. L. and G. J. F. Heigenhauser. Effects of hydrogen ions on metabolism during exercise. In: *Energy Metabolism in Exercise and Sport*, edited by D. R. Lamb and C. V. Gisolfi. Dubuque,IA: W.C.Brown and Benchmark, 1992, p. 107-148.

20. Jones, N. L., J. R. Sutton, R. Taylor, and C. J. Toews. Effect of pH on cardiorespiratory and metabolic responses to exercise. *J. Appl. Physiol.* 43: 959-964, 1977.

21. Newsholme, E. A. and B. Crabtree. Theoretical principles in the approaches to control of metabolic pathways and their application to glycolysis in muscle. *J. Mol. Cell. Cardiol.* 11: 839-856, 1979.

22. Parolin, M. L., A. Chesley, M. P. Matsos, L. L. Spriet, N. L. Jones, and G. J. F. Heigenhauser. Regulation of human skeletal muscle phosphorylase and pyruvate dehydrogenase during maximal intermittent exercise. *Am J Physiol* submitted for pub. 1998.

23. Phillips, S. M., H. J. Green, M. A. Tarnopolsky, and S. M. Grant. Increased clearance of lactate after short-term training in men. *J. Appl. Physiol.* 79: 1862-1869, 1995.

24. Putman, C. T., N. L. Jones, E. Hultman, M. G. Hollidge-Horvat, A. Bonen, D. R. McConachie, and G. J. F. Heigenhauser. Effects of short-term submaximal training in humans on muscle metabolism in exercise. *Am. J. Physiol.* 275: E132-E135, 1998.

25. Putman, C. T., N. L. Jones, L. C. Lands, T. M. Bragg, M. G. Hollidge-Horvat, and G. J. F. Heigenhauser. Skeletal muscle pyruvate dehydrogenase activity during maximal exercise in humans. *Am. J. Physiol.* 269: E458-E468, 1995.

26. Putman, C. T., L. L. Spriet, E. Hultman, M. I. Lindinger, L. C. Lands, R. S. McKelvie, G. Cederblad, N. L. Jones, and G. J. F. Heigenhauser. Pyruvate dehydrogenase activity and acetyl group accumulation during exercise after different diets. *Am. J. Physiol.* 265: E752-E760, 1993.

27. Sahlin, K. NADH and NADPH in human skeletal muscle at rest and during ischaemia. *Clin. Physiol.* 3: 477-485, 1983.

28. Sahlin, K. NADH in human skeletal muscle during short-term intense exercise. *Pflugers Arch.* 403: 193-196, 1985.

29. Sahlin, K., A. Katz, and S. Broberg. Tricarboxylic acid cycle intermediates in human muscle during prolonged exercise. *Am. J. Physiol.* 259: C834-C841, 1990.

30. Spriet, L. L., M. I. Lindinger, G. J. F. Heigenhauser, and N. L. Jones. Effects of alkalosis on skeletal muscle metabolism and performance during exercise. *Am. J. Physiol.* 251: R833-R839, 1986.

31. Spriet, L. L., M. I. Lindinger, R. S. McKelvie, G. J. F. Heigenhauser, and N. L. Jones. Muscle glycogenolysis and H^+ concentration during maximal intermittent cycling. *J. Appl. Physiol.* 66: 8-13, 1989.

32. Stansbie, D. Regulation of the human pyruvate dehydrogenase complex. *Clin. Sci. Mol. Med.* 51: 445-452, 1976.

33. Timmons, J. A., T. Gustafsson, C. J. Sundberg, E. Jansson, and P. L. Greenhaff. Muscle acetyl group availability is a major determinant of oxygen deficit in humans during submaximal exercise. *Am. J. Physiol.* 274: E377-E380, 1998.

34. Timmons, J. A., T. Gustafsson, C. J. Sundberg, E. Jansson, E. Hultman, L. Kaijser, J. Chwalbinska-Moneta, D. Constantin-Teodosiu, I. A. Macdonald, and P. L. Greenhaff. Substrate availability limits human skeletal muscle oxidative ATP regeneration at the onset of ischemic exercise. *J. Clin. Invest.* 101: 79-85, 1998.

35. Timmons, J. A., S. M. Poucher, D. Constantin-Teodosiu, I. A. Macdonald, and P. L. Greenhaff. Metabolic responses from rest to steady state determine contractile function in ischemic skeletal muscle. *Am. J. Physiol.* 273: E233-E238, 1997.

36. Timmons, J. A., S. M. Poucher, D. Constantin-Teodosiu, V. Worrall, I. A. Macdonald, and P. L. Greenhaff. Increased acetyl group availability enhances contractile function of canine skeletal muscle during ischemia. *J. Clin. Invest.* 97: 879-883, 1996.

37. Timmons, J. A., S. M. Poucher, D. Constantin-Teodosiu, V. Worrall, I. A. Macdonald, and P. L. Greenhaff. Metabolic responses of canine gracilis muscle during contraction with partial ischemia. *Am. J. Physiol.* 270: E400-E406, 1997.

38. Wilson, D. F. Factors affecting the rate and energetics of mitochondrial oxidative phosphorylation. *Med. Sci. Sports Exerc.* 26: 37-43, 1994.

39. Wilson, D. F. Energy metabolism in muscle approaching maximal rates of oxygen utilization. *Med. Sci. Sports Exerc.* 27: 54-59, 1995.

Chapter 18

Cross-Species Studies of Glycolytic Function

Peter W. Hochachka

Department of Zoology, University of British Columbia, Vancouver, B.C., V6T 1Z4, Canada

Key words: glycogenolysis, glycolysis, lactate metabolism, enzyme diffusion, substrate diffusion, metabolic regulation, glycolytic regulation

Abstract: Researchers probing the functional properties of glycogen (glucose) fermentation to lactate typically work within either one of two theoretical frameworks or models. The first assumes that the cell is analogous to a watery bag of enzymes, while the second assumes that three dimensional order and structure constrain the behaviors of glycolytic intermediates, of glycolytic enzymes, and of integrated glycolytic pathway functions per se. The former approach has been quite successful in accounting for many glycolytic functions but has not been able to satisfactorily explain a hallmark property of the pathway: namely, that large scale change in pathway flux is reflected in only modest changes in concentrations of pathway intermediates. Despite being composed of very different kinds of enzymes, the pathway is remarkably homeostatic by criterion of stability of concentrations of its intermediates in different metabolic states. The view of the cell as a system in which enzyme, substrate, and modulator mobilities are constrained by intracellular structures, the second framework above, posits intracellular perfusion or convection as a means for increasing rates of enzyme-substrate encounter and as an explanation for how high glycolytic pathway fluxes and homeostasis of pathway intermediates can be sustained simultaneously.

1.   TWO THEORETICAL APPROACHES CHARACTERIZE THE METABOLIC REGULATION FIELD

Over the last 3-4 decades, two general frameworks (we shall term them models I and II) accounting for metabolic regulation have dominated thinking in the field (1-5, 7-12, 15-23, 28). These two views can be nicely illustrated by considering the vertebrate phosphagen system (18). Model I assumes (i) that the total acid-extractable pool of Cr + PCr (termed tCr) occurs in aqueous solution and is fully accessible to creatine phosphokinase, CPK, (ii) that solution chemistry rules apply globally in muscle cells in vivo, and (iii) that the main CPK-phosphagen function is to 'buffer' ATP concentrations during large scale changes in muscle work and in ATP turnover rates. Model II hypotheses, on the other hand, consider (i) that the structural organization of phosphagen containing cells physically constrains tCr, (ii) that solution chemistry rules may apply in vivo mainly to localized PCr/Cr pools, and (iii) that intracellularly localized CPK isoforms in vivo create complex and possibly directional pathways of PCr and Cr metabolism - forming so-called creatine shuttles in metabolism (35). Model I considers the cell essentially as a watery bag of enzymes in which simple solution chemistry rules apply; Model II sees the cell as a highly structured system with intracellular ultrastructure incorporating constraints on metabolic processes and in the extreme imposing 3D order on metabolic function. *The polarization illustrated by these two views extends throughout the metabolic regulation field* and has caused the field to progress along two surprisingly independent paths with minimal communication between them. This peculiar phenomenon can be well illustrated by reviewing recent contributions by these two different approaches to current understanding of how the glycolytic pathway functions under various physiological and metabolic conditions.

2.   MODEL I – NEW DEVELOPMENTS FROM CROSS SPECIES STUDIES OF LACTATE METABOLISM AND GLYCOLYTIC FUNCTION

Most researchers in this area have been working with the Model I framework above and admittedly have enjoyed significant success. A minimal list of important 'Year 2000' insights into glycolytic function arising from comparative studies includes the following:

In fish white muscle (WM), which is uniformly composed of fast twitch oxidative glycolytic (FOG) fibers, phosphagen function and glycolysis are frequently stoichiometrically linked (2,15). Under steady state conditions (glycolytic ATP synthesis rates = cell ATPase rates), lactate and H^+ are produced in a 1:1 stoichiometry. In MRS studies, this is evident as dropping intracellular pH. In fact, this effect probably dominates the CPK system, since in particularly advantageous systems (homogenous fiber types such as tuna white muscle) there is an inverse relationship between [lactate] and [PCr]. Under these conditions, the interaction between glycolysis and the phosphagen system can be described simply as the former driving the latter; i.e., H^+ generated by glycolysis serving to drive CPK to the right (H^+ + PCr + ADP ----> ATP + Cr). During early stages of high intensity exercise requiring active glycolytic contributions to ATP generation, H^+ concentration is stable but [ADP] rises into the Km(ADP) range for phosphoglycerate and pyruvate kinases (PGK and PK, respectively) and this is thought to be the main stoichiometric interaction between the two ATP yielding pathways. A similar ADP-based interaction is thought to occur in heart metabolism during preferential glucose (vs free fatty acid, FFA) utilization in mammals (20).

Another interesting feature of glycolysis in fish FOG fibers is the apparent 'spring like' function of anaerobic glycolysis. Although this was suspected in many earlier studies, recent studies have quantified the main fates of lactate following anaerobic bursts of WM work. What these show is that most of the lactate formed during burst work is reconverted to muscle glycogen in situ during recovery (11,32). In fact, supplying ATP to drive this process may be the main function of WM mitochondrial metabolism during WM recovery from intense bursts of swimming (29).

Because in many fish species WM mass is large (60% or more of total body mass) while blood volume is small, there may be strong selective pressure to avoid WM lactate movement into the plasma compartment; i.e. there may be strong selective pressure to avoid sky rocketing plasma lactate concentrations. That may be why fish WM appear to have an active transport mechanism for lactate, which in vivo can transport lactate into WM cells against concentration gradients and can thus counteract diffusion of WM lactate into the plasma (37).

Like in other ectotherms, in most fishes body temperature is determined by the environmental temperature. Catalytic, regulatory, and structural properties of enzymes are highly temperature sensitive; hence, it is not surprising to find temperature-linked 'performance' alleles. Fundulus, a species which thrives over a broad thermal range, is a favorite species in these studies. In northern cold waters, this species expresses a northern or 'cold' LDH gene and a 'cold' LDH promoter (this situation could be viewed as two alleles but probably only one haplotype). Southern warm water populations of *Fundulus* express a 'warm' LDH allele and a 'warm' LDH promoter (again, two alleles but probably one haplotype). Both the catalytic properties of the enzyme, and the amounts synthesized and maintained under steady state conditions, can be fine-tuned so as to compensate LDH function for the thermal environment in which the animal finds itself (31).

For some years now it has been known that the amount of LDH and pyruvate kinase (PK) present per g of muscle tissue scales with body mass: i.e., larger fish have more enzyme per g of WM than do small fish and this is expressed also in terms of the capacity to support burst swimming by anaerobic glycogenolysis. At least in some species, the regulation of this scaling phenomenon is now known to occur at the transcriptional level. In these cases, steady stage concentrations of mRNA for enzymes such as PK also increase with body mass (6). What is not known is how information on body size is sensed and then how it is trasduced down to the transcriptional level.

The capacity for large magnitude change from low to high activity states is one of the hallmark characteristics of the glycolytic pathway (over 100 fold activation of glycolytic flux is routinely achievable in skeletal muscles of many species). How increasing enzyme-substrate encounter rates for enzyme reactions in the glycolytic pathway are achieved during such large scale transitions from low to high fluxes has been a difficult problem. Traditionally, Model I views of this problem (1-5,7-10,28) assume increasing diffusion-based enzyme-substrate (and for regulated steps, enzyme-modulator) encounters to account for increasing pathway fluxes. However, even though the glycolytic path is composed of enzymes with quite different catalytic and regulatory properties, the empirical observation is that the intermediates of the pathway are remarkably homeostatic during muscle work. Whereas glycolytic flux may increase by over 100 fold, the concentrations of intermediates change by only about 2-3 fold (15,21). Under test tube conditions, with high concentrations of 'near equilibrium' enzymes, small changes in substrate/product ratios allow large enough changes to accommodate the in vivo behavior (33). However, because high concentrations of substrate for a given reaction step in glycolysis means high concentrations of product for the preceding enzyme in the pathway, it has not been possible to expand these mechanisms into realistic in vivo (multienzyme) settings (6). While this quantitative discordance between change in pathway fluxes and change in concentrations of intermediates was first noted for the glycolytic path, it is worth noting that it is now known to apply to over 60 intermediates in other pathways of carbohydrate, fat, and amino acid metabolism (16), as well as to molecular O_2. In fact, even if O_2 delivery correlates well with work (15,22,23), 1H MRS studies show constant %MbO_2 (i.e., constant intracellular [O_2]) over broad ranges of aerobic metabolism and work both for skeletal muscle (30) and heart (24).

Thus the relative homeostasis of pathway intermediates during large magnitude changes in pathway fluxes is general but it has remained a poorly explained (or even unexplained) paradox in research dominated by Model I approaches (15,21). This is a point of departure for Model II approaches, which take a different tack and assume changing intracellular perfusion as the main means for achieving changes in enzyme substrate encounter rates (and hence changes in net forward flux) for enzymes in pathways such as glycolysis.

3. MODEL II: INTRACELLULAR STRUCTURE IMPLIES REQUIREMENT FOR AN INTRACELLULAR PERFUSION SYSTEM

The main difference between the Model 1 or traditional approach to metabolic regulation and Model II is the emphasis placed upon intracellular order and structure. Three different lines of evidence are usually relied upon and in all three cases it is less a matter of *favoring intracellular perfusion and more a matter of not favoring diffusion as the dominant means for regulating enzyme–substrate encounter* (including cytochrome oxidase – O_2 encounter). First and most fundamental is the structural argument: ultrastructural, histochemical, and cytochemical studies do not indicate the cell as a static bag of substrates and enzymes, but rather a 3D membrane bound system filled with complex organelles, motors, membranes, cables, trabeculae, and channels. Rather than a static, dead-still solution (as would be required for formal application of laws of diffusion), the internal medium is very much 'alive' in the sense that movement is the rule of thumb (38,39), movement of organelles, of particles, and of cytosol (so called cytoplasmic streaming at rates of up to 2-3 μm per sec (38)). In contrast to what might be expected of a bag of enzymes and substrates, over a half-century of research has clearly concluded that many metabolic pathways and their component enzymes are restricted to specific cell compartments and numerous so called soluble enzymes show intracellular binding to specific intracellular sites. Order and structure is the name of the game, as far as the literature on cell ultrastructure is concerned, and it is not a diffusion-dominated game. Take away the order and the system behaviour falls apart; sometimes function is lost completely. A good recent example of this comes from genetic studies of Drosophila flight muscle metabolism. While earlier studies had shown that ALD, GAPDH, and GPDH colocalize mainly at Z-discs, Wojtas et al. (40) used clever genetic manipulations (that influenced binding but not overall catalytic activities) to show that mislocating these enzyme activities in the cytosol rather than correctly bound to Z-discs would render

Drosophila flightless – a dramatic demonstration that even if all three enzymes are expressed at high activities, their 3D organization is part and parcel of in vivo regulated function of the pathway.

Second is the argument on macromolecular functional constraints. As we might expect from the above (and indeed find), the intracellular mobilities of enzymes and of carrier proteins such as Mb are not equivalent to those in simple aqueous solutions. For example, intracellular diffusibility estimates for Mb in the cytosol range from as low as 1/10th that found in simple solutions (25) to values of about ½ that in simple solution (36). Interestingly, the latter MRS estimate is for rotational diffusion, while the former is for translational diffusion and the two parameters may change independently. These are instructive data since myoglobin facilitated diffusion of O_2 is considered by traditional models to be crucial to O_2 transfer especially at high work rates. It is unclear how these traditional models deal with the observation that transgenic mice appear to show no debilitating effects of myoglobin gene knockout (13). In any event, a combination of recent studies suggests that Mb facilitated diffusion may be less helpful to traditional O_2 diffusion models than previously thought. Just as Mb appears to be less mobile within the cytosol than previously believed, so also are cytosolic enzymes such as aldolase, PGK, CPK, glycogen phosphorylase and hexokinase apparently rather restricted in their intracellular mobility – again this picture is not easily compatible with the concept of the cell as a bag of enzymes whose functions are determined mainly by self-diffusion and substrate diffusion at appropriate rates (15,16). With enzyme and myoglobin translational mobilities reduced to only 1/10th that expected in aqueous solutiion, diffusion of macromolecules becomes a highly inefficient means for assisting in enzyme – substrate encounter (or in the case of myoglobin, for assisting O_2 flux through the cytosol).

Third is the argument on metabolite mobility: because of the complexity of the internal milieu, the translational mobility even of simple molecules may be restricted compared to simple solutions and this is especially true in the mitochondrial matrix. For example (18), studies with ^{14}C-labeled Cr show that CPK is unable to readily equilibrate the entire pool of PCr + Cr in fish white muscle (fast twitch fibers). At the same time, parallel ^{1}H MRS studies show that in human muscle in vivo the intracellular behaviour of Cr is highly constrained (14). One set of studies, focussing on the methyl hydrogens (34), show that Cr mobility is metabolic state dependent: 3-4 fold less mobile in ischemic fatigue than in muscle at rest. Another set of studies focussing on the methylene protons (27) found that the methylene protons only in PCr were MRS visible; on PCr conversion to Cr during muscle work, the methylene protons become MRS invisible (in simple solutions MRS cannot distinguish these in PCr and Cr). Taken together these data supply powerful evidence that the behaviour of metabolites in vivo may be much more precisely regulated (and certainly much more constrained) than previously expected. Another recent study showed that 3 factors (viscosity, binding, and interference from cell solids) could account for translational diffusion of a metabolite-sized analogue in cytosol being decreased to only 27% that observed in water (26). As in the MRS studies, these workers also demonstrated mobilites that were state dependent: during osmotic stress (2 fold cell volume increase), when metabolism is known to be increased, there is a correlated (if unexplained) 6 fold! increase in the apparent translational diffusion coefficient, while rotational diffusion remained constant. The complex and metabolic state-dependent diffusion behavior of metabolite-sized molecules would not readily facilitate enzyme-substrate encounters as required for simple solution models of regulated cell function.

Given these constraints, we and others consider diffusion by itself to be an inadequate, inefficient, and minimally regulatable means of delivering carbon substrates and oxygen to appropriate enzyme targets in the cell under the variable conditions and rates that are required in vivo. Instead, we favor an hypothesis (38,39) – almost required by a structured and ordered internal milieu – of an intracellular convection or perfusion system as an elegantly simply resolution of the problem of how substrates (including O_2) and enzymes are brought together. From our present point of view, the key advantage of this model is that it easily explains how enzymes and substrates can be brought together and how reaction rates can occur at widely varying rates with minimal change in substrate concentrations – this feature, first clearly demonstrated for the glycolytic path and now known to hold for O_2 as well as for over 60 intermediates in pathways of carbohydrate, fat, and amino acid catabolism (16), is the empirical starting point of the paradox in this whole field (15,16) that to our minds has never been satisfactorily explained to this day by anyone else anywhere else (for O_2 or for any other intermediate in mainline metabolism). As in the perfusion of organs/tissues such as muscle, rates of intracellular metabolic reactions by this model are simple products of intracellular perfusion rates: the greater the perfusion rates the greater the enzyme-substrate encounter rate and the greater the metabolic rates with no concomitant changes in substrate concentrations required. At our current level of understanding, we cannot specify the nature of intracellular perfusion systems: are enzymes perfusing pools of substrate, or are substrates perfusing targeted enzymes? For our purposes, either system would work equally well. In this view, during osmotic activation of metabolic rate, the 6 fold increase in metabolite mobility observed (but not explained) could well represent a similarly large increase in intracellular convection. In the case of the MRS data, a 4 fold change in Cr mobility in hypometabolic ischemic muscle (34) may well represent a similar change in intracellular convection (this is viewed as a coarse but dominant control, which to be sure need not rule out other fine tuning control mechanisms, the kinds that have so far absorbed much of metabolic research).

Parenthetically, we might add that for O_2 transport, this view places the function of a half O_2 saturated, randomly distributed Mb (24,30) into an entirely different perspective where the fundamental purpose of an intracellular Mb may be to equalize $[O_2]$ everywhere in the cytosol – this would assure that intracellular convection would always be delivering similar amounts of O_2 per unit volume of cytosol to cytochrome oxidases (and would simultaneously minimize or even destroy intracellular O_2 gradients). While this model is consistent with the minimal intracellular O_2 gradients in muscle cells proposed by the Honig, Connett, and Gayeski work (8-10), it takes on a quite a different meaning. Finally, the concept of an intracellular perfusion system supplies purpose and meaning to intracellular movements (motor driven or otherwise induced cytoplasmic streaming) which have been pretty well ignored by traditional metabolic biochemists to this time. If accepted, the concept of intracellular convection modifies our overall view to include an intracellular component to the chain of convective and diffusive steps in the overall path of O_2 from air to mitochondria.

4.   OVERVIEW

From the above discussion, it will be evident that the research into glycolytic function, and metabolic regulation in general, has progressed along two independent research paths each of which has been undeniably successful. Because of the different experimental requirements and different experimental designs, different laboratories often specialize in either Model I or Model II research approaches usually quite in isolation one from the other. That is why I have referred to these two research paths as 'two solitudes'. Sometimes, as in my own case, a kind of schizophrenia envelopes the scene, wherein the same individual researcher may work within Model I boundaries in some studies and in Model II frameworks in others.

In considering the concept of intracellular convection, early pioneers in this field (Clegg, Coulson and Wheatley, to mention three (see literature in ref. (38 & 39)) may be prone to over-enthusiastic pressing of their case; this is understandable, since it seems to explain so much previously puzzling data so easily. Nevertheless, there clearly remain critical functions that are largely or solely diffusion based, so the understandable over-enthusiasm with which Model II proponents minimize the importance of diffusion in energy metabolism puts them at risk of throwing the baby out with the bathwater. To finally assemble a model which can realistically explain a realistic working range of metabolic systems what seems to be required for the future is an opening up of channels of communication between the above two very differing views of metabolic regulation.

REFERENCES

1. Allen, P.S., G.O.Matheson, G.Zhu, D. Gheorgiu, R.S.Dunlop, T.Falcomer, C. Stanley, and P.W.Hochachka. Simultaneous 31P Magnetic Resonance spectroscopy of the soleus and gastrocnemius in Sherpas during graded calf muscle exercise. *Am. J. Physiol.* 273: R999-R1005, 1997.

2. Arthur, P.G., T.G.West, R.W. Brill, P.M.Schulte and P.W.Hochachka. Recovery metabolism in tuna white muscle: rapid and parallel changes of lactate and phosphocreatine after exercise. *Can. J. Zool.*, 70: 1230-1239. 1992.

3. Atkinson, D.E. *Control of Metabolic Processes* (Ed. Cornish-Bowden, A. an M.L. Cardenas), Plenum Press, N.Y., pp. 11-27, 1992.

4. Balban, R.S. Regulation of oxidative phosphorylation in the mammalian cell. *Am. J. Physiol.* 258: C377-C389, 1990.

5. Betts, D.F. and D.K. Srivastava (1991) The rationalization of high enzyme concentrations in metabolic pathways such as glycolysis. *J. Theoret. Biol.* 151: 155-167, 1991

6. Burness, G.P., S.C.Leary, P.W.Hochachka, and C.D.Moyes. The molecular basis for allometric scaling of enzyme activity. *Am. J. Physiol.*, in review stages

7. Connett, R.J. Analysis of metabolic control: new insights using scaled creatine kinase model. *Am. J. Physiol.* 254: R949-959, 1988.

8. Connett, R.J. and C.R. Honig. Regulation of VO₂max. Do current biochemical hypothesis fit in vivo data? *Am. J. Physiol.* 256, R898-R906, 1989.

9. Connett, R.J., C.R. Honig, T.E.J. Gayeski, and G.A. Brooks. Defining hypoxia. *J. Appl. Physiol.* 63: 833-842, 1990.

10. Connett, R.J., T.E. Gayeski and C.R. Honig. Energy sources in fully aerobic rest-work transitions: a new role for glycolysis. *Am. J. Physiol.* 248: H922-H929, 1985.

11. Dobson, G.P. and P.W. Hochachka. Role of glycolysis in adenylate depletion and repletion during work and recovery in teleost white muscle. *J. Exp. Biol.* 129: 125-140, 1987..

12. Dobson, G.P., W.S. Parkhouse, J.M. Weber, E. Stuttard, J. Harman, D.H. Snow, and P.W. Hochachka (1988) Metabolic changes in skeletal muscle and blood in greyhounds during 800 m track sprint. *Am. J. Physiol.* 255: R513-R519, 1988.

13. Garry, D.J., G.A.Ordway, J.N.Lorenz, N.B.Radfor, E.R.Chin, R.W.Grange, R.Bassel-Duby, and R. S. Williams.. Mice without myoglobin. *Nature* 395: 905-906, 1998.

14. Hanstock, C.C., R.B. Thompson , M.E.Trump , D. Gheorghiu , P.W. Hochachka, P.S. Allen (1998) Characterisation of the TE-dependence for the Cr / PCr methyl resonance in resting human medial gastrocnemius muscle. *Magn. Resonance Med.*, in submission stages.

15. Hochachka, P.W. (1994) *Muscles and Molecular and Metabolic Machines*. CRC Press, Boca Raton, FL pp 1-157.

16. Hochachka, P.W. Two research paths to probing the roles of oxygen in metabolic regulation. *Br. J. Med. Biol. Res.*, 32: *in press*.

17. Hochachka, P.W. and G.O.Matheson. Regulation of ATP turnover over broad dynamic muscle work ranges. *J. Appl. Physiol.*. 73: 570-575, 1992.

18. Hochachka, P.W. and M.K.P. Mossey . Does muscle creatine phosphokinase have access to the total pool of phosphocreatine and creatine? *Amer. J. Physiol.*, 274:R868-R872, 1998.

19. Hochachka, P.W., M. Bianconcini, W.S. Parkhouse, and G.P. Dobson. Role of actomyosin ATPase in metabolic regulation during intense exercise. *Proc. Natl. Acad. Sci. USA*, 88: 5764-5768, 1991.

20. Hochachka, P.W., C.M.Clark, J.E.Holden, C.Stanley, K.Ugurbil, and R.S.Menon. 31P MRS of the Sherpa heart: A PCr/ATP signature of metabolic defense against hypobaric hypoxia. *Proc. Natl. Acad. Sci.* USA 93: 1215-1220, 1996.

21. Hochachka, P.W., McClelland G.B., Burness, G.P., J.F.Staples, and R.K.Suarez. Integrating metabolic pathway fluxes with gene-to-enzyme expression rates. *Comp. Biochem. Physiol.* B 120: 17-26, 1998..

22. Hogan, M.C., P.G. Arthur, D.E. Bebout, P.W. Hochachka, and P.D. Wagner. The role of O_2 in regulating tissue respiration in dog muscle working in situ. *J. Appl. Physiol.* 73: 728-736, 1992.

23. Hogan, M.C., S.S.Kurdak and P.G.Arthur. Effect of gradual reduction in O_2 delivery on intracellular homeostasis in contracting skeletal muscle. *J. Appl. Physiol.* 80, 1313-132, 1996.

24. Jelicks, L.A. and B.A.Wittenberg. 1H NMR studies of sarcoplasmic oxygenation in the red cell perfused rat heart. *Biophys. J.* 68: 2129-2136, 1995.

25. Juergens, K.D., T. Peters, and G. Gros. Diffusivity of myoglobin in intact. *Proc. Natl. Acad. Sci. USA* 91: 3829-3833, 1994.

26. Kao, H.P., J.R.Abney, and A.S.Verkman. Determinants of the translational mobility of a small solute in cell cytoplasm. *J. Cell. Biol.* 120: 175-184, 1993.

27. Kreis, R., B.Jung, J.Felblinger, J.Slotboom and C. Boesch. Creatine signals in localized 1H_MR spectra of human skeletal muscle vary linearly with muscular phosphocreatine. *Proc. Intl. Soc. Magn. Res. Med* p385, 1998.

28. Matheson, G.O. P.S. Allen, D.C. Ellinger, C.C. Hanstock, D. Gheorghiu, D.C. McKenzie, C. Stanley, W.S. Parkhouse, and P.W. Hochachka, (1991) Skeletal muscle metabolism and work capacity: a 31P-NMR study of Andean natives and lowlanders. *J. Appl. Physiol.*, 70: 1963-1976.

29. Moyes, C.D., P.M.Schlute, and P.W. Hochachka. Recovery metabolism of trout white muscle: role of the mitochondria. *Am. J. Physiol.*, 262: R295-R304, 1992.

30. Richardson, R.S., E.A.Noyszewski, K.F.Kendrick, J.S.Leigh, and P.D.Wagner. Myoglobin O_2 desaturation during exercise. Evidence of limited O_2 transport. *J. Clin. Invest.* 96: 1916-1926, 1996.

31. Schulte P M., M.Gomez Chiarri, and D.A. Powers. Structural and functional differences in the promoter and 5'flanking region of Ldh-B within and between populations of the teleost Fundulus heteroclitus. *Genetics* 145:759-769, 1997.

32. Schulte, P.M., C.D. Moyes, and P.W. Hochachka. Integrating metabolic pathways in post-exercise recovery of white muscle. *J. Exp. Biol.*, 166: 181-195, 1992.

33. Staples, J.F. and R.K.Suarez. Honeybee flight muscle phosphoglucoseisomerase: matching enzyme capacities to flux requirements at a near-equilibrium reaction. *J. Exp. Biol.* 200:1247-1254, 1997.

34. Trump, M.E., P.S.Allen, D.Gheorghiu, C.C.Hanstock, and P.W.Hochachka. 1H-MRS evaluation of the phosphocreatine-creatine (PCr/Cr) pool in human muscle. *Proc. Intl. Soc. Magn. Res. Med.* p 1337, 1997.

35. Wallimann, T. 31P-NMR-measured creatine kinase reaction flux in muscle: a caveat! *J. of Muscle Res. and Cell Mot.* 17: 177-181, 1996.

36. Wang, D., U. Kruetzer,, Y. Chung, and T. Jue. Myoglobin and hemoglobin rotational diffusion in the cell. *Biophys.* J. 73: 2764-2770, 1997.

37. Wang Y. P.M. Wright, G.J.F. Heigenhauser, and C.M. Wood. Lactate transport by rainbow trout white muscle: Kinetic characteristics and sensitivity to inhibitors. American *Journal of Physiology* 272: R1577-R1587, 1997.

38. Wheatley, D.N. Diffusion theory, the cell, and the synapse. *Biosystems* 45, 151-163.1998.

39. Wheatley D.N. and J.S. Clegg. What determines the metabolic rate of vertebrate cells. *Biosystems* 32: 83-92. 1994.

40. Wojtas, K., N. Slepecky, L. von-Kalm and D. Sullivan. Flight muscle function in Drosophila requires colocalization of glycolytic enzymes. *Molecular Biology of the Cell.* 8: 1665-1675, 1997.

Chapter 19

Hypoxia Induces Cell-Specific Changes in Gene Expression in Vascular Wall Cells: Implications for Pulmonary Hypertension

Kurt R. Stenmark, Maria Frid, Raphael Nemenoff*, Edward C. Dempsey, and Mita Das
Department of Pediatrics, Developmental Lung Biology Laboratory and Department of Medicine, *University of Colorado Health Sciences Center, Denver, CO 80262, USA*

Key words: hypoxia, fibroblast proliferation, SMC proliferation, protein kinase C, mitogen activated protein kinase

Abstract: Mammals respond to reduced oxygen concentrations (hypoxia) in many different ways at the systemic, local, cellular and molecular levels. Within the pulmonary circulation, exposure to chronic hypoxia has been demonstrated to illicit increases in pulmonary artery pressure as well as dramatic structural changes in both large and small vessels. It has become increasingly clear that the response to hypoxia in vivo is differentially regulated at the level of specific cell types within the vessel wall. For instance, in large pulmonary blood vessels there is now convincing evidence to suggest that the medial layer is made up of many different subpopulations of smooth muscle cells. In response to hypoxia there are remarkable differences in the proliferative and matrix producing responses of these cells to the hypoxic environment. Some cell populations proliferate and increase matrix protein synthesis, while in other cell populations no apparent change in the proliferative or differentiation state of the cell takes place. In more peripheral vessels, the predominant proliferative changes in response to hypoxia in the pulmonary circulation occur in the adventitial layer rather than in the medial layer. Here again, specific increases in proliferation and matrix protein synthesis take place. Accumulating evidence suggests that the unique responses exhibited by specific cell types to hypoxia in vivo can be modeled in vitro. We have isolated, in culture, specific medial cell populations which demonstrate significant increases in proliferation in response to hypoxia, and others which

Hypoxia: Into the Next Millennium,
Edited by R. C. Roach, *et al.* Kluwer Academic/Plenum Publishing, New York, 1999.

231

exhibit no change or, in fact, a decrease in proliferation under hypoxic conditions. We have also isolated and cloned several unique populations of adventitial fibroblasts. There is good evidence that only certain fibroblast populations are capable of responding to hypoxia with an increase in proliferation. We have begun to elucidate the signaling pathways which are activated in those cell populations that exhibit proliferative responses to hypoxia. We show that hypoxia, in the absence of serum or mitogens, specifically activates select members of the protein kinase C isozyme family, as well as members of the mitogen-activated protein kinase (MAPK) family of proteins. This selective activation appears to take place in response to hypoxia only in those cells exhibiting a proliferative response, and antagonists of this pathway inhibit the response. Thus, there appear to be cells within each organ that demonstrate unique responses to hypoxia. A better understanding of why these cells exist and how they specifically transduce hypoxia-mediated signals will lead to a better understanding of how the changes in the pulmonary circulation take place under conditions of chronic hypoxia.

1.   INTRODUCTION

In response to generalized hypoxia, all mammalian species exhibit systemic responses that are designed, in general terms, to decrease cellular oxygen need and dependence and to increase tissue oxygen supply. Though these responses to hypoxia have been known almost since Joseph Priestley's demonstration in 1774 of the deleterious effects of a burning candle on a mouse in a bell jar, only recently have we begun to understand at the molecular, cellular and tissue level how animal cells sense when oxygen concentration is limiting and respond to the crisis. For instance, work over the past decade has demonstrated the cellular and molecular events which mediate the increase in breathing that is noted in response to hypoxia. We know this response is neuronal in nature and depends on rapid inhibition of conductance through potassium channels, as well as on the relatively fast induction of the gene encoding tyrosine hydroxylase, the rate limiting step in the synthesis of the neurotransmitter dopamine in type I cells in the carotid body (12,57). Further, we have a much better understanding of the mechanisms contributing to the increase in erythrocyte mass, which was first attributed to the low partial pressure of oxygen at high altitude by Viault in 1890. We now know in detail the molecular mechanisms which elicit erythropoietin production (12,13,57). In fact, work on this problem provided the essential groundwork for our current understanding of how hypoxia elicits a variety of changes in virtually all cells of the body (12,13,30,35).

Alterations in oxygen tension elicit equally important physiologic responses at the organ and tissue level. Exposure to chronic hypoxia causes pulmonary hypertension in most mammalian species. The pulmonary hypertension is associated with changes in vascular tone and is nearly always associated with significant structural changes within the pulmonary vascular bed (65,66). Furthermore, during the development of chronic pulmonary hypertension, marked changes in the phenotype of endothelial, smooth muscle and fibroblast cell populations occur. However, the cellular and structural changes observed in pulmonary hypertension vary significantly depending on the age, as well as duration, and degree of hypoxic exposure and the presence of associated abnormalities such as chronic inflammation or high pulmonary blood flow (17,18). It is now clear that the vascular responses to hypoxia involve complex cell-cell interactions which are mediated by the release of growth factors, cytokines, biological messengers, and by changes in the composition of interstitial and basement membrane matrix proteins (41,42,66). It is also evident that the cellular responses to local decreases in oxygen concentration are heterogeneous between and even among the cell populations that comprise the vessel wall. Dramatic differences in the proliferative, matrix producing and secretory phenotype of different cells along the longitudinal axis of the vessel wall, as well as at a specific site, have been observed (8,21,23,72). There is also evidence demonstrating that the response of a particular gene to hypoxia *in vivo* is differentially regulated at the level of specific cell types and regions within the tissue (49). Thus, up- or downregulation of specific gene expression by unique or specialized cells within a tissue may influence the overall organ or tissue response to local changes in oxygen concentration. An understanding of the changes that take place in cells in the vascular wall when exposed to decreases in oxygen concentration and the mechanisms which cause them are thus critical for a better understanding of the pathophysiology of many vascular disorders. This knowledge is also necessary for developing better treatments for the vascular complications associated with global or local hypoxic exposure.

The purpose of this report is to briefly review the changes that decreased oxygen concentration exerts on endothelial cells, smooth muscle cells (SMC) and fibroblasts. Evidence is presented demonstrating that generalized alveolar hypoxia exerts unique and differential effects on the heterogeneic subpopulations of cells that comprise the intima, media and adventitia of the pulmonary vessel wall. Data are discussed suggesting that while all cells sense hypoxia, the functional response observed is directed by the presence or absence of unique downstream signaling molecules and transcription factors in unique cell subpopulations.

2. HYPOXIA-INDUCED CHANGES IN ENDOTHELIAL CELL GENE EXPRESSION

Among the numerous cell types in which either tolerance and/or adaptation to hypoxia are likely crucial for survival are the vascular endothelial cells. Thus, a great deal of attention has been given to the endothelial cells' response to low levels of oxygen. Within the lung, pulmonary arterial endothelial cells are continually exposed to low levels of oxygen (PO2 40-45 Torr) due to the low oxygen content of mixed venous blood even under normal conditions. During hypoxia exposure, the endothelial cells may be exposed to even lower levels (PO2 < 25 Torr) and under conditions of blood flow obstruction (e.g. thrombosis), oxygen tensions less than 5 torr can be seen. It is therefore not surprising that the endothelial cell has probably developed unique ways to respond to environmental hypoxia which enable its survival as well as its ability to contribute to the maintenance of vascular and tissue homeostasis. It is also clear, however, that changes in endothelial cell phenotype in response to hypoxia can contribute to the pathogenesis of the disease process.

In response to hypoxia, a number of genes have been shown to be induced in endothelial cells from various vascular beds (see Table 1). As suggested above, changes in these gene products may participate in adaptive as well as maladaptive responses. For instance, induction of factors such as endothelin 1 and PDGF may affect not only vascular tone but also influence the proliferative state of underlying SMC (41,42). In this context, it is also clear that hypoxia effects gene expression in smooth muscle cells of factors that also influence vascular tone (e.g., hemeoxygenase 1). These gene products may exert significant influence on endothelial cell gene expression. Thus, as described by Kourembanas et al., there is a complex interaction between endothelial cells and SMC that exists in the chronically hypoxic microenvironment and contributes to changes in tone and structure under hypoxic conditions (41). Many other dramatic changes occur in endothelial cell protein expression and function under hypoxic conditions. These include changes in permeability, as well as striking changes in the production of factors that have profound effect on the interaction with circulating blood cells (39,63,73,74). Significant increases in adhesion molecule production (ICAM-1) as well as in IL-1α, IL-8 and IL-6 have been described in hypoxic endothelial cells. Not only can an inflammatory response be observed, which is secondary to binding of platelets and neutrophils to the hypoxically activated endothelium, but recent experiments from the Stern laboratory also demonstrate that hypoxic environments can cause an increase in fibrin deposition (73). Thus, at a local level, hypoxia has a profound impact on nearly all functions of the endothelial cell.

Hypoxia Induces Cell-Specific Changes in Gene Expression in
Vascular Wall Cells: Implications for Pulmonary Hypertension

235

Table 1. Hypoxia-Induced Genes in Endothelial Cells

Process	Gene Product
Glucose Transport	Glucose transporter 1, 2, 3
Glycolysis	Lactate dehydrogenase A
	Phosphofructokinase L and 1
	Enolase A
	Glyceraldehyde-3-phosphate-dehydrogenase
	Non-neuronal enolase
Growth Factors	Vascular endothelial growth factor
	Transforming growth factor-β
	Platelet derived growth factor
Vasomotor Regulation	Endothelin 1
	Inducible nitric oxide synthase
	Hemeoxygenase 1

One wonders how the endothelial cell, which is in the position to direct so many important events within the vessel wall, has evolved to be able to adapt to the hypoxic environment. Endothelial cells, whether from the microvasculature, aorta or pulmonary artery, maintain viability during prolonged hypoxic exposure much better than a number of nonendothelial cell types including fibroblasts and SMC (Fig. 1). When deprived of oxygen, endothelial cells, like other cells but perhaps in a more efficient way, respond with rapid stimulation of glucose utilization by nonoxidative routes. The well known Pasteur effect is an increase in glycolysis upon inhibition of mitochondrial respiration. Because the ATP yield from the glycolytic pathway is 18-fold lower than that from the Krebs oxidative pathway, the rate of glucose consumption must increase substantially during hypoxic stress. This is usually achieved in two ways. There is an increase in glucose transport as well as an induction of the glycolytic enzymes. Increases in the glucose transporter (GLUT-1) have been demonstrated in endothelial cells *in vivo*, as well as in cultured cells (45). In addition, increases in glycolytic enzymes have also been observed in endothelial cells (12,30,33). The effect of hypoxia on expression on glycolytic enzymes does vary between cells from different vascular beds and may contribute to differences in stress adaptation. Further, endothelial cells express a unique set of hypoxia inducible proteins which are not observed in other cells of the vessel wall under conditions of extreme hypoxia that may also contribute to survival of the endothelium (33,34). Studies in the Farber laboratory have demonstrated that cultured endothelial cells exposed to acute or chronic hypoxia upregulate a specific set of proteins termed hypoxia associated proteins (HAPS) that are distinct from other previously described stress proteins and which are unique to the endothelial cell (33,34). These proteins are uniquely expressed in response to hypoxia not to other general cell stresses. Two of the HAPS have been identified as the glycolytic enzymes, glyceraldehyde-3-phosphate dehydrogenase (GAPDH) and nonneuronal endase (NNE). Preliminary work suggest that HAPS may be regulated differently from other hypoxia responsive genes. The HAPS, may be related to the relative unique hypoxia tolerance of endothelial cells.

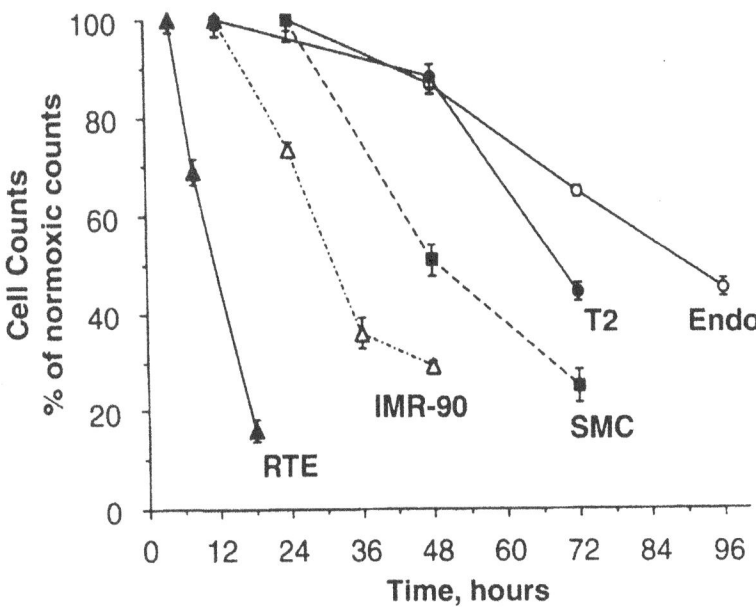

Figure 1. Endothelial cells exhibit the greatest tolerance to hypoxic stress. When exposed to 0% oxygen, cell survival was greatest in endothelial cells (Endo, SMC = smooth muscle cells, IMR-90 = fetal lung fibroblasts, T2 = alveolar type II cells, RTE = renal tubular epithelial cells; from Graven and Farber, 33).

The mechanism(s) through which hypoxia exerts its effects on endothelial gene expression has received much recent attention. Current evidence suggests that most of the presumably essential adaptive responses to hypoxia exhibited by endothelial cells are mediated mainly through the transcription factor called hypoxia inducible factor (HIF) (12,13,57). Changes in endothelial expression known to be regulated by the HIF transcription factor include gene glycolytic enzymes, the glucose transporter GLUT-1, VEGF-receptor expression, hemeoxygenase (HO), endothelin and PDGF. However, as mentioned, there are other changes in cellular function which are triggered by exposure to low concentrations of oxygen. These changes, which include upregulation of adhesion molecules followed by leukocyte and platelet adhesion, as well as fibrin deposition, appear to be the result of increased tissue factor expression and are clearly less beneficial to the organism and appear to underlie hypoxia-mediated tissue dysfunction (73). Importantly, Yan et al. have demonstrated that in contrast to hypoxia-induced adaptive responses that appear to be subject mostly to regulation by HIF-1, those responses that could be considered maladaptive (thrombogenesis and inflammation) appear to be under control of other transcription factors, most notably early growth response gene product (Egr-1) (73) (Fig. 2). Thus, hypoxia appears to activate several distinct types of host response mechanisms in the hypoxemic milleu. Both HIF dependent and HIF-independent changes in gene expression (Egr-1, AP-1) must be considered when considering therapies for hypoxia-induced vascular dysfunction.

Recent studies also raise the possibility that the response to hypoxic stress exhibited by endothelial cells within the pulmonary circulation may not be equal or homogeneous. This idea is raised by the recent observations of Levin et al. (44) demonstrating that the expression of endothelial cell-derived tissue plasminogen activator (tPA) protein is restricted to the endothelium of discrete groups of vessels within the lung. Interestingly, bronchial arteries show consistent immunostaining for this protein in mouse and primate lung, whereas vessels in brain, heart, and kidney rarely show expression of this protein. It also appears that tPA is present only in a small fraction of small vessels of the pulmonary circulation (7-30 micron diameter), whereas it is not observed in the capillaries or larger pulmonary arteries. Conditions associated with acute pulmonary inflammation increased expression of tPA antigen in a very heterogeneous manner. These studies support the idea that there are distinct subsets of endothelial cells within the bronchial and pulmonary arterial circulation. Further, these endothelial cell subpopulations appear to possess unique abilities to express proteins in response to hypoxic or inflammatory stimuli.

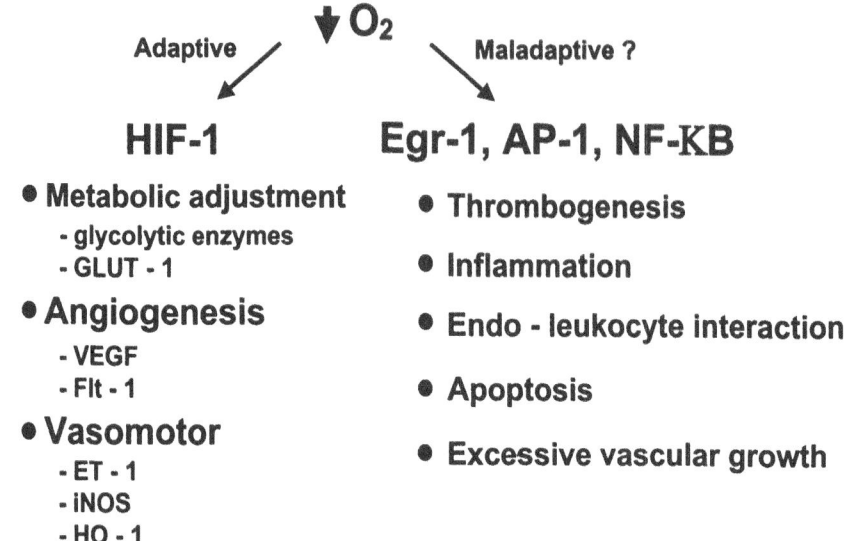

Figure 2. Vascular cell responses to hypoxia are mediated through HIF dependent and independent pathways.

3.   HETEROGENEITY IN THE SMC RESPONSE TO HYPOXIA

3.1   In-Vivo Evidence for SMC Heterogeneity

Experimental evidence supporting the concept of phenotypic heterogeneity of vascular SMC initially emerged from studies analyzing the expression of muscle- specific contractile and cytoskeletal proteins in the systemic circulation. These studies demonstrated unique differences between SMC at different locations along the longitudinal axis of the arterial tree as well as in distinct arterial layers (i.e. intima versus media) of injured animal or atherosclerotic human vessels (28,48). Recent studies, analyzing the expression of contractile proteins, or using electron microscopy to evaluate morphological appearance and relative microfilament content have demonstrated that heterogeneity of SMC phenotype also exists at specific sites within the media of both the systemic and pulmonary circulations (3,31).

In the bovine species, using routine histochemical techniques, we observed SMC in the media of the large elastic pulmonary and systemic arteries that varied in arrangement pattern, orientation, tropoelastin mRNA expression and proliferative indices. Subsequently, we systematically analyzed SMC phenotype in bovine pulmonary and systemic arterial media using a broad panel of antibodies against muscle-specific proteins that are believed to be reliable markers of smooth muscle cell phenotype (α-SM-actin, SM-myosin, calponin, desmin, high molecular weight caldesmon, and metavinculin). We demonstrated the existence of a very complex site-specific heterogeneity in the structure and cell phenotype of SMC in the vascular media of pulmonary and systemic arteries. Based on morphological appearance and immunobiochemical characteristics, we demonstrated the presence of at least four phenotypically distinct SMC subpopulations in the mature arterial media (27). Interestingly, we found that different subtypes of cells existed in an almost compartmentalized fashion within the vascular media. In the subendothelial space, we observed cells which were small and irregular in appearance, and found that these cells lacked expression of contractile and cytoskeletal proteins traditionally associated with the "differentiated" SM phenotype. Within the middle media, we identified spindle-shaped cells oriented circumferentially. These cells expressed most SM markers, although they lacked expression of alternatively spliced products of SM-myosin heavy chain (SM-α isoform), vinculin (metavinculin), and caldesmon (150 kDa caldesmon). In the outer media, two very different cell subtypes were observed. One cell type was oriented in a longitudinal or spiral pattern along the vessel and was characterized by a highly differentiated phenotype (i.e. expressed all SM markers analyzed, including the alternatively spliced products of the contractile and cytoskeletal proteins mentioned above). Recently, we have demonstrated that this cell phenotype also expresses the SM-B isoform of the myosin heavy chain. This isoform is characterized by the presence of a unique 7-amino acid insert in the head region of the molecule, exhibiting high ATPase activity (67). Studies have shown that this isoform of myosin is expressed in greater amounts in fast, phasic than in slow, tonic smooth muscle, thus implying that the presence of such cells could confer unique functional properties to the vessel wall (46). Another population of cells, oriented circumferentially, did not express any of the SMC markers tested.

To evaluate the possibility that the cell subtypes observed in mature vascular media represented distinct cell lineages, and were not simply the result of temporal and transient modulation of a single phenotype, the developmental differentiation pathways of these specific cell populations were evaluated from early fetal life to maturity (27). The data demonstrated that the unique medial SMC subpopulations identified in the mature arterial media progressed along very distinct differentiation pathways during development. Importantly, we found that subpopulations of cells which expressed markers of a differentiated phenotype appeared rather early in development (120 days of gestation) and expanded by active proliferation during the fetal period. This observation further supported the idea that the different cell subpopulations in the vascular media were derived from separate unique cell lineages (68). The data, like those of Owens et al. (54), also suggest that modulation of the SMC phenotype from "contractile" to "synthetic" is not necessarily required for proliferation to occur. Thus, we have suggested that the existence of heterogenic SMC subpopulations in the mature media was the result of the presence of different subsets of cells progressing along distinct differentiation pathways during development. These observations are consistent with those in avian models of vascular development where unique SMC precursors have been shown to exist and give rise to functionally distinct cells within the vascular wall (68).

3.2   In Vivo Evidence For Unique Responses of Specific SMC Subpopulations to Hypoxia

The idea that specific subsets of arterial SMC contribute selectively to the vascular response to injury is supported by a substantial body of experimental evidence demonstrating that pathological lesions in atherosclerosis, restenosis and hypertension in humans (as well as the neointima in injured animal vessels) are composed mainly of cells with certain nonmuscle-like characteristics (20,58,59). The absence or paucity of muscle-specific markers in these cells was, in the past, usually attributed to a process of "phenotypic modulation" of a differentiated medial SMC type during its proliferation and migration into the intimal space. However, the identification of cells with nonmuscle-like characteristics in the normal mature vascular media in studies by several investigators, including our own, suggested that pathological lesions in the arteries could also originate via expansion of a subset of relatively "undifferentiated" or "immature" medial cells. For example, Holifield et al. suggested that the intimal thickening seen after balloon injury in canine arteries is the result of selective proliferation of a subset of nonmuscle-like cells in the arterial media (37). Recent studies by Murry et al., demonstrating monoclonality of atherosclerotic plaques in human arteries, also raised the possibility of participation of unique subsets of medial cells in the pathologic response of the vessel wall to injury (52).

In our laboratory we found marked heterogeneity in the proliferative and matrix-producing responses of the pulmonary medial SMC to the stimuli associated with hypoxic pulmonary hypertension (27,72). Using double-label immunofluorescence staining, we showed that phenotypically unique SMC subpopulations in bovine pulmonary arteries demonstrated markedly different proliferative responses to hypoxia-induced pulmonary hypertension. Quantitative analysis demonstrated that at every post-hypoxic time point studied, greater than 95% of the proliferation occurred within a SMC subpopulation lacking expression of a muscle-specific marker, metavinculin, whereas a population of SMC expressing metavinculin remained quiescent. These findings argue that the population of metavinculin-negative cells is functionally distinct from another, metavinculin-positive population of SMC.

3.3   In Vitro Evidence for SMC Heterogeneity and Unique Responses to Hypoxia

Evidence for the existence of phenotypically distinct and functionally unique SMC subpopulations within the arterial wall also comes from now fairly extensive *in vitro* studies. Initial observations in the systemic circulation of two populations of SMC with markedly different morphologies and growth patterns, one isolated from the neointima of injured rat carotid arteries, and the other from the unmanipulated tunica media, supported the hypothesis that the arterial wall may be composed of different SMC types (55,58). Also raised was the possibility that neointima originates via expansion of a small pre-existing medial SMC population with enhanced potential for proliferation and extracellular matrix protein synthesis, rather than simply by phenotypic modulation of the overall medial SMC population. Villaschi et al. recently demonstrated that two morphologically and functionally distinct SMC types could be isolated from different compartments of the vascular media at the same site in the normal rat aorta (69). Aortic medial SMC (MSMC) were isolated from the media after removal of the intima and adventitia. Aortic intimal SMC (ISMC) were isolated from the luminal side of everted rat aortas by scraping. MSMC were spindle-shaped, grew in the hill-and-valley pattern traditionally described for differentiated vascular SMC, and expressed α-SM-actin and SM-myosin. Conversely, ISMC displayed a polygonal or epitheloid shape, grew mainly as a monolayer and expressed α-SM-actin, but not SM-myosin, and were negative for Factor VIII-antigen. ISMC produced large amounts of a laminin- and type IV collagen-rich extracellular matrix which had a very unique and characteristic pericellular distribution. Contractile responses to endothelin differed significantly between the two SMC populations. Interestingly, the ISMC isolated from the normal rat arteries exhibited characteristics extremely similar to those reported for neointimal cells isolated from injured carotid arteries (69).

Studies using cloning techniques have also provided strong experimental evidence for the existence of phenotypically unique and stable SMC subpopulations within the rat and human arterial media. Gabbiani's group cloned four cell subtypes from the normal rat arterial media, which differed markedly in morphological and biochemical characteristics (9). The biological features of these cell subpopulations were distinct and were non-interchangeable over time in culture, suggesting that they were derived from different SMC precursors. Two of these cell clones were very similar to the cells previously isolated by others (37,69) and described above. One cell subtype exhibited a distinct "epitheloid" or "rounded" morphology and grew as a monolayer at confluence. These cells had high thymidine incorporation in response to serum stimulation compared to other clones. Another clone of cells exhibited a spindle-like morphology and a hill-and-valley pattern of growth at confluence. These cells were less reactive to mitogenic stimuli. The clonal populations exhibited striking resemblance to cell subpopulations which could be cultured from experimentally induced intimal thickening. Again, the results strongly suggested the possibility that the SMC population observed in response to at least balloon-induced endothelial injury *in vivo* was derived mainly from SMC belonging to a specific pre-existing cell subpopulation.

Since most previous studies had been performed in rodent vessels, which have a rather simple structure compared to human vessels, we performed cell culture studies using pulmonary and systemic arteries of a large mammalian species (the bovine), with the goal of isolating and maintaining in culture heterogeneous arterial SMC subpopulations that exhibited unique characteristics similar to those observed *in vivo* (26). We succeeded in isolating four phenotypically unique SMC populations, each exhibiting distinct morphological and biochemical characteristics (26). The isolated cell populations could be broadly split into two major categories, one exhibiting smooth muscle characteristics and the other "nonmuscle-like" features. Interestingly, the cell subpopulations isolated from the bovine species demonstrated many morphological, biochemical and functional characteristics similar to cell subpopulations derived from the normal rat arterial media. As was the case with the rat cells, the observed morphological and biochemical differences were maintained by the distinct cell populations over multiple passages in culture. None of the cell populations were observed to undergo a modulation into another phenotype, again supporting the possibility that they represented distinct cell lineages.

Cells exhibiting unique morphological and biochemical characteristics also differed significantly with respect to their proliferative responses to growth-promoting stimuli (25,26). We found that, in general, the "nonmuscle-like" cell subpopulations exhibited markedly enhanced growth capabilities under serum-stimulated conditions compared to "differentiated" SMC populations. Moreover, nonmuscle-like cells exhibited the capacity to grow in plasma-based media, whereas the differentiated SMC remained quiescent under these conditions. We also found among the nonmuscle-like cell populations specific subsets of cells that proliferated autonomously, similar to embryonic aortic cells previously described by Cook et al. (14).

Since *in vivo* studies have demonstrated selective proliferative responses of arterial SMC to hypoxia-induced pulmonary hypertension, we examined the possibility that distinct cell subpopulations isolated from the normal arterial media would also exhibit different responses to hypoxia *in vitro*. Indeed, we found that only specific cell populations proliferated in response to hypoxia (in general, the nonmuscle-like cells), whereas differentiated SMC were growth-inhibited under hypoxic conditions (Fig. 3 & 4) (25).

Differential contractile responses of pulmonary and systemic vessels to similar stimuli (e.g., hypoxia) also support the idea of SMC diversity (6,7,71). Even within the pulmonary vascular bed, differences in the responses to hypoxia between large conduit and small resistance pulmonary arteries are observed. For example, hypoxia has been shown to constrict resistance pulmonary arteries while causing biphasic responses in conduit arteries. Questions have arisen regarding the cellular basis for this variability. Madden et al. found that vascular SMC isolated from resistance pulmonary arteries constricted in response to hypoxia, whereas those from conduit pulmonary arteries and the systemic cerebral circulation did not (47). The constrictor response to hypoxia was associated with an increase in intracellular calcium. This information suggested that the differential response of the vessels was intrinsic based on the differences in the vascular SMC themselves. Recent work by Archer suggests that this characteristic is the preferential occurrence of an O_2-sensor and O_2-sensitive potassium channels in SMC of resistance-size vessels. The lack of hypoxia-induced K+ channel inhibition or membrane depolarization (or both) in systemic arteries may account for the absence of hypoxic vasoconstriction in the systemic beds (6).

In attempts to explain the differences in reactivity to hypoxia and other stimuli between proximal and distal arteries, Archer et al. and Weir et al. have carried out a series of studies evaluating K+ channel distribution in SMC from large and small pulmonary vessels (6,7,71). SMC from the pulmonary artery were shown to contain various types of K+ channels

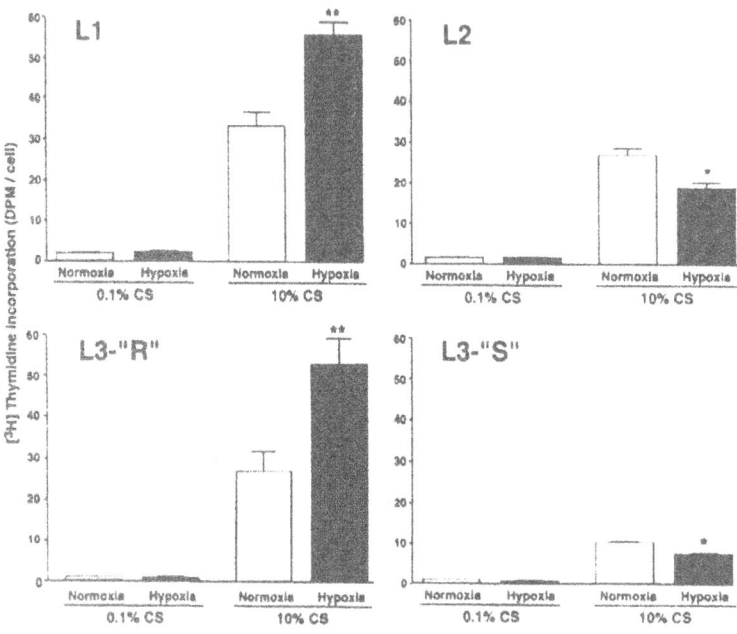

Figure 3. Effects of hypoxia on SMC proliferation are subpopulation specific. In the presence of serum, hypoxia (3% O2) stimulates proliferation only in two cell types (L1 and L3 - "R"). These cell populations are characterized by a less differentiated phenotype than that exhibited by hypoxia unresponsive cells L2 and L3 - "S" (Frid et al., 25).

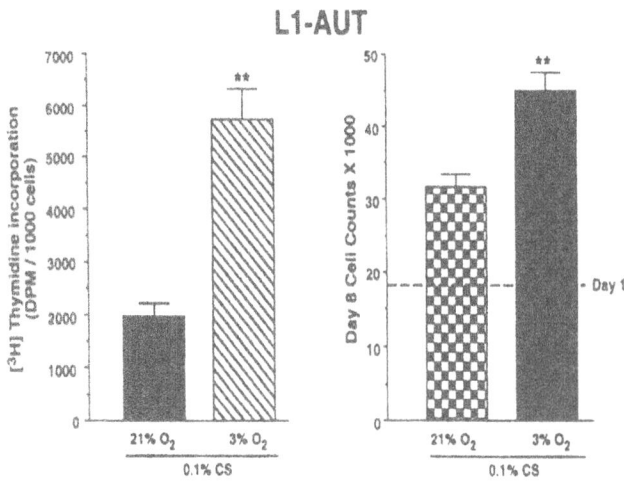

Figure 4. Hypoxia stimulates proliferation in the absence of serum in a unique subpopulation of cells (L1-Aut) that exhibit autonomous growth capabilities (Frid et al., #25).

Differential contractile responses of pulmonary and systemic vessels to similar stimuli (e.g. hypoxia) also support the idea of SMC diversity (6,7,71). Even within the pulmonary vascular bed, differences in the responses to hypoxia between large conduit and small resistance pulmonary arteries are observed. For example, hypoxia has been shown to constrict resistance pulmonary arteries while causing biphasic responses in conduit arteries. Questions have arisen regarding the cellular basis for this variability. Madden et al. found that vascular SMC isolated from resistance pulmonary arteries constricted in response to hypoxia whereas those from conduit pulmonary arteries and the systemic cerebral circulation did not (47). The constrictor response to hypoxia was associated with an increase in intracellular calcium. This information suggested that the differential response of the vessels was intrinsic based on the differences in the vascular SMC themselves. Recent work by Archer, suggests that this characteristic is the preferential occurrence of an O_2-sensor and O_2-sensitive potassium channels in SMC of resistance size vessels. The lack of hypoxia-induced K+ channel inhibition or membrane depolarization or both in systemic arteries may account for the absence of hypoxic vasoconstriction in the systemic beds (6).

In attempts to explain the differences in reactivity to hypoxia and other stimuli between proximal and distal arteries, and Archer et al. and Weir et al. have carried out a series of studies evaluating K+ channel distribution in SMC from large and small pulmonary vessels (6,7,71). SMC from the pulmonary artery were shown to contain various types of K channels including K_{ca}, delayed rectifier (K_{DR}), and K_{ATP}-gated channels, and that one channel type was often dominant in a specific cell. K_{ca} channels are activated by depolarization and by increases in $[Ca_2+]i$ and thus tend to restore membrane potential toward basal levels when vasoconstrictors cause depolarization. K_{DR} channels control resting membrane potential in pulmonary SMC and appear to be the hypoxia-inhibited K+ channels involved in hypoxic pulmonary vasoconstriction. The authors found that the relative distribution of these electrophysiologically distinguishable cells varied in vessels along the longitudinal axis of the pulmonary artery in a manner that was consistent with the overall response exhibited to hypoxia. For example, "K_{DR}" cells constituted 65% of the SMC in distal rat pulmonary arteries but only 15% of cells in the proximal pulmonary artery. "K_{ca}" cells constituted 15% of the cells in the proximal PA but only 3% of those from the distal PA. To confirm the cellular observations, radiolabeled K+ channel ligand studies were performed to evaluate the number of ion channels in large amounts of homogenized vascular tissue. These studies confirmed that the K_{ca} channel number was significantly enhanced in conduit versus resistance pulmonary arteries (6,7). Thus, the presence of diverse electrophysiological cell types within and between vascular segments may contribute to regional differences in vascular reactivity to stimuli that influence tone via modulation of K+ channels, such as hypoxia and NO.

3.4   Distinct Signaling Pathways are Involved in Conferring Unique Growth and Functional Properties to SMC Subpopulations

The remarkable differences in proliferative and matrix protein synthetic responses to similar stimuli between different medial SMC subpopulations suggest that the membrane receptor and/or intracellular signaling pathways controlling these responses may be quite different in these cells. As mentioned above, different SMC subpopulations have been shown to exhibit unique electrophysiological properties, and thus responses to hypoxia, that are due to differences in the types of K+ channels expressed on the cell membrane. In addition, cells demonstrating activation of K_{ca} channels and hyperpolarization in response to endothelin and α-thrombin, were found to exhibit an epitheliod morphology and enhanced growth capacity compared to cells with a spindle morphology, which depolarized in response to the same stimuli (53). Other studies have demonstrated differences in the relative proportion or types of receptors for mitogenic and/or vasoconstrictor agents on different SMC lines (59). Differences in the contribution of the receptor tyrosine kinase and the G-protein-coupled pathways to growth have been shown to vary between vascular SMC isolated from different species. Studies in our laboratory have demonstrated that the cells isolated from the subendothelial space, which exhibit markedly enhanced growth potential utilize a pertussis toxin-sensitive G-protein coupled pathway (Gi) that does not appear to contribute to growth in the other cell types present in the bovine arterial wall (2). Additional studies using stable transfection have shown that over-expression of specific G-proteins in vascular cells significantly changes the functional responses of the cell to external stimuli (36).

Even in the absence of obvious receptor or membrane differences, cells could exhibit different responses to similar stimuli based on the presence of and/or differential activation of downstream effector pathways. This concept has recently been nicely demonstrated by Bornfeldt et al., who showed that the mitogen-activated protein kinase pathway can mediate either growth inhibition or proliferation in different human vascular SMC types, depending on the availability of specific downstream mitogen-activated protein kinase

(MAPK) targets (10). They showed that some human vascular SMC expressed the inducible form of cyclooxygenase (COX-2), whereas other SMC do not. They showed in SMC which expressed COX-2, that activation of MAPK served as a negative regulator of proliferation, whereas in SMC lacking COX-2, MAPK activation, as classically described, led to proliferation. In cells expressing COX-2, PDGF-induced MAPK activation led to cytosolic phospholipase A_2 activation, PGE_2 release, and subsequent activation of the cAMP-dependent protein kinase (PKA), which acts as a strong inhibitor of SMC proliferation. Thus, the biological outcome in response to similar stimuli, at least those mediated by MAPK, is highly dependent on downstream enzymes expressed by the cell. Since different SMC express different downstream enzymes, the diversity in the response to similar stimuli might be expected. It is interesting that the only subpopulations of SMC that appear to exhibit enhanced proliferative responses to hypoxia, in the absence of exogenous mitogens or serum, are those that demonstrate constituitive activation of extracellular signal regulated kinase (Erk) 1 and 2.

Another intracellular signaling pathway that exerts a wide variety of effects on different cell processes is the protein kinase C pathway. Numerous isozymes of PKC have been identified and have been demonstrated to be both developmentally regulated and cell-specific. Thus, the presence of specific PKC isozymes and their susceptibility to activation could confer unique properties to different cell types. Since PKC activation can contribute to a general pattern of overall enhanced growth capacity, we tested whether the cell subpopulations susceptible to hypoxic growth stimulation in our studies would exhibit different patterns of PKC isozyme expression than those SMC that were growth-inhibited by hypoxia. Further, since Dempsey et al. had previously shown that the α-isozyme of PKC (a calcium-dependent isoform) is an important determinant of hypoxic growth capacity (17), we compared the level of expression of PKC-α isoform in the two medial SMC subtypes and found that nonmuscle-like cells had increased levels of immunodetectable PKC-α compared to the nonproliferative differentiated SMC (19). This pattern of isozyme expression was paralleled by increased whole cellular PKC catalytic activity in the hypoxia-sensitive compared to hypoxia-insensitive cells. Thus, distinct arterial cell subpopulations, similar to those observed *in vivo*, were isolated and maintained in culture and demonstrated unique differences in the signaling mechanisms that appear to contribute to their unique growth responses.

4.   FIBROBLAST RESPONSES TO HYPOXIA

4.1   In Vivo Studies

In animal models, the earliest and most dramatic structural changes following hypoxic exposure are found in the adventitial compartment of the vessel wall (38,66). Resident adventitial fibroblasts exhibit early and sustained increases in proliferation that exceed those observed in endothelial or smooth muscle cells (8,50). In addition, early and dramatic changes in extracellular matrix protein synthesis occur (23). These include early upregulation of collagen, fibronectin, and tropoelastin mRNA's followed by a subsequent increased deposition of each of these proteins. These changes in the proliferative and matrix-producing phenotype of the fibroblast are accompanied by appearance of α-SMC actin, in at least some of the cells in the adventitial compartment, indicating a modulation of fibroblasts to myofibroblasts (65). The fibroproliferative changes in the adventitia are ultimately associated with luminal narrowing and progressive decrease in the ability of the vessel wall to respond to vasodilating stimuli (22). In humans with hypoxic-associated forms of pulmonary hypertension, adventitial changes can be dramatic and even predominate. For instance, even the earliest pathologic descriptions of persistent pulmonary hypertension of the newborn (PPHN) pointed out significant adventitial thickening (51). Dramatic adventitial changes have also been observed in the lung vessels of young infants dying of high-altitude-induced pulmonary hypertension (64). Similar, though less dramatic changes are seen in the adventitial compartment of infants with cyanotic forms of congenital heart disease that are complicated by pulmonary hypertension.

The possibility that hypoxia acts directly (or in unique ways) on the adventitial fibroblast in the setting of chronic hypoxic pulmonary hypertension is raised by previously well documented observations that reduced oxygen tension (anoxia/hypoxia) results in profound changes in fibroblast physiology and metabolism. Cellular anoxia represents a biochemical state distinct from hypoxia, yet still represents a normal physiological condition present during wound healing (5). Since a response quite different from that seen with hypoxia is induced in anoxic fibroblasts, these cells must possess the unique ability to activate a different, possibly overlapping set of genes to cope with these different environmental conditions (4). As noted above, the activity of several different transcription factors is known to be influenced by low oxygen tensions. In cells that are stressed by oxygen deprivation, nuclear factor-κB (NF-κB) activity increases as a result of phosphorylation and subsequent degradation of inhibitory κBIκB)40In other cells, low oxygen tensions induce the transcription of multiple members of the bZIP (basic/leucine zipper domain) superfamily (75), result in nuclear accumulation of p53 (32), or induce the activity of hypoxia-inducible factor 1 (HIF-1) (62). Estes et al (24) demonstrated that one DNA-binding activity induced in hypoxic, anoxic, and cobalt-treated fibroblasts recognizes secondary anoxia-responsive element (SARE), and has electrophoretic mobility similar to that of HIF-1. It has also been demonstrated that a second, more prominent SARE binding activity, termed the anoxia-inducible factor (AIF), is also induced in anoxic fibroblasts. Two-dimensional gel analysis indicated that AIF is a heterodimer composed of 61- and 52-kDa subunits and is likely to arise from post-translational modification of a heterodimeric SARE binding complex present in aerobic cells. Identification of a mammalian anoxic response element has interesting implications. This element may prove useful in gene therapy regimens for targeting expression to physiological situations in which functional anaerobiosis exists, such as during wound healing. Interestingly, deregulation of genes normally expressed during anoxia is often also seen in cancer cells, regardless of their state of oxygenation (4). Thus, understanding the molecular basis of the mammalian anoxic regulatory pathway in fibroblasts and how similar genes become constitutively activated in malignancy, or perhaps in simply pathophysiologic states, may further lead to unique approaches to therapeutic intervention in settings of vascular disease complicated by hypoxia.

4.2   Signal Transduction Pathways in Hypoxic Stimulated Fibroblast Proliferation

Protein phosphorylation appears to be crucial for expression of many hypoxic-inducible genes. Inhibition of tyrosine kinase pathways has been shown to inhibit many HIF-inducible genes. One important target, perhaps crucial for proliferation, is the mitogen-activated protein kinase (MAPK) family of enzymes. Many studies have demonstrated that the MAPK's p44 (Erk 1) and p42 (Erk 2) are crucial to proliferation in response to growth factors in a variety of cell types (61,70). The growth factors, via their cell surface receptors, initiate a series of events culminating in the phosphorylation of ras-GDP to the active form ras-GTP. In turn, ras then activates raf, which activates MEK (MAPK/Erk Kinase). MEK very specifically activates Erk 1 and Erk 2 by tyrosine and threonine phosphorylation. Active Erks are proline directed, serine-threonine kinases which then can 1) phosphorylate cytoplasmic proteins, and 2) translocate to the nucleus where they activate transcription factors such as Elk-1 and activate genes involved in proliferation such as c-fos.

Recent work from Rodney Rhoades lab and Marc Hershenson's lab has shown that Erk-mediated signaling is also important in stress-induced proliferation via H_2O_2 in pulmonary arterial SMC and airway SMC, respectively (1,76). Work in Hela cells demonstrates that hypoxia can induce c-fos expression and that this expression is dependent on MAPK direct activation of Erk-1. We therefore sought to determine whether Erk 1 and 2 mediated the proliferation in pulmonary arterial adventitial fibroblasts induced by hypoxic stress. In order to separate the proliferative effects of hypoxia from those of growth factors and cytokines, we performed experiments in growth arrested, serum deprived cells. Under these conditions, hypoxia induced an increase in DNA synthesis above normoxic levels, as measured by ^{3}H-thymidine incorporation, in pulmonary artery adventitial fibroblasts as early as 24 hours after exposure (Fig. 4). Continued exposure to hypoxia for three days resulted in increased cell density compared to cultures maintained in normoxic atmosphere (11). Thus, the proliferative stimulus of hypoxia is both early and sustained. Interestingly, we found that when systemic adventitial fibroblasts, isolated from the aortas of the same animals, were assayed for hypoxic induction of DNA synthesis, only 25% of the cultures demonstrated hypoxia-induced increases in DNA synthesis.

We also wanted to determine whether the proliferative effect of hypoxia on adventitial fibroblasts was dependent on oxygen concentration. We compared levels of DNA synthesis under oxygen concentrations ranging from 1% to 20%. We found that 3% oxygen stimulated DNA synthesis maximally whereas 1% oxygen did not increase DNA synthesis. Hypoxic-induced proliferation was associated with an increase in Erk 1/Erk 2 activity, as measured by ability of immuno-complexes to incorporate ^{32}P label onto EGF-receptor peptides, a known substrate for Erk activity. Hypoxia induced a transient increase in Erk activity, peaking at 10 minutes and returning to basal levels at 30-45 minutes. The peak represented a 2.5-fold increase in activity which was 25% of the activity detected under maximal stimulation by serum. Transient increases in Erk activity have been reported with growth factor-induced proliferation of other cell types, usually peaking at 5 minutes and returning to basal at 15 minutes. Importantly, an increase in Erk activity was again noted at 24 and 72 hours in cells that remained exposed to hypoxic conditions. We also demonstrated that interruption of the Erk signaling pathway, by inhibition of ras activation or inhibition of MEK activation, abrogated the ability of hypoxia to stimulate DNA synthesis, and also abolished the increase in cell density noted with sustained hypoxia under serum-deprived conditions. Thus, it appears that the ability of hypoxia to stimulate proliferation in adventitial fibroblasts under serum-deprived conditions is at least partially dependent on the Erk signaling pathway.

These results are in complete agreement with the effects of hypoxia on Hela cells and human osteoblastic cells.

In addition to the "classic" forms of MAP kinase, families of related protein serine/threonine kinases exist in cells, and are referred to as the stress-activated protein (SAP) kinases. These kinases, consisting of at least two homologues, c-Jun NH2-terminal kinase (JNK) and p38 MAP kinase are strongly activated by environmental stress, including heat shock and ultraviolet (UV) irradiation, cytokines (TNF, IL-1) and toxins (lipopolysaccharide). Recent studies have also demonstrated that exposure of adventitial fibroblasts to acute hypoxia (1%) activates both JNK and p38 MAP kinase (60). Peaks of activity 6 and then 24 hours following the activation of Erk 1 and 2 were observed. Activation of these kinases may be involved in proliferation. In addition, they may also be involved in adventitial fibroblast apoptosis that we have observed in response to 1% O2.

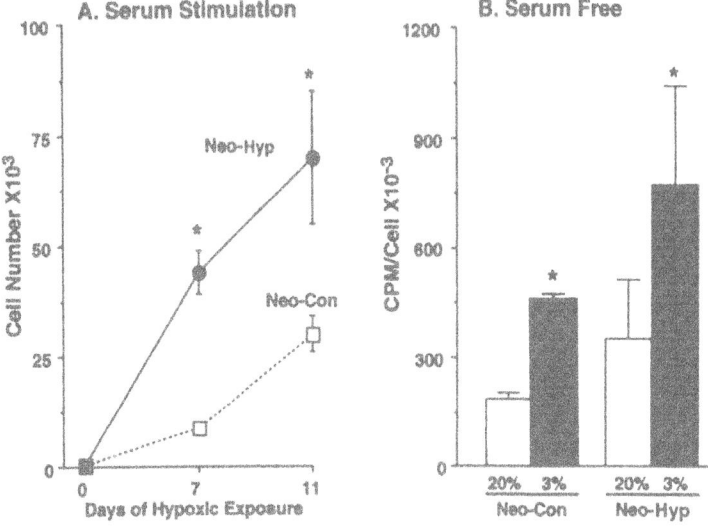

Figure 5. Hypoxia stimulates proliferation in adventitial fibroblasts. Fibroblasts were isolated from control neonatal animals (Neo-Con 15d of age) or from neonatal animals exposed to 14 days of hypoxia (Neo-Hyp, 15d of age). Hypoxia induces an increase in fibroblast proliferation in the presence or absence of serum. Responses in fibroblasts from chronically hypoxic animals were consistently greater than those from control animals.

4.3   Fibroblast Heterogeneity: Hypoxia Induces Proliferation Only in a Subset of Adventitial Fibroblasts

In addition to the developmentally regulated and site- or organ-specific differences in fibroblast phenotype that have been well documented, there is a growing body of literature documenting the existence of phenotypic heterogeneity within the resident fibroblast population of a given tissue at a specified developmental stage. The extensive diversity of this intra-site heterogeneity includes differences in proliferative potential, synthesis of matrix molecules, production and response to growth factors, synthesis of matrix degrading enzymes, phagocytic activity and the presence of specific receptors and/or antigenic determinants at the cell surface (For review, see 29,56).

To examine the possibility that several unique pulmonary artery adventitial fibroblast populations exist and thus contribute in unique ways to the vascular remodeling process, we used limited dilution and clonal expansion strategies to try and establish pure, stable subpopulations of adventitial fibroblasts. We found that subpopulations of fibroblasts could be distinguished not only on the basis of their light microscopic appearance (i.e., rounded or epitheloid vs. traditional elongated spindle shape), but also on the basis of their cytoskeletal protein expression. Subpopulations with a rounded appearance did not express SM-specific α-actin in culture (15). In contrast, there was significantly brighter immunostaining with SM-specific α-actin antibody in fibroblast subpopulations demonstrating a spindle-like appearance. Marked differences in proliferative potential of different fibroblast clones were also documented. In general, cells exhibiting a spindle-like appearance tended to demonstrate far greater growth potential to serum or peptide mitogens than did the rounded cells. We also found that certain clones of fibroblasts expressed extremely high levels of type I and III collagen mRNA compared to other clones. In most, but not all instances, cells that exhibited a high growth potential also exhibited a high potential for collagen synthesis. On the other hand, elastin mRNA levels were significantly elevated in only one relatively slow growing clone of adventitial fibroblasts.

We also sought to determine if differences in the proliferative response of hypoxia existed between fibroblast clones. We found that there are subsets of fibroblasts which are highly sensitive to growth promoting effects of hypoxia and subsets which are resistant (16). Susceptibility to the growth promoting effects of hypoxia was not predictable on the basis of morphology or growth potential in serum. Collectively, these *in vitro* findings strongly support the idea that distinct subpopulations of fibroblasts exist within the pulmonary artery adventitia and may contribute selectively to the adventitial thickening observed in response to chronic hypoxia.

Changes in the relative proportion of different fibroblast subsets may have profound effects not only on the adventitial remodeling but on the whole vessel wall. It is possible that alteration in the relative proportion of different fibroblast subsets with different capabilities for matrix protein and soluble growth factor production, might be expected to influence the behavior of adjacent SMC or endothelial cells (dynamic reciprocity, see above). It is clear that there is continuous feedback of information between cell and matrix such that the extracellular matrix in contact with the cells is itself a product of cellular activity (by virtue of biosynthesis, degradation, and modification of matrix macromolecules), and that the extracellular matrix influences various fundamental aspects of cell behavior, such as the deposition of matrix itself, cell proliferation and the pattern of gene expression and cell migration. Activation of a fibroblast subset secreting unique matrix molecules and soluble factors may thus have an influence on neighboring SMC or epithelial cells that is not exhibited under normal conditions.

5.   SUMMARY

The arterial media and adventitia are no longer thought to be comprised of homogeneous populations of SMC and fibroblasts (respectively) but rather of a mosaic of subtypes of cells with unique biochemical and functional characteristics. With regard to the changes in structure the pulmonary circulation is known to undergo in response to chronic hypoxia, there is convincing evidence to suggest that unique subtypes of cells participate selectively by virtue of their unique proliferative and matrix producing responses to hypoxia. These responses appear dependent on the activation by hypoxia of critical protein phosphorylation steps involving both PKC and MAPK. The reasons these pathways are activated by hypoxia in only certain cell subpopulation remains a mystery at present but is the subject of intense investigation. Solving the issues of how and why hypoxia activates proproliferative signaling in only select cell populations will lead to a greater understanding of chronic hypoxic pulmonary hypertension.

REFERENCES

1. Abe M.K., S. Kartha, A.Y. Karpova, J. Li, P.T. Liu, W-L Kho, and M.B. Hershenson. Hydrogen peroxide activates extracelluar signal-regulated kinase via protein kinase C, Raf-1, and MEK1. *Am. J. Respir. Cell Mol. Biol.* 18: 562-569, 1998.

2. Aldashev A.A., M.G. Frid, R. Nemenoff, and K.R. Stenmark. Unique growth capabilities of phenotypically distinct SMC subpopulations are controlled by different signaling pathways. *Am. J. Respir. Crit. Care Med.* 153(4):A577, 1996.

3. Allen K.M., and S.G. Haworth. Cytoskeletal features of immature pulmonary vascular smooth muscle cells: the influence of pulmonary hypertension on normal development. *J. Pathol.* 158: 311-317, 1989.

4. Anderson G.R., D.L. Stolerand, and L.A. Scarcello. Normal fibroblasts responding to anoxia exhibit features of the malignant phenotype. *J. Biol. Chem.* 264: 14885-14892, 1989.

5. Anderson G.R., C.M. Volpe, C.A. Russo, D.L. Stoler, and S.M. Miloro. The anoxic fibroblast response is an early stage wound healing program. *J Surg. Res.* 59: 666-674, 1995.

6. Archer S.L., J.M.C. Huang, H.L. Reeve, V. Hampl, S. Tolarova, E. Michelakis and E.K. Weir. Differential distribution of electrophysiologically distinct myocytes in conduit and resistance arteries determines their response to nitric oxide and hypoxia. *Circ. Res.* 78: 431-442, 1996.

7. Archer S.L. Diversity of phenotype and function of vascular smooth muscle cells. *J. Lab. Clin. Med.* 127: 524-529, 1996.

8. Belknap J.K., E.C. Orton, B. Ensley, and K.R. Stenmark. Hypoxia increases bromodeoxyuridine labeling indices in bovine neonatal pulmonary arteries. *Am. J. Respi.r Cell Mol. Biol.* 16:366-371, 1997.

9. Bochaton-Piallat M-L., P. Ropraz, F. Gabbiani, and G. Gabbiani. Phenotypic heterogeneity of rat arterial smooth muscle cell clones. *Arterioscler. Thromb. Vasc. Biol.* 16: 815-820, 1996.

10. Bornfeldt K.E., J.S. Campbell, H. Koyama, G.M. Argast, C.C. Leslie, E.W. Raines, E.G. Krebs, and R. Ross. The mitogen-activated protein kinase pathway can mediate growth inhibition and proliferation in smooth muscle cells. *J. Clin. Invest.* 100:875-885, 1997.

11. Bouchey D., R. Nemenoff, and K.R. Stenmark. Hypoxia activates extracellular-signal regulated kinase (Erk) and induces proliferation in adventitial fibroblasts from the neonatal bovine main pulmonary artery (MPA-Fibs). *Am. Soc. Cell Biol.* 1998; (Submitted).

12. Bunn H.F. and R.O. Poyton. Oxygen sensing and molecular adaptation to hypoxia. *Physiol. Rev.* 76: 839-885, 1996.

13. Bunn H.F., J. Gu, L.E. Huang, J-W. Park and H. Zhu. Erythropoietin: a model system for studying oxygen-dependent gene regulation. *J. Exp. Biol.* 201: 1197-1201, 1998.

14. Cook C.L., M.C.M. Weiser, P.E. Schwartz, C.L. Jones, R.A. Majack. Developmentally timed expression of an embryonic growth phenotype in vascular smooth muscle cells. *Circ. Res.* 74:189-196, 1994.

15. Das M., E..C Dempsey, and K.R. Stenmark. Selective subpopulations of pulmonary artery adventitial fibroblasts exhibit unique proliferative and apoptotic capabilities. *FASEB J.* 12(4):A339:1971, 1998.

16. Das M., K.R. Stenmark, and E.C. Dempsey. Hypoxia stimulates growth of selective subsets of pulmonary artery adventitial fibroblasts. *FASEB J.* 11:A557, 1997.

17. Dempsey E.C., D.B. Badesch, E.L. Dobyns, and K.R. Stenmark. Enhanced growth capacity of neonatal pulmonary artery smooth muscle cells in vitro:Dependence on cell

size, time from birth, insulin-like growth factor 1, and auto-activation of protein kinase C. *J. Cell Physiol.* 160: 469-481, 1994.

18. Dempsey E.C., M. Das, M.G. Frid, and K.R. Stenmark. Unique growth properties of neonatal pulmonary vascular cells: importance of time- and site-specific responses, cell-cell interaction, and synergy. *J. Perinatol.* 16: S2-S11, 1996.

19. Dempsey E.C., M.G. Frid, A.A. Aldashev, and K.R. Stenmark. Heterogeneity in the proliferative response of bovine pulmonary artery smooth muscle cells to mitogens and hypoxia: importance of protein kinase C-α1. *Can. J. Physiol. Pharmacol.* 75: 936-944, 1997.

20. Desmouliere A., and G. Gabbiani. The cytoskeleton of arterial smooth muscle cells during human and experimental atheromatosis. *Kidney Internatl.* 37: S87-S89, 1992.

21. Durmowicz A.G., M.G. Frid, J.D. Wohrley, and K.R. Stenmark. Expression and localization of tropoelastin mRNA in the developing bovine pulmonary artery is dependent on vascular cell phenotype. *Am. J. Respir. Cell Mol. Biol.* 14: 569-576, 1996.

22. Durmowicz A.G., E.C. Orton, and K.R. Stenmark. Progressive loss of vasodilator responsive component of pulmonary hypertension in neonatal calves exposed to 4,570m. *Am. J. Physiol.* 265: H2175-2183, 1993.

23. Durmowicz A.G., W.C. Parks, D.M. Hyde, R.P. Mecham, and K.R. Stenmark. Persistence, re-expression, and induction of pulmonary arterial fibronectin, tropoelastin and type I procollagen mRNA expression in neonatal hypoxic pulmonary hypertension. *Am. J. Pathol.* 145: 1411-1420, 1994.

24. Estes S.D., D.L. Stoler, and G.R. Anderson. Anoxic induction of a sarcoma virus-related VL30 retrotransposon is mediated by a cis-acting element which binds hypoxia-inducible factor 1 and an anoxia inducible factor. *J. Virol.* 69:6335-6341, 1995.

25. Frid M.G., A.A. Aldashev, E.C. Dempsey, and K.R. Stenmark. Smooth muscle cells isolated from discrete compartments of the mature vascular media exhibit unique phenotypes and distinct growth capabilities. *Circ. Res.* 81: 940-952, 1997.

26. Frid M.G., E.C. Dempsey, A.G. Durmowicz, and K.R. Stenmark. Smooth muscle cell heterogeneity in pulmonary and systemic vessels. *Arterioscler. Thromb. Vasc. Biol.* 17:1203-1209, 1997.

27. Frid M.G., E.P. Moiseeva, and K.R. Stenmark. Multiple phenotypically distinct smooth muscle cell populations exist in the adult and developing bovine pulmonary arterial media in vivo. *Circ. Res.* 75:669-681, 1994.

28. Frid M.G., O.Y. Printseva, A. Chiavegato, E. Faggin, M. Scatena, V.E. Koteliansky, P. Pauletto, M.A. Glukhova, and S. Sartore. Myosin heavy-chain isoform composition and distribution in developing and adult human aortic smooth muscle. *J. Vasc. Res.* 30:279-292, 1993.

29. Fries K.M., T. Blieden, R.J. Looney, G.D. Sempowski, M.R. Silvera, R.A. Willis, R.P. Phipps. Evidence of fibroblast heterogeneity and the role of fibroblast subpopulations in fibrosis. *Clin. Immunol. Immunopathol.* 72(3):283-292, 1994.

30. Gleadle J.M. and P.J. Ratcliffe. Hypoxia and the regulation of gene expression. *Molec. Med. Today* 4: 122-129, 1998.

31. Glukhova M.A., A.E. Kabakov, M.G. Frid, O.I. Ornatsky, A.M. Belkin, D.N. Mukhin, A.N. Orekhov, V.E. Koteliansky, and V.N. Smirnov. Modulation of human aorta smooth muscle cell phenotype: a study of muscle-specific variants of vinculin, caldesmon, and actin expression. *Proc. Natl. Acad. Sci. USA.* 85:9542-9546, 1988.

32. Graeber T.G., J.F. Peterson, M. Tsai, K Monica, A.J. Fornace, Jr., and A.J. Giaccia. Hypoxia induces accumulation of p53 protein, but activation of a G1-phase checkpoint by low-oxygen conditions is independent of p53 status. Mol. Cell Biol. 14:6264-6277, 1994.

33. Graven K.K., and H.W. Farber. Endothelial hypoxic stress proteins. *Kidney Internatl.* 51: 426-437, 1997.

34. Graven K.K., L.H. Zimmerman, E.W. Dickson, G.L. Weinhouse, and H.W. Farber. Endothelial cell hypoxia associated proteins are cell and stress specific. *J. Cell Physiol.* 157: 544-554, 1993.

35. Guillemin K., and M.A. Krasnow. The hypoxic response: huffing and HIFing. *Cell* 89: 9-12, 1997.

36. Higashita R., L. Li, V. Van Putten, Y. Yamamura, F. Zarinetchi, L. Heasley, R.A. Nemenoff. Gα16 mimics vasoconstrictor action to induce smooth muscle α-actin in vascular smooth muscle cells through a Jun-NH2-terminal kinase-dependent pathway. *J. Biol. Chem.* 272: 25845-25850, 1997.

37. Holifield B., T. Helgason, S. Jemelka, A. Taylor, S. Navran, J. Allen, C. Seidel. Differentiated vascular myocytes: are they involved in neointimal formation? *J. Clin. Invest.* 97:814-825, 1996.

38. Jones R., and L. Reid. Vascular remodelling in clinical and experimental pulmonary hypertensions. In: *Pulmonary Vascular Remodeling.* edited by JE Bishop, JT Reeves, GJ Laurent eds: London: Portland Press; 1995:47-115.

39. Karakurum M., R. Shreeniwas, J. Chen, D. Pinsky, S-D Yan, M. Anderson, K. Sunouchi, J. Major, T. Hamilton, K. Kuwabara, A. Rot, R. Nowygrod, and D. Stern. Hypoxic induction of interleukin-8 gene expression in human endothelial cells. *J. Clin. Invest.* 93: 1564-1570, 1994.

40. Koong A.C., E.Y. Chen, and A.J. Giaccia. Hypoxia causes the activation of nuclear factor kappa B through the phosphorylation of I kappa B alpha on tyrosine residues. *Cancer Res.* 54:1425-1430, 1994.

41. Kourembanas S., P.A. Marsden, L.P. McQuillan, and D.V. Faller. Hypoxia induces endothelin gene expression and secretion in cultured human endothelium. *J. Clin. Invest.* 88: 1054-1057, 1991.

42. Kourembanas S., R.L. Hannan and D.V. Faller. Oxygen tension regulates the expression of the platelet-derived growth factor-B chain gene in human endothelial cells. *J. Clin. Invest.* 86: 670-674, 1990.

43. Lee S., and B.L. Fanburg. Glycolytic activity and enhancement of serotonin uptake by endothelial cells exposed to hypoxia/anoxia. *Circ. Res..* 60: 653-658, 1987.

44. Levin E.G., L. Santell, and K.G. Osborn. The expression of endothelial tissue plasminogen activator in vivo: a function defined by vessel size and anatomic location. *J. Cell. Sci.* 110: 139-148, 1997.

45. Loike J.D., L. Cao, J. Brett, S. Ogawa, S.C. Silverstein, and D. Stern. Hypoxia induces glucose transporter expression in endothelial cells. *Am. J. Physiol.* 263:C326-C333, 1992.

46. Low R.B., and S.S. White. Lung smooth muscle differentiation. *J. Cell. Biochem.* 1997; (In Press).

47. Madden J.A., M.S. Vadula, and V. Kump. Effects of hypoxia and other vasoactive agents on pulmonary and cerebral artery smooth muscle cells. *Am. J. Physiol.* 263; L384-L393, 1992.

48. Majesky M.W., S.M. Schwartz. Smooth muscle diversity in arterial wound repair. *Toxicol. Pathol.* 18: 554-559, 1990.

49. Marti H.H., and W. Risau. Systemic hypoxia changes the organ-specific distribution of vascular endothelial growth factor and its receptors. *Proc. Natl. Acad. Sci.* 95:15809-15814, 1998.

50. Meyrick B., and L. Reid. Hypoxia and incorporation of [3H]-thymidine by cells of the rat pulmonary arteries and alveolar wall. *Am. J. Pathol.* 96:51-70, 1979.

51. Murphy J.D., M. Rabinovitch, J.D. Goldstein, L.M. Reid. The structural basis of persistent pulmonary hypertension of the newborn infant. *J. Pediatr.* 98:962-967, 1981.
52. Murry C.E., C.T. Gipaya, T. Bartosek, E.P. Benditt, and S.M. Schwartz. Monoclonality of smooth muscle cells in human atherosclerosis. *Am. J. Pathol.* 151(3):697-706, 1997.
53. Neylon C.B., P.V. Avdonin, R.J. Dilley, M.A. Larsen, V.A. Tkachuk, and A Bobik. Different electrical responses to vasoactive agonists in morphologically distinct smooth muscle cell types. *Circ. Res.* 75:733-741, 1994.
54. Owens G.K., S.M. Vernon, C.S. Madesn. Molecular regulation of smooth muscle cell differentiation. *J. Hypertens.* 14: S56-S64, 1996.
55. Pauletto P., A. Chiavegato, L. Giuriato, M. Scatena, E. Faggin, A Grisenti, R. Sarzani, M.V. Paci, D. Fulgeri, A.L. Rappelli, A.C. Pessina, and S. Sartore. Hyperplastic growth of aortic smooth muscle cells in renovascular hypertensive rabbits is characterized by the expansion of an immature cell phenotype. *Circ. Res.* 74: 774-788, 1994.
56. Phipps R.P. *Pulmonary Fibroblast Heterogeneity.* Boca Raton, FL: CRC Press, Inc.; 1992:1-336.
57. Ratcliffe P.J., B.L. Ebert, J.D. Firth, J.M. Gleadle, P.H. Maxwell, M. Nagao, J.F. O'Rourke, C.W. Pugh and S.M. Wood. Oxygen regulated gene expression: erythropoietin as a model system. *Kidney Internatl.* 51: 514-526, 1997.
58. Schwartz S.M., D. deBlois, E.R.M. O'Brien. The intima: soil for atherosclerosis and restenosis. *Circ. Res.* 77:445-465, 1995.
59. Schwartz S.M., L. Foy, D.F. Bowen-Pope, and R. Ross. Derivation and properties of platelet-derived growth factor-independent rat smooth muscle cells. *Am. J. Pathol.* 136:1417-1428, 1990.
60. Scott P.H., A. Paul, C.M. Belham, A.J. Peacock, R.M. Wadsworth, G.W. Gould, D. Welsh, and R. Plevin. Hypoxic stimulation of the stress-activated protein kinases in pulmonary artery fibroblasts. *Am. J. Respir. Crit Care Med.* 158: 958-962, 1998.
61. Segal R.A., and M.E. Greenberg. Intracellular signalling pathways activated by neurotrophic factors. *Ann. Rev. Neurosci.* 19:463-489, 1996.
62. Semenza G.L., and G.L. Wang. A nuclear factor induced by hypoxia via de novo protein synthesis binds to the human erythropoietin gene enhancer at a site required for transcriptional activation. *Mol. Cell. Biol.* 12:5447-5454, 1992.
63. Shreeniwas R., S. Koga, M. Karakurum, D. Pinsky, E. Kaiser, J. Brett, B.A. Wolitsky, C. Norton, J Plocinski, W. Benjamin, D.K. Burns, A. Goldstein, and D Stern. Hypoxia-mediated induction of endothelial cell interleukin-1a. *J. Clin. Invest.* 90: 2333-2339, 1992.
64. Siu G.J., Liu Y.H., X.S. Chang, I.S. Anand, E. Harris, P. Harris, D. Heath. Subacute infantile mountain sickness. *J. Pathol.* 155:61-70, 1988.
65. Stenmark K.R., A.G. Durmowicz, and E.C. Dempsey. Modulation of vascular wall cell phenotype in pulmonary hypertension. In: *Pulmonary Vascular Remodeling.* edited by Bishop JE, Reeves JJ, Laurent GJ, eds: London, U.K: Portland Press; 1995.
66. Stenmark K.R., and R.P. Mecham. Cellular and molecular mechanisms of pulmonary vascular remodeling. *Ann. Re.v Physiol.* 59:89-144, 1997.
67. Stiebellehner L., M. Gnanasekharan, M. Frid, R.B. Low, and K.R. Stenmark. Smooth muscle myosin heavy chain SM-B isoform expression is increased in newly muscularized arteries of patients and animals with severe pulmonary hypertension. *Am. J. Respir. Crit. Care Med.* 157(3):A589, 1998.
68. Topouzis S., and M.W. Majesky. Smooth muscle lineage diversity in the chick embryo. *Dev. Biol.* 178:430-445, 1996.
69. Villaschi S., R.F. Nicosia, and M.R. Smith. Isolation of a morphologically and functionally distinct smooth muscle cell type from the intimal aspect of the normal rat

aorta. Evidence for smooth muscle cell heterogeneity. *In vitro Cell. Dev. Biol Animal* 30A:589-595, 1994.

70. Waskiewicz A.J., and J.A. Cooper. Mitogen and stress response pathways: MAP kinase cascades and phosphatase regulation in mammals and yeast. *Current Opinion Cell Biol.* 7:798-805, 1995.

71. Weir E.K., H.L. Reeve, D.N. Cornfield, M. Tristani-Firouzi, D.A. Peterson, S.L. Archer. Diversity of response in vascular smooth muscle cells to changes in oxygen tension. *Kidney Internatl.* 51:462-466, 1997.

72. Wohrley J.D., M.G. Frid, E.C. Orton, J.K. Belknap, and K.R. Stenmark. Hypoxia selectively induces proliferation in a specific subpopulation of smooth muscle cells in the bovine neonatal pulmonary arterial media. *J. Clin. Invest.* 96:273-281, 1995.

73. Yan S-H, Y.S. Zou, Y. Gao, C. Zhai, N. Mackman, S.L. Lee, J. Milbrandt, D. Pinsky, W. Kisiel, and D. Stern. Tissue factor transcription driven by Egr-1 is a critical mechanism of murine pulmonary fibrin deposition in hypoxia. *Proc Natl. Acad. Sci.* 95:8298-8303, 1998.

74. Yan S-F, S. Ogawa, D.M. Stern and D.J. Pinsky. Hypoxia-induced modulation of endothelial cell properties: regulation of barrier function and expression of interleukin-6. *Kidney Internatl.* 51: 419-425, 1997.

75. Yao K-S, S. Xanthoudakis, T. Curran, and P.J. O'Dwyer. Activation of AP-1 and of a nuclear redox factor, Ref-1, in the response of HT29 colon cancer cells to hypoxia. *Mol. Cell Biol.* 14:5997-6003, 1994.

76. Zhang J., N. Jin, Y. Liu, R.A. Rhoades. Hydrogen peroxide stimulates extracellular signal-regulated protein kinases in pulmonary arterial smooth muscle cells. Am. J. Respir. Cell. Mol. Biol. 19:324-332, 1998.76. Zhang J, N Jin, Y Liu, RA Rhoades. Hydrogen peroxide stimulates extracellular signal-regulated protein kinases in pulmonary arterial smooth muscle cells. *Am J Respir Cell Mol Biol.* 19:p324-332, 1998.

Chapter 20

Oxygen and Placental Vascular Development

John C.P. Kingdom and Peter Kaufmann
Department of Obstetrics & Gynecology, University of Toronto and Maternal-Fetal Medicine Division, Suite 775B Mount Sinai Hospital, 600 University Avenue, Toronto M5G 1X5, Ontario, Canada and Department of Anatomy, University of Technology, Aachen, Germany

Key words: embryogenesis, vasculogenesis, fetal-placental circulation, intrauterine growth restriction, placenta-like growth factor, placenta

Abstract: Human embryogenesis takes place in a hypoxic environment because the trophoblast shell excludes entry of maternal blood. The first fetal-placental villi develop as trophoblast sprouts. These are invaded by allantoic mesoderm to form secondary villi and are transformed, by vasculogenesis, into tertiary villi. The placental barrier to maternal blood is gradually breached between 8-12 weeks of gestation, due to invasion of placental-bed uteroplacental spiral arteries by the extravillous trophoblast (EVT). Placental oxygen tension thus rises and a phase of branching angiogenesis continues until 24 weeks. Thereafter a gradual shift takes place favoring non-branching angiogenesis. Gas-exchanging terminal villi thus form which are essential for rapid fetal growth and development of a high-flow, low-resistance fetal-placental circulation.

Inadequate invasion of the uteroplacental spiral arteries by EVT results in placental ischemia and the development of obstetrical complications - pre-eclampsia and/or intrauterine growth restriction (IUGR). Placental villi often show evidence of continued branching angiogenesis, as is the case with anemic pregnancy, and pregnancy at high altitude. These structural alterations may reflect continued hypoxia-driven activity of vascular endothelial growth factor (VEGF). By contrast, a minority of severe early-onset IUGR pregnancies exhibit reduced fetal-placental blood flow with elongated maldeveloped villous capillaries. Placenta-like growth factor (PlGF) expression is increased while trophoblast proliferation is reduced, suggesting "hyperoxia" in the placental villous tree. IUGR may thus have two phenotypes

– a more common hypoxic and a rarer hyperoxic type. While this concept is gaining acceptance, we have no insight as to the initiating mechanism(s).

1.   INTRODUCTION

The birth of a healthy infant at term is dependent upon normal placental development. Conversely, disordered placentation is responsible for a wide range of pregnancy complications, ranging from miscarriage (embryonic death) through second trimester fetal death, and the classic 3rd trimester complications of pre-eclampsia, intrauterine growth restriction (IUGR) and abruption (premature placental separation (34). Placentation begins with implantation of the blastocyst beneath the uterine epithelium and differentiation into embryonic and extra-embryonic tissues (13). A maternal uteroplacental circulation is gradually established in tandem with a fetoplacental circulation. Close co-ordination of the development of these circulations is essential to meet the rising fetal demands for oxygen. Any disturbance of the balance between these circulations will alter intra-placental oxygen content. An increasing body of literature supports the concept that villous development depends upon local oxygen conditions (36) and in turn that disturbed placental oxygenation is a feature of many pathological situations. This overview will discuss the physiologic role of oxygen in placental development, and the role of both hypoxia and hyperoxia in mediating disordered placental function.

2.   EARLY PLACENTAL DEVELOPMENT

The extra-embryonic layer forms the trophoblast around the embryo, from which the extravillous trophoblast (EVT) cells proliferate and begin to invade the maternal vessels of the uterine stroma (14). In the early part of the first trimester, the EVT has a greater proliferative than invasive potential; a trophoblast "shell" thus accumulates around the embryo, ensuring that organogenesis takes place in a hypoxic environment. Ultrasound-guided placement of oxygen electrode studies during the first trimester have elegantly demonstrated a gradient between maternal decidua and placenta in the early first trimester, which disappears by 12-14 weeks (58). Following the completion of embryogenesis, at 10 post-menstrual weeks, the EVT assumes a more invasive phenotype, surrounding and invading the maternal spiral arterioles. The functional shell begins to open, allowing maternal blood to enter the lacunae, or primitive intervillous space (28). The invasive nature of EVT reduces the number of layers separating maternal and fetal blood to three: villous trophoblast, stroma and fetoplacental vascular endothelium. The resultant direct contact of maternal blood with the villous syncytiotrophoblast of the intervillous space gives the term hemochorial placentation.

The development of placental villi during the first trimester is illustrated in Figure 1. Cytotrophoblast proliferates to form sprouts, or primary villi, and are transformed via the proximal invasion of stroma (allantoic mesoderm) into secondary villi. Vasculogenesis, the de novo formation of blood vessels (57), then takes place within the stroma, transforming secondary into tertiary villi. These primitive capillaries become connected to the umbilical cord vessels to establish a primitive fetoplacental circulation by 8 weeks of post-menstrual gestation. By definition these villi are poorly-vascularized, and umbilical artery Doppler studies during the first trimester show the typical features of a high-resistance circulation, characterized by absent end-diastolic flow velocity (AEDFV) – Figure 2 (16). These immature villi are not yet capable of effective oxygen transfer, but this is not critical since the intervillous space is not perfused by oxygenated maternal blood.

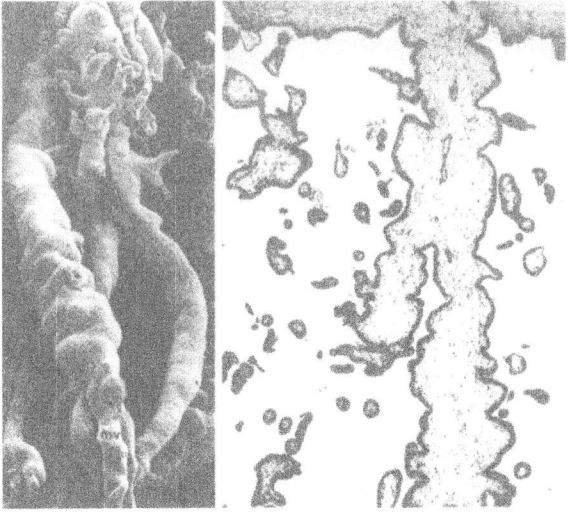

Figure 1. Scanning electron micrograph (left panel – x105) and corresponding plastic section (right panel) demonstrating human placental villous tree development at 6 weeks of post-menstrual gestation. Villous tree elaboration begins with the formation of trophoblast sprouts (S), budding off an immature intermediate villus. The latter become invaded centrally by mesoderm to form secondary villi. The plastic section (right panel – x75) indicates the poor vascularization of these villi – continued vasculogenesis, followed by branching angiogenesis will transform these villi into their more mature counterparts as gestation advances. From Castellucci et al. (7) with permission.

3.   THE SECOND TRIMESTER

Uteroplacental blood flow increases during the second trimester, due to progressive transformation of the spiral arteries by the EVT. By 24 weeks of gestation the uteroplacental spiral arteries have been transformed into wide non-muscularized vessels, producing a low-resistance system. Uteroplacental blood flow is now regulated by maternal perfusion pressure. Serial Doppler studies of the proximal uterine arteries show a progressive rise in diastolic velocities during the second trimester, such that the early diastolic notch of the non-pregnant state normally disappears by 24 weeks of gestation (Figure 3a & b).

Parallel changes occur in the fetoplacental circulation, with serial Doppler studies of the umbilical artery showing a progressive rise in end-diastolic velocities (20). Histologically, the tertiary villi are transformed into immature intermediate villi (IIV) by a process of branching angiogenesis (7). Thus, typical cross-sections of IIV show several vessel profiles. IIV are the "growth zone" of the villous tree. They continue to proliferate, leaving behind increasing generations of stem villi as shown in Figure 4. The latter differentiate from IIV through a process of vascular remodeling of the central vessels to stem artery and vein, and a parallel regression of the peripheral capillaries. New sprouts go through the differentiation process described in the first trimester.

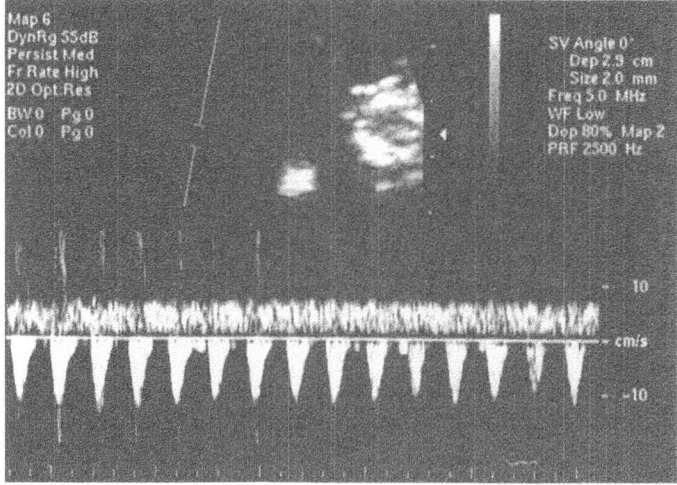

Figure 2. Umbilical cord pulsed-Doppler waveforms at 10 weeks of post-menstrual gestation. The upper channel shows continuous flow velocity in the umbilical vein, returning blood to the embryonic heart via the ductus venosus. The lower panel shows the umbilical artery waveform, characterized by systolic jets of flow, but absence of flow velocity at the end of diastole. This waveform indicates high distal vascular resistance in the immature villi. Diastolic flow progressively rises as gestation advances in tandem with increased vascularization and differentiation of the villi.

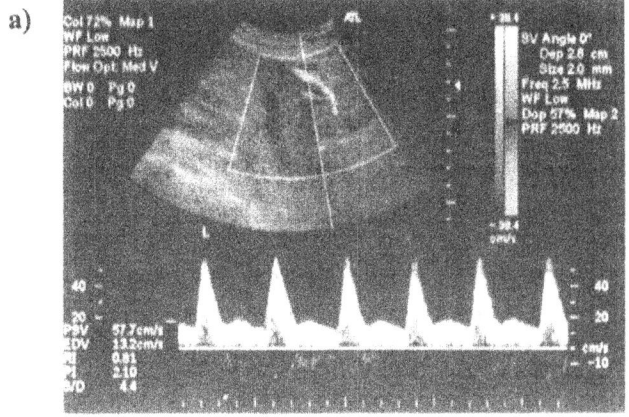

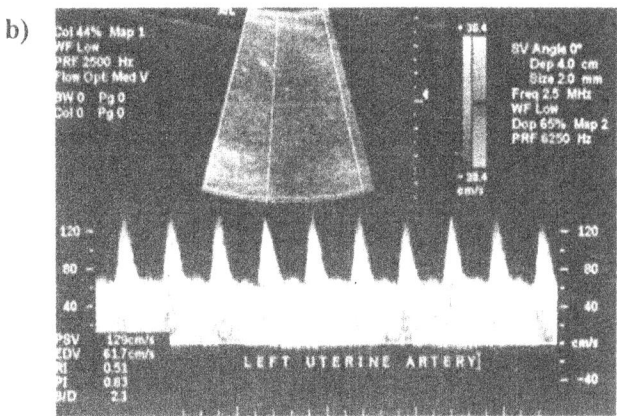

Figure 3. Uterine artery pulsed-Doppler waveforms at 10 weeks (a) and 22 weeks (b) of gestation. Note the increase in diastolic velocities as gestation advances, together with loss of the early diastolic notch. These changes are brought about by the invasive properties of the extravillous trophoblast, transforming the spiral artery branches of the uterine arteries into low-resistance vessels. The pregnancy is at risk of pre-eclampsia and/or IUGR when this transformation has not taken place by 22 weeks.

4.   THE THIRD TRIMESTER

From the onset of fetal viability, at around 24-26 weeks of gestation, a developmental switch occurs in the IIV, which transform into their mature intermediate villi (MIV) counterparts shown in the lower panel of Figure 4. The third trimester, from 26 weeks until normal delivery (at 38-41 weeks), is thus characterized by development of the peripheral gas-exchanging villi (25) . This 3rd phase of placental vascular growth is dominated by non-branching angiogenesis within the capillaries of the MIV. The rapid rate of elongation of MIV capillaries proceeds faster than growth of the actual villus, such that capillary loops "prolapse" laterally to produce bulges known as terminal villi. Fetoplacental capillaries within terminal villi are pushed towards the maternal surface of the syncytiotrophoblast and the resultant minimal diffusion distance between maternal and fetal blood is known as the vasculo-syncytial membrane (26, 46).

The formation of terminal villi thus depends upon a final phase of predominantly non-branching angiogenesis. Their production increases placental capillary volume to around 80ml by term, representing 25% of fetoplacental blood volume. The total surface area of fetal capillaries available for diffusional exchange within terminal villi is estimated to be 13m^2 (41).

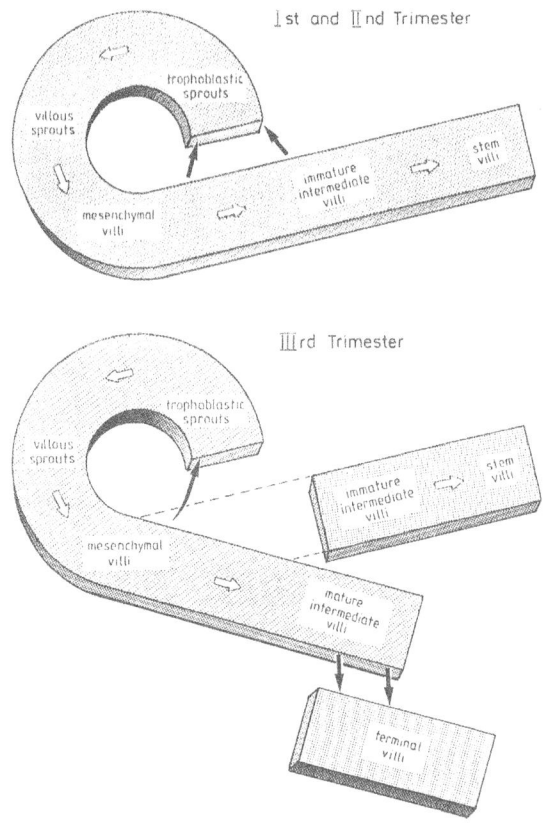

Figure 4. Diagrammatic representation of the shift in development of the human placental villous tree as gestation advances. In the first and second trimesters (upper panel), newly-generated villous sprouts are destined to form the proximal villi, containing muscularized arteries and veins. Differentiation of the immature intermediate villi into their mature counterparts results in a shift towards production of terminal villi (lower panel). From Castellucci et al. (7) with permission.

5. GROWTH FACTORS AND PLACENTAL VILLOUS DEVELOPMENT

A number of growth factors and their receptors are known to be expressed in the human placenta, the best-studied to date being vascular endothelial growth factor (VEGF) (10). In the human placenta, VEGF is expressed in villous (trophoblast and stromal Hofbauer cells) and maternal decidual cells during the first trimester (11, 24). Total VEGF can be detected in maternal plasma at 6 weeks of gestation and rises to a peak at the end of the first trimester, in parallel with hCG (15). Villous trophoblast VEGF expression appears to decline as pregnancy advances and has been confirmed by Western and Northern blotting studies (12). VEGF transcription is increased under hypoxic conditions. This is in part mediated by hypoxia-inducible factor (HIF) 1-alpha, for example in the hypoxic murine retina (51). VEGF (60) and HIF-1 alpha (59) mRNA are increased in hypoxic trophoblast in-vitro.

Secreted VEGF mediates its actions via two 2 tyrosine kinase receptor isoforms, VEGF-R1 (flt-1) and VEGF-R2 (KDR) (57). VEGF-R2 binding by VEGF induces endothelial cell proliferation and thus angiogenesis, while binding to VEGF-R1 stimulates endothelial nitric oxide synthase (eNOS) and leads to inhibition of cytotrophoblast proliferation (1). VEGF induces branching angiogenesis in vitro, as demonstrated in the chick chorio-allantoic membrane (40), and in the avascular cornea assay (62). These data suggest that VEGF acting via VEGF-R2 may be responsible for the extensive branching angiogenesis found in IIV during the second trimester.

Placenta-like growth factor (PlGF) shares 53% sequence homology with VEGF (44). Synthesis appears localized to the villous and extravillous trophoblast, which is in contrast to VEGF (11). PlGF acts exclusively through the receptor VEGF-R1, though may in part mediate its angiogenic activity by forming heterodimers with VEGF (6). The quality of angiogenesis induced by PlGF differs from VEGF in two ways. First, PlGF expression is stimulated by oxygen which is opposite to VEGF (32), and second, it appears to induce non-branching angiogenesis (40). Placental PlGF mRNA and protein levels both increase as gestation advances, which is in contrast to VEGF (32). This gradual shift in balance from the actions of VEGF to PlGF may explain the change in villous angiogenesis to a non-branching type necessary for the formation of terminal villi.

6.   OXYGEN DELIVERY AND PLACENTAL
PATHOLOGY

Uteroplacental blood flow, which is dependent upon transformation of spiral arteries by EVT cells, is deficient in pregnancies complicated by pre-eclampsia and/or intrauterine IUGR (33). Before the advent of Doppler ultrasound, radio-isotope studies demonstrated a 30-50% reduction in uteroplacental blood flow in such pregnancies (48) and more recently, magnetic resonance imaging has been employed to demonstrate qualitative differences (18). With the aid of color Doppler imaging the proximal uterine artery can be visualized (2) thereby obtaining reproducible waveforms. Bilateral high-resistance flow velocity waveforms with early diastolic notches are associated with fetal death, IUGR and pre-eclampsia (for comprehensive reviews see (9, 61)). Gelfoam embolization studies of the uterine arteries in pregnant sheep show that bilateral notched high-resistance waveforms are associated with a 50% reduction in uteroplacental blood flow (49). Oxygen delivery into the placental intervillous space is thus significantly impaired in the presence of bilateral abnormal uterine artery Doppler waveforms.

The concept of "placental hypoxia" in pre-eclampsia and/or IUGR was established long before the advent of Doppler ultrasound. Tenney and Parker in 1940 and subsequent workers (reviewed in (36)) described increased numbers of proliferating villous cytotrophoblast cells in histological sections of placentas from pregnancies complicated by pre-eclampsia at term. Fox (17) developed this concept by culturing villous explants under hypoxic conditions, establishing the link between villous cytotrophoblast proliferation and hypoxia. Similar, though perhaps more homogeneous, findings have been observed in situations where placental oxygen delivery is reduced: pregnancy at high altitude (4, 26) and maternal anemia (30). In each of these situations the increased villous vascularization resulting from chronic placental hypoxia will further reduce fetoplacental vascular impedance as pregnancy advances (Figure 5). Umbilical artery Doppler waveforms are typically normal in late-gestation pre-eclampsia. The same is true for late-gestation IUGR, which is likewise associated with impaired uteroplacental vascular development (8, 50). These pregnancies may have accelerated sonographic maturation of the placenta (19, 55) a finding which is associated with a 30% increase in capillary volume fraction (3).

Early-onset IUGR is a severe form of placental insufficiency resulting in perinatal death or iatrogenic delivery before 34 weeks of gestation. Umbilical artery Doppler is characterized by reduced, absent, or even reversed end-diastolic flow velocity (31), i.e. waveforms quite similar to those found during normal early placental development (Figures 1 & 2) indicating elevated fetoplacental vascular resistance for this later period of gestation (47). The underlying pathology of increased vascular resistance must reside either in the stem arteries (increased vasomotor tone) or in the vascular arrangement of the capillaries within gas-exchanging villi (reviewed in (35)). Stereologic 2-dimensional studies of placental structure have indicated a reduction in the elaboration of the peripheral gas-exchanging parts of the villous tree in early-onset IUGR (21, 27). To address this subject in more detail we employed scanning electron microscopy of peripheral villi and corrosion cast specimens of their capillaries, to clarify a severe defect in villous development characterized by reduced numbers of non-branched capillaries (38). This difference is summarized in Figure 5 (upper panel). In parallel we employed immunohistochemistry and transmission electron microscopy to compare villous structure in early-onset IUGR with ARED in the umbilical arteries with gestation age-matched control placentas (43). Terminal villi in the IUGR cases were characterized by reduced numbers of proliferating cytotrophoblast, with excess numbers of overlying syncytiotrophoblast nuclei. Since syncytial fusion is thought to focally retard apoptosis in the syncytiotrophoblast (23) we interpreted these findings as representing accelerated trophoblast aging.

The combination of arrested trophoblast turnover and failure to evoke an adaptive angiogenic response, led us to speculate that these villi had been exposed to a higher than normal (more arterialized) oxygen tension – a situation which we termed placental "hyperoxia" (43). That this self-perpetuating situation could arise in the face of uteroplacental ischemia is superficially hard to understand until one appreciates that the catabolic severely-IUGR fetus (with reduced activity) is surviving with minimal oxygen consumption (53). Fractional extraction of oxygen from the intervillous space is greatly reduced with ARED in the umbilical arteries, such that uteroplacental venous blood has a 30% higher oxygen content than under normal circumstances (52). Early-onset IUGR and abnormal umbilical artery Doppler is very uncommon in unselected pregnancies (45) while between 5-10% of such pregnancies are often conventionally assigned as IUGR based on birthweight centiles (the correct term for the latter is small-for-gestational age). The pathology of ARED, and thus the phenomenon of placental hyperoxia, is thus the exception to the rule that the placenta adapts to reduced uteroplacental blood flow (34). Thus a new category of fetal hypoxia may exist, termed "post-placental" hypoxia, to indicate that the defect in fetal oxygenation exists at the level of the fetoplacental circulation, rather than the intervillous space. These categories are shown in Figure 6 (36).

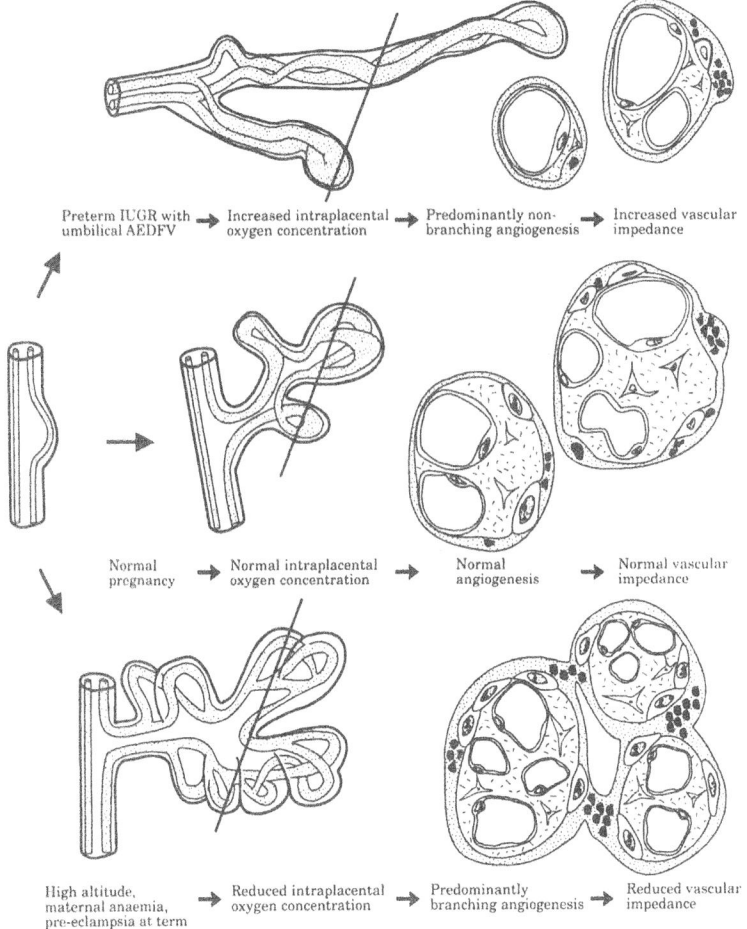

Figure 5. Pathways of villous angiogenesis according to villous oxygenation. The oblique lines across the villi refer to the position of the cross sections shown to the right. Adaptive angiogenesis and trophoblast proliferation result from either pre-placental or uteroplacental hypoxia (lower panel). By contrast, failure of villous development will further inhibit angiogenesis because the intra-placental hypoxic drive for villous growth is reduced (upper panel). Placentas from IUGR pregnancies at 26-32 weeks show this type of villous maldevelopment and the corresponding immature umbilical artery Doppler waveform as in Figure 2. From Kingdom & Kaufmann (36) with permission.

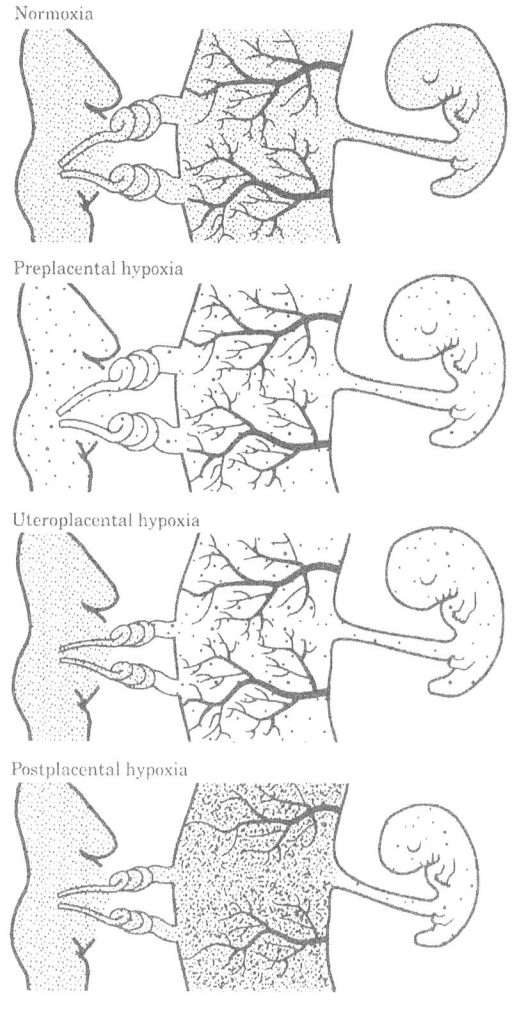

Figure 6. The origins of fetal hypoxia according to villous development and placental oxygenation. The degree of point shading symbolizes the degree of oxygenation. The coiled vessels depict the uterine arteries supplying the intervillous space of the placenta. These are drawn smaller in the lower 2 panels to indicate reduced uterine artery blood flow, illustrated by Doppler ultrasound in Figure 3a. From Kingdom & Kaufmann (36) with permission.

7. MOLECULAR EVIDENCE FOR PLACENTAL HYPEROXIA

Human villous explants cultured in increasing (0-40%) oxygen conditions display upregulation of PlGF and inhibition of VEGF mRNA's respectively (32). This same group has demonstrated increased protein and mRNA expression of placenta growth factor (PlGF) in early-onset IUGR with ARED in the umbilical arteries. We previously noted reduced immunohistochemical expression of trophoblast VEGF expression in these pregnancies (42).

From a clinical standpoint, the consolidation of the hypoxia-hyperoxia model of IUGR (Figure 5) has important implications. First, that fetal hypoxia in the presence of ARED in the umbilical arteries is not due to impaired uteroplacental blood flow. Attempts to dilate the maternal circulation (5) may be misguided, since improved villous oxygenation may further inhibit any drive towards further villous development (54). Supplemental maternal oxygen therapy appears to improve perinatal survival (29), though again on theoretical grounds this would be expected to further damage the placenta. Perhaps the benefits of improved fetal oxygenation predominate over ongoing placental damage (37).

8.   STILL A CIRCULAR AGRUMENT

Despite the advancing evidence to support hyperoxia in severe IUGR, including descriptive molecular methods, at present no initiating event has been proposed . We currently have little understanding of the factor(s) which regulate the critical stages of human placental villous development, for example the mid-gestation switch from immature to mature intermediate villi (7). The latter involves two distinct processes: inhibition of vasculogenesis, and a switch to non-branching angiogenesis.

An alternative way of viewing early-onset IUGR is as the tail end of early reproductive loss which begins as "anembryonic" pregnancy loss in the first trimester (39). Many of these losses appear to occur around the time of transition from the vitelline (yolk sac) to umbilical (chorio-allantoic) circulation, suggesting that some fundamental failure of allantoic vasculogenesis, and/or mesoderm-trophoblast interaction (which leads to the vascularization of primitive villi). Whilst the molecular hierarchy of these events cannot be solved in human tissues it is possible to learn from rodent models of placentation (13). This is especially true for the mouse since transgenic knock-out technology permits targeted disruption of specific genes to unravel the key molecular events at critical stages of placentation (22, 56). Such studies will in future fuel hypothesis-driven research addressing the possibility that pregnancy loss or disease due to failure of normal villous may be caused by disordered gene expression/function upstream of vascular development.

9. SUMMARY

• placental vascular development proceeds through an orderly sequence of vasculogenesis: branching angiogenesis followed by a final phase of predominantly non-branching angiogenesis

• this process is mediated by oxygen-sensing growth factors, and is thus critically dependent upon intra-placental oxygenation status

• this process is thus sensitive to the balance between oxygen entry from mother into the placenta and it's extraction by the fetus, and as such both hypoxic and hyperoxic situations could arise

• severe villous maldevelopment presenting as IUGR with ARED in the umbilical arteries may represent the tail end of a spectrum of disordered angiogenesis

• the study of genes critical for successful murine chorio-allantoic development may lead to a greater understanding of the pathology of post-implantation pregnancy failure

ACKNOWLEDGEMENTS

The authors are grateful to; Medical Research Council (UK), Tommy's Campaign (UK), Action Research (UK), Scottish Hospitals Endowment Research Trust (UK), European Biomed Program and the Samuel Lunenfeld Research Institute, Toronto, Canada, for supporting their placental research.

REFERENCES

1. Ahmed, A., C. Dunk, D. Kniss, and M. Wilkes. Role of VEGF receptor-1 (Flt-1) in mediating calcium-dependent nitric oxide release and limiting DNA synthesis in human trophoblast cells. *Lab Invest* 76: 779-791, 1997.
2. Bower, S., S. Bewley, and S. Campbell. Improved prediction of preeclampsia by two-stage screening of uterine arteries using the early diastolic notch and color Doppler imaging. *Obstet Gynecol* 82: 78-83, 1993.
3. Burton, G.J. and E. Jauniaux. Sonographic, stereological and Doppler flow velocimetric assessments of placental maturity. *Br J Obstet Gynaecol* 102: 818-825, 1995.
4. Burton, G.J., O.S. Reshetnikova, A.P. Milovanov, and O.V. Teleshova. Stereological evaluation of vascular adaptations in human placental villi to differing forms of hypoxic stress. *Placenta* 17: 49-55, 1996.
5. Cacciatore, B., E. Halmesmaki, R. Kaaja, K. Teramo, and O. Ylikorkala. Effects of transdermal nitroglycerin on impedance to flow in the uterine, umbilical, and fetal middle cerebral arteries in pregnancies complicated by preeclampsia and intrauterine growth retardation. *Am J Obstet Gynecol* 179: 140-145, 1998.
6. Cao, Y., H. Chen, L. Zhou, M.K. Chiang, B. Anand-Apte, J.A. Weatherbee, Y. Wang, F. Fang, J.G. Flanagan, and M.L. Tsang. Heterodimers of placenta growth factor/vascular

endothelial growth factor. Endothelial activity, tumor cell expression, and high affinity binding to Flk-1/KDR. *J Biol Chem* 271: 3154-3162, 1996.

7. Castellucci, M., M. Scheper, I. Scheffen, A. Celona, and P. Kaufmann. The development of the human placental villous tree. *Anat Embryol (Berl)* 181: 117-128, 1990.

8. Chang, T.C., S.C. Robson, J.A. Spencer, and S. Gallivan. Identification of fetal growth retardation: comparison of Doppler waveform indices and serial ultrasound measurements of abdominal circumference and fetal weight. *Obstet Gynecol* 82: 230-236, 1993.

9. Chappell, L. and S. Bewley. Pre-eclamptic toxaemia: the role of uterine artery Doppler. *Br J Obstet Gynaecol* 105: 379-382, 1998.

10. Cheung, C.Y. Vascular endothelial growth factor: possible role in fetal development and placental function. *J Soc Gynecol Investig* 4: 169-177, 1997.

11. Clark, D.E., S.K. Smith, D. Licence, A.L. Evans, and D.S. Charnock-Jones. Comparison of expression patterns for placenta growth factor, vascular endothelial growth factor (VEGF), VEGF-B and VEGF-C in the human placenta throughout gestation. *J Endocrinol* 159: 459-467, 1998.

12. Cooper, J.C., A.M. Sharkey, D.S. Charnock-Jones, C.R. Palmer, and S.K. Smith. VEGF mRNA levels in placentae from pregnancies complicated by pre- eclampsia [see comments]. *Br J Obstet Gynaecol* 103: 1191-1196, 1996.

13. Cross, J.C. Formation of the placenta and extraembryonic membranes [In Process Citation]. *Ann N Y Acad Sci* 857: 23-32, 1998.

14. Cross, J.C., Z. Werb, and S.J. Fisher. Implantation and the placenta: key pieces of the development puzzle. *Science* 266: 1508-1518, 1994.

15. Evans, P.W., T. Wheeler, F.W. Anthony, and C. Osmond. A longitudinal study of maternal serum vascular endothelial growth factor in early pregnancy. *Hum Reprod* 13: 1057-1062, 1998.

16. Fisk, N.M., N. MacLachlan, C. Ellis, Y. Tannirandorn, H.M. Tonge, and C.H. Rodeck. Absent end-diastolic flow in first trimester umbilical artery [letter]. *Lancet* 2: 1256-1257, 1988.

17. Fox, H. Effect of hypoxia on trophoblast in organ culture. A morphologic and autoradiographic study. *Am J Obstet Gynecol* 107: 1058-1064, 1970.

18. Francis, S.T., K.R. Duncan, R.J. Moore, P.N. Baker, I.R. Johnson, and P.A. Gowland. Non-invasive mapping of placental perfusion. *Lancet* 351: 1397-1399, 1998.

19. Grannum, P.A., R.L. Berkowitz, and J.C. Hobbins. The ultrasonic changes in the maturing placenta and their relation to fetal pulmonic maturity. *Am J Obstet Gynecol* 133: 915-922, 1979.

20. Hendricks, S.K., T.K. Sorensen, K.Y. Wang, J.M. Bushnell, E.M. Seguin, and R.W. Zingheim. Doppler umbilical artery waveform indices--normal values from fourteen to forty-two weeks. *Am J Obstet Gynecol* 161: 761-765, 1989.

21. Hitschold, T.P. Doppler flow velocity waveforms of the umbilical arteries correlate with intravillous blood volume. *Am J Obstet Gynecol* 179: 540-543, 1998.

22. Hunter, P.J., B.J. Swanson, M.A. Haendel, G.E. Lyons, and J.C. Cross. Mrj encodes a DnaJ-related co-chaperone that is essential for murine placental development. *Development* 126: 1247-1258, 1999.

23. Huppertz, B., H.G. Frank, J.C. Kingdom, F. Reister, and P. Kaufmann. Villous cytotrophoblast regulation of the syncytial apoptotic cascade in the human placenta. *Histochem Cell Biol* 110: 495-508, 1998.

24. Jackson, M.R., E.W. Carney, S.J. Lye, and J.W. Ritchie. Localization of two angiogenic growth factors (PDECGF and VEGF) in human placentae throughout gestation. *Placenta* 15: 341-353, 1994.

25. Jackson, M.R., T.M. Mayhew, and P.A. Boyd. Quantitative description of the elaboration and maturation of villi from 10 weeks of gestation to term. *Placenta* 13: 357-370, 1992.
26. Jackson, M.R., T.M. Mayhew, and J.D. Haas. On the factors which contribute to thinning of the villous membrane in human placentae at high altitude. I. Thinning and regional variation in thickness of trophoblast. *Placenta* 9: 1-8, 1988.
27. Jackson, M.R., A.J. Walsh, R.J. Morrow, J.B. Mullen, S.J. Lye, and J.W. Ritchie. Reduced placental villous tree elaboration in small-for-gestational-age pregnancies: relationship with umbilical artery Doppler waveforms. *Am J Obstet Gynecol* 172: 518-525, 1995.
28. Jaffe, R., E. Jauniaux, and J. Hustin. Maternal circulation in the first-trimester human placenta--myth or reality? *Am J Obstet Gynecol* 176: 695-705, 1997.
29. Johanson, R., S.W. Lindow, C. van der Elst, Z. Jaquire, S. van der Westhuizen, and A. Tucker. A prospective randomised comparison of the effect of continuous O2 therapy and bedrest on fetuses with absent end-diastolic flow on umbilical artery Doppler waveform analysis. *Br J Obstet Gynaecol* 102: 662-665, 1995.
30. Kadyrov, M., G. Kosanke, J. Kingdom, and P. Kaufmann. Increased fetoplacental angiogenesis during first trimester in anaemic women. *Lancet* 352: 1747-1749, 1998.
31. Karsdorp, V.H., J.M. van Vugt, H.P. van Geijn, P.J. Kostense, D. Arduini, N. Montenegro, and T. Todros. Clinical significance of absent or reversed end diastolic velocity waveforms in umbilical artery. *Lancet* 344: 1664-1668, 1994.
32. Khaliq, A., C. Dunk, J. Jiang, M. Shams, X. Li, C. Acevedo, H. Weich, M. Whittle, and A. Ahmed. Hypoxia Down-Regulates Placenta growth factor whereas Fetal Growth Restriction Up-Regulates Placenta growth factor Expresion: Molecular Evidence for "Placental Hyperoxia" in Intrauterine Growth Restriction. *Laboratory Investigation* 1999.(In Press)
33. Khong, T.Y., F. De Wolf, W.B. Robertson, and I. Brosens. Inadequate maternal vascular response to placentation in pregnancies complicated by pre-eclampsia and by small-for-gestational age infants. *Br J Obstet Gynaecol* 93: 1049-1059, 1986.
34. Kingdom, J. Adriana and Luisa Castellucci Award Lecture 1997. Placental pathology in obstetrics: adaptation or failure of the villous tree? *Placenta* 19: 347-351, 1998.
35. Kingdom, J.C., S.J. Burrell, and P. Kaufmann. Pathology and clinical implications of abnormal umbilical artery Doppler waveforms. *Ultrasound Obstet Gynecol* 9: 271-286, 1997.
36. Kingdom, J.C. and P. Kaufmann. Oxygen and placental villous development: origins of fetal hypoxia. *Placenta* 18: 613-621, 1997.
37. Kingdom, J.C., C.H. Rodeck, and P. Kaufmann. Umbilical artery Doppler--more harm than good? *Br J Obstet Gynaecol* 104: 393-396, 1997.
38. Krebs, C., L.M. Macara, R. Leiser, A.W. Bowman, I.A. Greer, and J.C. Kingdom. Intrauterine growth restriction with absent end-diastolic flow velocity in the umbilical artery is associated with maldevelopment of the placental terminal villous tree. *Am J Obstet Gynecol* 175: 1534-1542, 1996.
39. Kurjak, A. and S. Kupesic. Parallel Doppler assessment of yolk sac and intervillous circulation in normal pregnancy and missed abortion [In Process Citation]. *Placenta* 19: 619-623, 1998.
40. Kurz, H., J. Wilting, K. Sandau, and B. Christ. Automated evaluation of angiogenic effects mediated by VEGF and PlGF homo- and heterodimers. *Microvasc Res* 55: 92-102, 1998.
41. Luckhardt, M., R. Leiser, J. Kingdom, A. Malek, R. Sager, C. Kaisig, and H. Schneider. Effect of physiologic perfusion-fixation on the morphometrically evaluated dimensions of the term placental cotyledon. *J Soc Gynecol Investig* 3: 166-171, 1996.

42. Lyall, F., A. Young, F. Boswell, J.C. Kingdom, and I.A. Greer. Placental expression of vascular endothelial growth factor in placentae from pregnancies complicated by pre-eclampsia and intrauterine growth restriction does not support placental hypoxia at delivery. *Placenta* 18: 269-276, 1997.

43. Macara, L., J.C. Kingdom, P. Kaufmann, G. Kohnen, J. Hair, I.A. More, F. Lyall, and I.A. Greer. Structural analysis of placental terminal villi from growth-restricted pregnancies with abnormal umbilical artery Doppler waveforms. *Placenta* 17: 37-48, 1996.

44. Maglione, D., V. Guerriero, G. Viglietto, P. Delli-Bovi, and M.G. Persico. Isolation of a human placenta cDNA coding for a protein related to the vascular permeability factor. *Proc Natl Acad Sci U S A* 88: 9267-9271, 1991.

45. Mason, G.C., R.J. Lilford, J. Porter, E. Nelson, and S. Tyrell. Randomised comparison of routine versus highly selective use of Doppler ultrasound in low risk pregnancies. *Br J Obstet Gynaecol* 100: 130-133, 1993.

46. Mayhew, T.M., M.R. Jackson, and P.A. Boyd. Changes in oxygen diffusive conductances of human placentae during gestation (10-41 weeks) are commensurate with the gain in fetal weight. *Placenta* 14: 51-61, 1993.

47. Morrow, R.J., S.L. Adamson, S.B. Bull, and J.W. Ritchie. Effect of placental embolization on the umbilical arterial velocity waveform in fetal sheep. *Am J Obstet Gynecol* 161: 1055-1060, 1989.

48. Nylund, L., N.O. Lunell, R. Lewander, and B. Sarby. Uteroplacental blood flow index in intrauterine growth retardation of fetal or maternal origin. *Br J Obstet Gynaecol* 90: 16-20, 1983.

49. Ochi, H., K. Matsubara, Y. Kusanagi, H. Taniguchi, and M. Ito. Significance of a diastolic notch in the uterine artery flow velocity waveform induced by uterine embolisation in the pregnant ewe. *Br J Obstet Gynaecol* 105: 1118-1121, 1998.

50. Olofsson, P., R.N. Laurini, and K. Marsal. A high uterine artery pulsatility index reflects a defective development of placental bed spiral arteries in pregnancies complicated by hypertension and fetal growth retardation. *Eur J Obstet Gynecol Reprod Biol* 49: 161-168, 1993.

51. Ozaki, H., A.Y. Yu, N. Della, K. Ozaki, J.D. Luna, H. Yamada, S.F. Hackett, N. Okamoto, D.J. Zack, G.L. Semenza, and P.A. Campochiaro. Hypoxia inducible factor-1alpha is increased in ischemic retina: temporal and spatial correlation with VEGF expression. *Invest Ophthalmol Vis Sci* 40: 182-189, 1999.

52. Pardi, G., I. Cetin, A.M. Marconi, P. Bozzetti, M. Buscaglia, E.L. Makowski, and F.C. Battaglia. Venous drainage of the human uterus: respiratory gas studies in normal and fetal growth-retarded pregnancies. *Am J Obstet Gynecol* 166: 699-706, 1992.

53. Pardi, G., I. Cetin, A.M. Marconi, A. Lanfranchi, P. Bozzetti, E. Ferrazzi, M. Buscaglia, and F.C. Battaglia. Diagnostic value of blood sampling in fetuses with growth retardation [see comments]. *N Engl J Med* 328: 692-696, 1993.

54. Poston, L. Nitrovasodilators--will they be useful in lowering uterine artery resistance in pre-eclampsia and intrauterine growth restriction? [comment]. *Ultrasound Obstet Gynecol* 11: 92-93, 1998.

55. Proud, J. and A.M. Grant. Third trimester placental grading by ultrasonography as a test of fetal wellbeing. *Br Med J (Clin Res Ed)* 294: 1641-1644, 1987.

56. Riley, P., L. Anson-Cartwright, and J.C. Cross. The Hand1 bHLH transcription factor is essential for placentation and cardiac morphogenesis. *Nat Genet* 18: 271-275, 1998.

57. Risau, W. Mechanisms of angiogenesis. *Nature* 386: 671-674, 1999.

58. Rodesch, F., P. Simon, C. Donner, and E. Jauniaux. Oxygen measurements in endometrial and trophoblastic tissues during early pregnancy. *Obstet Gynecol* 80: 283-285, 1992.

59. Seligman, S.P., T. Nishiwaki, S.S. Kadner, J. Dancis, and T.H. Finlay. Hypoxia stimulates ecNOS mRNA expression by differentiated human trophoblasts. *Ann N Y Acad Sci* 828: 180-187, 1997.
60. Taylor, C.M., H. Stevens, F.W. Anthony, and T. Wheeler. Influence of hypoxia on vascular endothelial growth factor and chorionic gonadotrophin production in the trophoblast-derived cell lines: JEG, JAr and BeWo. *Placenta* 18: 451-458, 1997.
61. Valensise, H. Uterine artery Doppler velocimetry as a screening test: where we are and where we go [editorial]. *Ultrasound Obstet Gynecol* 12: 81-83, 1998.
62. Ziche, M., D. Maglione, D. Ribatti, L. Morbidelli, C.T. Lago, M. Battisti, I. Paoletti, A. Barra, M. Tucci, G. Parise, V. Vincenti, H.J. Granger, G. Viglietto, and M.G. Persico. Placenta growth factor-1 is chemotactic, mitogenic, and angiogenic. *Lab Invest* 76: 517-531, 1997.

Chapter 21

Vascular Growth in Hypoxic Skeletal Muscle

Hans Hoppeler

Department of Anatomy, University of Bern, Bühlstrasse 26, CH-3000 Bern 9, Switzerland

Key words: muscle, capillaries, hypoxia, growth factors, morphometry, VEGF

Abstract: The critical role of skeletal muscle capillaries is the supply of oxygen to skeletal muscle fibers during conditions of maximal aerobic work. The supply of substrates under these conditions is not limited by the vascular bed but rather by the capacity of the sarcolemmal transporter systems. Because of this dominant role of oxygen supply in muscle tissue, hypoxia has generally been considered to be an important stimulus for capillary neo-formation in skeletal muscle. Early morphometric work seemed to indicate that animals exposed to permanent hypoxia had in fact a significantly improved vascular supply in muscle tissue. Later work questioned these early findings and it was concluded that hypoxia per se was not a sufficient stimulus for capillary neo-formation but that additional stimuli such as cold-exposure needed to be present. In humans exposed to severe hypoxia during simulated or real ascents to Mt. Everest an increase in capillary density was in fact found. However, this increase could be shown to result from a reduction of muscle fiber volume and not from capillary growth. Broadly compatible results were obtained in animal experiments in which changes in capillarity were assessed in muscles with limited blood supply which were exposed to chronic electrical stimulation. Recently we have shown that endurance exercise training in humans results in a rise in mRNA of vascular endothelial growth factor (VEGF) only when carried out vigorously and in hypoxia. These results indicate that molecular techniques will allow in the near future to delineate the role played by hypoxia in capillary neo-formation.

1.   INTRODUCTION

The capillary network serves as a bed for the exchange of respiratory gases, substrates and waste products of tissue cells. While oxygen transport is critically dependent on the quantity of erythrocytes present in peripheral capillaries, substrates are carried in the plasma space. A particular situation of muscle capillaries arises from the fact that the metabolic needs of skeletal muscle tissue varies by as much as 2 orders of magnitude between the resting state and maximal muscle activation. Clearly therefore, the design of the capillary network must be such that it can accommodate the metabolic demand of muscle cells during the state of maximal work such as during locomotion at a pace eliciting maximal oxygen uptake (VO_2max) of the organism.

2.   FUNCTIONAL ROLE OF CAPILLARIES

What is the critical function that the capillary network must perform under limiting conditions of maximal aerobic exercise? Comparative studies indicate that the critical function is the supply of oxygen to muscle cells (36). As there are only very limited stores of oxygen in the muscles of most vertebrates muscle activity depends on the steady supply of oxygen in quantities matching mitochondrial oxidation. Substrate supply from capillaries is generally not critical to muscle aerobic work. Muscle cells contain considerable stores of carbohydrates in the form of glycogen as well as triglycerides in the form of small lipid droplets (IMCL = intramyocellular lipid) in the vicinity of mitochondria which can both be used during periods of muscle work.

The intracellular substrate stores are utilized during muscle activities exceeding some 30% of maximal aerobic work. At these intensities (an easy walk for a healthy human) the upper limit of the transport capacity for substrates into muscle cells is reached, likely due to limitation of the transfer processes through the sarcolemma (35, 29). When substrate stores are depleted during long term exercise they are replenished at low rates during periods of rest of the organism.

3.   ASSESSING CAPILLARIES

Krogh has modeled the critical function of capillaries, oxygen supply to muscle tissue, as early as 1919 (19). He assumed muscle capillaries to supply a cylindrical tissue unit surrounding a straight and unbranched circular capillary tube. As a consequence it has become customary to morphometrically quantify muscle capillarity by estimating the number of capillary profiles observed per unit area of muscle (or muscle fiber) on cross-sections of muscle tissue. This estimate is usually designated "capillary density" $N_A(c,f)$. Another frequently used estimate of capillarity is the number of capillaries per number of fibers or "capillary-to-fiber ratio" $N_N(c,f)$. The advantage of the latter estimate is that it avoids problems related to tissue shrinkage, which may distort capillary density estimates. The drawback of capillary-to-fiber ratios is that they can not provide information on diffusion distance or capillary geometry.

Advanced morphometric techniques are available which allow for estimating muscle tissue capillarity by measuring capillary length, $J_V(c,f)$, taking into account that capillaries are branched and do not run a course parallel to muscle fibers (15, 26). It has been established that capillary length density, $J_V(c,f)$, can be considered to be the functionally relevant morphometrical estimate of capillarity. It allows for calculating both capillary volume and capillary surface area per volume of muscle fiber (14). Classically, $J_V(c,f)$ is determined from a set of sections taken both parallel and transverse to the muscle fiber axis (26). Alternatively, it may be sufficient to estimate $N_A(c,f)$ and to consider sarcomere length to calculate $J_V(c,f)$ at least when comparisons are made within the same species (22). An unbiased estimate of muscle capillary length and surface density can in principle be obtained by using sections that are not oriented with regard to the muscle fiber axis (Isotropic Uniform Random or IUR sections; see 36). In theory this approach should be preferred because it yields bias-free estimates of capillary parameters. The disadvantage of the methodologically "clean" approach is that it increases sampling variation. Hence, the labor of sectioning tissue and counting may be increased dramatically for a given accuracy. The IUR method may therefore not be practical in many situations.

An additional consideration when estimating capillarity relates to capillary luminal dimensions. Although most mammals seem to have very similar capillary cross-sectional dimensions, there are instances in which capillary diameter may change as a function of experimental procedures (16). Under these conditions $J_V(c,f)$ can not be considered a sufficient descriptor of capillarity. In these cases it is necessary to calculate capillary volume and surface densities from $J_V(c,f)$, taking capillary diameter into account. By contrast, any morphometric approach based on IUR sections would directly estimate volume and surface densities correctly.

4.　　CAPILLARY PLASTICITY WITH HYPOXIA

4.1　　The early experiments

Valdivia reported 1958 (34) an increased skeletal muscle capillarity in Andean guinea pigs compared to lowland controls. Similar reports appeared on rats (5) and dogs (2). These results led to the general notion of hypoxia as a specific factor enhancing skeletal muscle capillarity. In 1983 Hochachka formulated an "interpretative hypothesis" stating that skeletal muscle capillarity in mammals was increased during exposure to permanent hypoxia in order to ensure adequate oxygen supply to mitochondria under conditions of reduced oxygen availability (10). This view was challenged subsequently by Banchero (3). Based on a critical review of the available literature he concluded that "skeletal muscle capillarity does not respond to simple normothermic hypoxia even when the muscle is active". As one of the confounding variables potentially responsible for differences in capillarity he identified cold-exposure for which a number of the early experiments had not controlled for.

4.2　　A special case for birds at altitude?

Recently, there have been reports on increases in capillarity in skeletal muscles of Andean coots (20), finches (25) and pigeons (23). These studies report increases in capillary tortuosity in high-altitude animals as well as an increase in capillary diameter in the case of the altitude pigeons. It would be tempting to speculate that the high aerobic demand of bird flight muscles might responsible for the altitude adaptations observed in these studies. However, a study by the same research team on pigeons caught wild in La Paz or at sea level did not show differences of either capillary density or orientation between the two conditions (24). It is thus currently unclear whether birds show a different adaptation potential to altitude stress than mammals.

4.3　　Humans exposed to severe hypoxia

In the early 90ies studies were published on changes in capillarity of subjects participating in real (12) or simulated (24) mountaineering expeditions to the Himalayas. During these expeditions (or their simulation) low-landers were exposed for several weeks to altitudes around 5000m (base camp) with excursions to altitudes in excess of 8000m. The dominant finding in these studies was a loss in muscle mass, muscle fiber size and muscle oxidative capacity. Capillary density in biopsies of M vastus lateralis was found to be increased. However, this increase was not due to capillary neo-formation but rather to a loss of fiber cross-sectional area. In absolute terms, total capillary length seemed unaltered by high-altitude exposure. It was thus found that a constant capillary length supplied a greatly reduced muscle oxidative capacity.

4.4   High-altitude residents

A number of studies have been conducted on permanent high-altitude residents. It was reasoned that the effect of hypoxia could be different for low-landers during a mountaineering expedition during which subjects were exposed to cold, stress and marginal nutritional supply then for high-altitude residents. Reports on Sherpas (18), Quechas from the high Andes (30) and residents of the City of La Paz of varied ethnic background (8) come to similar conclusions. All these high-altitude populations show a significant reduction of muscle oxidative capacity and a concomitant proportional reduction in capillary density. This reduction of capillarity is brought about by a decrease in capillary to fiber ratio. It is found that permanent high-altitude residents have muscle fibers, which are similar in size than those of low-landers but with a capillary supply reduced in proportion to the reduction of mitochondria in these muscles. In contrast to low-landers acutely exposed to hypoxia, permanent high-altitude residents therefore show no signs of an improved capillary supply with regard to muscle oxidative demand.

4.5   Ischemia

Peripheral vascular disease is also characterized by a situation of severe (local) hypoxia of skeletal muscle tissue. Reports on skeletal muscle adaptations in patients are conflicting. An increase in muscle oxidative capacity is observed in some studies (1, 17). Others report decreases in oxidative enzymes (6, 9) possibly in cases with severe blood flow restrictions. We have characterized the response of skeletal muscle to peripheral arterial insufficiency in rat extensor digitorum longus muscle. Arterial insufficiency was induced by ligation of the common iliac artery; activity by chronic low frequency stimulation (13). Interestingly, ligation of the common iliac artery alone had no effect on capillarity or muscle oxidative capacity (measured as volume density of mitochondria). If ligation was combined with chronic stimulation a 33% reduction in muscle mass was observed. However, both absolute volumes of mitochondria and total capillary length were maintained in these muscles, by a corresponding increase in capillary and mitochondrial densities in ligated stimulated muscles. These observations support the notion that hypoxia per se does not necessarily provoke muscle tissue adaptations. Changes in muscle capillarity and oxidative capacity seem to depend on the presence of activity in addition to hypoxia.

4.6   Exercise training in severe hypoxia

The unexpected result of a decrease of skeletal muscle oxidative capacity with continuous high-altitude exposure in humans begged the question of the role of "hypoxia" in triggering adaptational events in endurance exercise training. It had generally (in many cases tacitly) been assumed that a key stimulus for muscle adaptational events was the local hypoxia incurred during heavy exercise (11). In order to study the effect of hypoxia as a trigger of skeletal muscle adaptation we therefore conducted studies in which subjects were exposed to severe (normobaric) hypoxia (4000 – 6300 m) only during exercise training. An initial set of experiments indicated that endurance exercise training in severe normobaric hypoxia led to the typical modification of skeletal muscle structure such as an increase in muscle oxidative capacity as well as in capillarity (7) while exercise training at the same absolute work intensities in normoxia had no measurable systemic or local effect on subjects. These experiments clearly indicated the importance of relative exercise intensity while substrate fluxes, similar under hypoxic and normoxic training conditions, appeared of negligible importance. The data of this and similar studies (32, 33) in which training sessions alone were done in hypoxia hinted at a number of specific effects hypoxia could have in skeletal muscle tissue when added to endurance exercise. The list of hypoxia specific effects of exercise training in hypoxia is currently based on circumstantial evidence – the functional consequences of these changes have not yet been delineated. Maybe the best-documented effect of training in hypoxia is an increase in the myoglobin concentration of the trained muscles (28, 32, 33, 37) not seen with training in normoxia in humans. A larger myoglobin concentration of muscles trained in hypoxia eventually coupled with an increase in capillarity (7, 37) can be conjectured to have the effect of a better supply of oxygen to muscle mitochondria. An adaptive feature effective in particular under hypoxic conditions. At a constant oxidative capacity of muscle one would expect subjects with these structural modifications to be able to maintain more of their normoxic VO_2max when exposed to hypoxia. A large myoglobin concentration and an increased capillarity is in fact a key functional feature of the mole rat, an animal adapted to living in hypoxic burrows (38). Compared to normal rats, mole rats have the same VO_2max in normoxia but a smaller decrease of this variable when exercised under hypoxia. A larger myoglobin concentration could also be of advantage in sports in which muscle activity interferes with blood supply such as during prolonged near isometric contractions. One would expect hypoxia trained muscle to be able to maintain tension longer due to larger on-board oxygen stores. This tenet has so far not been tested in humans, results from diving mammals would be compatible with this contention.

4.7 Molecular mechanisms responsible for vascular growth

The role of the physiological stimuli related to angiogenesis in skeletal muscle have recently been reviewed extensively (16). Important players in angiogenesis are various angiogenic growth factors such as vascular endothelial growth factor (VEGF), basic fibroblast growth factor (bTGF) and transforming growth and factor- ß_1 (TGF-ß_1). Looking at the mRNA responses of these growth factors immediately after exercise in rats it is found that all of them increase transiently at least two-fold over a period of 4 hours (4). This response is intensity dependent and can further be increased by hypoxia at least with regard to VEGF. Although the precise angiogenic role of these factors in exercise remains elusive hypoxia seems to be capable of modulating the VEGF response (31).

We have recently conducted experiments to separate the effects of training intensity and hypoxia (37) To this end 4 groups of subjects were trained. Two groups were trained at a high intensity (approximately 75% of VO_2max) and two groups at a low intensity (50% of VO_2max). From both the high and low intensity groups one trained in normoxia, while the other trained in hypoxia (equivalent to an altitude of 4000m). Biopsies taken before and after 6 weeks of endurance training (30min/day; 5 days/week) were analyzed using quantitative PCR (27). We found an elevation of hypoxia inducible factor 1 (hif-1) independent of work intensity in all subjects that trained under hypoxia. However, mRNA concentration for VEGF (and for myoglobin), were elevated only in the group that trained under hypoxia at a high work intensity. This lends support to the notion that exercise and hypoxia have an additive effect on VEGF response (4).

5. CONCLUSIONS

The bulk of evidence currently available indicates that hypoxia without additional stressors such as exercise or cold has little effect on skeletal muscle capillarity. However, local hypoxia in working muscle is likely one (of several) factors responsible for vascular growth with chronic exercise training. Exercise in (severe) hypoxia affects skeletal muscle tissue specifically promoting adaptations that facilitate oxygen transfer under hypoxic conditions such as an increase in capillarity and myoglobin. The tools of modern biology start to unravel the components of the molecular mechanism responsible for these modifications.

REFERENCES

1. Aengquist, K. A. and A. Sjoestroem. Intermittent claudication and muscle fiber fine structure: morphometric values on mitochondrial volumes. *Ultrastruct. Pathol.* 1: 461-470, 1980.
2. Banchero, N. Capillary density of skeletal muscle in dogs exposed to simulated altitude. *Proc. Soc. Exp. Biol. Med.* 148: 435-439, 1975.
3. Banchero, N. Cardiovascular responses to chronic hypoxia. *Annu. Rev. Physiol.* 49: 465-476, 1987.
4. Breen, E., E. C. Johnson, H. Wagner, H. M. Tseng, L. A. Sung, and P. D. Wagner. Angiogenic growth factor mRNA responses in muscle to a single bout of exercise. *J. Appl. Physiol.* 81: 355-361, 1996.
5. Cassin, S., D. Gilbert, C. E. Bunnell, and E. M. Johnson. Capillary development during exposure to chronic hypoxia. *Am. J. Physiol.* 220: 448-451, 1971.
6. Clyne, C. A. C., H. Mears, and R. O. Weller. Calf muscle adaptation to peripheral vascular disease. *Cardiovasc. Dis.* 19: 507-512, 1985.
7. Desplanches, D., H. Hoppeler, M. T. Linossier, C. Denis, H. Claassen, D. Dormois, J. R. Lacour, and A. Geyssant. Effects of training in normobaric hypoxia on human muscle ultrastructure. *Pflügers Arch.* 425: 263-267, 1993.
8. Desplanches, D., H. Hoppeler, L. Tüscher, M. H. Mayet, H. Spielvogel, G. Ferretti, B. Kayser, M. Leuenberger, A. Grünenfelder, and R. Favier. Muscle tissue adaptation of high-altitude natives to training in chronic hypoxia or acute normoxia. *J. Appl. Physiol.* 81: 1946-1951, 1996.
9. Henriksson, J., E. Nygaard, J. Andersson, and B. Eklof. Enzyme activities, fiber types and capillarization in calf muscles of patients with intermittent claudication. *Scand. J. Clin. Lab. Invest.* 40: 361-369, 1980.
10. Hochachka, P. W., C. Stanley, J. Merkt, and J. Sumar Kalinowski. Metabolic meaning of elevated levels of oxidative enzymes in high altitude adapted animals: An interpretive hypothesis. *Respir. Physiol.* 52: 303-313, 1983.
11. Holloszy, J. O. and E. F. Coyle. Adaptations of skeletal muscles to endurance exercise and their metabolic consequences. *J. Appl. Physiol.* 56: 831-838, 1984.
12. Hoppeler, H., H. Howald, and P. Cerretelli. Human muscle structure after exposure to extreme altitude. *Experientia* 46: 1185-1187, 1990.
13. Hoppeler, H., O. Hudlicka, E. Uhlmann, and H. Claassen. Skeletal muscle adaptations to ischemia and severe exercise. *Clin. J. Sport Med.* 2: 43-51, 1992.
14. Hoppeler, H., O. Mathieu, E. R. Weibel, R. Krauer, S. L. Lindstedt, and C. R. Taylor. Design of the mammalian respiratory system. VIII. Capillaries in skeletal muscle. *Respir. Physiol.* 44: 129-150, 1981.
15. Hoppeler, H., O. Mathieu-Costello, and S. R. Kayar. Mitochondria and microvascular design. In: *The Lung: Scientific Foundations*. Crystal, R. G.; West, J. B.; Barnes, P. J.; Cherniack, N. S.; Weibel, E. R. (editors), Raven Press, New York, 1467-1477, 1991.

16. Hudlicka, O. Is physiological angiogenesis in skeletal muscle regulated by changes in microcirculation? *Microcirc.* 5: 5-23, 1998.

17. Jansson, E., J. Johansson, C. Sylven, and L. Kaijser. Calf muscle adaptation in intermittent claudication. Side-differences in muscle metabolic characteristics in patients with unilateral arterial disease. *Clin. Physiol.* 8: 17-29, 1988.

18. Kayser, B., H. Hoppeler, H. Claasen, and P. Cerretelli. Muscle structure and performance capacity of Himalayan Sherpas. *J. Appl. Physiol.* 70: 1938-1942, 1991.

19. Krogh, A. The number and distribution of capillaries in muscle with calculations of the oxygen pressure head necessary for supplying the tissue. *J. Physiol.* (London) 52: 409-415, 1919.

20. Léon-Velarde, F., J. Sanchez, A. X. Bigard, A. Brunet, C. Lesty, and C. Monge. High altitude tissue adaptation in Andean coots - Capillarity, fibre area, fibre type and enzymatic activities of skeletal muscle. *J. Comp. Physiol.* B 163(1): 52-58, 1993.

21. MacDougall, J. D., H. J. Green, J. R. Sutton, G. Coates, A. Y. P. Cymerman, and C. S. Houston. Operation Everst-II - Structural adaptations in skeletal muscle in response to extreme simulated altitude. *Acta Physiol. Scand.* 421-427, 1997.

22. Mathieu-Costello, O. Muscle capillary tortuosity in high altitude mice depends on sarcomere length. *Respir. Physiol.* 76: 289-302, 1989.

23. Mathieu-Costello, O. and P. J. Agey. Chronic hypoxia affects capillary density and geometry in pigeon pectoralis muscle. *Respir. Physiol.* 109: 39-52, 1997.

24. Mathieu-Costello, O., P. J. Agey, and H. Normand. Capillary geometry in flight muscle of pigeons native and flying at altitude. *Respir. Physiol.* 103: 187-194, 1996.

25. Mathieu-Costello, O., P. J. Agey, L. Wu, L. Hazelwood, J. M. Szewczak, and R. E. MacMillen. Increased fiber capillarization in flight muscle of finch at altitude. *Faseb J.* 10: A645, 1996.

26. Mathieu, O., L. M. Cruz Orive, H. Hoppeler, and E. R. Weibel. Estimating length density and quantifying anisotropy in skeletal muscle capillaries. *J. Microsc.* 131: 131-146, 1983.

27. Puntschart, A., K. Jostarndt, H. Hoppeler, and R. Billeter. An efficient polymerase chain reaction approach for the quantitation of multiple RNAs in human tissue samples. *PCR Meth. Appl.* 3: 232-238, 1994.

28. Reynafarje, B. Myoglobin content and enzymatic activity of muscle and altitude adaptation. *J. Appl. Physiol.* 17: 301-305, 1962.

29. Romijn, J. A., S. Klein, E. F. Coyle, L. S. Sidossis, and R. R. Wolfe. Strenuous endurance training increases lipolysis and triglyceride-fatty acid cycling at rest. *J. Appl. Physiol.* 75: 108-113, 1993.

30. Rosser, B. W. and P. W. Hochachka. Metabolic capacity of muscle fibers from high-altitude natives. Eur. *J. Appl. Physiol.* 67: 513-517, 1993.

31. Shweiki, D., A. Itin, D. Soffer, and E. Keshet. Vascular endothelial growth factor induced by hypoxia may mediate hypoxia-initiated angiogenesis. *Nature* 359: 843-845, 1992.

32. Terrados, N., E. Jansson, C. Sylven, and L. Kaijser. Is hypoxia a stimulus for synthesis of oxidative enzymes and myoglobin? *J. Appl. Physiol.* 68: 2369-2372, 1990.

33. Terrados, N., J. Melichna, C. Sylven, E. Jansson, and L. Kaijser. Effects of training at simulated altitude on performance and muscle metabolic capacity in competitive road cyclists. *Eur. J. Appl. Physiol.* 57: 203-209, 1988.

34. Valdivia, E. Total capillary bed in striated muscle of Guinea pigs native to the Peruvian mountains. *Amer. J. Physiol.* 194: 585-589, 1958.

35. Vock, R., H. Hoppeler, H. Claassen, D. X. Y. Wu, R. Billeter, J. M. Weber, C. R. Taylor, and E. R. Weibel. Design of the oxygen and substrate pathways. VI. Structural basis of intracellular substrate supply to mitochondria in muscle cells. *J. Exp. Biol.* 199: 1689-1697, 1996.

36. Vock, R., E. R. Weibel, H. Hoppeler, G. Ordway, J. M. Weber, and C. R. Taylor. Design of the oxygen and substrate pathways. V. Structural basis of vascular substrate supply to muscle cells. *J. Exp. Biol.* 199: 1675-1688, 1996.

37. Vogt, M. Hypoxie und Diät als Beeinflussungsvariablen trainingsbedingter Adaptationsprozesse in der menschlichen Skelettmuskulatur. *Dissertation*, pp 1-160, 1999.

38. Widmer, H. R., H. Hoppeler, E. Nevo, C. R. Taylor, and E. R. Weibel. Working underground: Respiratory adaptations in the blind mole rat. *Proc. Natl. Acad. Sci.* USA 94: 2062-2067, 1997.

Chapter 22

Recent Advances in Human Physiology at Extreme Altitude

John B. West

Department of Medicine, University of California San Diego, La Jolla, California 92093-0623, USA

Key words: extreme altitude, maximal oxygen uptake, acclimatization, work capacity, extreme hypoxia, alveolar P_{CO_2}

Abstract: There have been recent advances in the physiology of extreme altitude, especially on the barometric pressure-altitude relationship, and pulmonary gas exchange. Until recently, the only direct measurement of barometric pressure on the summit of Mt. Everest was the value of 253 Torr obtained in October 1981. During the 1997 NOVA Everest expedition, another measurement was made with a hand-held barometer and, after calibration, the value was within approximately 1 Torr of the previous measurement. In addition, weather balloons released at approximately the same time in the vicinity of Mt. Everest gave values that agreed closely. In 1998, a large series of measurements of barometric pressure were made using a weather probe placed on the South Col of Everest (altitude 7,986 m). The mean pressure in May was 283.7 Torr which agrees well with the measurements made just above the South Col in October 1981. The new data fit closely with the Model Atmosphere Equation $P_B = \exp (6.63268 - 0.1112h - 0.00149h^2)$ where h is in km. The conclusion is that on days when the mountain is usually climbed during May and October, the summit pressure is 251-253 Torr. The inspired P_{O_2} is therefore 43 Torr and these data clarify expected pulmonary gas exchange on the summit. Sixty-three measurements of alveolar P_{O_2} for barometric pressures of 300 to 253 Torr from the Silver Hut and AMREE field expeditions gave a mean value for P_{O_2} of 35 Torr. Therefore for this value the alveolar P_{CO_2} cannot be greater than 8 Torr under steady-state, conditions when the respiratory exchange ratio (R) is 1. When R is less than 1, the alveolar P_{CO_2} must be even lower.

1.   INTRODUCTION

There have been advances in our knowledge about the physiology of extreme altitude during the last three years, particularly on the relationship between barometric pressure and altitude. These new data have implications for gas exchange at very high altitude, notably on the summit of Mt. Everest.

Barometric pressure is a critical factor at extreme altitude because it determines the inspired PO_2 and this is the starting point for the oxygen cascade to the mitochondria where the oxygen is utilized. It is a remarkable fact that the barometric pressure near the summit of Mt. Everest (altitude 8,848 m) is so low that the inspired PO_2 is very near the limit for human survival.

Until recently, only one direct measurement of barometric pressure on the summit of Mt. Everest was available. This was obtained by Dr. Christopher Pizzo on October 24, 1981 during the American Medical Research Expedition to Everest (AMREE), and the value was 253 Torr (7). In spite of being only one measurement, this value has been used by several investigators. For example, it was the pressure selected for the "summit" in Operation Everest II (2). It would clearly be desirable to have more data on barometric pressure at extreme altitude, and two studies in the last three years have provided this.

2.   1997 NOVA EVEREST EXPEDITION

The scientific objectives of this expedition which took place in the spring of 1997 included measurement of neuropsychological function at extreme altitude, imaging of the brain before and after the expedition, and some cardiopulmonary studies. We were not aware of the expedition until the last minute but just managed send a hand-held barometer in time in the hope that a measurement could be made on the summit. This was done by David Breashears at 7:00 a.m. local time on May 23, 1997. The instrument was a Pretel Alti Plus K2 Barometer (Groupe Pretel Claix, France) which we had used on a number of occasions up to altitudes of 5000 m. However we had not had an opportunity to calibrate it for the pressures and the temperatures expected near the summit.

When the barometer was returned to the University of California San Diego, it was calibrated against a mercury column at a temperature of -20° C. The barometer was carried in Breashears' backpack and therefore was exposed to the ambient temperature though this was not measured. However data from weather balloons (see below) indicated that the temperature at the altitude of the summit was about -22° C.

The reading made by Breashears was 346 mbar, and when this was corrected according to the calibrations carried out in our laboratory at the same pressure and a temperature of -20° C., the corrected pressure was found to be 252.5 Torr (5). This was therefore in close agreement with the value obtained by Pizzo in 1981.

3. SIMULTANEOUS MEASUREMENTS FROM WEATHER BALLOONS

Weather balloons (radiosondes) are released from many meteorological stations throughout the world at 0000 and 1200 UTC (Universal Coordinated Time) every day. There are 14 stations in the general vicinity of Mt. Everest (27° 59' N and 86° 56' E) all between 22° and 38° N and between 74° and 95° E. These data can be retrieved by professional meteorologists and this was done for us by Laurence G. Riddle of the Scripps Institution of Oceanography, UCSD, for balloons released at 0000 UTC on May 23, 1997. This corresponded to 5:40 a.m. Nepalese time and so was within 1.5 hours of when Breashears made his measurement.

Each balloon records barometric pressure, temperature and humidity, at altitudes up to about 30,000 m, and wind direction and velocity can also be obtained by following the path of the balloon. We obtained altitudes for barometric pressures of 150, 200, 250, 300, 400, 500, and 700 mbar from each balloon and thus obtained the relationship between barometric pressure and altitude for each station. The barometric pressure at an altitude of 8848 m was then obtained by interpolation and the results are shown in Figure 1. Note that at Gorakhpur, just southwest of Everest, the pressure at 8,848 m altitude was 254 Torr. The corresponding pressures for the two closest stations to the southeast and northeast of Everest were 253 and 252 Torr respectively. Thus these weather balloon data agree well with the direct measurement made by Breashears.

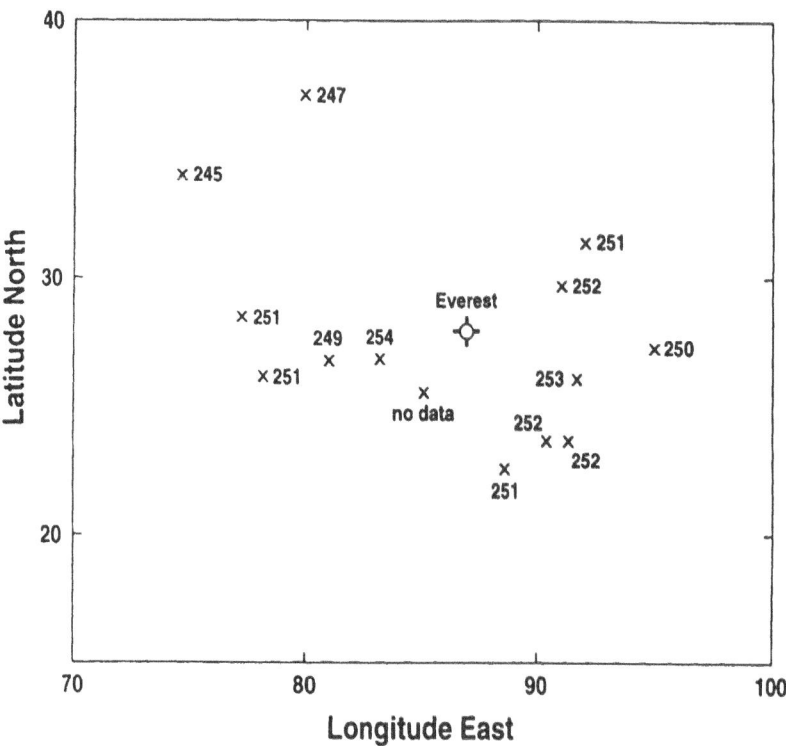

Figure 1. Barometric pressures (Torr) at an altitude of 8848 m in the vicinity of Mt. Everest at 0000 UTC on May 23, 1997 as determined from weather balloons. Note that the stations nearest to the Everest summit gave barometric pressures close to 253 Torr. The values therefore agreed well with measurement of 252.5 made on the summit by the 1997 NOVA Expedition. From West (5).

An interesting feature of these data is that the summit of Mt. Everest was in a high pressure area. This is more clearly seen in Figure 2 which shows the altitudes for a pressure of 300 mbar in the vicinity of Mt. Everest at the same time. Note that the Everest summit is close to a center of a high pressure area. It is not surprising that the pressure is relatively high on a day selected for climbing to the summit because climbers choose days when the weather is fine. It is interesting that Pizzo's measurement of 253 Torr on October 24, 1981 was also made on an unusually fine day. In fact the temperature directly measured on the summit was -9° C. which was exceptionally warm for this altitude.

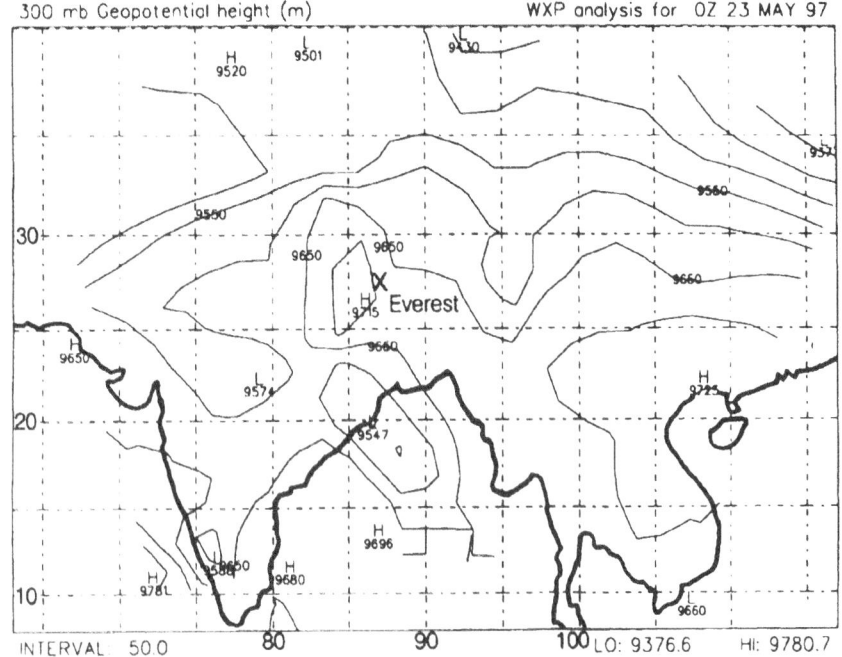

Figure 2. Altitudes for a pressure of 300 mbar (225 Torr) in the vicinity of Mt. Everest at 0000 UTC on May 23, 1997 as determined from weather balloons. Note that Everest was near the center of a high pressure system. From West (5).

4. BAROMETRIC PRESSURES ON THE SOUTH COL OF EVEREST (7,986 M) IN THE SUMMER OF 1998

The Media Laboratory of the Massachusetts Institute of Technology (MIT) has developed sophisticated weather probes which measure barometric pressure, temperature, wind speed, and degree of lightness or darkness, and transmit the data to orbiting satellites. One of these probes was placed on the South Col of Everest (altitude 7986 m) in early May 1998. Barometric pressure was measured with a Motorola sensor (MPX 5100AP, Motorola, Schaumburg, IL) which can operate at temperatures down to -40° C. The resulting data were posted on a web site (http://janson.media.mit.edu/weather/14836). Up to 30 measurements of pressure each day were available from May 4 to August 26.

The results showed that the mean barometric pressures for May, June, July, and August respectively were 283.7, 285.5, 286.3, 286.9 Torr respectively (5). The increase in pressure from May to July is in line with the known seasonal changes at this altitude (7). The highest pressures are seen in July and August, and the lowest pressures in January. May and October are at approximately the same height on the descending limbs of the plot of pressure against month (see Figure 3 of West et al. (5)). Therefore we are justified in comparing pressures made in these months.

Barometric pressures were measured during AMREE at Camp 5 which was about 60 m above the South Col (altitude 8,050 m). Six measurements of pressure were made between October 12 and October 25, 1981, and the mean value was 283.6 Torr (7). There is therefore good agreement with the pressure of 283.7 measured in May 1998 although the slightly greater height of camp 5 would be expected to cause a reduction in pressure of about 2 Torr.

5.   RELATIONSHIP BETWEEN BAROMETRIC PRESSURE AND ALTITUDE ON MT. EVEREST

These new data allow us to determine the relationship between barometric pressure and extreme altitude on Mt. Everest with much more confidence. During AMREE, barometric pressures were measured at altitudes of 5,400, 8,050, and 8,848 m (summit). The means for these altitudes are shown by open circles in Figure 3. The figure also shows the new measurement made by the 1997 NOVA Everest Expedition on the summit (8,848 m), and the mean pressure at an altitude of 7,986 m made by the MIT study (crosses). The equation of the line was determined from the AMREE data points and additional data from many high altitude stations, the altitudes of which are accurately known (4). This Model Atmosphere equation is $P_B = \exp(6.63268 - 0.1112h - 0.00149h^2)$ where P_B is in Torr and h is km. Table 1 summarizes the barometric pressures measured by the three studies cited here, and shows how well these are fitted by the Model Atmosphere equation.

It should be emphasized that the two measures of 253 Torr on the summit obtained by the AMREE and NOVA studies represent the barometric pressures on fine days when a high pressure system is present. The mean barometric pressure at an altitude of 8,848 m in May and October at this latitude as obtained by weather balloons is about 251 Torr. Since climbers only attempt to reach the summit on fine days, we can conclude that the barometric pressure on the summit when the mountain is usually climbed is between 251 and 253 Torr.

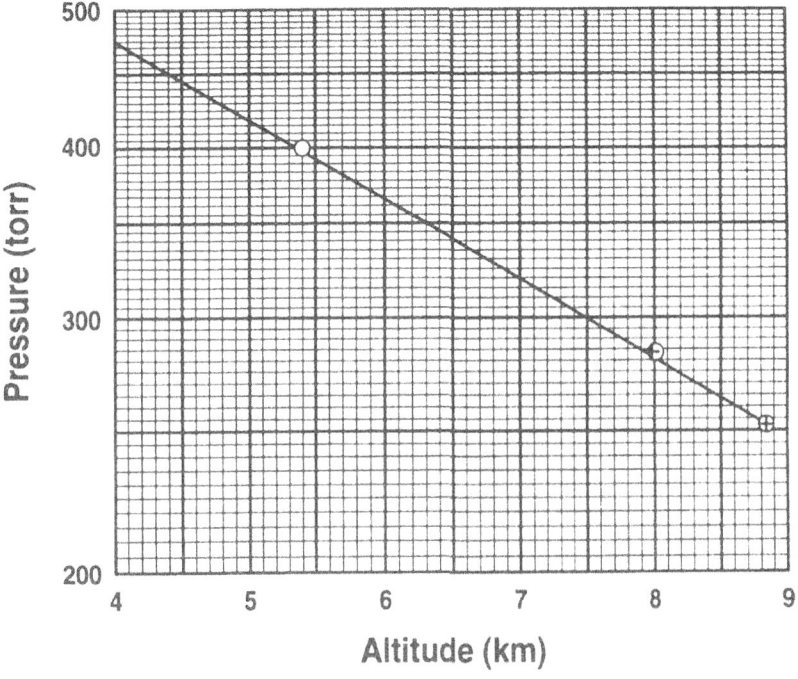

Figure 3. Barometric pressure-altitude relationship at extreme altitudes on Mt. Everest. The circles show data from the 1981 American Medical Research Expedition to Everest. The cross at the extreme right is the data point from the 1997 NOVA Expedition. The cross at an altitude of 7986 m is from the MIT study. The line corresponds to the Model Atmosphere Equation: $P_B = \exp(6.63268 - 0.1112\,h - 0.00149\,h^2)$ where P_B is in Torr and the altitude is in km. From West (5).

Table 1. Barometric pressures (Torr) on Mt. Everest. From West (5).

Altitude, m	AMREE	NOVA	MIT	Model Atmosphere Equation
8,848 (Summit)	253	253		253
8,050	284			282
7,986			284	284
5,400	400			399

6. IMPLICATIONS FOR PULMONARY GAS EXCHANGE ON THE EVEREST SUMMIT

We now have considerable confidence that the PO_2 of moist inspired gas on the summit is 43 Torr and this has important implications for pulmonary gas exchange. Figure 4 shows an oxygen-carbon dioxide diagram with alveolar gas values for acclimatized subjects from sea level to extreme altitude. Most of the data were collected by Rahn and Otis (3) with additional points from two field expeditions, the Silver Hut expedition (1) and AMREE (6). Note that as the altitude increases, both the PO_2 and the PCO_2 fall. The alveolar PO_2 falls because of the decrease in inspired PO_2 as altitude increases. The alveolar PCO_2 falls because of increasing hyperventilation. When the barometric pressure falls below about 300 Torr, corresponding to an altitude of about 7,500 m, the alveolar PO_2 shows no further change but is defended at a value between and 30 and 40 Torr.

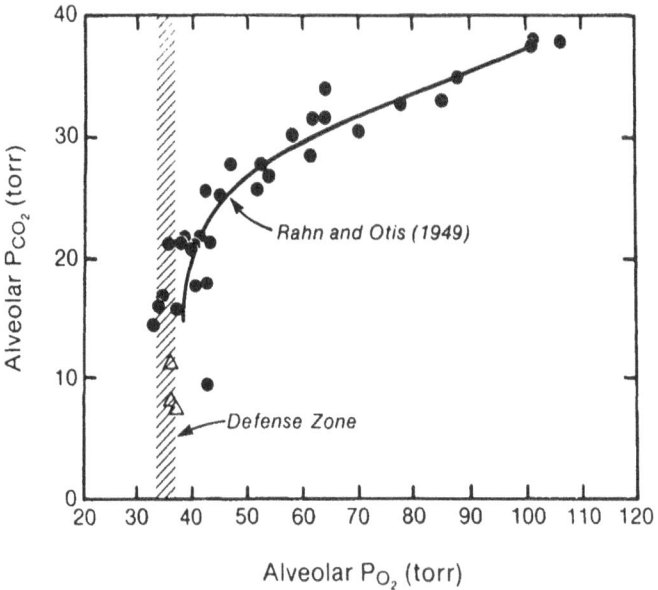

Figure 4. Oxygen-carbon dioxide diagram showing values of alveolar PO_2 and PCO_2 in acclimatized subjects at high altitude. Sea level is top right and the Everest summit is at bottom left. Most of the data were collected by Rahn and Otis (3). Note that above a certain altitude (about 7,500 m) there is no further fall in alveolar PO_2 and this is defended at a value between 30 and 40 Torr. From West et al. (6).

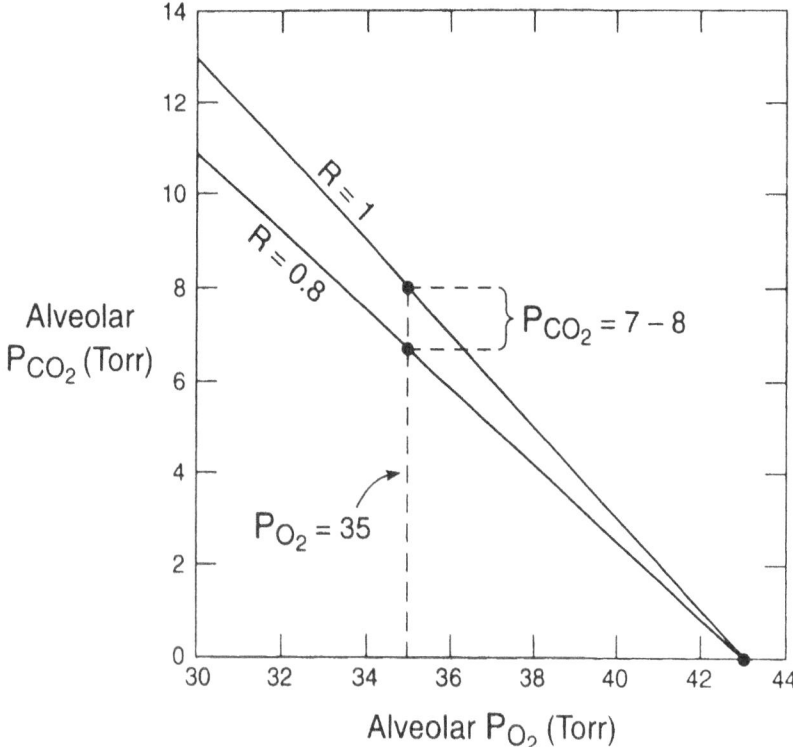

Figure 5. Oxygen-carbon dioxide diagram showing respiratory exchange ratio (R) lines for an inspired P_{O_2} of 43 Torr on the summit of Mt. Everest. Note that if the alveolar P_{O_2} is defended at a value of 35 Torr, the P_{CO_2} cannot be higher than 8 Torr under steady-state conditions.

Additional information on the alveolar P_{O_2} at extreme altitude is available by analyzing the data from the Silver Hut and AMREE field expeditions. A total of 63 alveolar P_{O_2} values were reported for barometric pressures between 300 and 253 Torr with a mean of 34.8 Torr, SD of 3.24, and SEM of 0.41. Figure 5 shows that if the alveolar P_{O_2} is 35 Torr, the alveolar P_{CO_2} cannot exceed 8 Torr under steady state conditions when the highest value of R is 1. This was the value obtained by Pizzo on the Everest summit during AMREE. Simulated ascents carried out in low pressure chambers such as Operation Everest II (2) tend to show higher values for alveolar P_{CO_2} probably because of lesser degrees of acclimatization to high altitude.

REFERENCES

1. Gill, M.B., J.S. Milledge, L.G. Pugh, and J.B. West. Alveolar gas composition at 21,000 to 25,700 ft. *J Physiol* (London) 163: 373-377, 1962.
2. Houston, C.S., A. Cymerman, and J.R. Sutton. *Operation Everest II: Biomedical Studies During a Simulated Ascent of Mt. Everest.* Natick, MA: U.S. Army Research Institute of Environmental Medicine, 1991.
3. Rahn, H., and A.B. Otis. Man's respiratory response during and after acclimatization to high altitude. *Am J Physiol* 157: 445-482, 1949.
4. West, J.B. Prediction of barometric pressures at high altitude with the use of model atmospheres. *J Appl Physiol* 81: 1850-1854, 1996.
5. West, J.B. Barometric pressures on Mt. Everest: new data and physiological significance. *J Appl Physio*l 86: 1062-1854, 1999.
6. West, J.B., P.H. Hackett, K.H. Maret, J.S. Milledge, and R.M. Peters Jr. Pulmonary gas exchange on the summit of Mount Everest. *J Appl Physiol* 55: 678-687, 1983.
7. West, J.B., S. Lahiri, K.H. Maret, R.M. Peters Jr, and C.J. Pizzo. Barometric pressures at extreme altitudes on Mt. Everest: Physiological significance. *J Appl Physiol* 54: 1188-1194, 1983.

Chapter 23

Operation Everest III (COMEX '97)
Effects Of Prolonged And Progressive Hypoxia On Humans During A Simulated Ascent To 8,848 M In A Hypobaric Chamber

Jean-Paul Richalet, Paul Robach, Sébastien Jarrot, Jean-Christophe Schneider, Nicholas P. Mason, Emmanuel Cauchy, Jean-Pierre Herry, Annick Bienvenu, Bernard Gardette and Claude Gortan
Association pour la Recherche en Physiologie de l'Environnement, Laboratoire Réponses cellulaires et fonctionnelles à l'hypoxie (EA 2363), U.F.R. Médecine, Université Paris Nord, Bobigny; Ecole Nationale de Ski et d'Alpinisme, Chamonix; COMEX S.A., Marseille, France

Key words: hypobaria, acclimatization, $\dot{V}O_{2MAX}$, acute mountain sickness

Abstract: Exposure to high altitude induces physiological or pathological modifications that are not always clearly attributable to a specific environmental factor: hypoxia, cold, stress, inadequate food. The principal goal of hypobaric chamber studies is to determine the specific effect of hypoxia. Eight male volunteers ("altinauts"), aged 23 to 37 were selected. They were first pre-acclimatized in the Observatoire Vallot (4,350m) before entering the chamber. The chamber was progressively decompressed down to 253 mmHg barometric pressure, with a recovery period of 3 days at 5,000m in the middle of the decompression period. They spent a total of 31 days in the chamber. Eighteen protocols were organized by 14 European teams, exploring the limiting factors of physical and psychological performance, and the pathophysiology of acute mountain sickness (AMS). All subjects reached 8,000m and 7 of them reached the simulated altitude of 8,848m. Three altinauts complained of transient neurological symptoms which resolved rapidly with reoxygenation. Body weight decreased by 5.4 kg through a negative caloric balance. Only four days after the return to sea-level, subjects had recovered 3.4 kg, i.e. 63% of the total loss. At 8,848m (n=5), PaO_2 was 30.6 ± 1.4 mmHg, PCO_2 11.9 ± 1.4 mmHg, pH 7.58 ± 0.02 (arterialized capillary blood). Hemoglobin concentration increased from 14.8±1.4 to 18.4±1.5 g/dl at 8,000m and recovered within 4 days at sea-level. AMS score increased rapidly at 6,000m and was maximal at 7,000m, especially for sleep. AMS was related to alteration in color vision and elevation of body temperature. $\dot{V}O_{2MAX}$ decreased by 59% at 7,000m. The

Hypoxia: Into the Next Millennium,
Edited by R. C. Roach, *et al.* Kluwer Academic/Plenum Publishing, New York, 1999.

297

purpose of this paper is to give a general description of the study and the time course of the main clinical and physiological parameters. The altinauts reached the "summit" (for some of them three consecutive times) in better physiological conditions than it would have been possible in the mountains, probably because acclimatization and other environmental factors such as cold and nutrition were controlled.

1.   INTRODUCTION

The exposure of humans to the environment of high altitude regions induces various physiological adjustments or pathological manifestations which are not always clearly attributable to one or another stressor associated with this particular milieu. Altitude hypoxia, cold, dryness of air, inadequate food or liquid intake, exhaustion and psychological stress are the main factors that could modify human physiology and behavior at high altitude. The first objective of hypobaric chamber studies is to isolate hypobaric hypoxia from the other stressors. The possibility to use advanced technology and sophisticated equipment as well as ethical and safety considerations give a clear advantage to chamber studies as compared to field studies when the effect of hypoxia is the main question. Paul Bert was the first scientist at the end of the last century to use a hypobaric chamber to study the effect of altitude hypoxia on himself (2) and was able to demonstrate that the well known effects of acute altitude exposure (dyspnea, tachycardia, dizziness) were due to the lack of oxygen and not to hypobaria alone. In 1946, the US Navy promoted a study called "Operation Everest" where four subjects were able to reach the standard altitude equivalent to Mount Everest (235 mmHg) after a 30-day period of confinement in a small chamber (3.3m x 3.3m x 2.3m) (4). In 1985, Operation Everest II was directed by Charles Houston, John Sutton and Allen Cymerman. It was a large scale investigation which produced a lot of new interesting data and allowed the formulation of new concepts in the field of high altitude physiology and medicine (5). Eight male subjects entered the chamber, six of them reached the "summit" (ambient pressure of 240 mmHg) after a 40 day stay in the chamber. In 1989, Operation Everest Turbo demonstrated the positive effects of pre-acclimatization in a hypobaric chamber before an expedition to Mount Everest (8). Six subjects (five male and one female) were intermittently exposed to equivalent altitudes up to 8,848m for 5 days and showed physiological and clinical signs of acclimatization.

The objectives of the present study were to use the advantages of chambers studies (pure hypobaric hypoxia, advanced technology, safety) to address some specific questions remaining unanswered by previous chamber or field studies.

2. SUBJECTS

Selection of subjects. Eighteen male subjects volunteered to take part in the study. We will call them " altinauts ", as a combination of altitude and astronauts. Nine were selected from various criterion: experience of mountaineering, maximal oxygen uptake, hypoxic ventilatory and cardiac response to hypoxia at rest and exercise, psychological profile and motivation, interest for science in general and high altitude physiology in particular. Eight subjects and one reserve entered the study for baseline normoxic studies. Finally, eight altinauts underwent the altitude chamber program. Their characteristics were as follows:

1. K.B. 23 yr old, male nurse, high level climber in the Alps, no altitude experience above Mont Blanc (4807m), lives in Chamonix (1035m), smokes 2 cig./day; height 180cm; weight 66.5 kg.
2. E.C. 37 yr old, medical doctor specialized in emergency medicine and mountain rescue, mountain guide, participated in various high altitude expeditions including ARPE scientific expedition to Mount Sajama (6542m) in 1991, reached the altitude of 8,760m without supplementary oxygen on Mount Everest in 1990, lives in Chamonix (1035m), occasional smoker; height 183cm; weight 77.2 kg.
3. G.D. 25 yr old, medical student (last year), has good mountaineering experience, climbed various summits in the Andes and reached the altitude of 6435m, lives in Toulouse (146m), non smoker; height 190cm; weight 80.2 kg.
4. J.F.F. 25 yr old, medical student (last year), has good mountaineering experience, climbed various summits in the Andes and reached the altitude of 6435m, lives in Toulouse (146m), non smoker; height 188cm; weight 82.7 kg.
5. M.G. 26 yr old, medical student (last year), has good mountaineering experience, climbed various summits in the Andes and reached the altitude of 6435m, lives in Toulouse (146m), non smoker; height 176cm; weight 72.2 kg.
7. G.S. 25 yr old, electrician, high level climber in the Alps, no altitude experience above 4100m, lives in Challes les Eaux (310m), smokes 4 to 5 cig. /day; height 177cm; weight 70.3 kg.
8. P.S. 25 yr old, skier, good climber in the Alps, has an experience of trekking in Nepal up to 5200m, lives in Servoz (815m), non smoker; height 172cm; weight 65.4 kg.
9. A. H. 27 yr old, master in law, regular climber, moderately trained as compared with the others, no experience of high altitude above 4300m, lives near Paris (60 m), non smoker; height 176cm; weight 80.3 kg.

3.   METHODS

3.1   Location and schedule of experiments

Subjects were studied at the COMEX S.A. facilities in Marseille, France. The hypobaric chamber consisted of three rooms - one spherical study room (diameter 5m, available volume 65 m^3) connected to a cylindrical living room with eight sleeping bunks and a table for meals (length 8 m, available volume 32 m^3) via an airlock room usable for toilet and shower (available volume 8 m^3) (Figure 1). Pressures in the living room and airlock on one side and in the study room on the other side were controlled independently by a computerized system. Food and drinks, urine and blood samples, and any necessary small object could be transferred between outside and inside the chamber via two airlock devices. Altinauts were constantly monitored through five video cameras and audio systems by two technicians who were continuously present to manage the chamber, day and night. During day time, a medical doctor was present in the control room. During night time, a doctor could be called at any time and be present on the site within 15 minutes. Oxygen masks were available at each bed, in the dining room and in the study room. A portable oxygen bottle with a mask was also available within the chamber, as well as an emergency pack usable by one of the subjects, a doctor trained in high-altitude emergencies. In case of severe problems necessitating emergency evacuation, a subject could be taken out of the chamber within 30 minutes from 8,848m equivalent altitude, and more quickly from lower altitudes.

Eighteen protocols were planned and executed by fourteen scientific teams from France, England and the Netherlands to study the effect of prolonged hypobaric hypoxia on various systems:

1. Role of hemoconcentration on aerobic performance, with related hydroelectrolytic hormones.
2. Alpha motoneuron excitability and recruitment of motor units.
3. Sensori-motor control and maximal performance of skeletal muscles.
4. Role of hemoconcentration on aerobic performance, with related hydroelectrolytic hormones.
5. Alpha motoneuron excitability and recruitment of motor units.
6. Sensori-motor control and maximal performance of skeletal muscles.

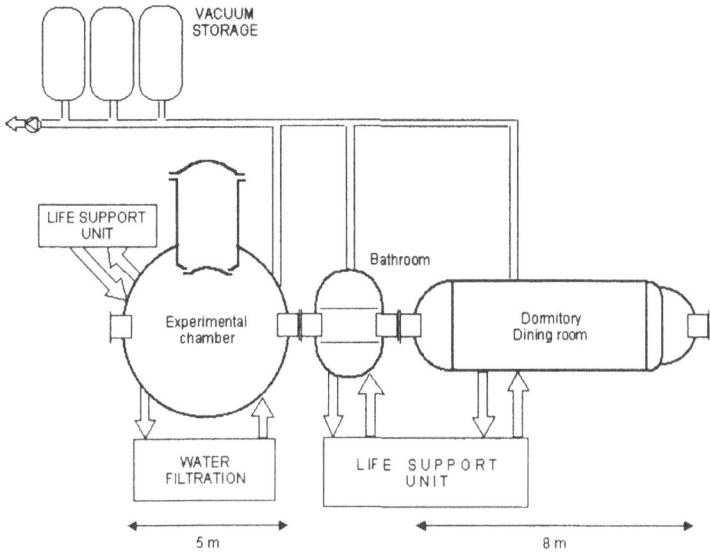

Figure 1. Plan of the hypobaric chambers at COMEX industries.

7. Role of hemoconcentration on aerobic performance, with related hydroelectrolytic hormones.
8. Alpha motoneuron excitability and recruitment of motor units.
9. Sensori-motor control and maximal performance of skeletal muscles.
10. Production of oxygen free radicals at rest and exercise.
11. Coordination during a simulated traverse climb of short duration.
12. Transport of oxygen and oxyhemoglobin dissociation curve.
13. Acclimatization and cardiac and ventilatory response to hypoxia, ventilatory response to CO_2.
14. Role of peripheral chemoreceptors on ventilatory acclimatization.
15. Defense responses of respiratory tract. Variation of cough frequency with altitude.
16. Role of NO, endothelin and eicosanoids in the pathophysiology of pulmonary hypertension. Effects of a supplementation with L-arginine.
17. Cardiac function evaluated by echocardiography. Formation of circulating bubbles.
18. Autoregulation of cerebral blood flow evaluated by transcranial Doppler.
19. Calcium and phosphate metabolism, with related hormones.
20. Measurement of energy expenditure and distribution of total body water by doubly labeled water.
21. Sensitivity of adipose tissue to various lipolytic or antilipolytic agents. Variation in body composition.

22. Psychological adaptation to prolonged hypoxia: cognitive and affective sensorimotor aspects.
23. Psychological adaptation to prolonged hypoxia: individual psychological profile, decision taking and solving group problems.
24. Determinants of food consumption: taste sensitivity, appetite and satiety.

Written informed consent was obtained from all subjects. The protocols were approved, after revision, by the ethical committee of the University Hospital of Marseille. Special recommendations from the committee were to restrict blood gases to arterialized capillary blood sampling, maximal exercise no higher than 7,000 m, dopamine infusion at a maximal dose of 3 µg/kg/min for protocol #8, avoid the use of CO breathing to measure plasma volume in protocol #1.

The schedule of experiments was as follows:

3.2   Basal normoxic measurements

Basal measurements were performed on the nine subjects within the chamber with open doors from March 10th to 16th.

3.3   Pre-acclimatization period

In order to shorten the time spent within the chamber, subjects were allowed to pre-acclimatize in the Alps, at Refuge des Cosmiques (3,650m) for one day and Observatoire Vallot (4,350m) for five days. During this period, free climbing activity was allowed and no scientific observation was performed. This period was planned, not only to allow a rapid entrance to the chamber at 5,000 m but also to test the ability of the subjects to withstand high altitude and community life in a hostile environment. During this period, subject #6 suffered from high altitude pulmonary edema (documented by X-ray after evacuation to Chamonix hospital). He was excluded from the study and the alternate subject (#9) was then fully included in the study.

3.4   Hypobaric chamber period

Subjects descended from Observatoire Vallot on April 1st at mid-day and entered the chamber on April 2nd at mid-day. They spend their first night in the chamber at 4500m then went up to 5,000m where they started the experimental procedures. The ascent profile is shown on Figure 2. The pressures were chosen as the real pressures for the latitude of Mount Everest (14), up to 253 mmHg for the altitude of 8,848m. Except in the last period of

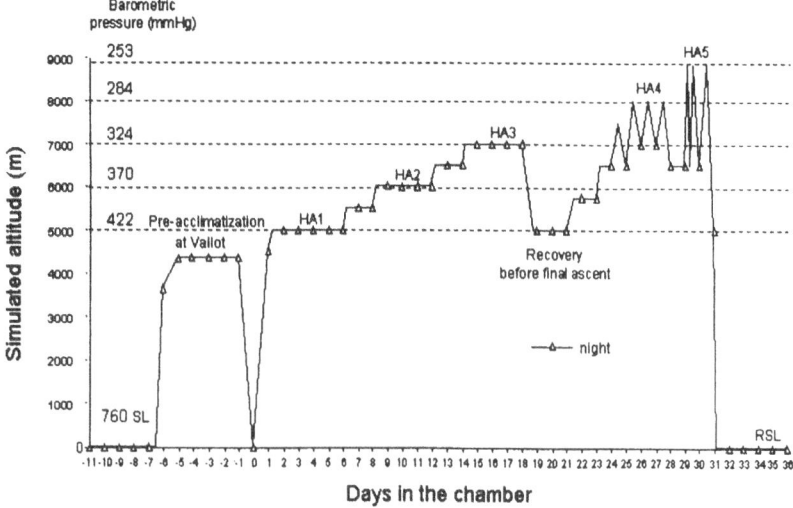

Figure 2. Simulated progression profile. SL, HA1 to HA5, RSL: periods of experimental studies.

ascent to the "summit", the pressure changes were performed early in the morning, before wake up and breakfast, within 15 minutes for an altitude difference of 500 m, 30 minutes for an altitude difference of 1000 m, and 90 minutes for an altitude difference of 1500 or 2348 m. At the lowest barometric pressure of 253 mmHg, the subjects spent 6 hours on day 30 and 4 hours on day 31. Experiments were performed at sea-level (SL), at 5,000m (HA1), 6,000m (HA2), 7,000m (HA3), return to 5,000m (RHA1), 8,000m (HA4), 8,848m (HA5) and after the return to sea-level (RSL). Subjects spent their last night in the chamber at 5,000m, after the last "summit" climb. During the days when no experiments were performed, altinauts were strongly encouraged to do some exercise on the treadmill or on the cycloergometer. Most of them did so (30 to 90 minutes per day), although their motivation decreased considerably with increasing altitude.

3.5   Recovery period

Altinauts left the chamber on May 2nd and underwent the RSL experiments until May 5th. This type of observation is quite unique: very few studies have explored the time course of physiological and psychological parameters after return to normoxic conditions.

Three subjects did not follow the complete schedule. One subject (#1) experienced neurological symptoms at 8,000m (day 25): while performing a cognitive test, he suddenly could hardly speak and write. These symptoms rapidly disappeared when he breathed pure oxygen, but a severe headache of migraine type could not be relieved by oxygen breathing and was not tolerated by the subject. A decision to evacuate the subject was taken and executed. Subsequent neurological examination, fundoscopy and cerebral magnetic resonance imaging were entirely normal. Subject #8 suffered from neurological symptoms at 8,848m (day 29): he felt dizzy and could not recognize his friends within the chamber and had the sensation of floating in the air. All signs disappeared with oxygen inhalation but the subject and his colleagues were still anxious and for safety reasons, subject #8 was evacuated from the chamber. Neurological examination and magnetic resonance imaging performed after evacuation were entirely normal. Subject #3 suffered from neurological symptoms at his second ascent to 8,848m (day 30): sudden pain in the back, paralysis of the left lower limb, with aphasia and facial paralysis. Symptoms disappeared rapidly with oxygen inhalation. He was brought down to 6,500 m where he felt perfectly well. He was kept under oxygen inhalation while his colleagues underwent their third ascent to 8,848m and stayed with them at 5,000m during the last night in the chamber. Neurological examination and magnetic resonance imaging performed after leaving the chamber were entirely normal. Altogether, 8 out of 8 altinauts reached 8,000m, 7 reached 8,848m among whom 5 reached the "summit" three times, one twice and another one only once. All altinauts, included those who left the chamber before time, underwent the protocols planned during the RSL period, the delay from leaving the chamber being respected. Subjects were not allowed to take medications except paracetamol for severe headache. One subject entered the chamber two days after a dental abscess evacuation and took antibiotics for 5 days within the chamber. Dexamethasone (8 mg IV) was given to subject #1 before evacuation on day 25. Despite strong discouragement against taking any medication for insomnia, sleeping pills (10 to 20 mg zolpidem) were occasionally given to some of the subjects in response to their strong demands and mainly to avoid a severe conflict between altinauts and the staff which could easily have jeopardized the study. As no sleep study was performed and as the plasma half life of zolpidem is 2.4 hours, this drug use was considered as having a potentially minimal influence on protocols performed the day after. However, any effect (mainly beneficial) cannot be excluded either on psychological or physical tests.

3.6   Environmental conditions

Pressure variations were continuously monitored in the chamber. Mean values for the altitudes where experiments were performed are shown in Figure 2. Variations in the chamber temperature are shown in Figure 3 (top). During experiments, temperature was, most of the time, kept between 18°C

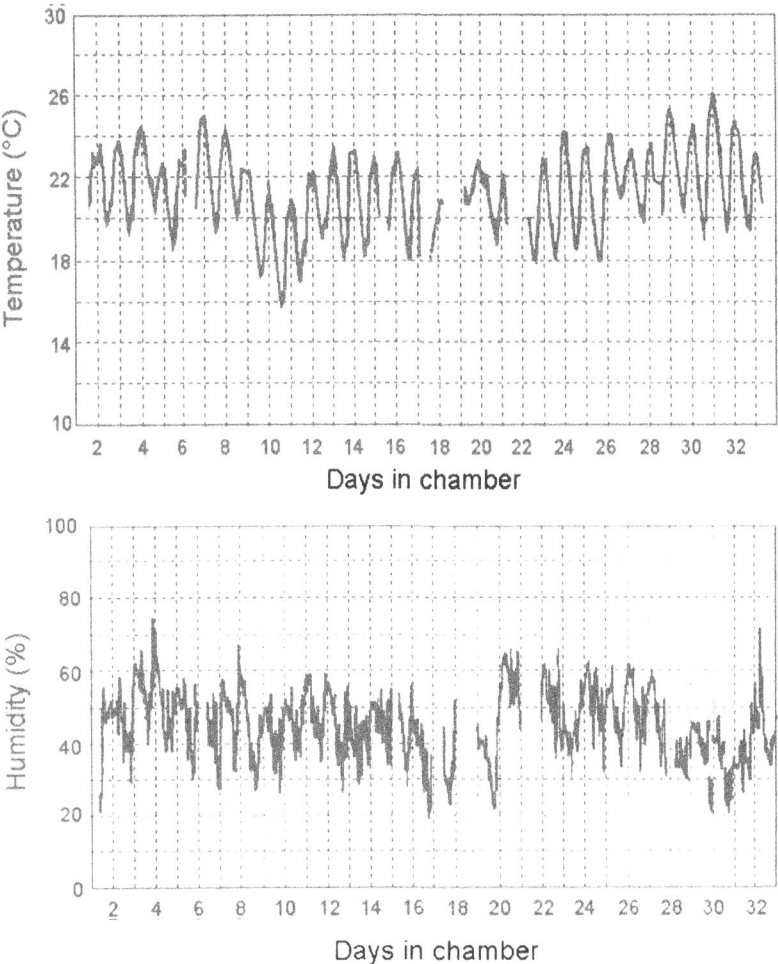

Figure 3. Variations of ambient temperature (top) and humidity (bottom) in the main experimental chamber.

and 24°C. Percentage of humidity in the chamber is shown in Figure 3 (bottom). It varied with outside ambient humidity and was mostly between 30 and 60 %. Day/night rhythm was maintained: altinauts woke up at 07:00 - 07:30 and went to bed between 22:00 and midnight. Ambient (dry) PiO_2 and $PiCO_2$ were monitored continuously and are shown on Figures 4.

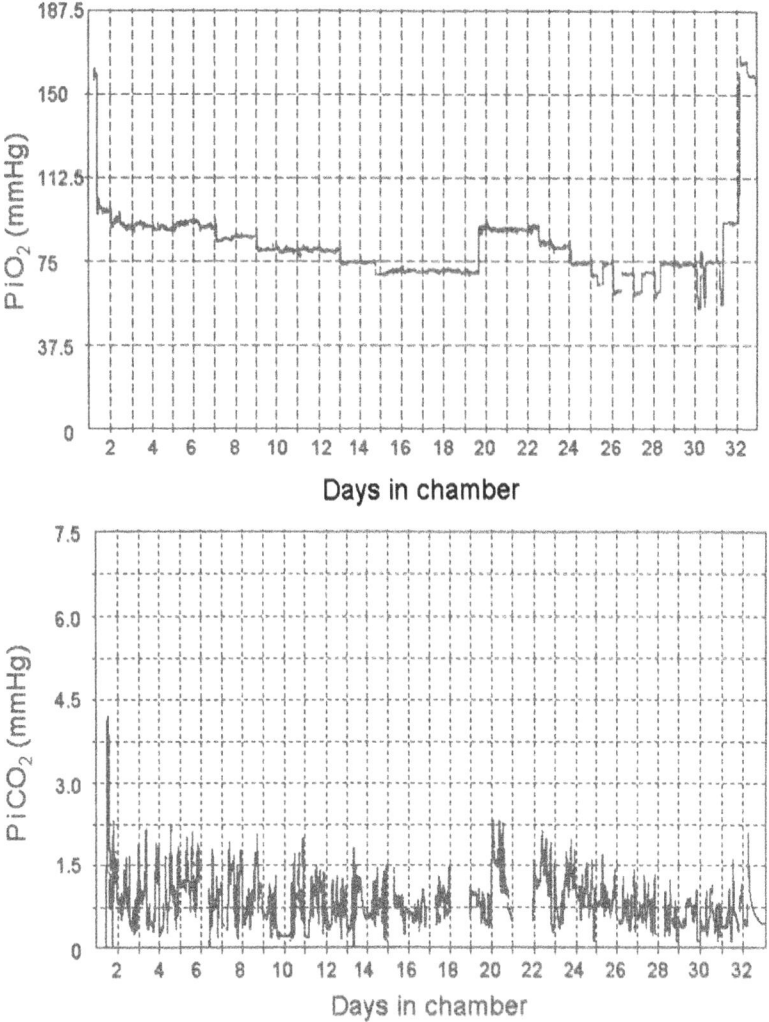

Figure 4. Variations of PO_2 (top) and PCO_2 (bottom) in ambient air (dry) of the main experimental chamber.

3.7   Investigators

They were no more than two investigators at the same time in the chamber. At very low barometric pressures (284 and 253 mmHg), they breathed pure oxygen for 30 minutes before entering the chamber in order to avoid decompression sickness. They were using supplemental oxygen at all altitudes. Oxygen supply was through a kind of space suit with a hood (not a mask). Exhaled gas was pumped directly from the hood. The possibility for leakage of oxygen to the chamber was thus minimal and the comfort of the investigator maximal. However, at the lowest barometric pressure of 253 mmHg, some leakage occurred for a short period, leading to discard values of blood gases taken in two subjects during this specific period.

4.   METHODS

Each protocol will be described in detail in other articles. The main purpose of the present paper is to give a general description of the study and the time course of the main clinical and physiological parameters. Daily questionnaire, body weighing and basal physiological parameters were recorded in the morning just after waking up, before breakfast, except at HA4 and HA5 were they were recorded after two to three hours of exposure to the corresponding altitude. Body weight was measured by a whole body scale ± 0.01 kg (Mettler-Toledo, type Sider 1-150, Switzerland). Body mass index was calculated as body weight / height^2 as an overall indication of fat proportion in body composition. Liquid and food intake were carefully measured daily by weighing all food and drinks entering and leaving the chamber, for each subject. Day time food intake, outside principal meals (breakfast, lunch, dinner) was noted by the subject himself by careful weighing using a table food scale within the chamber (Kern, model 440-53, Prolabo, France). Twenty four hour urine was collected and weighed daily, outside the chamber. Acute mountain sickness (AMS) score (Lake Louise Consensus, (12)) was self recorded (headache: 0 to 3; gastrointestinal symptoms: 0 to 3; fatigue/weakness: 0 to 3; dizziness/lightheadedness: 0 to 3), as well as an evaluation of insomnia, ataxia and dyspnea (each coded from 0 to 3). Rectal temperature was taken every morning before getting up. Heart rate, systemic arterial pressure and transcutaneous arterial saturation were measured daily in the morning before breakfast (Hewlett Packard, model Viridia M3). Color vision was evaluated at the same time by an anomaloscope, as an objective measurement of AMS (9). The color vision index presented here for each individual is the variation from the sea-level basal value. Blood hemoglobin concentration was obtained through peripheral venous blood sampling and measured by a CO-oximeter (Chiron Diagnostics, model 270). The CO-oximeter was kept inside the chamber and was calibrated for each chamber pressure. Blood gases were measured from arterialized capillary blood obtained from an ear lobe previously heated with capsaicin cream. The blood gas analyzer (Chiron Diagnostics, model 348) was outside the chamber and capillary blood samples were passed through an air lock and analyzed within 2 minutes after sampling. Maximal oxygen uptake was measured using a step by step progressive exercise regime on a cycloergometer (Monark) until exhaustion. Ventilation, oxygen and CO_2 concentrations were analyzed using a Medical Graphics system (CPX/D

Cardiopulmonary exercise system, Minneapolis, MN), modified for low partial pressures of O_2 and with a more powerful gas pumping system for high altitudes. The apparatus was kept within the chamber and functioned perfectly up to 7,000 m.

4.1　Statistics

Values presented are mean±standard deviation. Analysis of variance with repeated measures was used to assess the significance of variations with time and altitude.

5.　RESULTS

Variations of each symptom forming part of the AMS score as well as the total AMS score, insomnia, ataxia and dyspnea scores are shown in Figure 5.

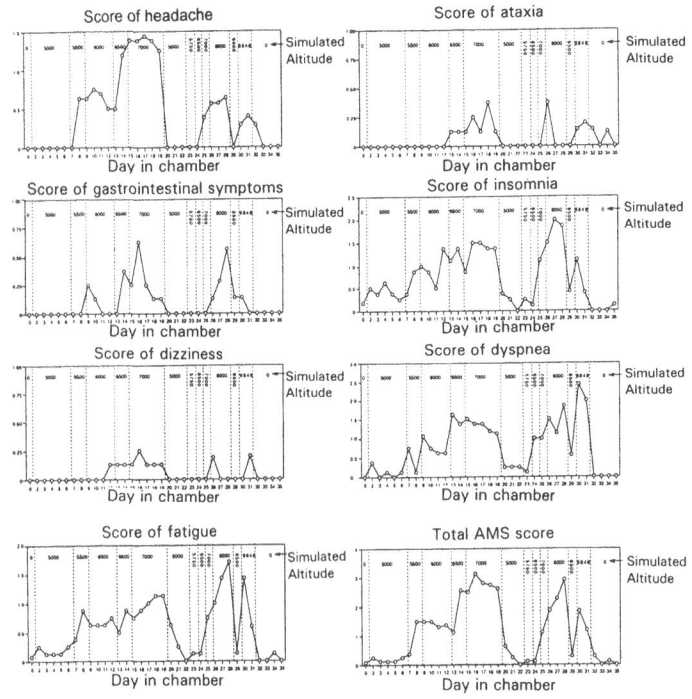

Figure 5. AMS score. Total score, and scores for headache, gastrointestinal, dizziness, fatigue, insomnia, ataxia and dyspnea. Mean values for the group. Standard deviations are not shown. n=8 except from day 27 to 32 where n=7. Note: the insomnia score at 8000m is for sleep at 7000m and the insomnia score at 8848m is for sleep at 6500m (see profile in Figure 2).

Total AMS score was almost zero at 5,000m thanks to the pre-acclimatization period on Mont Blanc. Symptoms appeared at 5,500m and 6,000m, were increased at 6,500m and maximal at 7,000m. During the recovery at 5,000m, AMS score went back to zero after 3 days, stayed very low upon re-ascent until 7,000m was reached again, peaked on the third ascent at 8,000m, but was lower during ascent to 8,848m. One subject still felt some symptoms one day after leaving the chamber (day 32). Among the four items included in the AMS score, the trend for each symptom was different. The headache score was zero at 5,000m, peaked at 7,000m and was relatively low at 8,000m and 8,848m. At 6,000m and 7,000m, there was a progressive decline with time due to clinical acclimatization. Gastrointestinal symptoms were zero up to 5,500m, increased on the first days at 6,000m, 7,000m then declined rapidly with time at a given altitude. However, it increased with the successive intermittent exposures to 8,000m. Fatigue increased with time and altitude up to 7,000m, progressively returned to zero after 3 days of recovery at 5,000m, then rose again with altitude and reached its maximum on the third exposure to 8,000m, whereas the exposure to 8,848m was better tolerated, probably because it was shorter. Dizziness score was very low during the whole period, peaked at 7,000m and showed only a small rise at 8,000 and 8,848m. Dyspnea score always showed a peak on the first day at a new altitude, progressively increasing with altitude with a peak at 6,500m, did not completely returned to zero on recovery at 5,000m, increased again with re-ascent and reached its maximum at 8,848m. Ataxia score was very low during the whole period except at 7,000m, on the first exposure to 8,000m and at both exposures to 8,848m. Some altinauts still complained of one of these symptoms one to three days after return to sea-level. Quality of sleep was already not perfect at 5,000m, progressively deteriorated with altitude up to 7,000m, took three days to restore on recovery at 5,000m, increased again and was lowest during the nights spent at 7,000m between days at 8,000m. Recovery after descent to sea-level was immediate.

Mean variations in body weight are shown in Figure 6. Body weight loss was maximal on day 29: 5.4 kg (7.3% of initial body weight, n=7). During the preacclimatization period on Mont-Blanc, 1.4 kg were already lost. Then, the loss was progressive up to 7,000m. As soon as the first day of recovery at 5,000m, 0.7 kg were recovered and 0.15 kg more within two more days. Re-ascent to 8,848m led to a further loss of 1.7 kg in 7 days. The individual maximal weight loss varied from 2.9 to 10.0 kg and was related to initial body mass index (r=0.877, p < 0.005). The rate of weight gain after return to sea-level was dramatically high: after 4 days of recovery, mean body weight increased by 3.4 kg, i.e. 63% of the total weight loss.

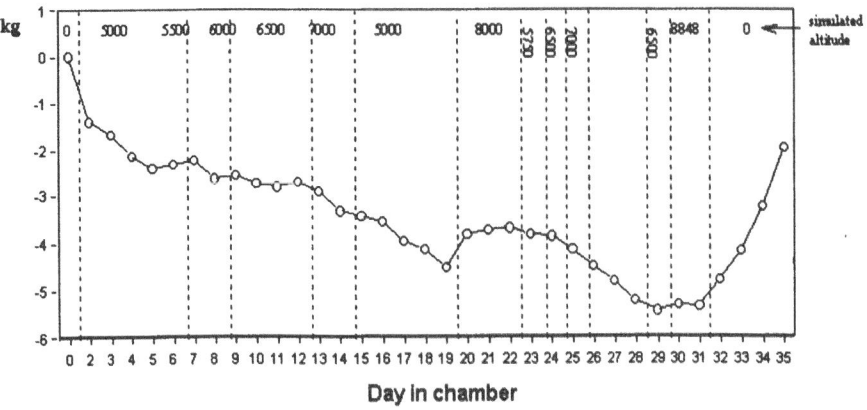

Figure 6. Mean variations in body weight. Standard deviations are not shown. n=8 except from day 27 to 32 where n=7.

Mean caloric input decreased by 11% at 5,000m, by 22% at 6,000m, by 44% at 7,000m, and by 55% at 8,000m (Westerterp et al., submitted).

Resting heart rate and transcutaneous arterial saturation are shown in Figure 7. SaO_2 decreased with altitude and increased with re-exposure to the same altitude, due to ventilatory acclimatization. The lowest mean resting SaO_2 was reached at 8,000m : 67.9 %. Heart rate increased with altitude, up to 7,000m and mirrored variations in SaO_2. No further increase was observed at 8,000m and 8,848m. During return to sea-level, some individuals showed values of heart rate lower than before entering the chamber.

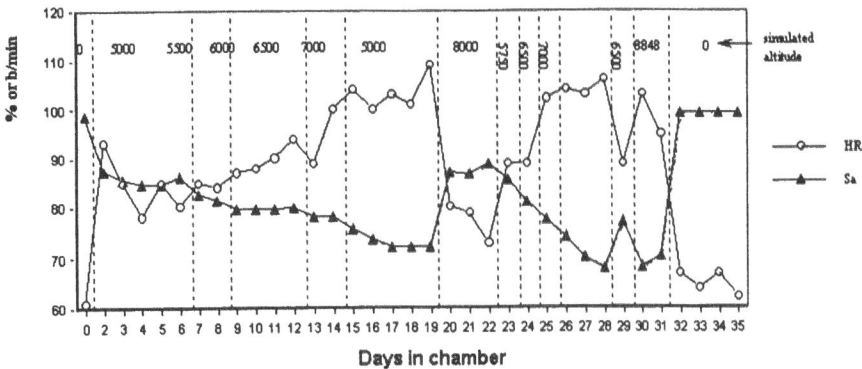

Figure 7. Mean resting heart rate and transcutaneous arterial saturation. Standard deviations are not shown. n=8 except from day 27 to 32 where n=7.

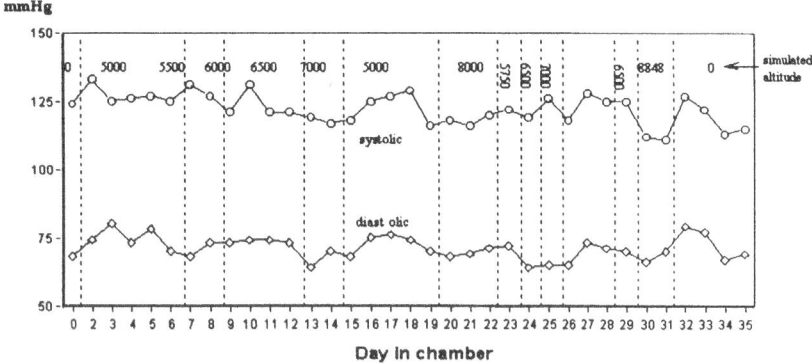

Figure 8. Variations of mean systolic and diastolic arterial pressures. Standard deviations are not shown. n=8 except from day 27 to 32 where n=7.

Systolic and diastolic arterial pressures are given on Figure 8. No significant variations were observed, neither in systolic nor in diastolic arterial pressures.

There was a progressive slight increase of rectal temperature with altitude, but the most striking observation was that temperature peaked at 7,000m in some subjects, with a concomitant rise in the clinical AMS score (Figure 9). The high values of rectal temperature were only seen when the AMS score was high (Figure 10).

Variation of color vision index in the red/green axis with altitude is shown on Figure 9. Color vision index decreased with altitude at and above 6,000 m, showing a slight relation with AMS: color vision index was lower when AMS was different from zero (significant when score equals 2 or 3).

As expected, maximal oxygen consumption decreased with altitude (Table 1): -44% at 5,000m, -58% at 6,000m and -59% at 7,000m. One subject refused to perform a maximal exercise test at 7,000m (n=7). Maximal performance recovered almost completely with return to sea-level (n.s. between SL and RSL). Resting values of PO_2, PCO_2 and pH in arterialized capillary blood at different altitudes are shown in table 1. At the lowest barometric pressure (253 mmHg), some oxygen enrichment occurred within the chamber during a short period and values of blood gases sampled in two subjects during this period were discarded. Hemoglobin concentration increased with altitude exposure. Four days after leaving the chamber it was not different from basal SL values (Table 1).

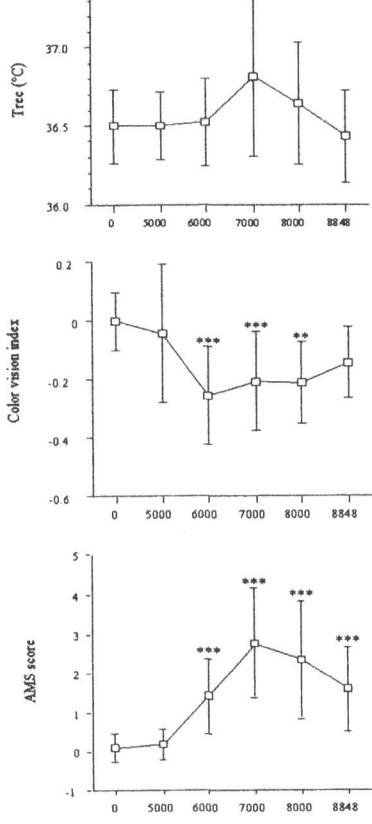

Figure 9. Variations of rectal temperature (Trec), Color vision index and AMS score with increasing altitude. Mean ± SD. Altitude vs sealevel: **, p< 0.01; ***, p<0.001. n= 8 except for 8848m where n=7.

From other protocols, we can select some observations already published. Nocturnal cough frequency and cough receptor sensitivity to citric acid challenge increased with altitude. This observation refutes the common hypothesis that altitude cough is due to cold, dry air and suggest that other mechanisms such as pulmonary interstitial edema might be involved (7).

Cognitive performance, evaluated by visual reaction time, Pegboard psychomotor test and number ordination test was not significantly altered below 8,000m, suggesting efficient compensatory mechanisms to hypoxic stress, at least below a certain threshold (1).

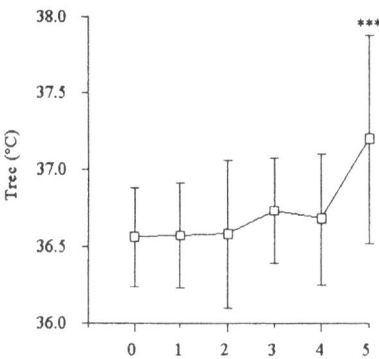

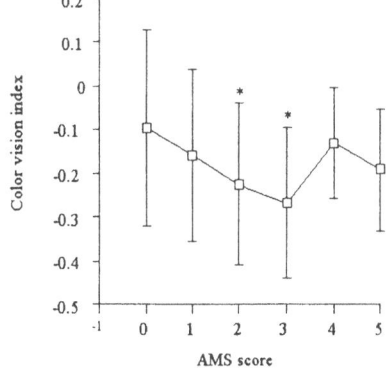

Figure 10. Variations of rectal temperature (Trec) and color vision index as a function of each individual level of AMS score. Mean ± SD. AMS score different from 0 vs AMS score = 0 : *, p< 0.05; ***, p<0.001.

6. COMMENTS

Detailed results of each protocol will be presented and discussed elsewhere. However, general observations and comments can be made. This operation was a great success, both from a scientific and from a human point of view. Approximately 80% of the expected studies have been completed. Seven out of eight altinauts reached the maximal equivalent altitude of Mount Everest. No major accident occurred. The only comparable study previously organized along similar lines was Operation Everest II (OEII) in 1985 (5). No major difference in the main clinical and physiological measured parameters was found between the two studies. However, some interesting variations resulted from the different profile of ascent.

Table 1. General characteristics of the subjects. Maximal oxygen uptake, resting blood gases and hemoglobin concentrations. Mean ± SD. BMI: body mass index. n=8, except + where n=7 and $ where n=5. γ: p<0.001, **: p<0.01, *: p<0.05 vs SL

Day in chamber	-10	2	10	17	26	30	35
Condition	SL	5,000	6,000	7,000	8,000	8,848	RSL
Age (yr)	26.6 ±4.3						
Height (cm)	180 ±6						
BMI (kg.m^{-2})	22.9 ±1.5						
Body weight (kg)	74.3 ±6.6	72.9 ±6.2*	71.6 ±6.0γ	70.4 ±5.8γ	69.8 ±5.8γ	70.2 ±5.4 γ	72.2 ±6.4 γ
VO$_{2,max}$ (ml/min/kg)	56.8 ±5.0	32.0 ±2.4γ	23.6 ±2.8γ	22.9 ±2.4γ	/	/	50.8 ±6.8
PO$_2$ (mmHg)	101.8 ±3.9	51.1 ±3.4γ	49.3 ±3.3γ	40.2 ±5.0γ	37.0 ±4.6γ	30.6 ±1.4$^{\$}$ γ	102.3 ±6.0
PCO$_2$ (mmHg)	40.3 ±3.1	27.5 ±1.4γ	19.8 ±2.0γ	18.0 ±2.6γ	14.3 ±2.1γ	11.9 ±1.4$^{\$}$ γ	31.6 ±2.1 γ
pH	7.41 ±0.03	7.47 ±0.02γ	7.51 ±0.02γ	7.49 ±0.02γ	7.57 ±0.02 γ	7.58 ±0.02$^{\$}$ γ	7.43 ±0.01

Pre-acclimatization at Observatoire Vallot allowed a much better clinical status at 5,000 m during OEIII than during OEII: symptoms of AMS appeared at 6,000 m only. However, with exposure above 7,000 m, headache, dyspnea and lethargy were similarly present in both Operation Everest II and III. Body weight loss, mainly due to dramatic decrease in food intake, was similar, although slightly less in OEIII: 7.3% vs 8.9% of initial body weight (10). A great care was given to the choice of palatable food that was every day adapted to the mood and cravings of the altinauts. This may explain part of the difference. The decrement in $\dot{V}O_{2MAX}$ was greater in OEIII than in OEII, at 5,000m and 6,000m. However, basal SL $\dot{V}O_{2MAX}$ was higher in the present study (56.8 ml/min/kg) than in OEII (51.2 ml/min/kg) and it has been suggested that subjects with higher $\dot{V}O_{2MAX}$ at SL may show a larger decrease at high altitude (3). The further decrease in $\dot{V}O_{2MAX}$ between 6,000 and 7,000m was insignificant, probably because the 7-day period of acclimatization between the two altitudes was efficient to minimize the effect of increasing altitude. After 1 to 3 days of recovery in normoxia, $\dot{V}O_{2MAX}$ was not different from baseline values when expressed in ml/kg/min (Table1), but significantly different (p<0.05) when expressed in l/min (results not shown), resulting from an incomplete recovery of body weight.

Blood gases were very similar in both OEII and the present study, including at extreme altitude (11). These values obtained in chamber (n=6 for OEII, n=5 for OEIII) were slightly higher than the value (n=1) obtained during the AMREE expedition in 1981 (13).

The speed of recovery from hypoxia when leaving the chamber was quite surprising, especially the gain of body weight (63% of total loss was regained in 4 days). Hemoglobin concentration also went back to sea-level values within four days. This rapid hemodilution effect of reoxygenation (or recompression) is concomitant with a great increase in plasma volume (Robach et al, submitted).

No clear variation of systemic blood pressure was observed along the stay in the chamber, suggesting that despite probable increased blood viscosity and adrenergic activity, there is no sensible increase in peripheral resistance.

The relation between severe AMS and raised body temperature was recently suggested (6) and confirmed in the present study. It may indicate that an inflammatory process is concomitant with the development of AMS. Color vision is slightly altered at high altitude, especially in subjects suffering from AMS. This observation confirms previous findings (9) and may help in providing an objective measurement in the evaluation of AMS. However no clear correlation was found between the variation in color vision index and the intensity of AMS evaluated by the subjective Lake Louise scoring system.

7. HOW DOES A CHAMBER STUDY DIFFER FROM FIELD CONDITIONS ?

The easy availability of palatable food, the absence of cold stress, the relatively low energy expenditure and absence of prolonged physical exercise, the absence of the dangers of climbing mountains and the confinement within a closed space, are factors which differ from field studies. The relative good clinical status of our altinauts throughout the study, their ability to withstand for a few hours extreme hypoxic conditions lead us to think that, in comparison with OEII experiment, the pre-acclimatization period in real mountain conditions and the recovery period at 5,000m before the final ascent may have had a beneficial physiological and psychological impact.

Brain function, as a whole, appeared to be maintained below 8,000m whereas physical performance is known to decline even at moderate altitudes. Hopefully, we can say that the brain is better than the muscle in compensating the lack of oxygen. However, at extreme altitudes, both are compromised, exposing the mountaineer to considerable dangers (Figure 11).

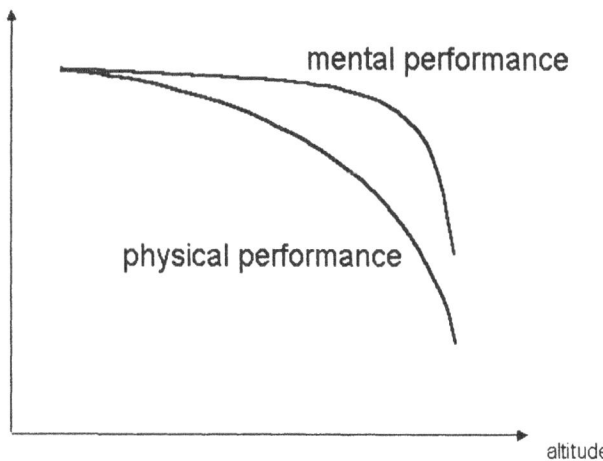

Figure 11. Schematic representation of the variations of mental and physical performance with altitude.

ACKNOWLEDGMENTS

We express our gratitude to all the administrative and technical crew of COMEX S.A. for its assistance to the investigators and to the altinauts during the whole experiment. This experiment was made possible by the attribution of grants from Région PACA and Ministère Jeunesse et Sports, France.

We are very grateful to the nine volunteers for their patience and courage throughout this exceptional experience: Kim Bodin, Emmanuel Cauchy, Guillaume Despiau, Jean-François Finance, Mathieu Gayet, Vincent Marchand, Guillaume Sabin, Philippe Serpollet and Alexandre Héritier.

REFERENCES

1. Abraini J.H., Bouquet C., Joulia F., Nicolas M., Kriem B. Cognitive performance during a simulated climb of Mount Everest: implications for brain function and central adaptive processes under chronic hypoxic stress. *Pflügers Arch. - Eur. J. Physiol.* 436: 553-559, 1998.
2. Bert P. La pression barométrique. Masson éd. Paris, 1878.
3. Cymerman A., Reeves J.T., Sutton J.R., Rock P.B., Groves B.M., Malconian M.K., Young P.M., Wagner P.D., Houston C.S. Operation Everest II: maximal oxygen uptake at extreme altitude. *J. Appl. Physiol.* 66: 2446-2453, 1989.
4. Houston C.S. Operation Everest. U.S. Naval Medical Bulletin. 46: 1783-1792, 1946.
5. Houston C.S., Sutton J.R., Cymerman A. and J.T. Reeves. Operation Everest II: man at extreme altitude. *J. Appl. Physiol.* 63: 877-882, 1987.

6. Maggiorini M., Bärtsch P., Oelz O. Elevated body temperature in severe acute mountain sickness (AMS). In *Hypoxia and Mountain Medicine*, J.R. Sutton, G. Coates and C. Houston eds. Queen City Printers Inc. Burlington, VT, 1992, p 311 (abstract n°62).

7. Mason N.P., Barry P.W., Despiau G., Gardette B., Richalet J.-P. Cough frequency and cough receptor sensitivity to citric acid challenge during a simulated ascent to extreme altitude. *Eur. Respir.* J. 13: 508-513, 1999.

8. Richalet J.-P., Bittel J., Herry J.-P., Savourey G., Le Trong J.L., Auvert J.F., Janin C. Use of a hypobaric chamber for pre-acclimatization before climbing Mount Everest. *Int J Sports Med.* 13, S216-S220, 1992

9. Richalet J.-P., Rutgers V., Bouchet P., Rymer J.-C., Kéromès A., Duval-Arnould G., Rathat C. Diurnal variations of acute mountain sickness, color vision and plasma cortisol and ACTH at high altitude. *Aviat. Space Envrion. Med.* 60 :105-111, 1989.

10. Rose M.S., Houston C.S., Fulco C.S., Coates G., Sutton J.R., Cymerman A. Operation Everest II: nutrition and body composition. *J. Appl. Physiol.* 65: 2545-2551, 1988.

11. Sutton J.R., Reeves J.T., Wagner P.D., Cymerman A., Malconian M.K., Rock P.B., Young P.M., Walter S.D., Houston C.S. Operation Everest II: oxygen transport during exercise at extreme simulated altitude. *J. Appl. Physiol.* 64: 1309-1321, 1988.

12. The Lake Louise Consensus on the definition and quantification of altitude illness. In: *Hypoxia and Mountain Medicine* , J.R. Sutton, G. Coates, C.S. Houston eds. Queen City Printers Inc. Burlington, VT, 1992, p 327-330.

13. West J.B., Hackett P.H., Maret K.H., Milledge J.S., Peters R.M. Jr., Pizzo C.J. Winslow R.M. Pulmonary gas exchange on the summit of Mount Everest. *J. Appl. Physiol.* 55: 678-687, 1983.

14. West J.B. Prediction of barometric pressure at high altitudes with use of model atmospheres. *J. Appl. Physiol.* 81: 1850-1854, 1996.

Chapter 24

Dynamic Cerebral Autoregulation At High Altitude

Benjamin D. Levine, Rong Zhang, Robert C. Roach
Institute for Exercise and Environmental Medicine, Presbyterian Hospital and University of Texas Southwestern Medical Center, Dallas, TX; IEEM and UT Southwestern, Dallas, TX; Copenhagen Muscle Research Center, Denmark and New Mexico Highlands University, Las Vegas, New Mexico, USA

Key words: cerebral blood flow, hemodynamics, transfer function

1. INTRODUCTION

Cerebral autoregulation is a dynamic process that is frequency dependent. In other words, the ability of local vascular control mechanisms to buffer changes in arterial pressure and keep cerebral blood flow (CBF) constant may be more or less effective depending on the time period, or frequency at which changes in blood pressure occur. Previous work in our laboratory (1) has described the cerebral circulation as a "high pass filter" with ineffective modulation of pressure induced changes in cerebral blood flow at high frequencies (>0.20 Hz, or faster than every 5 seconds). Over these short time periods, the biophysical properties of the cerebral circulation, including cerebrovascular impedance, conductance, and inertia of the blood column predominate, and changes in blood pressure are transmitted directly into changes in CBF. In contrast, at lower frequencies (<0.07 Hz, or slower than every 13 seconds), autoregulation is more effective and the relationship between arterial blood pressure and CBF is inherently non-linear with little quantitative dependence of flow on pressure. When autoregulation fails, for example as is seen in patients with malignant hypertension, the upper limit of autoregulation may be breached, resulting in over perfusion of the brain and cerebral edema. This mechanism may be specifically relevant for the illnesses of high altitude such as acute mountain sickness and high altitude cerebral edema.

At high altitude, the factors that govern the distribution of blood flow to the brain are radically altered. Hypoxia causes vasodilation that is proportionate to the reduction in arterial oxygen content. Conversely, hypocapnia, as a result of hyperventilation causes cerebral vasoconstriction. Despite extensive study, whether the combination of these two potent metabolic stimuli to the cerebral circulation results in a significant change in autoregulation remains unclear. Moreover, whether autoregulation is altered to a greater or lesser degree at specific frequencies is entirely unknown.

2.   THE AIM

Therefore the specific aim of this project was to examine the frequency components of autoregulation in subjects well acclimatized to high altitude. We hypothesized that acute altitude exposure would result in profound cerebral vasodilation, and impairment of autoregulation. With acclimatization however, we hypothesized that the combination of increased arterial O_2 content and progressive hypocapnia would restore CBF towards normal, with restoration of normal autoregulation.

3.   METHODS

Eleven healthy members of the Danish Medical Research Expedition to the Andes, 4 women/7men were studied as part of this project. All the subjects had resided for > 1 month at Chacaltaya, Bolivia (5,200m), and all had fully recovered from a successful summit of Huyana Potosi (6,088 m). No subject had any signs or symptoms of acute mountain sickness. CBF (transcranial Doppler - DWL), and arterial pressure (ABP, applanation tonometry - Collin), were recorded on a beat-by-beat basis during 6 min quiet, spontaneous respiration, during which ventilation, end-tidal carbon dioxide ($ETCO_2$), and SaO_2 (pulse oximetry) were monitored. After resampling at 1Hz to create an equidistant time series, spectral analysis was performed (Welch method) and the transfer function calculated between CBF and ABP. Coherence (strength of association) and gain (magnitude of association) at frequencies <0.07 Hz were used as indices of autoregulation. A detailed set of experiments examining cardiovascular regulation during: controlled frequency breathing; the Valsalva maneuver; hand grip exercise;

and lower body negative pressure were also performed. Only the data for dynamic cerebral autoregulation are reported here.

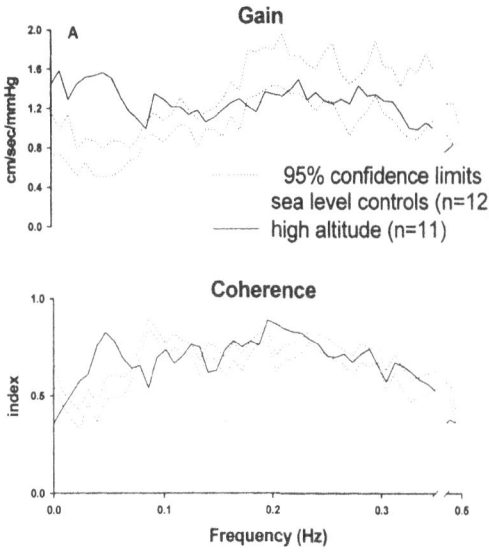

Figure 1. Top panel displays the *gain* or magnitude of association (equivalent in concept to the slope of a linear regression), and the bottom panel shows the *coherence* or strength of association (equivalent in concept to the r^2 of a linear regression) between arterial pressure (the input variable) and cerebral blood flow velocity (the output variable) at frequencies ranging from 0 to 0.5 Hz. Dotted lines represent the 95% confidence limits for a group of normal subjects of similar age and gender to the study subjects, previously reported in reference 1. Solid lines represent the transfer function data from the present experiment.

4.   RESULTS

SaO$_2$ and ETCO$_2$ were low (range: 84-91% and 21-27 mmHg respectively) as expected. Baseline and acute studies have not yet been performed, so data are compared to a group of normal controls of similar age and gender, previously reported from our laboratory. Figure 1 shows that coherence and gain were markedly increased at low frequencies compared to controls suggesting increased dependence of CBF on ABP. Thus for any given change in arterial blood pressure, there was a substantially greater change in cerebral blood flow in the subjects acclimatized to high altitude, compared to normal controls. No differences were noted at higher frequencies suggesting that the biophysical properties of the cerebral circulation were unchanged.

5.   CONCLUSION

High altitude impairs dynamic cerebral autoregulation, probably as a function of hypoxia induced vasodilation even after prolonged and successful acclimatization.

6.   IMPLICATION

We speculate that this impairment may be even greater with acute high altitude exposure compared to baseline in these subjects. Such an impairment in autoregulation could be a significant risk factor for the development of acute mountain sickness or high altitude cerebral edema, if the cerebral circulation is relatively unprotected from increases in blood pressure such as that caused by exercise.

REFERENCES

1. Zhang, R., J. H. Zuckerman, C. A. Giller, and B. D. Levine. Transfer function analysis of dynamic cerebral autoregulation in humans. *Am J Physiol* 274: H233-H241, 1998.

Chapter 25

Kangchenjunga 1998
A Venture Undertaken With "Medical Expeditions"

Annabel Nickol and David Collier
Department of Medicine, Newport Hospital, Gwent, and Division of Pharmacology, St Bartholomew's and The Royal London School of Medicine and Dentistry, Charterhouse Square, London, UK

Key words: chemoreceptor, nitric oxide, endothelin, appetite, leptin, infection, sensory function, age, gender, cough, ciliary function, respiratory training, eye, oxidative stress.

Abstract: The article describes the research carried out on the recent Kanchenjunga Medical Expedition to Eastern Nepal during the post-monsoon season of 1998. Twenty-two projects are described, under the general functional headings of respiratory, cardiovascular, hormonal, sensory and neurological and infection and immunity.

1. INTRODUCTION

In September of 1998 "Medical Expeditions" embarked upon its second major Himalayan venture, this time to Kangchenjunga, the third highest mountain in the world, situated in the far east of Nepal. It forms part of a majestic chain of mountains which straddle the border with Sikkim and can be seen across the tea plantations from Darjeeling. Medical Expeditions is a charitable organization made up of enthusiasts of high altitude medicine and mountains. This latest enterprise was borne of the success and ongoing enthusiasm which just didn't die down following our first research expedition to Everest in 1994. Our research team on Kangchenjunga was large with over 20 personnel in the field and many more contributing in some vital way back home. The research program included a well-balanced blend of work following on from Everest, and entirely new ideas. Our trekkers and climbers acted as volunteers for the research, lured by the descriptions of the trek. This promised to take us, over two weeks, from the beautiful lush green rice paddy fields around Basantipur, through bamboo and rain forest, up into the foothills, and finally to the high glaciers and mountains. One of our strengths at Medical Expeditions is the large numbers of trekkers involved, who come out in small staggered groups to Pang Pema base camp, situated at 5000m. This not only adds a most welcome diversity of skills to the party, but also enables us to study large numbers of people where this is indicated, and to look for correlation between projects which are not always expected. The commitment of the trekkers to the research is borne out by the fact that over 90% of them attended sea level pre-expedition data collecting week ends, collected daily simple data measurements whilst on the trek and took part in many of the studies taking place at base camp. During the expedition a small climbing team led by Chris Comerie attempted Kangchenjunga by the Boardman-Tasker route, successfully climbing to above the North Col, and another party climbed a new route on Ramtang, a 6700m peak. Below is a brief resume of the projects undertaken.

2.   RESPIRATORY

2.1   Airway Defense (Peter Barry, Andrew Pollard, Sarah Bakewell, Kate Wilson, Roger McMorrow, David Williams and Nigel Hart)

Debilitating dry cough is a familiar problem at high altitude, and previous work by this group has shown cough threshold, as determined by inhalation of varying concentrations of citric acid, to be reduced at high altitude. Twice daily inhaled serevent or nedocromil sodium was found to diminish altitude related lowering of cough threshold compared to placebo, although this change was not significant, suggesting that they may have a role in prophylaxis of high altitude cough (1).

Nasal muco-ciliary clearance has been shown to decline on ascent to high altitude, as demonstrated by measuring the time taken for saccharin, placed in the nostril, to be tasted. The current study aimed to find out if this decrement in muco-ciliary function could be prevented by nasal moistening. Nasal moistening using a saline spray four times a day (n=15) was compared with a control group (n=25), and although muco-ciliary clearance with altitude was reduced only in the control group, and not in the intervention group, the difference between the two groups did not quite reach statistical significance (p=0.07) (14).

It has been speculated that normal subjects exposed to cold and hypoxia may develop increased bronchial reactivity, and that these airway changes may be involved in some way in hypoxic cough. Bronchial reactivity was investigated using varying concentrations of inhaled histamine. There was no significant difference in the concentrations of histamine required to cause a 20% fall in FEV_1 at altitude compared with sea level but the fall in FEV_1 was greater at sea level than at altitude for the highest concentration of histamine inhaled (7).

2.2   **Inspiratory Muscle Training** (Lee Romer, Rick and Gill Havely and Alison McConnell)

Ventilation is significantly increased on ascent to high altitude, and marked dyspnea is often noticed. The effect of inspiratory muscle training using a "POWERbreathe" was investigated. Subjects were randomized either to the intervention group (30 inspiratory efforts of 50% max inspiratory muscle strength, twice daily from 8 weeks prior to departure and for the duration of the trek) or control group (no respiratory muscle training). On ascent to high altitude the control group was found to have a significant reduction in both inspiratory and expiratory muscle strength, and in inspiratory muscle endurance. In contrast the experimental group demonstrated a small increase in inspiratory muscle strength at altitude compared to pre-training. They suffered from a smaller decline in inspiratory muscle endurance than the control group, but still demonstrated the same decrease in expiratory muscle strength as the control group. Base line and transitional dyspnoea indices were carried out for both groups. The level of dyspnoea experienced by the trained group was marginally less than that of the control group. The functional significance of these observations is not yet clear.

2.3   **Ventilatory Control** (David Collier, Annabel Nickol, Henriette van Ruiten, Jim Milledge, David Williams and Chris Wolff)

Peripheral chemoreceptors are known to detect and respond rapidly to second by second oscillations in arterial CO_2 generated by the ventilatory cycle, and so are candidates for an important role in ventilatory acclimatization (4, 5). Peripheral chemoreceptor function was studied in volunteers exercising gently on a bicycle ergometer by measuring the ventilatory response to small inhaled pulses of CO_2 given either early in every breath (thought to augment arterial CO_2 oscillations), or late in every breath (thought to dampen CO_2 oscillations). At sea level under normoxic conditions a ventilatory response to the timing of CO_2 pulses was observed, with ventilation being significantly greater with early than late pulses. This response was completely abolished by isobaric hypoxia at sea level (equivalent to the P_IO_2 at Pang Pema base camp). This result is interesting because it demonstrates an aspect of ventilatory control likely to be mediated by the peripheral chemoreceptors which is impaired on exposure to acute hypoxia (steady-state responses to inhaled carbon dioxide are of course increased during exposure to acute hypoxia). At base camp pre-acclimatization (days 0-3) ventilation was greater with early pulses, although this difference was not significant, but after a period of acclimatization there was a highly significant ventilatory response to the timing of CO_2 pulses. This work shows that sensitivity of the peripheral chemoreceptor to a dynamic signal is present at sea level, abolished by acute hypoxia but then gradually restored and even heightened during acclimatization. This response may be important in ventilatory acclimatization during the first few weeks at high altitude. The time-course of the restoration of responsiveness to fast changes in carbon dioxide may be related to the subjective improvement in exercise performance that is experienced over the first 7-10 days after gradual ascent to 5000m. Results from the British Mount Everest Medical Expedition showed that steady-state acclimatization was almost complete within 1-2 days of arrival at base camp (arterialized capillary and end-tidal PCO2's did not fall further with extra time at base camp), largely due to a gentle ascent rate. The restoration of responsiveness to the timing of CO2 pulses, however, is not complete until several more days have elapsed at 5000m (3, 9).

3.   CARDIOVASCULAR

3.1   Systemic Circulation (David Collier, Richard Weller, Mukul
         Agarwal, Nigel Benjamin, and Pablo Forte)

Nitric oxide (NO) is an important vasodilator formed in many tissues, including the vascular endothelium. It is synthesized from the amino acid L-arginine by a family of enzymes, the nitric oxide synthases, through the l-arginine-nitric oxide pathway. We have developed sensitive and specific methods for measuring the activity of the L-arginine nitric oxide system in humans (6, 8). This method relies on the administration of trace amounts of the stable isotope 15N labeled L-arginine (which is not radioactive) with the measurement of urinary excretion of 15N. This method is independent of the dietary intake of nitrate and is completely specific for the L-arginine-nitric oxide pathway. Use of this method has shown large differences in nitric oxide synthesis in patients with essential hypertension compared with controls (6).

We have recently shown that blood pressure in healthy trekkers and climbers increases during ascent to high altitude (2). Although this observation may have been confounded by the pressor effect of reduced daytime temperature with increased altitude, the increase in blood pressure seen was much greater than that recognized by a large cohort study from BUPA. One possible cause of the increase in blood pressure at high altitude is a reduction in the synthesis of nitric oxide from L-arginine. This study aims to answer this question.

3.2   Peripheral Circulation (Henriette van Ruiten and H Daanen)

When the extremities are exposed to an extreme cold environment there is an initial vaso-constriction followed by vaso-dilatation, so called "cold induced vasodilatation" or CIVD. This opening and closing of blood vessels is seen as an important protective mechanism against the occurrence of local cold injuries. CIVD in the finger exposed to water at 0oC has previously been found to be reduced during initial exposure to high altitude. It was not certain whether this is due to the effect of hypoxia or lowered core body temperature. This study confirmed the presence of CIVD, and also showed that core temperature was actually higher at altitude, suggesting that it is hypoxia per se which is responsible for this phenomenon. In subjects who were well acclimatized to 5000m and had spent time at extreme altitude, CIVD increased again towards normal sea level values demonstrating the restoration of a protective mechanism against cold injury (13).

3.3   Electrical Impedance in the Thorax (Nick Mason, Mukul Agarwal, Jim Milledge, A Wilson, David Williams and B Brown)

Pulmonary impedance measurements were made in subjects at sea level, on initial arrival at base camp, and in a limited number of subjects before and during oxygen therapy. This may enable changes in lung water to be estimated.

3.4   Systemic and Pulmonary Circulation (Nick Cruden, D Newby, David Webb)

Endothelin-1 is a potent vasoconstrictor peptide, which is secreted by endothelium both basely and in response to various stimuli including hypoxia. Levels are thought to be elevated at high altitude, and may be implicated in the development of pulmonary hypertension and possibly HAPE. Elevated endothelin-1 levels may be secondary to increased production, in which case big endothelin-1 levels will also be elevated, or to reduced clearance. Both endothelin-1 and big endothelin-1 levels were measured in subjects at sea level and during sojourn at high altitude.

4.   METABOLIC

4.1   The Role Of Female Hormones In Acclimatization (Debby Miller and Liz Bowen)

All trekkers and climbers completed twice-daily AMS scores, and recorded daily oxygen saturation. Resting end-tidal CO_2 measurements were made both at sea level and on initial arrival at 5000m. Menstrual and contraceptive histories were taken, and the day of peak luteinizing Hormone was determined using urinary dipsticks to indicate the day of ovulation. This data will be compared in men, and women at different phases of their menstrual cycle, taking the oral contraceptive pill or on depo-provera.

4.2   Leptin at altitude (Matthias Tschoep)

Leptin has been described as an "obese gene" product which was discovered in 1994. It is thought to be important in the regulation of body weight and energy balance, acting as a signal to the brain and several other peripheral organs and endocrine sub-systems regarding energy stores of the body. It is speculated that changes in leptin levels may occur at high altitude since weight loss at extreme altitude and changes in appetite are known to occur, and furthermore impairment of reproductive function and reduced growth and adult height are known to occur in high altitude populations. A highly sensitive immunoassay using monoclonal antibodies and biotin-streptavidin technology has recently been developed. This has enabled leptin to be measured in conditions where levels are known to be very low such as in anorexia nervosa or in cachectic individuals. Leptin levels were determined both at sea level and during sojourn at high altitude, and may play a role in the pathophysiology of hypoxia induced endocrine disorders.

4.3 Appetite and Anthropometrics (Sandra Green, David Collier, Mike Richards and Damian Bailey)

Daily questionnaires and visual analogue scores were completed regarding appetite and satiety during the trek. Weights and detailed anthropometrics were recorded at staggered intervals prior to and during the expedition. In addition electrical impedance allowed the estimation of body fat composition. We are interested in the observation made on the British Mount Everest Medical Expedition in 1994 that women did not lose any weight after reaching 5300m, whereas men continued to lose weight at this altitude. We hypothesize that changes in appetite and therefore energy intake may be more important than any alteration in food absorption or energy utilization.

5. SENSORY AND NEUROLOGICAL

5.1 Judgement of vertical and horizontal and body sway (Martin Rosenberg, Jim Milledge, Gwilym Rivett and David Collier)

It is widely known that many aspects of cognitive and other neurological function is adversely affected by high altitude. Several aspects of these changes were studied. **Judgement of horizontal and vertical** was investigated by asking subjects to rotate an electronically controlled arm until it was exactly horizontal or vertical. This was carried out in a darkened environment 20 times, and the mean error (unsigned) from the true positions determined for each subject. There was found to be a small but highly significant increase in error at high altitude.

Postural sway was measured using a pressure sensitive plate in a darkened space. Subjects were studied under four conditions: eyes closed, eyes open with central fixation on a single light emitting diode (LED), eyes open with attention to peripheral vision (four LEDs on at the periphery of vision), and with attention to both central and peripheral vision (all five LEDs on). All of the LED's were mounted on an "H" shaped frame, the centre of which was 1.2 m from the subject. At sea level fixation on either the single central LED, or on all 5 LED's significantly reduced postural sway, as expected. The four peripheral LED's did not improve body sway at sea level. Of the 28 subjects studied at both sea level and 5000m and shown to have increases in sway at altitude, which was highly significant under all conditions except using peripheral vision alone. It is uncertain whether these changes can be attributed to changes in the vestibular apparatus or more central higher centers (11).

5.2 Movement Detection Thresholds at altitude (Diana Depla and Mark Howarth)

Reduced perception of movement in the peripheral visual field is known to occur at high altitude. This phenomenon was studied on arrival at high altitude and after a period of acclimatization, with and without supplementary oxygen in both cases. Preliminary results suggest that short term oxygen therapy works very effectively at restoring peripheral vision loss secondary to hypoxia.

5.3 Motor Function (Eli Silber)

Fine motor function deteriorates at altitude, but little is known about the effects of age and acclimatization. Nine-hole pegboard tests were performed on 46 subjects at sea level and at base camp. The results show that there is a decline in fine motor co-ordination at altitude, and that those over 50 appear particularly susceptible. Difference between those tested within 24 hours of arrival at base camp and after this period suggest that acclimatization is important in optimizing fine motor function.

5.4   Headache (Eli Silber, Andrew Pollard and David Murdoch)

A detailed questionnaire was carried out to fully characterize features of headache at high altitude, and to assess whether any individuals are at particular risk of developing high altitude headaches, e.g.: those known to suffer from migraine. Results of this study are still being collated.

5.5   Acupuncture in the prophylaxis of acute mountain sickness (Paul Richards)

Acupuncture at specific points has been shown to reduce nausea and headache under sea level conditions, but has never to our knowledge been investigated in the prophylaxis or treatment of acute mountain sickness. As there was only one investigator trained to apply the acupuncture, members of only one of several trekking parties received the intervention and their acute mountain sickness and oxygen saturations were compared with those from the other ascent groups. Although the "control" and intervention subjects had similar ascent profiles, the acupuncture group showed significantly worse AMS scores and lower oxygen saturation than their untreated counterparts. Because the intervention and control groups were not randomly selected, bias may be the most plausible explanation of the results (10).

5.6   Autonomic Function (Mark Howarth and Diana Depla)

Autonomic function was studied in the eye by performing pupillometry both at sea level and high altitude, pre and post acclimatization. A topical agent was given which is known to interfere with the autonomic function of the eye, and pupillometry performed before and half an hour after this. It is hypothesized that the parasympathetic system is down regulated at high altitude. This study may help to throw light on this hypothesis, and to determine whether this effect in the eye is mediated centrally or at the motor end plate.

6.   INFECTION AND IMMUNITY

6.1   Oxidative stress during heavy exercise at sea level and high altitude (Damian Bailey and Mike Richards)

Increased incidence of gastro-intestinal and respiratory infections is common amongst trekking parties ascending to high altitude. This is likely to be due mainly to exposure to new unfamiliar pathogens, but may be contributed to by hypoxia induced changes in immune function.

A number of biochemical processes which are thought to be affected by high altitude and are important in maintaining effective immunity were studied. These included changes in glutamine concentrations, changes in free radical induced cell damage and anti-oxidant status. These results will be correlated against acute mountain sickness scores and infective episodes, which were documented on a twice daily basis.

6.2   Markers of Infection and High Altitude Illness (Lance Jennings, Warren and Leonie Dellow, Andrew Pollard, David Collier and David Murdoch)

A further large-scale epidemiological study investigated the incidence and pathological etiology of both clinical and sub-clinical respiratory tract infections. Daily respiratory symptoms were recorded. Attempts to identify pathogens involved were made by taking serum samples for respiratory titres, respiratory secretions and nasal and throat swabs pre and post expedition and at specific points in the trek. This study will provide interesting data not only on the types of respiratory pathogens acquired in this part of Nepal by western trekkers, but also on the spread of infection as trekkers in well defined groups meet and separate from other parties.

7.   CLOSED CIRCUIT OXYGEN DELIVERY SYSTEM
(Ullrich Steiner, R Fischer, K Voll And R Huber)

A new closed circuit breathing system was tested in both normal volunteers and patients with suspected HACE or HAPE at Pang Pema base camp. It comprises a tight fitting facemask, breathing bag, CO2 absorber and carbon fiber oxygen cylinder. It was found to function reasonably well and to have the advantage of being lighter than conventional systems at 4.5 kg (12).

8.   SUMMARY

We hope this brief synopsis gives a flavor of the extent of our research program. Some of it has already been presented at meetings in the UK, and at "Hypoxia '99", and we are looking forward to publishing full papers in the near future.

Medical Expeditions obtained a number of small grants to assist in funding this research. We are particularly grateful for the help of David Williams and The University of Liverpool for financial support. Research leaders of the expedition can be contacted for further information: David Collier (djcollier@mds.qmw.ac.uk), Andrew Pollard (apollard@csi.com). Annabel Nickol (annabel.nickol@virgin.net) and Jim Milledge (jmilledge@cix.co.uk).

REFERENCES

1. Bakewell, S.E., N.D. Hart, C.M. Wilson , R. McMorrow, D. Collier, D. Williams, and P.W. Barry. A randomized , double blind placebo controlled trial of the effect of inhaled nedocomil sodium or salbutamol zinafoate on the citric acid cough threshold in subjects traveling to high altitude (Abstract). In: *Hypoxia: Into the Next Millennium*, edited by R.C. Roach, P.D. Wagner and P.H. Hackett. New York: Kluwer Academic/Plenum Publishers, 1999, p. 362.
2. Collier, D.J., C.J. Collier, and M. Rosenberg. Blood pressure during ascent to high altitude in man (Abstract). In: *Hypoxia. Women at Altitude*. Burlington: Queen City Printers, 1995, p. 13-14.
3. Collier, D.J., A. Nickol, J.S. Milledge, A.K. Datta, C.J. Collier, and C.B. Wolff. Dynamic chemosensitivity to carbon dioxide increases with acclimatization to chronic hypoxia in man. *J Physiol* 487P: 109-110, 1999.
4. Cunningham, D.J.C., M.G. Howson, and S.B. Pearson. The respiratory effects in man of altering the time profile of alveolar carbon dioxide and oxygen within each respiratory cycle. *J Physiol* 234: 1-28, 1973.
5. Datta, A.K., and A. Nickol. Dynamic chemoreceptiveness studied in man during moderate exercise breath by breath. *Adv Exp Med Biol* 393: 235-238, 1995.
6. Forte, P., M. Copland, L.M. Smith, E. Milne, J. Sutherland, and N. Benjamin. Basal nitric oxide synthesis in essential hypertension. *Lancet* 349: 837-842, 1997.
7. Hart, N.D., C.M. Wilson , S.E. Bakewell, R. McMorrow, D. Collier, D. Williams, M.R. Miller, and A.J. Pollard. Changes in airway responsiveness induced by chronic exposure to hypoxia

(Abstract). In: *Hypoxia: Into the Next Millennium*, edited by R.C. Roach, P.D. Wagner and P.H. Hackett. New York: Kluwer Academic/Plenum Publishers, 1999, p. 386.

8. Macallan, D., L. Smith, J. Ferber, E. Milne, G.E. Griffin, N. Benjamin, and M.A. McNurlen. Measurement of nitric oxide synthesis in man by L[15N]-arginine; application to response to vaccination. *Am J Physiol* in press, 1999.

9. Nickol, A.H., D.J. Collier, J.S. Milledge, H. van Ruiten, and C.B. Wolff. The ventilatory response to timed pulses of CO2 during acclimatization to hypoxia (Abstract). In: *Hypoxia: Into the Next Millennium*, edited by R.C. Roach, P.D. Wagner and P.H. Hackett. New York: Kluwer Academic/Plenum Publishers, 1999, p. 417.

10. Richards, P. The use of acupuncture in the prophylaxis and treatment of altitude induced headache and nausea (Abstract). In: *Hypoxia: Into the Next Millennium*, edited by R.C. Roach, P.D. Wagner and P.H. Hackett. New York: Kluwer Academic/Plenum Publishers, 1999, p. 424.

11. Rosenberg, M.E., J.S. Milledge, G. Rivett, and D.J. Collier. Effect of altitude on the perception of vertical and horizontal and on sway (Abstract). *J Physiol* in press, 1999.

12. Steiner, U., R. Fischer, K. Voll, and R. Huber. Closed circuit oxygen delivery system (Abstract). In: *Hypoxia: Into the Next Millennium*, edited by R.C. Roach, P.D. Wagner and P.H. Hackett. New York: Kluwer Academic/Plenum Publishers, 1999, p. 431.

13. van Ruiten, H., and H.A.M. Daanen. Cold induced vasodilatation at altitude (Abstract). In: *Hypoxia: Into the Next Millennium*, edited by R.C. Roach, P.D. Wagner and P.H. Hackett. New York: Kluwer Academic/Plenum Publishers, 1999, p. 436.

14. Wilson, C.M., S.E. Bakewell, R. McMorrow, N.D. Hart, D. Collier, D. Williams, and P.W. Barry. Impairment of nasal mucociliary clearance may be reduced by intermittent moistening of the nasal passages (Abstract). In: *Hypoxia: Into the Next Millennium*, edited by R.C. Roach, P.D. Wagner and P.H. Hackett. New York: Kluwer Academic/Plenum Publishers, 1999, p. 440.

Chapter 26

Why Does the Exercise Cardiac Output Fall During Altitude Residence and Is It Important?

John T. Reeves

Professor Emeritus of Medicine, Pediatrics, Family Medicine, University of Colorado Health Sciences Center, Denver, USA

Key words: exercise, work, exertion, cardiac output, chronic hypoxia, exercise limitations

1.   INTRODUCTION

"..... on Pike's Peak the rate of introduction of oxygen into the body (could) *not keep the oxygen tension in the blood reaching the tissues sufficient during moderately severe work; in Oxford the limits of oxygen supply were determined by the capacity of the circulation to transport oxygen to the tissues"* Douglas, Haldane, Henderson, Schneider 1913 (see reference (12).

Mountaineers have long known that the ability to climb decreases with increasing altitude, but physiologists are not agreed on why. Douglas et al. (12) suggested that oxygen transport at altitude differed from sea level. In the first half of this century physiologists were concerned primarily with documentation that altitude limited oxygen transport. In the second half they tried to identify limitations within the various links of the oxygen transport chain. They have agreed on the primary importance of the respiratory links (ventilation and diffusion) which are limitations at altitude, but the role of the circulatory link is not so clear. Below, perspectives are presented from two physiologists (Dr. Peter D. Wagner, and Dr. Loring B. Rowell) who have spent their professional careers considering O_2 transport and its limitations. As we prepare for their discussion at the end of this century, we may ask, "What do we know, and when did we know it?"

2.   EARLY HISTORICAL BACKGROUND

Margaria reported in 1930 (20) that student volunteers using a bicycle ergometer in an altitude chamber, had decreasing capacity for work with increasing altitude, but O_2 uptake was not measured. Dill and his colleagues (11) reported for the first time the reduction in maximal oxygen uptake at high altitude, Figure 1.

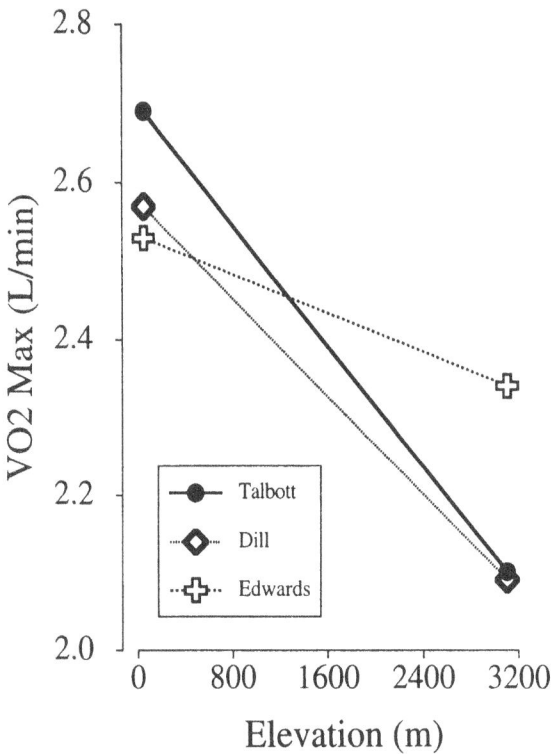

Figure 1. Fall in $\dot{V}O_{2MAX}$ from sea level (Boston) to 3100 m (10150 feet, Leadville, CO) in 3 subjects as reported by Dill et al. (11).

Each of the three subjects *"pushed himself to the limit at sea level (Boston) and at 10,000 ft (Leadville, 3100 m, P_B~530 mm Hg). The high lactate concentrations in the most exhausting experiments.....furnished evidence that each....reached the limit of his oxygen intake...."* The amount of the decrease from sea level ranged from 8% in Edwards to 22% in

Talbott. Dill commented on the oxygen transport chain: *"The supply of oxygen to the tissues is dependent on a large number of factors, chief among which are (a) circulation rate, (b) oxygen capacity of the blood, and (c) oxygen saturation of arterial blood"*. Dill had not measured cardiac output, but this deficiency was rectified in the 1935 Chilean expedition, an expedition in which Dill played a crucial role (37). Christensen (6) confirmed Dill's findings of a reduction in $\dot{V}O_{2MAX}$ at 'Quilcha, Chile (17,500 ft, P_B~401 mm Hg). And he and Forbes (7), using Grollman's acetylene method, suggested the cardiac output was also reduced at altitude, but felt that maximum ventilation, not cardiac output was limiting oxygen uptake. Dill did not agree; he felt that limitations in cardiac output were key to the fall in $\dot{V}O_{2MAX}$ at altitude (10).

There the cardiac output question stood, until the classical 'Silver Hut'expedition, planned by Sir Edmund Hillary and Griffith Pugh (37), and led by Pugh where he and 6 others resided over 6 months in 1960-1, on the Mingbo Glacier in Nepal (25). Their findings of *"falling arterial oxygen saturation during exercise at 1,200 kg-m/min was clear evidence of failure of (pulmonary) oxygen diffusion.....and the falling heart rate at 1,200 kg-m/min could not rise above 17 liters/min at this altitude"* (5800 m ~ 19,000 feet, P_B 380 mm Hg) (37). Pugh (24) commented, *"The output for a given work intensity was comparable with the output with the same work intensity at sea level, but the maximum output was reduced......"* *"The only evidence that cardiac output.....was not just limited by the limitation of work capacity due to other factors, was the leveling off of the heart-rate:work-rate curve. (23)."*

Whether cardiac output was limiting oxygen uptake or vice-versa was not an easy matter to establish. All parts of the oxygen transport system are interconnected, which was Dr. Bates point in his humorous exchange with Dr. McDonald, in 1965 at the Queen's University Conference (4):

Dr. D.A. McDonald: *"Dr. Bates, do you think champion swimmers develop large (pulmonary diffusing) capacities? Perhaps it could explain my own disappointments."*

Dr. D.V. Bates: *"If all of these are right (diffusing capacity, training, hemoglobin, capacity to increase cardiac stroke volume), I should think you would have a good chance at a bronze medal, Dr. McDonald!"* From the discussion following Dr. Bates paper (4) on lung diffusion as a limiting factor in exercise.

3.   BACKGROUND FOR PETER D. WAGNER

Clues to the role of cardiac output in limiting oxygen transport at altitude reside in a comparison of maximal cardiac output values in acute, versus chronic, hypoxia, but that comparison has been slow to materialize. That resting cardiac output in acute hypoxia was higher than that after acclimatization (Pikes Peak, CO) was first demonstrated by Grollman (13), but he did not study exercise on the Peak. Pugh had recognized that for a given sub-maximal work intensity, values of heart rate and cardiac output were higher in acute hypoxia than when the subjects were altitude acclimatized (24). He also knew that maximal cardiac output was reduced at altitude, but he had not measured maximal cardiac output at sea level with acute hypoxia. Stenberg et al. (32), using subjects decompressed for about one hour, were the first to show that although $\dot{V}O_{2MAX}$ was reduced in the chamber at ~4000 m, maximal values for heart rate, stroke volume and cardiac output were unchanged, as shown in Figure 2, but they did not study chronic hypoxia nor did they comment on the difference between acute and chronic hypoxia.

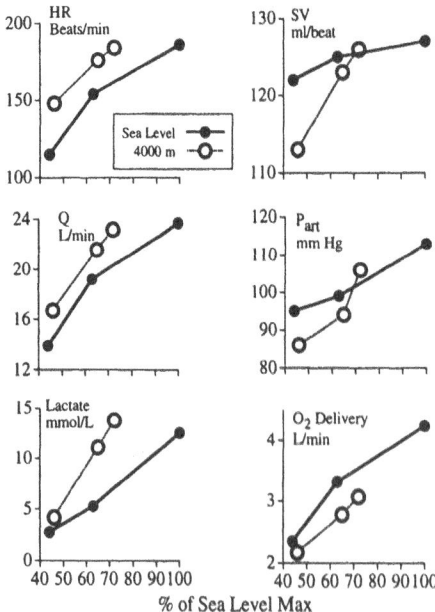

Figure 2. Measurements from Stenberg et al. (32) showing exercise measurements to maximal effort at sea level and within an hour of decompression to the equivalent of 4000 m. Maximal heart rate (HR) stroke volume (SV), cardiac output (Q) and lactate are not different between sea level normoxia and acute altitude hypoxia. At maximal effort, mean arterial pressure (Part) and arterial oxygen delivery (O$_2$ Delivery) were not maintained at sea level values.

The comparison of maximal cardiac output values in acute, versus chronic, hypoxia, came into focus with Grover's review in the 1967 Natick, MA conference (14). He collected prior studies which showed for submaximal exercise (as Grollman had shown at rest), that cardiac output at a given oxygen uptake actually rose above sea level values during the first few days at altitude, and then fell to and even below sea level values as acclimatization proceeded, Figure 3.

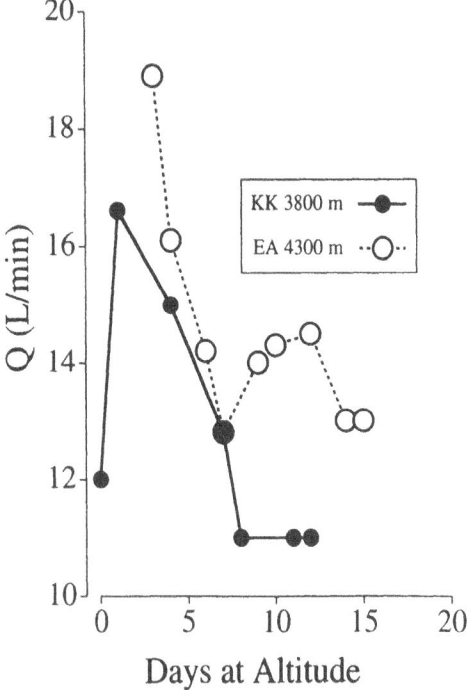

Figure 3. Measurements of sub maximal cardiac output (Q) in subjects EA from Asmussen and Consalazio at 4300 m (2) and subject KK from Klausen at sea level and 3800 m (19). Cardiac output is highest soon after arrival and then falls to a nadir by 10 days to two weeks.

Using his own data and those of Vogel et al. (34), Grover emphasized the remarkable findings for maximal effort, that with acute hypoxia heart rate, stroke volume, and cardiac output were the same as during maximal effort at sea level, but the $\dot{V}O_{2MAX}$ fell. Apparently, with acclimatization $\dot{V}O_{2MAX}$ did not change from arrival, but something had happened to decrease drastically maximal values for cardiac output, heart rate and stroke volume.

An extensive and active discussion followed Grover's presentation (14), but none of the discussants commented on the difference in maximal cardiac output between acute and chronic hypoxia. Dr. Herb Hultgren came closest to the mark, by commenting *"on the concept that cardiac performance limits maximal work capacity at high altitude.*" He concluded by saying, "*Certainly there is no evidence that under strenuous exertion at high altitude acute cardiac dilation or failure has been observed clinically, and there is no evidence that prolonged heavy work at high altitude has any unfavorable effect upon the heart. So it would seem that the heart is capable of delivering the blood that is necessary but perhaps the signal from the periphery for more cardiac output is deficient.*" Although as often occurs, the discussion did not center on the points Grover had made, there were important comments by Dr. Maurice Visscher relating to the role of the sympathetics in maximal performance, as noted below.

If there were any doubts that with acute exposure to altitude, the heart rate, stroke volume, and cardiac output were all maintained at sea level values, those doubts surely were dispelled by the study, Figure 4, in the Duke University altitude chamber in 1984, organized by Peter Wagner (36). The eight volunteers included R.B. (Brownie) Schoene and Rob Roach, and

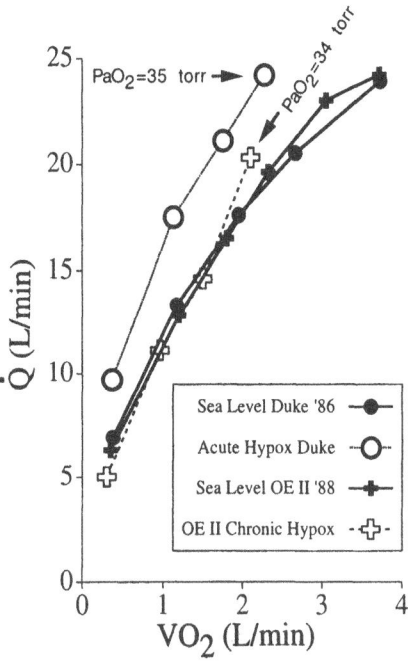

Figure 4. Measurements of cardiac output (Q) and oxygen uptake ($\dot{V}O_2$) from rest to maximal effort at sea level and during acute hypoxic exposure in the chamber at Duke University from Wagner et al. (36), compared with measurements at sea level and during chronic hypoxia from Operation Everest II (OE II: (16, 26, 33). By coincidence, the arterial oxygen pressures (PaO_2) at maximal effort were similar at altitude with acute (Duke study) and chronic (OE II) hypoxia. The relation of Q to $\dot{V}O_2$ was nearly identical in the two studies at sea level, but for the same $\dot{V}O_2$ and the same $\dot{V}O_{2MAX}$, Q was higher with acute than with chronic hypoxia.

also two women. They exercised to maximal effort at sea level, and then repeatedly at 5, 10 and 15 thousand feet in the chamber (36). It was a massive study which required substantial commitment from both subjects and investigators. The findings were that for a given oxygen uptake, heart rate, stroke volume, and cardiac output were higher with acute altitude exposure, than at sea level. But the maximal oxygen uptake was reduced. Thus, while the $\dot{V}O_{2MAX}$ fell at 15,000 feet (~4500 m), the cardiac output, heart rate, and stroke volume at maximal effort (Figure 4), were maintained at sea level values.

The focus of the 1984 study in the Duke altitude chamber was pulmonary gas exchange, but as is so often true in science, when something new is well done, new information and new questions emerge. Wagner surely went into that study with the idea that at maximal effort, the mixed venous blood would have the same low PO_2 both at sea level and at altitude. But that was not the case. The mixed venous PO_2 at $\dot{V}O_{2MAX}$ was less at 15,000 feet than at sea level. Wagner proposes that with brief altitude exposure, the muscle diffusing capacity didn't change, but the leg was capable of doing less work. If so, and from the Fick law of diffusion, venous blood draining the exercising leg must have a lower PO_2 at altitude than at sea level. He subsequently helped me to a better understanding (see appendix), and he continues to wrestle with these concepts (35).

The 1984 Duke study was an important precursor to the 1985 giant collaboration, Operation Everest II, (OE II) organized by Charles Houston, John Sutton and Allen Cymerman (18), and conducted in the United States Army altitude chambers at Natick, MA. At sea level, the OE II data and those of the Duke study were nearly identical (Figure 4). Coincidentally, (or perhaps by good planning) one of the altitudes studied in OE II (P_B=349, P_IO_2 =63 mm Hg) gave similar PaO_2 values to those found at 15,000 feet at Duke. Using all available data, Wagner has sought a unifying explanation, which he likely will argue.

3.1   QUOTE FROM P.D. WAGNER

"With increasing altitude, the influence of cardiac output and hemoglobin concentration falls, while that of ventilation, lung and muscle diffusing capacity progressively increases until at P_B = 253 (mm Hg), $\dot{V}O_{2MAX}$ is independent of cardiac output and hemoglobin." (35)

4.   BACKGROUND FOR LORING B. ROWELL

The above discussion may not be 'playing from a full deck', where at least some of the missing cards are: 1, a greater capacity of the exercising muscle mass to receive blood than the heart can pump, 2, the limitation of the heart's pumping capacity, 3, the exercise requirement to increase, or at least maintain, arterial pressure, 4, the problems of distributing the available flow (between organs and within muscle), and 5, the role of the autonomic nervous system, and particularly the sympathetics, in some of these processes.

4.1   Relative limitations in muscle and cardiac pumping.

Consider, for sea level subjects, cardiac limitation in relation to the heart's pumping capacity. In 1961 Åstrand and Saltin (3) showed that the addition of arm exercise to maximal leg exercise did not increase oxygen uptake, which suggested to them that limitations in the circulation provided a ceiling to oxygen uptake, which was then *"independent of the mass of muscle employed in the exercise as soon as it exceeds a certain mass"*. In reviewing the field, Rowell concludes (28), *"When additional muscles are activated at $\dot{V}O_{2MAX}$, arterial pressure is maintained by vasoconstriction in active muscle"*. The amount of maximally activated muscle which the heart can supply *"is unknown but may be 50% of the total mass"*. Increasing inspired oxygen (17) or raising hemoglobin concentration (27) increases $\dot{V}O_{2MAX}$, which suggested that muscle metabolism is not limiting, but implicated limitation by the heart.

Rowell (28) considers that the evidence does not sustain the symmorphosis hypothesis of Weibel and Taylor which holds that the oxidative capacity of muscle is closely matched to the transport capacity of the cardiovascular system. Rather, an arterial baroreflex *"is essential to the normal rise in sympathetic nervous activity and arterial pressure at the onset of exercise, ... and to prevent arterial hypotension (29)"*. If sympathetic tone is increased at altitude and also if the transport capacity is reduced, then the mismatch between capacity of muscle to use oxygen and that of the heart to deliver should become greater.

The issue is not new, but was raised following Dr. Grover's paper (14). Dr. Maurice Visscher's comment, which though directed at maximal heart rate at altitude, was relevant to the general circulation: *"quite obviously it (maximal heart rate) is a critical factor in determining ..... maximal work capacity at high altitude, ... and I wondered whether there might be some change in the setting of reflex regulatory mechanisms. I wonder whether it might not be central nervous system rather than peripheral tissue effect."*

Sympathetic activation might, indeed, be needed with hypoxia, if the hypoxia has a propensity to augment flow and thus overwhelm the pumping capacity of the heart. When Rowell et al. (31) used one leg exercise, to reduce the amount of exercising muscle, flow to the leg was higher in acute hypoxia than normoxia, and much higher than predicted for two leg exercise in normoxia. The authors speculated that muscle flow during exercise in hypoxia can "*rise.....without apparent limit when the mass of active muscle is too small to overwhelm the heart*". If so, with maximal effort by a large muscle mass, some central control will be needed. "*....the blood pressure is maintained by baroreflex-mediated vasoconstriction in the active muscle which must be the primary target of increased sympathetic neural activity and the source of noradrenaline*" (30). If the sympathetic nervous system rises to the occasion during acute hypoxia, what is its activity during chronic hypoxia, and what are the effects on blood pressure?

4.2   Arterial pressure and the possible role of the sympathetics

The increase in catecholamines as first reported by Cunningham et al. (9) during altitude exposure has been repeatedly confirmed (22, 38). With regard to ambulatory blood pressure, Wolfel et al. (38) utilized 24 hour monitoring of pressure by cuff and found that the resting levels increased above sea level values over the first few days at 4300 m to a plateau that was maintained during a three week stay. The increase in blood pressure had a time course similar to that for 24 hour urinary excretion norepinephrine (Figure 5).

With regard to exercise blood pressure, Bender et al. (5) reported that the exercise-related increase in blood pressure was similar during normoxia and during acute hypoxia, but for a given oxygen uptake, pressures were higher after 19 days at 4300 m (Figure 6). Not shown in Figure 6 was the return to sea level values of blood pressure, when the acclimatized subjects breathed an oxygen mixture simulating sea level PO_2. With acclimatization, norepinephrine release from the leg increased both at rest and during exercise, and the net release correlated strongly with arterial norepinephrine levels (Figure 7, (22)). Such data are compatible with, but not proof of, sympathetic neural activation and a sympathetically mediated increase in blood pressure at high altitude.

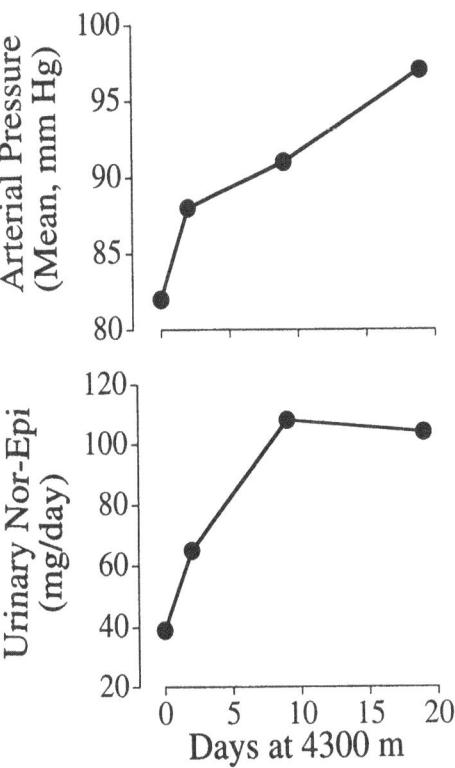

Figure 5. Measurements at sea level and over 19 days on Pikes Peak at 4300 m of ambulatory mean arterial pressure (top panel) and 24 hour urinary norepinephrine (Nor-epi, bottom panel) excretion as reported by Wolfel et al. (38). Pressure was recorded automatically every 20 minutes during the waking hours on the days shown. Similar time course for increases in pressure and norepinephrine excretion is suggested.

But, does the presumptive activation of the sympathetics at altitude impact the cardiac output during acclimatization? If the sympathetics mediate the reported (8) venoconstriction at altitude, then they could contribute to the well known decrease in plasma volume. Of interest, plasma volume decrease (15), norepinephrine net release, 24 hour urinary norepinephrine excretion, and arterial pressure - all are little changed from sea level with acute hypoxia or on arrival at 4300 m, but the changes become progressively greater with ventilatory acclimatization. From the coincident time course, Asano et al. (1) have speculated that ventilatory acclimatization and sympathetic activation may be related to each other. If so, the speculative possibility exists that the activation of sympathetics contribute to a reduction of plasma volume, which in turn, contributes to the lowering of cardiac output with acclimatization. Perhaps Rowell will comment on such a

possibility, and whether it provides understanding to the control of maximal
cardiac output after acclimatization.

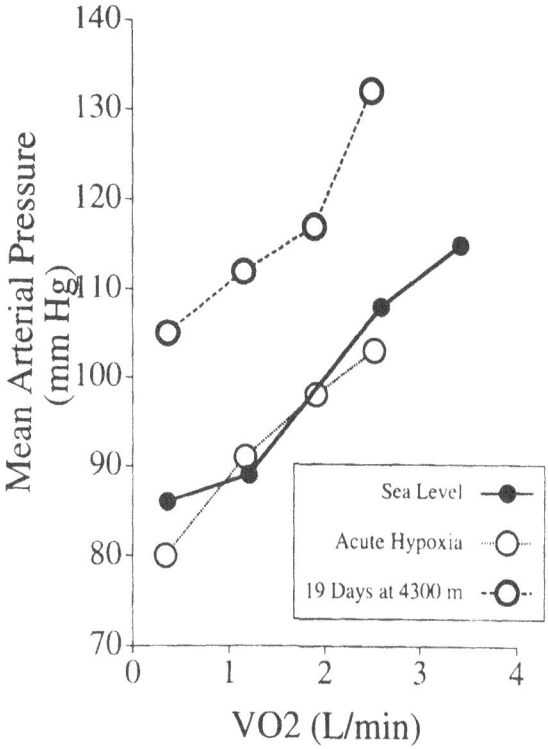

Figure 6. Directly recorded mean intra-arterial pressure at rest and during exercise to
maximal effort at sea level and, on the same day, during acute decompression to simulate the
altitude of Pikes Peak at 4300 m. Also shown for the same subjects are the higher pressures
observed after 19 days residence at 4300 m. Not shown is the return of pressure to sea level
values when on day 19 the subject breathed for a few minutes a high oxygen mixture to give a
PaO_2 equivalent to sea level. Data are from Bender et al. (5).

4.3   Distribution of available flow

Regarding flow distribution within muscle, Rowell (28) has taken issue
with Wagner's analysis with regard to the inhomogeniety of flow and the
diffusional effects of conditioning. *"Two crucial assumptions in Wagner's
analysis are that in humans at $\dot{V}O_{2MAX}$, $Q/\dot{V}O_2$ (muscle) heterogenicity and
both perfusional and diffusional shunting are negligible. It is clear that
muscle perfusion per unit mass during exercise is heterogeneous. What is
not known is the extent of $Q/\dot{V}O_2$ mismatching."* Rowell also has suggested
that exercise conditioning would increase diffusional transport in a way

which differs from that of Wagner. If maximal cardiac output is reduced at altitude and if sympathetic activity is increased (both of which could alter both $Q/\dot{V}O_2$ and diffusion), then Rowell has additional questions about the adequacy of Wagner's model at altitude.

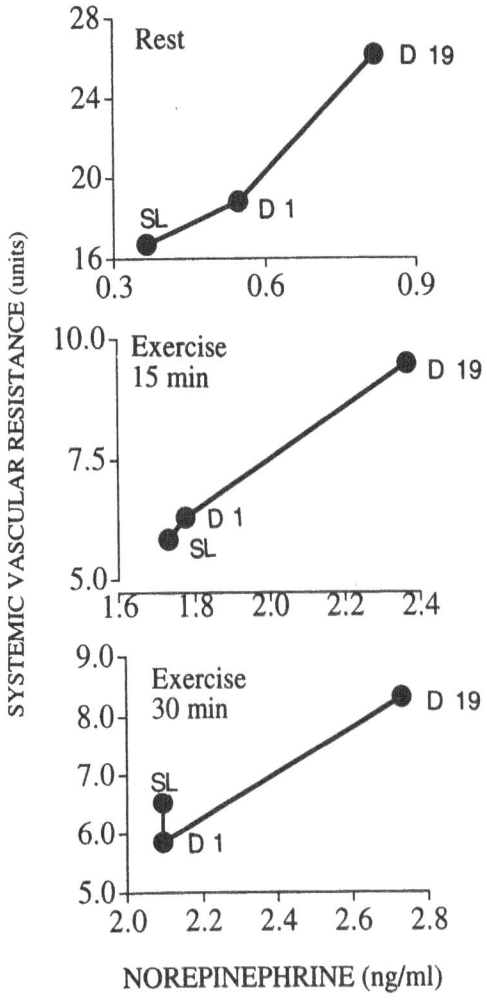

Figure 7. Relation of systemic vascular resistance to blood levels of norepinephrine in 7 subjects at rest (top panel), and after 15 (middle panel) and 30 (bottom panel) min of exercise (to give a $\dot{V}O_2$ of 37 ml/kg/min). Indicated are measurements at sea level (SL), the day of arrival at 4300 m (D1), and after 19 days residence at 4300 m (D19). Data are from Mazzeo et al. (21).

Regarding flow distribution between organs, Rowell is concerned that for maximal effort at altitude insufficient attention has been directed, for example, to the liver, an organ which is essential for the metabolic energy of exercise. For example, circulating lactate levels during maximal exercise are much higher during acute than during chronic altitude exposure. Maximal lactate levels in the acute hypoxia of the Duke chamber were 10.2 mmol/L (36), whereas for similar $\dot{V}O_{2MAX}$ and arterial PO_2 in OE II, lactate was 4.7 mmol/L (33). At issue is whether the decrease in lactate (popularly known as the lactate paradox) with acclimatization reflects altered flow distribution within muscle, between organs, or is independent of the flow changes.

4.4   QUOTE FROM LORING B. ROWELL:

"The ability of humans to raise cardiac output is not sufficient to supply oxygen to more than a fraction of the active muscle during exhausting exercise" (28). *"The crucial problem of keeping muscle blood flow in check by vasoconstriction (i.e., to avoid the potential for muscle vasodilation to outstrip cardiac pumping capacity is great at sea level and is even greater in* (acute) *hypoxia where active muscle vasodilation is greater per unit of* $\dot{V}O_2$*"*. L.B. Rowell (Personal communication)

5.   CONCLUSION

It may be too much to expect for our discussants to answer the question: Why does the exercise cardiac output fall during altitude residence and is it important? But each comes at the question from a different point of view and it is just possible that all of us will learn something. Clearly, the joy in life comes from the journey, not just the destination.

6.   APPENDIX: A PERSONAL NOTE

On October 30, 1985, during the conduct of OE II, we had just completed the '20,000 ft' measurements in our subjects in the US Army research chamber Natick. My diary for that day records my first confrontation with some of the above problems:

"Having the whole day with no other responsibilities, then I could begin the data analysis. So I started off by asking questions of the data - The only way I know how to proceed. The first question I asked was, 'how did the tissues function at 20,000 ft, P_B =347 compared to sea level?' I found that (mixed venous) PO_2 fell linearly with exertion (expressed as) $\dot{V}O_2$ as a % of max) and that at 20,000 ft all of the data fell below that for sea level. The lowest (mixed venous) PO_2 at sea level was between 15 and 20 mm Hg, but at 20,000 ft a value of 10 m Hg was reached.

"Peter Wagner said that he had observed the same thing in the acute experiment at Duke. I was a little distressed because now our finding was not so novel and further my thought (had been) *that the lower PO₂ meant greater tissue extraction as a result of some tissue adaptation. If Peter et al. had seen it after only a few hours at 15,000 feet then it could hardly be a tissue adaptation. Being at a loss for an explanation, I turned to Peter again and he indicated that because of the lower V̇O₂ₘₐₓ at high altitude the PO₂ would be reduced more in the venous blood. Of course, that was the explanation. It simply followed the laws of diffusion:*

Tissue diffusion capacity = O₂ uptake (Max) / PO₂₍capillary₎ - Ø, where Ø can be assumed to be the PO₂ in the cellular mitochondria. If the tissue diffusing capacity remains the same, then tissue capillary PO₂ will fall as the Max V̇O₂ falls. Very nice!"

REFERENCES

1. Asano, K., R.S. Mazzeo, R.E. McCullough, E.E. Wolfel, and J.T. Reeves. Relation of sympathetic activation in man at 4300 meters altitude. *Aviat Space Environ Med* 68: 104-110, 1997.
2. Asmussen, E., and C.F. Consolazio. The circulation in rest and work on Mount Evans (4,300 m). *Am J Physiol* 132: 555-563, 1941.
3. Astrand, P.O., and B. Saltin. Maximal oxygen uptake and heart rate in various types of muscular exercise. *J Appl Physiol* 16: 977-981, 1961.
4. Bates, D.V., J.B.L. Gee, L.G. Bentivoglio, and E. Mostyn. Diffusion as a limiting factor in oxygen transport across the lung. In: *Proceedings International Symposium Cardiovascular and Respiratory Effects of Hypoxia*, edited by J.D. Hatcher and D.B. Jennings. New York: Hafner Publishing, 1966.
5. Bender, P.R., B.M. Groves, R.E. McCullough, R.G. McCullough, S.Y. Huang, A.J. Hamilton, P.D. Wagner, A. Cymerman, and J.T. Reeves. Oxygen transport to exercising leg in chronic hypoxia. *J Appl Physiol* 65: 2592-2597, 1988.
6. Christensen, E.H. Sauerstoffaufnahmane und respiratorische Functionen in Grossem Höhen. *Skand Arch Physiol* 76, 1937.
7. Christensen, E.H., and W.H. Forbes. Der Kreislauf in grossen Höhen. *Skand Arch Physiol* 76: 75-89, 1937.
8. Cruz, J.C., R.F. Grover, J.T. Reeves, J.T. Maher, and A. Cymerman. Sustained venoconstriction in man supplemented with CO2 at high altitude. *J Appl Physiol* 40: 96-100, 1976.
9. Cunningham, W.L., E.J. Becker, and F. Kreuzer. Catecholamines in plasma and urine at high altitude. *J Appl Physiol* 20: 607-610, 1965.
10. Dill, D.B.*Life Heat, and Altitude. Physiological Effects of Hot Climates and Great Heights.* Cambridge, MA: Harvard University Press, 1938.
11. Dill, D.B., H.T. Edwards, A. Follings, S.A. Oberg, A.M. Pappenheimer, and J.H. Talbott. Adaptations of the organism to changes in oxygen pressure. *J Physiol (London)* 71: 47-63, 1931.

12. Douglas, C.G., J.S. Haldane, Y. Henderson, and E.C. Schneider. Physiological observations made on Pike's Peak, Colorado, with special reference to adaptation to low barometric pressures. *Proc Roy Soc London (Series B)* 203: 185-318, 1913.

13. Grollman, A. Physiological variations in the cardiac output of man VII. The effect of high altitude on the cardiac output and its related functions: an account of experiments conducted on the summit of Pike's Peak, Colorado. *Am J Physiol* 93: 19-40, 1930.

14. Grover, R.F. Influence of high altitude on cardiac output response to exercise. In: *Biomedical Problems of High Terrestrial Elevations*, edited by A.H. Hegnauer. Washington, DC: US Army Medical Research and Development Command, 1969, p. 223-247.

15. Grover, R.F., M.A. Selland, R.G. McCullough, T.E. Dahms, E.E. Wolfel, G.E. Butterfield, J.T. Reeves, and J.E. Greenleaf. Beta-adrenergic blockade does not prevent polycythemia or decrease in plasma volume in men at 4300 m altitude. *Eur J Appl Physiol* 77: 264-270, 1998.

16. Groves, B.M., J.T. Reeves, J.R. Sutton, P.D. Wagner, A. Cymerman, M.K. Malconian, P.B. Rock, P.M. Young, and C.S. Houston. Operation Everest II: Elevated high altitude pulmonary resistance unresponsive to oxygen. *J Appl Physiol* 63: 521-530, 1987.

17. Hill, A.V., C.N.H. Long, and H. Lupton. Muscular exercise, lactic acid, and the supply and utilization of oxygen. *Proc Roy Soc London (Series B)* 97: 155-167, 1924.

18. Houston, C.S., J.R. Sutton, and A. Cymerman. Operation Everest II: Man at extreme altitude. *J Appl Physiol* 63: 877-882, 1987.

19. Klausen, K. Cardiac output in man at rest and work during and after acclimatization to 3800m. *J Appl Physiol* 21: 609-616, 1966.

20. Margaria, R. Die Arbeitsfahgkeit des Menchen by vermindertem Luftdruck. *Arbeits-physiologie* 2: 261-272, 1930.

21. Mazzeo, R.S., P.R. Bender, G.A. Brooks, G.E. Butterfield, B.M. Groves, J.R. Sutton, E.E. Wolfel, and J.T. Reeves. Arterial catecholamine response during exercise with acute and chronic high altitude exposure. *Am J Physiol* 261: E419-E424, 1991.

22. Mazzeo, R.S., G.A. Brooks, G.E. Butterfield, D.A. Podolin, E.E. Wolfel, and J.T. Reeves. Acclimatization to high altitude increases muscle sympathetic activity both at rest and during exercise. *Am J Physiol* 269: R201-R207, 1995.

23. Pugh, L.G. Animals in high altitude: Man above 5,000 meters-mountain exploration. In: *Handbook of Physiology: Adaptation to the Environment*, edited by D.B. Dill. Washington, DC: American Physiological Society, 1964, p. 861-868.

24. Pugh, L.G. Cardiac output in muscular exercise at 5,800 m (19,000 ft). *J Appl Physiol* 19: 441-447, 1964.

25. Pugh, L.G., M.B. Gill, S. Lahiri, J.S. Milledge, M.P. Ward, and J.B. West. Muscular exercise at great altitude. *J Appl Physiol* 19: 431-440, 1964.

26. Reeves, J.T., B.M. Groves, J.R. Sutton, P.D. Wagner, A. Cymerman, M.K. Malconian, P.B. Rock, P.M. Young, and C.S. Houston. Operation Everest II: Preservation of cardiac function at extreme altitude. *J Appl Physiol* 63: 531-539, 1987.

27. Rowell, L.B. Human cardiovascular adjustments to exercise and thermal stress. *Physiol Rev* 54: 75-159, 1974.

28. Rowell, L.B. *Human Cardiovascular Control.* New York: Oxford University Press, 1993.

29. Rowell, L.B. Neural control of muscle blood flow: importance during dynamic exercise. *Clin Exp Pharmacol Physiol* 24: 117-125, 1997.

30. Rowell, L.B., and J.R. Blackmon. Human cardiovascular adjustments to acute hypoxaemia. *Clin Physiol* 7: 349-376, 1987.

31. Rowell, L.B., B. Saltin, B. Kiens, and N.J. Christensen. Is peak quadriceps blood flow in humans even higher during exercise with hypoxemia? *Am J Physiol* 251: H1038-H1044, 1986.
32. Stenberg, J., B. Ekblom, and R. Messin. Hemodynamic response to work at simulated altitude, 4000m. *J Appl Physiol* 21: 1589-1594, 1966.
33. Sutton, J.R., J.T. Reeves, P.D. Wagner, B.M. Groves, A. Cymerman, M.K. Malconian, P.B. Rock, P.M. Young, S.D. Walter, and C.S. Houston. Operation Everest II. Oxygen transport during exercise at extreme simulated altitude. *J Appl Physiol* 64: 1309-1321, 1988.
34. Vogel, J.A., J.E. Hansen, and C.W. Harris. Cardiovascular responses in man during exhaustive work at sea level and high altitude. *J Appl Physiol* 23: 531-539, 1967.
35. Wagner, P.D. A theoretical analysis of factors determining VO2 MAX at sea level and altitude. *Respir Physiol* 106: 329-343, 1996.
36. Wagner, P.D., G.E. Gale, R.E. Moon, J.R. Torre-Bueno, B.W. Stolp, and H.A. Saltzman. Pulmonary gas exchange in humans exercising at sea level and simulated altitude. *J Appl Physiol* 61: 260-270, 1986.
37. West, J.B. *High Life. A History Of High-Altitude Physiology And Medicine*. New York: Oxford University Press, 1998.
38. Wolfel, E.E., M.A. Selland, R.S. Mazzeo, and J.T. Reeves. Systemic hypertension at 4,300 m is related to sympathoadrenal activity. *J Appl Physiol* 76: 1643-1650, 1994.

Chapter 27

International Consensus Group on Chronic Mountain Sickness

Fabiola Leon-Velarde, Chair and John T. Reeves, Secretary
Professor of Physiology, Departmento de Fisiologia/Instituto de Investigaciones de la Altura,
Universidad Peruana Cayetano Heredia, Lima and ARPE/Paris XIII, France and Professor
Emeritus of Medicine, Pediatrics, Family Medicine, University of Colorado Health Sciences
Center, Denver, USA

Key words: polycythemia, Monge's disease, CMS

The Chronic Mountain Sickness (CMS) Consensus Group was established in 1998 in Matsumoto Japan in order to clarify issues surrounding CMS. Millions of people who live at high altitude are at risk for CMS, but the disorder is poorly understood. The Consensus Group hopes to lay the foundation for better understanding of description, pathogenesis, and treatment by developing consensus among interested scientists from many countries.

A meeting of the CMS Consensus Group was held during the 11th International Hypoxia Symposium, at Jasper Park Lodge, Alberta, Canada, March 2, 1999. The following report describes the results of that meeting. For further information about the CMS study group, please contact the group secretary, Dr. John T. Reeves.

Present: Yasuhiro Arain, Chiba University, Chiba, Japan; Ge Ri-Li, Shinshu University, Matsumoto, Japan and Qinghai Province, China; Tomonobu Koizumi, Shinshu University, Matsumoto Japan; Toshio Kobayashi, Shinshu University, Matsumoto, Japan; Shigeru Masuyama, Chiba University, Chiba, Japan; Aibek Ashirbaev, Kumptor Medical Center, Bishkek, Kyrgyz Republic; Ingrid Asmus, University of Colorado, Denver, USA; John T. Reeves, University of Colorado, Denver, USA; Fabiola Leon-

Velarde, Cayetano Heredia University, Lima, Peru and ARPE/ Paris XIII, France; Jean-Paul Richalet, ARPE/Paris XIII, France.

1. The booklet "Chronic Exposure to Hypoxia in Human Beings - Criteria and Classification of CMS" was extracted for publication from the published "Proceedings of the Third World Congress on Mountain Medicine and High Altitude Physiology, 1998 in Matsumoto, Japan. The booklet as well as the full text of the Proceedings allowed a wider dissemination of the discussions of the International Consensus Group on CMS and was the basis for the second meeting. The committee expressed its appreciation to the organizers of the Matsumoto Congress for this effort, and also for their donation of any proceeds to the John Sutton Foundation, which will promote the Hypoxia Symposia.

2. Fabiola Leon-Velarde, who chaired the first meeting, was again chosen as the chair of this, the second meeting of the Consensus Group.

3. The minutes of the Matsumoto meeting of the Consensus Group were reviewed and approved. However, there was further discussion of the recommendations for criteria of CMS as developed at that meeting. Ri-Li asked that pulmonary hypertension and high altitude heart disease be considered for inclusion in the CMS criteria. Asmus indicated that her preliminary data from Leadville, Colorado (3000 m) indicated a poor relationship between the criteria proposed in Matsumoto and the level of the blood hematocrit. Masuyama indicated that the criteria previously used by workers in Bolivia, China, and Peru were not identical, and that James Lynch was currently conducting work in Nepal, but did not comment on the criteria being used. Also, Masuyama indicated there was as yet no agreement as to what should be done about including persons with some pulmonary parenchymal disease, or about cut-off of normal levels of hemoglobin and hematocrit. The Chair then turned the discussion to the issue as to how to proceed.

4. The Chair and Richalet suggested that a world-wide organized approach was needed to collect information to serve as a basis for establishing better criteria and definitions. There was general agreement and the following steps were proposed.

4a) Key articles published in Chinese need to be disseminated through their publication in English. Several thousand persons living at high altitude in the Qinghai Province and in Tibet have been examined, but the details of this experience is not generally known outside China. Ri-Li agreed to get some of these articles translated into English for submission to an English journal. One suggested possibility was to work with the editors of the Journal of Wilderness and Mountain Medicine.

4b) Establish a format for an international data base. An issue was how broad the data base should be. One possibility was to restrict data entry to those clinical and laboratory aspects thought currently to be part of the CMS syndrome. The second possibility considered was to expand data entry to include chronic illnesses or disorders associated with residence at high altitude. Restricting data entry to CMS has the advantage of a more focused and more manageable data base, but the disadvantage was discussed that at present there is only a very general definition for the CMS syndrome. Enlarging the scope of the data base to include chronic disorders associated with altitude residence, would be less likely to exclude potentially important information, but would entail a much larger data base. After considerable discussion, it was agreed that the data base should be inclusive, not exclusive. It would then begin to define illnesses/disorders among high altitude populations. Given the current divergence of opinion about the nature of CMS, the dearth of information in general about illnesses among high altitude residents, the large populations residing at altitude world-wide, and the possible interest of the World Health Organization (WHO) in the problem, the Consensus Group recommended an expanded data base. While such an undertaking would appear formidable, a group consisting of the Chair and I. Asmus would begin to assemble for discussion the format of such a data base. It would then be presented for review at the next International Society of Mountain Medicine (ISMM) meeting in Arica, Chile in the year 2000.

4c) Concurrently with 4b, above, Asmus will establish a retrospective data base for information already collected in individual persons. The Chair, the Bolivian group (unfortunately not present in Jasper) and Ri-Li as well as Asmus already collectively have thousands of persons who have been examined. Assembling these data will be a very large task and Asmus was pleased to accept any help from the other participants in the group. The data in 4c should help with the format of the data base as envisioned in 4b, above.

4d) Masuyama suggested that at the next meeting of the ISMM that typical case reports should be presented by investigators from the various regions of the world. The suggestion was well received by the committee because such presentations, well done, would allow better understanding of the medical problems at altitude in general, and CMS in particular. (The Secretary suggests that the Chair appoint someone to organize this endeavor.)

5. The group agreed that the WHO should be informed of the formation, intent, and activities of the Consensus Group on CMS. The WHO could provide expert advice, support, and even financial assistance to the effort. The secretary agreed to draft a letter to be submitted to the Chair and to be reviewed and (if he agrees) signed by Carlos Monge for submission to WHO.

Chapter 28

A Tribute to Niels Lassen
December 7th, 1926 - April 30th, 1997

John W. Severinghaus

Professor Emeritus, Anesthesiology, University of California San Francisco, California 94123-0542 USA

Key words: cerebral blood flow

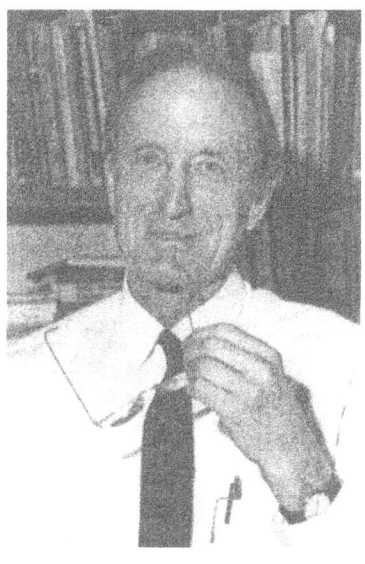

Niels Lassen died in Copenhagen of pancreatic carcinoma at 71. He was the premier leader in the field of quantitation of cerebral blood flow (CBF). Immediately after finishing medical school, he and Ole Munck introduced the use of radioactive isotopes for CBF measurement. With David Ingvar, he was the first to use collimated radioactive extracranial counting after intracarotid injection of the radioactive isotope [85]Krypton or [133]Xenon dissolved in saline to localize regions of high or low cerebral flow. His mathematician wife Edda Sveinsdotter developed programming methods and much technical support. Functional brain mapping was pioneered by Lassen using, finally, a 254 detector system. With Bo Siesjo and David Ingvar, he founded the International Cerebral Blood Flow meetings and later the Journal of Cerebral Blood Flow and Metabolism. From 1962 to 1996 he was chairman of the department of clinical physiology and nuclear medicine at Bispebjerg Hospital in Copenhagen. Niels' command of English was better than mine, elegant,

Hypoxia: Into the Next Millennium,
Edited by R. C. Roach, *et al.* Kluwer Academic/Plenum Publishing, New York, 1999.

355

witty and creative. The terms "luxury perfusion" and "ischemic penumbra" are his.

We first met in 1955 at NIH during his year with Seymour Kety. His interest in brain acid base balance was a major attraction for my choice of Copenhagen for my first sabbatical in 1964-5. Elinor, our 4 children and I arrived in late June, thinking we had a house waiting for us. Not so, and Niels, Edda and 4 children invited us to stay in their small house in Klampenborg for the two days it took to arrange a dwelling. Much floor sleeping, more by the Lassen than the Severinghaus family, I recall.

We decided to test whether falling Pco_2 constricted cerebral vessels directly, i.e. in the arterial walls, or indirectly, later when tissue Pco_2 fell, delayed by the 2 minute washout time constant. The test was to suddenly hyperventilate to a Pco_2 of 20 mmHg while watching a CO_2 analyser output of the expired air, and frequently sample jugular bulb blood oxygen as a proxy for CBF. Niels was the expert at needling the internal jugular bulb. When it was my turn to breathe, he had trouble finding blood, and suddenly one side of my tongue was numb and paralyzed. Niels was more worried than I, coming to visit twice a day, until both sensation and motor control came back on the 3rd day. The study was a success, showing a 25 sec time constant for the fall of jugular venous O_2 saturation, implying a direct arterial wall effect of CO_2.

In June, 1971, Niels, Edda, and their son Anders joined Elinor, Wendy, Jeff and me in a camping bike trip around Gotland. Niels was an inveterate adventurer, always looking for an excuse for a remote location science trip. He suggested LaPaz, Bolivia, where a CBF lab had been set up by Jean Coudert with French government support. The team in La Paz in 1972 consisted of Niels, with Søren Sørensen and Marianne Anker, Coudert, Mario Paz-Zamora the cardiologist who later became minister of health, the local doctors and helpers, my elder son and daughter as photographers, and me. In Quechua natives on the Altiplano CBF was not elevated, despite continued hypoxemia and normal or acidic CSF. This anomaly remains unexplained. As at sea level, CBF was inversely proportional to Hct.

One morning in Copenhagen, while I was showering, Niels called to say I was supposed to be lecturing to a group of WHO Anesthesia trainees. He had come to listen. He started the lecture, which was appropriate since he knew more about it than I did. I got there by bike in about 15 min, finished the lecture, using a blackboard to draw graphics. The students said they understood me much better without my usual slides.

Niels joined our UCSF group again in 1990, with Danish colleagues Bjorn Sperling and Jorgen Jensen. To explain the gradual fall of CBF with days to weeks at altitude, we tested whether an adaptation of the acute hypoxic increase of CBF occurs in normals during acclimatization to altitude. We faulted the hypothesis, finding a steeper than normal response to acute isocapnic hypoxia after 3-5 days at 3810m altitude. It was one of Niels' last publications (JAP, Apr 1996).

Lassen served on the Danish Medical Research Council and the Royal Danish Academy of Science. He received honorary degrees from Lund, Copenhagen, Lille and Toulose. He won the Novo Award and Anders Jahres Medical Award, the Lundbeck Foundation's Research Award, Johan M. Klein's Award, the Soriano Award, the Mogens Fog Award and, just before his death, the Lifetime Achievement Award from the International Society of Cerebral Blood Flow and Metabolism. I told him of this action by telephone when he was too ill to visit.

Niels Lassen was ever enthusiastic, and although fatally afflicted, wanted to mount another trip to Bolivia to test whether cerebral metabolic rate of oxygen in newcomers gradually decreases to the levels found in natives of altitude by Peter Hochachka's group. Niels' associates in Copenhagen, Olaf Paulsen, Rob Roach and Tom Hornbein tackled that question during the 1998 Danish expedition to LaPaz, a sort of Everest III trip.

We miss his keen intelligence, charm, enthusiasm, wit, sparkle, imagination, skill and insight, and are ever grateful for his career of new discovery and leadership.

Niels Lassen: A Bibliography Selected From More Than 400 Original Research Articles.

Lassen, N. A. Increase of cerebral blood flow at high altitude: its possible relation to AMS. *Int J Sports Med* 13 Suppl 1: S47-8, 1992.

Lassen, N. A. Is central chemoreceptor sensitive to intracellular rather than extracellular pH? *Clin Physiol* 10: 311-9, 1990.

Lassen, N. A., L. Friberg, J. Kastrup, D. Rizzi, and J. J. Jensen. Effects of acetazolamide on cerebral blood flow and brain tissue oxygenation. *Postgrad Med* J 63: 185-7, 1987.

Lassen, N. A., and A. M. Harper. Letter: High-altitude cerebral oedema. *Lancet* 2: 1154, 1975

and

Andersen, A. R., P. Tfelt-Hansen, and N. A. Lassen. The effect of ergotamine and dihydroergotamine on cerebral blood flow in man. *Stroke* 18: 120-3, 1987.

Friberg, L., J. Kastrup, D. Rizzi, J. B. Jensen, and N. A. Lassen. Cerebral blood flow and end-tidal PCO2 during prolonged acetazolamide treatment in humans. *Am J Physiol* 258: H954-9, 1990.

Harvey, T. C., M. E. Raichle, M. H. Winterborn, J. Jensen, N. A. Lassen, N. V. Richardson, and A. R. Bradwell. Effect of carbon dioxide in acute mountain sickness: a rediscovery. *Lancet* 2: 639-41, 1988.

Heuser, D., J. Astrup, N. A. Lassen, and B. E. Betz. Brain carbonic acid acidosis after acetazolamide. *Acta Physiol Scand* 93: 385-90, 1975.

Jensen, J. B., B. Sperling, J. W. Severinghaus, and N. A. Lassen. Augmented hypoxic cerebral vasodilation in men during 5 days at 3,810 m altitude. *J Appl Physiol* 80: 1214-8, 1996.

Jensen, J. B., A. D. Wright, N. A. Lassen, T. C. Harvey, M. H. Winterborn, M. E. Raichle, and A. R. Bradwell. Cerebral blood flow in acute mountain sickness. *J Appl Physiol* 69: 430-3, 1990.

Krasney, J. A., J. B. Jensen, and N. A. Lassen. Cerebral blood flow does not adapt to sustained hypoxia. *J Cereb Blood Flow Metab* 10: 759-64, 1990.

Lou, H. C., N. A. Lassen, and B. Friis-Hansen. Low cerebral blood flow in hypotensive perinatal distress. *Acta Neurol Scand* 56: 343-52, 1977.

Postiglione, A., T. Bobkiewicz, E. Vinholdt-Pedersen, N. A. Lassen, O. B. Paulson, and D. I. Barry. Cerebrovascular effects of angiotensin converting enzyme inhibition involve large artery dilatation in rats. *Stroke* 22: 1363-8, 1991.

Schroeder, T., S. Vorstrup, N. A. Lassen, and H. C. Engell. Noninvasive xenon-133 measurements of cerebral blood flow using stationary detectors compared with dynamic emission tomography. *J Cereb Blood Flow Metab* 6: 739-46, 1986.

Sorensen, S. C., N. A. Lassen, J. W. Severinghaus, J. Coudert, and M. P. Zamora. Cerebral glucose metabolism and cerebral blood flow in high-altitude residents. *J Appl Physiol* 37: 305-10, 1974.

Vorstrup, S., B. Brun, and N. A. Lassen. Evaluation of the cerebral vasodilatory capacity by the acetazolamide test before EC-IC bypass surgery in patients with occlusion of the internal carotid artery. *Stroke* 17: 1291-8, 1986.

Vorstrup, S., H. C. Engell, H. Lindewald, and N. A. Lassen. Hemodynamically significant stenosis of the internal carotid artery treated with endarterectomy. Case report. *J Neurosurg* 60: 1070-5, 1984.

Vorstrup, S., K. E. Jensen, C. Thomsen, O. Henriksen, N. A. Lassen, and O. B. Paulson. Neuronal pH regulation: constant normal intracellular pH is maintained in brain during low extracellular pH induced by acetazolamide--31P NMR study. *J Cereb Blood Flow Metab* 9: 417-21, 1989.

Vorstrup, S., O. B. Paulson, and N. A. Lassen. Cerebral blood flow in acute and chronic ischemic stroke using xenon- 133 inhalation tomography. *Acta Neurol Scand* 74: 439-51, 1986.

Wang, Q., O. B. Paulson, and N. A. Lassen. Effect of nitric oxide blockade by NG-nitro-L-arginine on cerebral blood flow response to changes in carbon dioxide tension. *J Cereb Blood Flow Metab* 12: 947-53, 1992.

Wang, Q., O. B. Paulson, and N. A. Lassen. Indomethacin abolishes cerebral blood flow increase in response to acetazolamide-induced extracellular acidosis: a mechanism for its effect on hypercapnia? *J Cereb Blood Flow Metab* 13: 724-7, 1993.

Chapter 29

Abstracts from the 11ᵗʰ International Hypoxia Symposium

High Altitude Doppler Echocardiography Estimation Of Systolic Pulmonary Artery Pressure Correlates Well With Its Invasive Measurement.

Allemann Y[1], Lepori M[2], Sartori C[2], Pierre S[3], Mélot C[3], Naeije R[3], Scherrer U[2], Maggiorini M[4]. University Hospital, Bern, Switzerland[1]; CHUV, Lausanne, Switzerland[2]; Erasmus University Hospital, Bruxelles, Belgium[3]; University Hospital, Zürich, Switzerland[4].

Background: An exaggerated, hypoxia-induced, vasoconstriction of the pulmonary arterial vascular bed is a hallmark of high altitude pulmonary edema (HAPE) and is thought to play a major role in its pathogenesis. All pathophysiologic studies of HAPE and conducted at high altitude have, so far, estimated systolic pulmonary artery pressure (SPAP) with Doppler-echocardiography (DE). Aim of the study: To demonstrate for the first time at high altitude, that DE-estimated values of SPAP correlate well with invasively (INV) measured SPAP and, consequently, to validate DE as an accurate and reproducible method for measuring SPAP at high altitude. Methods: SPAP was measured using right heart catheterization and estimated by DE at 4559 m in 17 healthy adults. Three women and 14 men aged 34 ± 8 years (mean±SD) were included in the study. Seven subjects had previously developed at least 1 episode of HAPE (HAPE-S group) and 4 were in acute HAPE during the determinations of SPAP. The 10 other subjects were known to be resistant to HAPE (HAPE-R group). Results:

	$SPAP_{DE}$ [mmHg]	$SPAP_{INV}$ [mmHg]	$Range_{DE}$ [mmHg]	$Range_{INV}$ [mmHg]	p (DE vs INV)
All (n = 17)	46 ± 14	47 ± 16	$31 - 75$	$31 - 84$	n.s.
HAPE-S (n = 7)	59 ± 11	62 ± 12	$48 - 75$	$48 - 84$	n.s.
HAPE-R (n = 10)	36 ± 04	36 ± 05	$31 - 41$	$31 - 43$	n.s.

DE: Doppler-Echocardiography; INV: invasive; All: all subjects; HAPE-S: HAPE-susceptible; HAPE-R: HAPE-resistant. Applied to all subjects, Spearman-Test showed a highly significant correlation ($r=0.87$; $p<0.0001$) between SPAPDE and SPAPINV values. Conclusions: For the first time at high altitude it is shown that DE-estimated SPAP, one of the most important pathophysiologic factors contributing to HAPE, correlates very well with its invasive measurement. Consequently, this study should definitively validate DE as an accurate and reproducible method for measuring SPAP at high altitude.

Burning-Hands-Burning-Feet And Chronic Mountain Sickness.
Appenzeller, O. , Thomas, P. K. London, UK., King, R. H. M. London, UK, Muddle, J. R. London, UK., Gamboa, J. Lima, Peru., Tapia, R. Cerro de Pasco, Peru., Vargas, M. Lima, Peru., Albuquerque, NM. 87122, USA.

OBJECTIVE. To characterize neurologic features in patients with chronic mountain sickness (CMS) including symptoms of "burning-hands-burning-feet" (BHBF). BACKGROUND. CMS (Monge's disease) denotes maladaptation in Andean natives to high altitude. Neurologic symptoms of CMS include headaches, tinnitus and dizziness. We have learned that BHBF occurs in Cerro de Pasco (CP). DESIGN/METHODS. Fifteen subjects living in CP, Peru (4338m.) were examined. Ten had classic symptoms of CMS, average hematocrit (HTC) 69% (range 60-78%). There were 5 controls average HTC 55% (range 49-60%) (p<0.005). Three sural nerve biopsies were performed and processed for light and electron microscopy, including morphometry in London. RESULTS. Eleven subjects had recurrent headaches (migraine with aura, migraine without aura or tension type headache). Five CMS patients had episodic "dizziness". Fourteen had sensory symptoms in their feet; in 9 CMS patients these were also present in their hands. They were described as burning (10) or tingling, intermittent in 8, continuous in 6. Reflex depression or loss, or distal cutaneous sensory impairment was found in 3. In 13 all symptoms disappeared on low altitude sojourn (3 hours to 3 days), symptoms recurring in CP but with considerable longer latency. Sural nerves showed a mild neuropathy with evidence of demyelination/remyelination and a reduction in the relative proportion of small myelinated fibers (<5mm). CONCLUSIONS. Typical symptoms and signs of CMS were present in those with high HCTs. We found BHBF to be common, and independent of CMS and documented this symptom complex as additional evidence of maladaptation to altitude in Andean natives. The rapid reversibility of BHBF on low altitude sojourn suggest an altitude associated metabolic rather than structural basis for these symptoms. Support. NMHEMC Research Foundation; Instituto de Investigationes de Altura Universidad Peruana Cayetano Heredia.

Lactate Concentration And Cardiac Output In High Altitude Natives During Exercise At 5250 m.
Araoz M., P.D. Wagner, G.Radegran, H. Wagner, H. Spielvogel, H. Søndergaard, J.A.L. Calbet. Instituto Boliviano de Biología de Altura, La Paz, Bolivia., University of California San Diego, USA., Copenhagen Muscle Research Centre, Denmark.

To assess the behavior of cardiac output (Q) and plasma lactate concentrations [La] during exercise in high altitude natives (HAN) at 5250 m, we studied 7 subjects born between 3600 and 4100 m. The following parameters were measured during graded exercise to maximum on a cycle ergometer and during one leg kicking exercise: [La] in femoral artery plasma (Radiometer ABL System 600); Q by acetylene inhalation (Sensor Medics V.Max) a) breathing ambient air (F_1O_2 = 0.208), b) breathing supplemental oxygen (F_1O_2 = 0.4), and c) after pharmacological vagal blockage (Glucopyrolate); femoral arterial pH (Radiometer ABL system 600). Results: No difference of [La] was found in HAN compared with values reported at sea level. No difference of Q was observed after pharmacological vagal blockage. During cycle ergometer exercise Q increased significantly with supplemental oxygen (p = 0.005). A significant difference of the slope <[La] versus Base excess> was observed between HAN and low altitude natives (LAN) after 6 weeks of acclimatization at 5250 m. (p = 0.00002). Conclusions: In this study the existence of the lactate paradox could not be verified. An increase in vagal nerve activity is apparently not responsible for the lower maximal heart rate and Q in HAN during exercise at 5250 m. HAN seem to have a more efficient buffer capacity than acclimatized LAN during exercise at 5250 m.

[1]presented as *Hot Topic in Mountain Medicine*; [2]presented as *Hot Topic in Hypoxia*; [3]*oral poster communication.*

Responsible Factors For Deterioration In Arterial Blood Gas Of Sherpa.

Arai, Yasuhiro[1], Nawang K. Sherpa[3], Yoshimasa Horie[1], Nobuaki Furuyama[2], Shigeru Masuyama[1], Takayuki Kuriyama[1], Department of Chest Medicine[1], Central Operation[2] Chiba University Kunde Hospital[3].

Gas exchange has been reported getting worse with aging in chronic hypoxic environment. Multiple regression analysis was done to identify responsible factors for the deterioration in gas exchange in Highlander Sherpa. Age, sex, dwelling altitude, living surroundings, past history, smoking history and pulmonary function were analyzed. Arterial blood gas on sitting position at rest was analyzed in 66 Sherpa people (25-57 years of age, 30 male, 36 female) who consulted or have lived near Kunde Hospital (3850m above sea level, PB=486 mmHg) in Khumbu area in Nepal. Pulmonary function test was performed in 54 subjects and questionnaire study was done in 38 subjects. Results; (1) pH was 7.431+/-0.027 (average±SD), $PaCO_2$ was 30.7+/- 2.9Torr, PaO_2 was 50.4+/-4.4Torr, and SaO_2 was 86.5+/-3.4%. (2)VC was 3.5+/-0.88l, %VC was 109+/-21%, FEV1.0 was 2.7+/-0.85l, FEV1.0% was 91+/-8.8%. (3) 6 people (15.8%) had past history of chest disease. (4) 6 people (15.8%) had smoking history. (5) 8 people (21.1%) had lived in highly smoky house. Multiple regression analysis revealed that such factors as age, sex, past history, dwelling altitude, and FEV1.0% were concerned in arterial blood gas deterioration in Sherpa. We concluded that multiple factors other than blunting in respiratory chemosensitivities should be taken into account when discussing gas exchange in residents in chronic hypoxic environment.

Treatment Of Altitude Sickness By Means Of Stationary Multiplace Hyperbaric Chamber (SMHC) At Kumtor Mine Site (4000 m).

Ashirbaev A.A., Le Roux J.M., Arstanbekova G.A., Kumtor Medical Clinic, 74 Kievskaya str., Bishkek, Kyrgyz Republic, 720000.

Objective: Acute mountain sickness (AMS) is common at Kumtor mine site (4000 m). The illness is managed by treatment with oxygen, acetazolamide, dexametazone, pain killers, nifedipine and descent. Portable hyperbaric chamber (e.g.Gamow bag) has been known among climbers. Since early 1998 we've been using SMHC. Methods: Evaluated protocols of 72 AMS patients (pts) of both sexes, 22-55 y. Average session time was 4-6 h, pressure 250 mbar. Protocol included baseline check, cbc, chest x-ray, Lake-Louise Questionnaire with follow ups after 24 h. All pts were divided into 3 categories, based on prevailence of certain symptoms: AMSG (general: headache, no sleep etc.) - 47 pts; AMSR (respiratory) - 16 pts; AMSC (cerebral) - 9 pts. Summary: I. Complete recovery of AMS–57 pts; II. Reccurent AMS -9 pts, mostly with neurological signs after 6-12 h: headache, dizziness etc. These pts additionally treated with acetazolamide, O_2, decadron etc. III. Six pts without effect, all with AMS-R (hape confirmed on chest x-ray). Pts were pressurized in the chamber with good effect, but rapidly deteriorated after release. With use of the chamber medical evacuations were reduced by 50% in comparison with 1997. Conclusion: SMHC has been very helpful treatment of AMS and for temporary stabilizing of HAPE pts, when descent was not immediately possible. With SMHC we treat most of the effects of altitude, therefore minimizing the need for evacuation off site. The treatment itself is harmless, as no gases or chemicals are added, and no time limits for treatment.

---

[1]presented as *Hot Topic in Mountain Medicine*; [2]presented as *Hot Topic in Hypoxia*; [3]*oral poster communication.*

Preliminary Data: Menstrual Status, Hormone Replacement Therapy And Hemoglobin Concentrations In Women Residing At 3100 m.
Asmus I, S Zamudio Ph.D., LG Moore Ph.D. University of Colorado, Denver CO.

Objective: We asked whether menopausal status or hormone replacement therapy (HRT) influence the development of polycythemia in women residing at high altitude. Methods: Women residing at 3100 m. for at least 6 months participated in a community survey which consisted of a questionnaire and measurements of height, weight, blood pressure, FEV_1, & FVC and SaO_2. Blood was drawn to assay hemoglobin, hematocrit, erythropoietin, ferritin, estradiol, progesterone and testosterone. Results: Post-menopausal women appear to have higher hemoglobin concentrations than premenopausal women regardless of age (see Table: data are presented as mean hemoglobin in g/dl ± SEM). Among post-menopausal women, HRT appeared to reduce hemoglobin concentrations in each age group. Analysis is continuuing to examine the relationship between menopause and HRT effects on circulating erythropoietin, estradiol, progesterone and testosterone. Conclusion: Hormone replacement therapy may aid in protecting postmenopausal women residents against the polycythemia of high altitude.

	Age 40-49	Age 50-59	Age 60-69	Age 70 +
Premeno w/o HRT	14.80±.21 n = 23	–	–	–
Postmeno w/o HRT	15.18 ±.43 n = 11	16.40 ±.96	16.34 ±.33 n = 8	16.7 ±.66 n = 5 n = 8
Postmeno w/ HRT	14.63 ±.78 n = 3	14.72 ±.29	15.5 ±.26 n = 16	14.45 ± 1.45 n = 5 n = 2

A Randomised, Double Blind, Placebo Controlled Trial Of The Effect Of Inhaled Nedocromil Sodium Or Salmeterol Xinafoate On The Citric Acid Cough Threshold In Subjects Travelling To High Altitude. [3]
Bakewell SE, Hart ND, Wilson CM, McMorrow R, Collier D, Williams D, Barry PB. Medical Expeditions. 19 Cambridge Road, Girton, Cambridge CB3 0PN, UK.

Debilitating dry cough is a common complaint at high altitude. The cause is unknown, but we postulated that it may be due to inflammatory changes in the lung. We have investigated the effect of two medicated inhalers on high altitude cough. Citric acid cough threshold (CACT) was measured at sea level and subjects randomised into four groups. They received either nedocromil sodium 4mg twice daily (Tilade, Rhone Poulenc Rorer), salmeterol xinafoate 50mcg twice daily (Serevent, Glaxo Wellcome), placebo two actuations twice daily, or no inhaler. They used the inhalers for two weeks prior to departure and for the duration of the trek to 5,000m. CACT was measured by inhaling increasing concentrations of nebulised citric acid (Easimist, Sonix, Lutterworth, UK). CACT is the lowest concentration of citric acid that provokes cough, if the next concentration also provokes cough. Paired data were obtained from 13 subjects taking nedocromil sodium, 10 taking salmeterol, and 22 controls (no inhaler or placebo). In the control group, the ratio of CACT at sea level compared with base camp, expressed as the geometric mean difference, is 1.66 (95% confidence intervals 1.04 to 2.64, p=0.035). In contrast, there is no significant change in CACT for the salmeterol (p=0.88) or Tilade (p=1.0) groups. There was no significant difference in the change in CACT between the treatment and placebo groups determined by analysis of variance (p=0.381). We have demonstrated a reduction in CACT on arrival at 5,000m in the

---

[1]presented as *Hot Topic in Mountain Medicine*; [2]presented as *Hot Topic in Hypoxia*; [3]*oral poster communication.*

control group that was not seen in the salmeterol or nedocromil sodium groups. However, the small numbers in the study mean that the hypothesis that salmeterol or tilade reduce high altitude cough is not proven. We thank the subjects, Medical Expeditions, Liverpool University, Glaxo Wellcome, Rhone Poulenc Rorer and Clement Clarke International.

Nasal Peak Inspiratory Flow During A Simulated Ascent To Extreme Altitude - Operation Everest III.

Barry PW , NP Mason, JP Richalet. ARPE, Laboratoire de Physiologie, UFR de Medicine, 93012 Bobigny, France.

INTRODUCTION: The upper respiratory tract warms and humidifies inspired air. At high altitude increased ventilation of cold, dry air overcomes this mechanism, leading to mucosal damage. Subjective nasal blockage and impaired nasal mucociliary function occurs at altitude (1). To measure this change and determine if it is due to the inhalation of cold, dry air we measured nasal peak inspiratory flow (NPIF) at altitude under controlled environmental conditions. METHODS: Seven subjects recorded NPIF, oral peak inspiratory and expiratory flow (OPIF, OPEF) using a modified turbine spirometer at sea level (SL) and simulated altitudes of 5000 and 8000m. Temperature was maintained between 16 and 26° C, and relative humidity between 30 and 60%. Results were analysed by linear modelling of spirometric measurements against altitude. RESULTS: NPIF increased by a mean of 16% (95% CI, 7-25%) between SL and 8000m. OPIF and OPEF increased by 47% (95% CI 36-58%) and 31% (95% CI 24-38%) respectively. Linear modeling gives an increase of 0.086 l/s per 1000m ascent for NPIF; 0.40 l/s per 1000m for OPIF. OPEF increased by 0.38 l/s per 1000m, consistent with previous reports. CONCLUSION: NPIF increases with altitude to a lesser extent than OPIF, suggesting flow limitation in the nose. This may be due to nasal blockage at altitude, and occurred despite controlled environmental conditions. The hypothesis that nasal dysfunction at altitude is due to the inhalation of cold dry air is not supported. Further studies are required to see if the reduction in NPIF limits performance at altitude. References: Barry PW, Mason NP, O'Callaghan C, Nasal mucocillary transport is impaired at altitude, Eur. Respir. J. (1997); 10: 35-37.

The Effect Of Protein Kinase C Inhibition On Canine Hypoxic Pulmonary Vasoconstriction.

Barman Scott A. , Ph.D. Department of Pharmacology and Toxicology, Medical College of Georgia, Augusta, Georgia, U.S.A.

The objective of this study was to determine the role of protein kinase C (PKC) in the canine pulmonary vascular response to hypoxia. Two experimental models were used: 1) the isolated blood perfused dog lung and, 2) isolated canine pulmonary arteries and veins. Pulmonary vascular resistances in the isolated dog lung were measured using vascular occlusion techniques, and isometric tension was measured in the isolated blood vessels via strain gauge transducers. In cyclooxygenase pretreated isolated dog lungs, hypoxic exposure to $95\%N_2/5\%$ CO_2 (PO_2 < 50 mm Hg) increased total pulmonary vascular resistance and capillary pressure by increasing precapillary resistance and postcapillary resistance. In isolated endothelial denuded pulmonary vessels, the same degree of hypoxia increased both pulmonary arterial and venous tension. The non-specific protein kinase C inhibitor calphostin C (10-7 M) blocked the pressor response to hypoxia, the specific protein kinase C isoform inhibitor GO 6976 (10-7 M; inhibitor of the a and b isoforms) partially blocked the hypoxic pressor response (50% inhibition), while the less specific PKC isoform inhibitor GO 6983 (10-7 M; inhibitor of the a, b, g, d, and z isoforms) had a greater effect on the hypoxic pressor response (80% inhibition) in both the isolated lung and the isolated blood vessels. Previous

[1]presented as *Hot Topic in Mountain Medicine*; [2]presented as *Hot Topic in Hypoxia*; [3]*oral poster communication.*

identification by this laboratory of specific protein kinase C isoforms in the canine pulmonary vasculature using western blots revealed the presence of the a, d, and i isoforms in both pulmonary arterial and venous smooth muscle cells. Collectively, these data indicate that the canine pulmonary vascular response to hypoxia may involve activation of protein kinase C, specifically PKCa and PKCd, and that isolated canine pulmonary blood vessels mimic the hypoxic vasoactive response that occurs in the intact pulmonary vasculature.

Recommended Changes In Lake Louise Acute Mountain Sickness (AMS) Scoring System.

Beazley M. , P. Hillenbrand, B. Johnson, P.J.G. Forster, A.D.Wright, C.H.E. Imray and Members of BMRES. The Medical School, University of Birmingham, Edgbaston, Birmingham B15 2TJ, U.K.

The Lake Louise scoring system is a useful grading of key symptoms of AMS in a standard format. We have previously made suggestions to improve the clarity of the wording. Our recent experience in a scientific study of cerebral oxygenation however showed that a better quantitation of CNS symptoms required the addition of the question of ataxia, which forms part of the clinical assessment rather than the self report score. We suggest ataxia is added to the self-report questionnaire and the same number of questions is offered regardless of the time of day. The criteria of a score of 3 or more indicating AMS, remains.

Headache a.m.
0 no headache
1 mild headache
2 moderate headache
3 severe headache

Appetite
0 normal appetite
1 loss of appetite
2 nausea
3 vomiting

Dizziness
0 not dizzy
1 mild dizziness
2 moderate dizziness
3 severe dizziness

Sleep
0 slept as well as usual
1 did not sleep as well as usual
2 woke many times; poor night's sleep
3 could not sleep at all

p.m. Co-ordination
0 no loss of balance
1 mild unsteadiness
2 moderate unsteadiness
3 difficulty standing

Supported by the Arthur Thomson Trust and Mount Everest Foundation

Autonomic Modulation Of Cerebral Blood Flow At Altitude. [3]

Bernardi L, Bandinelli G, Passino C, Spadacini G, Bonfichi M, Arcaini L, Malcovati L, Boiardi A, Keyl C, Schneider A, Feil P, Greene E.R. Univ. Pavia-IRCCS S.Matteo, Pavia, S. Maria Nuova Hosp. Florence, IRCCS Besta, Milan, Italy, Univ. Regensburg, Germany, Highlands Univ., Las Vegas, NM, USA.

The effects of autonomic modulation on CBF at altitude are unknown. To assess the importance of autonomic modulation in determining altitude-induced changes in CBF we compared beat-to- beat changes in RR interval (RR), systolic and diastolic blood pressure (SBP and DBP, by Colin tonometry), CBF (transcranial Doppler velocimetry in the middle cerebral artery), CO_2, oxygen saturation (SaO_2) and respiration in 12 subjects at baseline (Kathmandu, 1000m, BL), upon arriving (HA1) at 5050m (Italian Pyramid Laboratory, Ev-K2-CNR, Lobuche, Nepal) after a 7-day ascent, and after 8 days at 5050m (HA2). Autonomic

---

[1]presented as *Hot Topic in Mountain Medicine*; [2]presented as *Hot Topic in Hypoxia*; [3]*oral poster communication.*

modulation on each signal was assessed by spectral analysis (0.03-0.15Hz: LF, marker of sympathetic activity; respiratory-synchronous fluctuations: HF, marker of parasympathetic activity on the heart and of mechanic effect of changes in stroke volume on the circulation). Compared to BL, HA1 decreased mean RR interval, SaO_2 and CO_2, and increased mean SBP, DBP, CBF and ventilation (all p<0.001). Autonomic modulation to the heart showed a reduced variability, determining a decrease in both HF (despite increase in ventilation) and slight decrease in LF. SBP-LF and DBP-LF remained unchanged, while SBP-HF and DBP-HF increased, due to increased ventilation (P<0.01). All these data indicated only mild signs of sympathetic activation. Conversely, CBF global variability increased (p<0.01), due to a similar increase (p<0.05) in both LF and HF. At HA2, all data remained altered, but, due to the effects of acclimatisation, showed a trend toward a return to BL results. During exposure to high altitude CBF is primarily affected by changes in respiratory gases; hypoxia overrides the effect of reduced CO_2 and appears responsible for the observed generalised amplification of CBF fluctuations, regardless of their origin, i.e. autonomic (LF) or mechanic (HF).

Reduced Hypoxic Ventilatory Response With Preserved Blood Oxygenation In Yoga Trainees And Himalayan Buddist Monks At Altitude: Evidence Of Different Adaptive Strategy?

Bernardi L, Feil P, Spadacini G, Bandinelli G, Passino C, Bonfichi M, Arcaini L, Malcovati L, Boiardi A, Keyl C, Schneider A, Greene ER. Univ. Pavia-IRCCS S.Matteo, Pavia, S.Maria Nuova, Hosp. Florence, IRCCS Besta, Italy, Univ. Regensburg, Germany, Highlands Univ., Las Vegas, NM, USA.

To assess whether practice of yoga generates a different adaptative strategy at high altitude (HA) we measured hypoxic ventilatory response (HVR), minute ventilation (V_E) and oxygen saturation (SaO_2, Ohmeda), in 12 western yoga trainees (age 43± 3 years, mean ± SEM, Y) and in 12 age-matched western controls (C), all born and living at sea-level, at baseline (Kathmandu, 1000m, BL), upon arrival at 5050m (Italian Pyramid Lab, Ev-K2-CNR, Lobuche, Nepal) after a 7-day ascent (HA1) and after 8 days at 5050m (HA2); similar data were obtained in 42 HA natives living at 3800-4200m, as comparative examples of prevalently active (32 sherpas, 28±1 years SH) vs contemplative (yoga/meditation-oriented, 10 Buddhist monks, 31±3 years, MK) lifestyles. At BL V_E and SaO_2 were similar in Y and C; HVR was lower in Y (-.78 ±.18 vs -2.03±.52 L/min/%SaO_2, p<0.05). At HA1, HVR remained lower in Y (-.85±.15 vs -2.81±.94 L/min/% SaO_2, p<0.05), but SaO_2 was similar in both groups (85.4±1.2 vs 85.8±.9%, p:ns). Only at HA2 was HVR increased (p<0.05) in Y compared to BL, but remained lower than in C (-1.75±.41 vs -3.65±.76, p<0.05); unlike in C, V_E did not increase in Y from BL to HA1; only at HA2 did V_E increase in Y compared to BL, reaching values similar to C. Similarly, MK had lower HVR compared to SH (-.41±.13 vs -2,07±.34, p<0.01); these values were similar to Y and C at HA1, respectively, whereas SaO_2 and V_E values were not different between groups. Practice of yoga (in western Y) or yoga-like meditative lifestyle (in MK) seems associated to reduced HVR and blunted/delayed increase in V_E at altitude, but without reduction of resting oxygen saturation, likely as a result of more efficient respiration.

[1]presented as *Hot Topic in Mountain Medicine*; [2]presented as *Hot Topic in Hypoxia*; [3]*oral poster communication.*

Renal Sensitivity To Vasopressin In Man After Six Days At High Altitude.
Bestle, M. H., L. J. Andersen, T. D. Poulsen, N. V. Olsen, I. L. Kanstrup and P. Bie.
Department of Clinical Physiology, Herlev Hospital and Department of Medical Physiology,
University of Copenhagen, Denmark.

Water balance - regulated through changes in plasma osmolality (pOSM) and plasma vasopressin (pAVP) - is often negative at high altitude. Previously we found that pAVP was reduced at high altitude despite an increased pOSM. However, the pAVP response to hypertonic saline infusion was not abolished at high altitude. Renal sensitivity to AVP is unchanged in acute hypobaric hypoxia (4 hours, PB=505 mmHg ~ 3500 meter above sea level). However, it remains unknown whether several days of hypoxia changes renal sensitivity to AVP. This study investigated the antidiuretic response to infusion of AVP in six male volunteers at sea level and after six days at high altitude (4559 meter above sea level). Water diuresis was induced by an oral water load (2% of body weight) and sustained by intermittent drinking. After 1 hour an infusion of AVP (5 pg/kg/min) was administered intravenously over 2 hours. In response to AVP, urine flow rate decreased at sea level from 15.5±1.0 to 2.9±1.0 ml/min and at high altitude from 15.9±2.0 to 2.8±0.9 ml/min (both p<0.05). Free-water clearance decreased (p<0.05) from 12.8±0.8 to -0.8±0.7 ml/min at sea level and from 13.1±1.8 to 0.9±0.7 ml/min at high altitude. The responses did not differ between sea level and high altitude. In conclusion, renal sensitivity to AVP is unchanged after several days at high altitude.

Ion Channel Inactivation In Hypoxia-Tolerant Neurons-- A Key To Surviving Anoxia? [2]
Bickler P.E. , L.T. Buck[1], and P. H. Donohoe. Department of Anesthesia, UCSF and [1]Dept. Zoology, Univ. Toronto.

Cerebral neurons from painted turtles (Chrysemys) survive anoxia 25,000 times longer than their mammalian counterparts. During 2h of anoxia, [Ca2$^+$]i in turtle neurons increases 20%, whereas [Ca2$^+$]i rises 5-20 fold in mammalian neurons in 5-10 minutes. We hypothesized that turtle neurons are able to avoid Ca2$^+$/glutamate excitotoxicity, which characterizes hypoxia-stressed mammalian neurons, in part by decreasing the activity of ion channels responsible for Ca2$^+$ influx, such as the NMDA type glutamate receptor. With cell-attached patch clamping we found that open probability of the NMDA receptor decreased about 40% after 90 min of anoxia, and with fura-2 fluorescence microscopy, we found that Ca2$^+$ influx via the NMDA receptor was reduced by 60%. The mechanism of inactivation might be phosphorylation/ dephosphorylation of the receptor. The turtle NMDA receptor is activated by protein kinase A, a process which usually involves the Ca2$^+$-dependent activation of PKA via calmodulin and cyclic AMP. While stimulating PKA resulted in receptor activation during both anoxic and normoxic conditions, inhibition of calmodulin only decreased receptor activity, suggesting that increases in [Ca2$^+$]i during anoxia are uncoupled from receptor activation. Furthermore, preventing calcium-dependent actin-NMDA receptor depolymerization did not prevent inactivation. NMDA receptor inactivation could be prevented by inhibiting protein phosphatase 1/2A, but not calcineurin (phosphatase 2b). Preventing receptor inactivation during anoxia with forskolin resulted in cell death (vital dyes), and histologic damage (cell damage in fixed sections). We conclude that NMDA receptor downregulated during anoxia is complex, and involves suppression of normal activation pathways and activation of inactivation mechanisms including dephosphorylation by protein phosphatase 1/2A. These findings may provide clues as to how to increase the hypoxia tolerance of mammalian neurons.

[1]presented as *Hot Topic in Mountain Medicine*; [2]presented as *Hot Topic in Hypoxia*; [3]*oral poster communication.*

Lifestyle Influences Hematological Adaptation To High Altitude In Himalayan Native And Western Populations.

Bonfichi, M., L. Bernardi, L. Malcovati, L. Arcaini, A. Balduini, C. Passino, G. Spadacini, P. Feil, C.Keyl, A.Schneider, A. Boiardi, G.Bandinelli, R.E. Greene, C. Bernasconi. IRCCS Policlinico S. Matteo -Univ. of Pavia, IRCCS Besta, Milan, UO SM Nuova, Florence, Italy; Univ, Regensburg, Germany, Highlands Univ. Las Vegas NM, USA.

To assess to what extent hematological parameters and non-genetic factors such as lifestyle might contribute to HA adaptation we measured (Coulter ATC8) Hemoglobin (Hb), Hematocrit (Ht), and soluble transferrin receptor (sTFR, from frozen blood samples, maintained in liquid nitrogen vapors) at baseline (Kathmandu, BL) and upon arrival at 5050m (Pyramid Italian Research Lab. Ev-K2-CNR Project) after 1-week ascent (HA1) and after 8 day sojourn at 5050m (HA2) in 24 western-sea-level residents (12 yoga trainees, Y, and 12 controls, C), 26 Sherpas (SH) and 13 Buddist monks (M), all living permanently at 3800-4500m. Y and M were considered as examples of contemplative lifestyle of their respective ethnic groups, as compared to C and SH, respectively. At HA1, Hb, Ht and sTFR increased to similar values in C and Y, but at HA2 there was no further increase in Y and Hb and Ht remained lower than C (Hb: 14.7±.6 vs 15.8±.9g/dl.p<0.05; Ht: 43.1 ±4.7 vs 47.3±3.1% p<0.05). M had Hb and Ht values lower than SH (Hb: 14.9±1.7 vs 16.4±1.5g/dl. p<0.01; Ht: 43.3±4.6 vs 49.7±5.1% p<0.001).; At HA2, C reached Hb and Ht values similar to SH, whereas Y reached values similar to M. Thus optimal chronic adaptation to HA in native Himalayan populations is achieved by only moderate increase in Hb and Ht in active subjects, or, in contemplative subjects, by values similar to those found at SL in western controls. Lifestyle (probably in addition to specific breathing techniques, which are part of everyday practice of both Y and M) is thus an important factor in determining the hematological pattern of adaptation to hypoxia induced by subacute or chronic exposure to high altitude.

Central Adaptative Processes Under Prolonged Hypoxic Stress During A Simulated Ascent Of Mount Everest : Operation Everest III (Comex ' 97).

Bouquet C., Richalet JP., Joulia F., Abraini JH. Laboratoire de Neurosciences Cellulaires et Intégratives, Université Henri Poincaré Nancy 1, Faculté des Sciences, BP 239, 54506 Vandoeuvre-Les-Nancy, cedex, France. A.R.P.E., Faculté de Médecine 93017 Bobigny France.

The psychosensorimotor and reasonning processes of eight subjects were investigated during a 31-day simulated climb of Mount Everest in a decompression chamber (Operation Everest III). Tests of visual reaction time, psychomotor hability (pegboard psychomotor test) and number ordination (Rey's test) were used. Subjects were compared to a control group evaluated at sea level during the same period. Repeated testing led to a learning effect in both the climbers and control subjects. Climbers performance increased up to an altitude of 5,500-6,500 m. Above this altitude, the climbers' psychomotor performance and mental efficiency deteriorated progressively, leading to significant differences in psychomotor ability and mental efficiency between control subjects and climbers (9 and 13 % respectively at 8,000 m and 17,5 and 16,5 % respectively at 8,848 m). 72 hours after the climbers had returned to sea level their mental performances were still significantly lower than those of control subjects (by approximately 10 %). In contrast, visual reaction time showed no significant changes in either climbers or control subjects. Number ordination can be considered as a task requiring working memory processes since such processes have been recently defined as the storage and manipulation of informations (whereas short-term memory would require only storage) and is thought to depend greatly of the prefrontal cortex. Motor hability, such as visual

[1]presented as *Hot Topic in Mountain Medicine*; [2]presented as *Hot Topic in Hypoxia*; [3]*oral poster communication.*

reaction time depend greatly of the basal ganglia system and is known requiring the implicite memory involved in sensorimotor learning. Since these two task are unequaly affected by hypoxia, our data mainly suggest that chronic hypoxic stress could alter explicit (working memory), rather than implicit (stimulus-response learning processes) memory and cortico-limbic rather than basal ganglia-sensorimotor system fonction. With grants from the Region Provence Alpes Cote d'Azur.

Hypophagia-Induced Hypometabolism In Anemic Or Hypoxemic Rats.

Bozzini CE, Norese, MF, Lezón CE. Department of Physiology, University of Buenos Aires, MT de Alvear 2142, Buenos Aires (1122), and Bio Sidus S.A., Argentina.

Several well-known biological responses occur in mammals to compensate hypoxic stress. These range between the reduction in O_2 consumption (VO_2) and energy production, by conforming aerobic metabolism to O_2 availability, and the increment of O_2 convection and extraction. We have previously shown that depression of appetite and hypophagia also occur in hypobaria-induced hypoxemia in young rats, with normal protein utilization for growth and consequent lowering of body growth rate. The present study was designed to test the hypothesis that reduced food intake drives the hypometabolic response to both anemic and hypoxemic forms of hypoxia. Episodes of anemia were created in adult male rats by either blood withdrawal through cardiac puncture (hemorrhagic anemia) or phenylhidrazine administration (hemolytic anemia). Hematocrit, VO_2 and food consumption were serially measured in all animals during either 7 days (acute experiments) or 17 days (chronic experiments). Positive correlations were found between the three parameters during developing of and recovery from anemia during each anemic episode. When the amount of food offered to non-anemic rats was equalized to that freely eaten by anemic rats, VO_2 dropped in the former to the level found in the latter. Both food intake and VO_2 were similarly affected during continuous exposure of rats to air maintained at 0.5 atm in a simulated altitude chamber. Hypobaria-induced changes in both parameters were not affected by either previous acclimation or transfusion-induced polycythemia, treatments that improved O_2 convective transport. Data thus confirmed the hypothesis. It is thus suggested that hypometabolism in mammals, which has been considered as an immediate, emergency-type response to hypoxia, can be considered as a response secondary to hypophagia because of depressed appetite. The recently reported raised serum leptin concentrations at high altitude associated with loss of appetite give support to the hypothesis.

Can Acute Mountain Sickness Be Induced By Exercise?

Bradwell AR, D Williams, M Beazley, CHE Imray and BMRES. The Medical School, University of Birmingham, Birmingham B15 2TJ, U.K.

Anecdotal reports of acute mountain sickness (AMS) occurring after severe exercise at altitude are well documented but studies comparing subjects ascending to altitude by foot or mechanised transport show similar incidence of AMS. However, severe exercise at altitude does produce arterial desaturation, which might increase cerebral hypoxia and hence provoke AMS. To assess the effect of exercise on cerebral oxygenation five men were studied (aged 25-38) on an exercise bicycle in Birmingham (150m) and at 3,450m after 4 days of acclimatisation. The test comprised gradually increasing workload to maximum heart rate, over a fifteen-minute period. Changes in regional oxygen saturation were assessed using continuous, non-invasive, near infra-red spectroscopy (NIRs). Criticon 2020 monitors were placed over the frontal cortex and soleus muscle whilst digital pulse oximetry was measured using an Ohmeda 3770. At sea level, there was no reduction in cerebral oxygen saturation at maximum exercise whilst, at altitude, four subjects showed between 5 and 25% reduction.

---

[1]presented as *Hot Topic in Mountain Medicine*; [2]presented as *Hot Topic in Hypoxia*; [3]*oral poster communication.*

The fifth subject showed no change at altitude but was a smoker, exercised least and had an anomalous response at sea-level. Cerebral oxygen saturation reduced progressively during the exercise test but the rate of fall increased above 85% maximum heart rate. Soleus muscle regional oxygen saturation reduced earlier and to a greater extent than that of the brain. Digital pulse oximetry paralleled the changes in cerebral oxygenation. In this preliminary study, severe exercise clearly leads to reduced cerebral oxygenation at altitude. It is known that arterial PO_2 falls on exercise at altitude because of oxygen diffusion-limitation in the lungs and increased extraction of oxygen by the muscles. It appears that dilatation of cerebral arteries cannot compensate for the increased arterial desaturation and may be aggravated by hypocapnia resulting from the hyperventilation of exercise. Thus, severe exercise at altitude increases cerebral hypoxia and when prolonged, could provoke or exacerbate AMS. Supported by the Arthur Thomson Trust and Mount Everest Foundation.

Women At Altitude: Free Radical Production And Vitamin E Status At 4300 m.
Bradford[1] S. , B. Braun[2], S. Zamudio[3], P. Rock[4], M. Traber[5], J. Liu[6], B. Ames[6], and G. Butterfield[2]. [1]University, Palo Alto, CA; [2]VA Health Care System, Palo Alto, CA; [3]University of Colorado, Denver, CO; [4]United State Army Research Institute for Environmental Medicine, Natick, MA; [5]Oregon State University, Corvallis, OR, and [6]University of California, Berkeley CA.

High altitude (HA) has been implicated in the generation of free radicals (FR), and possible increased need for anti-oxidant nutrients such as Vitamin E (VitE) (Simon-Schnass, J. Nutr. 122:778-781, 1992). To evaluate the effect of HA (4301m) exposure on FR production and VitE status, 15 healthy, eumenorrheic women ([All data as Mean±SD] 23±4 yrs; 157.5±8.02cm; 70.6±11.76 kg) were studied over 12 days both at sea level (SL) and HA while consuming a diet replete in VitE (20.3±3.6 mg/d). Energy intake was sufficient to maintain bd wt. Eight women, randomly assigned, were treated with prazosin (6 mg/d), an a-adrenergic blocking agent administered in conjunction with the larger study in which this study of FR was imbedded. Resting plasma samples were drawn on Days 1 and 12 at SL, and Days 1, 3 and 12 at altitude. Samples were separated, frozen at -20°C and later analyzed for malonyldialdehyde (MDA) and a- and g- tocopherol concentrations. Repeated measures two way ANOVA (p>0.05) indicated no significant difference between blocked and unblocked subjects for the parameters measured and in subsequent analyses data were pooled. Repeated measures one-way ANOVA (p>0.05) confirmed that MDA levels were significantly higher on day 3 at HA (127.2±35.4 pmol/ml) than at SL (109.4±27.7 pmol/ml) or on Day 1 (104.2±33.4 pmol/ml) or Day 12 (107.7±20.1 pmol/ml) at HA. a-tocopherol concentration appeared to rise with time at HA, being 26.5±6.7 uM on Day 12 at HA and 25.0±9.7 uM on Day 1, although the increase did not reach statistical significance (p=0.07), nor were the means significantly different from SL (23.0±5.2 uM). g-tocopherol concentration did not change with HA exposure as compared to SL, nor did it change with time of HA exposure. Thus, although HA may transiently increase FR production, as indicated by increased circulating MDA, there was no measurable negative effect of this increase on short term VitE status, as monitored by blood concentrations, in these women exposed to HA for 12 days. There is no apparent need to increase dietary VitE at HA when the diet is adequate. Supported in part by DOD grant #DAMD 17-95-C5110.

[1]presented as *Hot Topic in Mountain Medicine*; [2]presented as *Hot Topic in Hypoxia*; [3]*oral poster communication*.

Women At Altitude: Glucoregulation During Exercise At 4300m And During Sea Level Exercise At The Same Absolute And Relative Intensity.

Braun[1] B , GE Butterfield[1], S Muza[2], RS Mazzeo[3], LG Moore[4]. [1]VA Health Care System, Palo Alto, CA, [2]US Army Res. Inst. of Envir. Med., Natick, MA, [3]U. of Colorado, Boulder CO, [4]U. of Colorado Health Sciences Center, Denver CO.

We hypothesized that the glucoregulatory hormone response to exercise at 4300m (HA) would be similar to sea level (SL) exercise at the same relative intensity. 16 women (21.7yr, 167cm, 62.2kg) were studied. VO_2peak decreased from 42.0 ml/kg/min at SL to 32.2 at HA. On 2 separate occasions, subjects performed 45' of cycle ergometry at 52.1% (SL50) and 64.8% (SL65) of SL-VO_2peak. After 10 days at HA, subjects cycled at 51.1% SL-VO_2peak (same absolute intensity as SL-50) which was 66.0% HA-VO_2peak (same relative intensity as SL-65). Arterial blood samples were collected at rest and at 15',30',45' of exercise and assayed for plasma concentrations of glucose (GLU), lactate (LAC), insulin (INS), cortisol (CORT) and catecholamines (CATS). Results were:

	SL50		SL65		HA	
	rest	exer.	rest	exer.	rest	exer.
LAC (mM)	0.36	1.73	0.53	3.60	0.60	3.44
INS (pM)	81	31	63	20	58	21
CORT (nM)	219	296	212	415	234	515

Results for CATS paralleled those for CORT. GLU fell in response to exercise at SL but rose at HA. The data indicate that the glucoregulatory environment at 4300m in women is similar to previous data from men (Roberts et al. 1996). Unlike men however, who increased carbohydrate use, women in this study decreased blood glucose use and RER values were lower (Braun et al., in review). In women, the hormonal environment may promote fatty acid use but the pronounced rise in CORT also suggests increased utilization of protein. Supported by DOD #DAMD17-95-C5110.

Aspirin Versus Diamox Plus Aspirin For Headache Prevention During Physical Activity At High Altitude.

Burtscher M., M. Philadelphy, R. Likar, W. Nachbauer. Dept. of Sports Sciences, Medical Unit, University of Innsbruck, Austria.

Headache is known to be the most predominant symptom in acute mountain sickness (AMS). Because inhibitors of prostaglandin synthesis are effective for therapy and prophylaxis of high-altitude headache (HAH), it can be assumed that prostaglandins contribute to the development of HAH. Aspirin prevents HAH when vigorous exercise is avoided. However, it has been suggested that low arterial oxygen saturation (SaO_2) during physical activity at high altitude may counteract this preventive effect. To test this hypothesis, we compared aspirin and aspirin plus Diamox for prophylaxis of HAH in a randomized, double-blind trial. 30 volunteers were randomized to the aspirin group (AG: 12 men, 4 women, mean age: 39, 22-58) and to the aspirin plus Diamox group (ADG: 11 men, 3 women, mean age: 32, 24-53). They were taken from an altitude of 600 m (Innsbruck) to an altitude of about 3000 m from where they ascended on skis to an altitude of 3800 m. Then they descended to a mountain hut (3480 m) and stayed there for 3 days. Diamox (125 mg) or placebo was given 12 hr and 2 hr before arrival and aspirin (320 mg) was administered 3 times at 4-hr intervals, beginning 2 hr before arrival at high altitude (3480 m). Headache scores (0-3), SaO_2, heart rate and blood gases were determined repeatedly at rest and during physical activity. Nine subjects (8 men, 1 woman) out of the AG (n=16) and none out of the ADG (n=14) developed headache between 5 and 10 hr after arrival at 3480 m (p<0.001). In

---

[1]presented as *Hot Topic in Mountain Medicine*; [2]presented as *Hot Topic in Hypoxia*; [3]*oral poster communication.*

these subjects, effective relief was achieved by administration of naproxen (550 mg). While ascending on skis, mean (+SD) SaO_2 of the AG was 76.9+4.1 % and that of the ADG 82.1+3.6 % (p=0.001). Resting SaO_2 of the AG about 5 hours after arrival at high altitude (3480 m) was 86.1+2.1 % and that of the ADG 88.3+2.4 % (p=0.01). Whereas SaO_2 values during physical activity were not different between subjects of the AG who got sick and those who did not, resting SaO_2 values differed significantly (84.7+1.3 vs. 87.9+1.3, p<0.001). HAH scores and resting SaO_2 values were negatively related within the AG (r = -0.8, p<0.01). In a previous study one year ago, we could demonstrate that in the absence of physical activity, aspirin clearly prevented HAH under similar conditions and despite similar resting SaO_2 values. In the present investigation, more than 50 % of the subjects of the AG developed headache despite aspirin intake, which would suggest that physical activity reduces the efficacy of aspirin to prevent HAH. In contrast, Diamox plus aspirin increased SaO_2 during rest and physical activity and prevented HAH. Thus we assume that physical activity may enhance the incidence of HAH, at least partly by increasing cyclooxygenase activity with decreasing oxygenation. Therefore, a higher aspirin dosage or Diamox plus aspirin might be considered for prevention of HAH during physical activity.

Beneficial Effects Of Short Term Hypoxia.[2]

Burtscher M[1], Tsvetkova AM[2], Tkatchouk EN[2], Brauchle G[3], Mitterbauer G[1], Gulyaeva NV[2], Kofler W[3], [1]Dept. of Sport Science, University of Innsbruck, A-6020 Innsbruck, Austria; [2]The Clinical Research Lab. of the Hypoxia Medical Academy, Moscow Russia; [3]Dept. of Social Medicine, University of Innsbruck, Austria.

Increased cardiorespiratory exercise responses when exposed to acute hypoxia are well known. During acclimatization to hypoxia, such over-responses diminish and seem even to be reduced in subsequent normoxia. These effects are therapeutically used by the application of normobaric short term hypoxia. However, the efficacy of short term hypoxia has not been studied in placebo-controlled experiments. 28 healthy and voluntary sports students of the University of Innsbruck were randomized to the Hypoxia Group (HG, 8 men, 6 women; aged (mean[SD]) 21.0[2.7] years) or to the Placebo Group (PG, 8 men, 6 women; aged 21.8[1.5] years) in a double blind fashion. After an incremental spiroergometric pre-test (Oxycon Alpha, Jaeger) participants underwent a 4 week breathing program (5 sessions per week). For the HG each session consisted of 3 to 7 hypoxic (11%-9% oxygen via face mask, HypoxiComplex HypO2, HypoMed) periods (3 to 6 min) with 3 to 5 min normoxic intervals. The PG inhaled normoxic air in the same way. Physical activity was standardized throughout the study. Incremental spiroergometric tests (50 watts increase each minute until exhaustion) were repeated five days and once again one month after completing the breathing program. Differences of mean values between groups were tested by Student's t-tests for independent samples and by ANOVA for repeated measurements. Performance and spiroergometric variables before the breathing program revealed no differences between the groups studied. Five days after the breathing program, however, differences between the HG and the PG were found for exercising heart rates at 150 watts (134.9[13.2] beats/min vs. 145.6[12.8] beats/min, p=0.04) and exercising minute ventilation at 150 watts (48.7[3.8] l/min vs. 53.7[7.9] l/min, p=0.045). Stroke volume determinations indicated that lower heart rates in the HG were compensated by an increased stroke volume (p=0.08). The double product (heart rate multiplied by systolic blood pressure) as an indirect measure for myocardial oxygen consumption was also reduced at 150 watts for the HG compared with the PG (19881±2068 vs. 21647±2224, p=0.04). Although these parameters still tended to be lower for the HG one month after completing the breathing program, differences did not reach significance. Such effects are similar to those observed after prolonged altitude exposure or due to beta-adrenoceptor blocking without, however, diminished maximum heart rates and performance.

---

[1]presented as *Hot Topic in Mountain Medicine*; [2]presented as *Hot Topic in Hypoxia*; [3]*oral poster communication.*

It is suggested that the repeated application of short term hypoxia reduces sympathoadrenergic exercise responses. Since the reduction of those responses enhances exercise tolerance and reduces mortality in patients with heart disease, short term hypoxia might be considered for therapeutic use.

Naproxen For Therapy Of High-Altitude Headache.

Burtscher M., M. Philadelphy, R. Likar, W. Nachbauer. Dept. of Sports Sciences, Medical Unit, University of Innsbruck, Austria.

Non-steroidal anti-inflammatory drugs like ibuprofen and aspirin were shown to be effective against high-altitude headache1-3. Whereas ibuprofen has been used therapeutically aspirin has been used prophylactically for high-altitude headache. We hypothesised that inhibitors of prostaglandin synthesis other than ibuprofen or aspirin may also be effective in the treatment of high-altitude headache. Therefore, we tested naproxen in a controlled experiment. 32 volunteers (20 males, 12 females, mean age 29, range 20-58) participated in a high-altitude experiment in July 1998. They were transported from Innsbruck (600 m) to an altitude of about 3000 m (bus, cable car) from where they ascended on skis to an altitude of 3800 m. Then they descended to a mountain hut (3480 m) and stayed there for 3 days. Participants were pre-treated with aspirin and diamox. When a headache score of 2 or higher (0=none, 1=mild, 2=moderate, 3=severe) was reported despite pre-treatment, naproxen (550 mg) was given. Scoring was repeated two hours after drug intake. Nutrition and physical activity were standardised throughout the study. 5 to 15 hours after arrival at high-altitude, 7 persons (4 males, 3 females, mean age 36, range 23-52) developed headache (score of 2 or higher) despite pre-treatment. Three of those subjects also complained of nausea. After naproxen (550 mg) therapy, complete relief of headache and nausea occurred in all patients within two hours (p=0.018). None of them needed further medication. No adverse effects were observed. These results support the hypothesis that inhibitors of prostaglandin synthesis other than ibuprofen or aspirin are also effective in the treatment of high-altitude headache. Pre-treatment was not fully sufficient probably due to the effects of low oxygen saturation (sometimes < 80 %) during physical activity at high altitude. Because additional inhibition of prostaglandin synthesis promptly relieved headache and nausea, a dosage-dependent effectiveness of those drugs on headache and the associated nausea can be assumed. Although not to go too high too fast remains the golden rule, in certain circumstances inhibitors of prostaglandin synthesis, preferably those with few gastrointestinal side effects, can offer sufficient headache relief at high-altitude.

Transient Cerebral Ischemia At Extreme Altitude During A Simulated Ascent Of Mount Everest.

Cauchy E. , P. Larmignat, J.P.Richalet. A.R.P.E. Laboratoire de Réponse Cellulaire et Fonctionnelles à l'Hypoxie, Bobigny ; D.M.T.M. Département de Médecine et de Traumatologie de Montagne Chamonix, France.

At high altitude transient neurological disorders are often seen but badly described. During a simulated ascent of Mount Everest by eight climbers in a hypobaric chamber (Operation Everest III, COMEX, 1997), three of them experienced problems promoting a transient cerebral ischemia. Clinical observation in the chamber allowed a better study of the location and circumstances of these problems. The first episode occurred on one of the subjects at 8000 m and looked like aura of Sylvien territory during a migraine attack. The symptoms disappeared in less than one hour with O_2. The CT scan, and the MRI, the evoked auditive potential and the vestibulary exam during the next 24 h were normal. The second

---

[1] presented as *Hot Topic in Mountain Medicine*; [2] presented as *Hot Topic in Hypoxia*; [3] *oral poster communication.*

episode occurred at 8848 m on an other subject and looked like a state of confusion without focalization. The symptoms disappeared in 45 min with O_2. The MRI was normal during the next 24 h. The third episode wich occurred at 8848 m as well on a third subject came from vertebro-basillary territory. The symptoms disappeared in less than 3 min with O_2. The MRI was normal during the next 24 h. No direct correlation has been reached between the appearance and the value of the following blood parameters: $PaCO_2$, PaO_2, pH, hematocrite, haemoglobinemia, nor with AMS results compared to the unaffected subjects. Nevertheless the analysis of the circumstances of the appearance allowed us to consider other hypotheses in addition to the hypocapnic vasoconstriction theory; a segmentary spastic theory of the accompanied migraine and the theory of clotting in the young subject (patent foramen ovale, mitral-valve prolapse), by migration of thrombi or gas emboli produced by the quick variation of pressure during experiences in a hypobaric chamber. The increase of intrathoracic pressure during effort with blocked respiration could play a role as well.

Can Excessive iNOS Induction Explain Much Of The Illness Of Acute Mountain Sickness?[1]

Clark I.A. , M. M. Awburn, W. B. Cowden, and K. A. Rockett*
Australian National University, Canberra, ACT 200, Australia and *University of Oxford, John Radcliffe Hospital, Oxford OX3 9DU, UK.

Our field of research is the pathogenesis of falciparum malaria, and the similarity of the severe manifestations seen in this disease and severe AMS, even though one is infectious and the other not, has intrigued us for some time. Histology, particularly of the brain, has remarkable similarities. Like the toxin released from the malaria parasite, hypoxia strongly generates the inducible form of nitric oxide synthase (iNOS). Our current experiments (done in collaboration with the Wellcome Trust Centre, Blantyre, Malawi), indicate, by immunohistochemistry, that iNOS is strongly upregulated in key locations in fatal cases of falciparum malaria. Nitrotyrosine, a footprint for the degree and extent of nitric oxide generation, is also greatly increased. We have also found that an inducer of inflammatory cytokines produces much more nitric oxide from human cells in vitro under hypoxic conditions. We therefore propose that these two diseases are similar because they are both systemic examples of hypoxia and inflammatory cytokines synergising to generate iNOS. In our malaria studies, this model has allowed us to rationalise the difference between falciparum malaria and the much milder vivax form, in which tissue hypoxia is absent. It could explain, in terms of whether or not low levels of inflammatory cytokines (from infection, cold stress, or extreme exertion) are present to synergise with hypoxia, the unpredictability of onset of severe symptoms of acute mountain sickness. Our model can be tested to explain many of the changes, central to both diseases, that severe AMS shares with falciparum malaria. It also provides a novel mechanism for acclimatisation as a climb proceeds.

Carbon Dioxide Or Oxygen At Altitude? Cutaneous, Muscle And Cerebral Oxygenation.

Clarke T, S Walsh, D Mole, T Harvey, J Morgan, S Brearey, C Imray and the BMRES. Dept. Vascular Surgery, Walsgrave Hospital, Coventry, CV2 2DX, UK.

Objectives: Supplemental oxygen is of proven benefit in the treatment of acute mountain sickness (AMS). CO_2 has been proposed as an alternative. The aim of this study was to assess the effects of CO_2, O_2 and CO_2/O_2 mix on cutaneous, peripheral and cerebral tissue oxygenation at sea-level and at 3450m. Methods: Twelve subjects (ten men), aged 24-53, were studied at 150m and one month later, the morning after ascent to 3,450m by cable car.

[1]presented as *Hot Topic in Mountain Medicine*; [2]presented as *Hot Topic in Hypoxia*; [3]*oral poster communication.*

Continuous non-invasive near infra-red spectroscopy (NIRs) was used to measure regional saturation (rSO_2). A Contron cutaneous oximeter was placed on right forearm ($CutO_2$). Probes from two Critikon 2020 monitors (Johnson and Johnson Medical UK) were placed on the right soleus muscle (Musc), and the other over the right frontal lobe (Cer). Results:

		Baseline	3%CO_2	O_2	O_2/CO_2
rSO_2Musc	150m	73.0(2.3)	73.2(2.2)	73.7(2.2)*	74.0(2.5)*	
rSO_2Musc	3450m	64.4(3.7)	68.9(3.6)*	70.3(3.6)*	71.2(3.9)*
rSO_2Cer	150m	69.9(2.6)	70.6(2.5)*	70.3(2.6)*	71.0(2.6)*	
rSO_2Cer	3450m	65.6(2.8)	66.7(3.2)*	68.8(2.9)*	70.2(3.8)*
$CutO_2$	3450m	5.3(1.7)	6.2(1.9)*	12.8(3.1)*	17.6(2.1)*

p<0.01 vs Baseline, Paired t test, Mean(SD).

Conclusion: This study confirms that CO_2 has a beneficial effect improving cutaneous, muscle and cerebral tissue oxygen saturation. The combination of CO_2 and O_2 appears to have a synergistic effect improving tissue oxygenation to a greater degree than either CO_2 or O_2 alone. Further investigation into a possible therapeutic role for the mix is indicated.

Moderate But Not Severe Hypoxia (H) Enhances The In Vitro Proliferation Of Tracheal Smooth Muscle Cells (TSMC).

Cogo A.L., M.C.Michoud, J.G.Martin. Meakins-Christie Laboratoires, McGill University, Montreal, Quebec, Canada, Institute of Respiratory Diseases, University of Ferrara, Italy.

Hypoxemia is known to induce pulmonary vascular remodeling in part due to vascular SMC proliferation. In vitro studies have focused on vascular SMC and no studies have examined the effect of H on in vitro proliferation of airway SMC. The aim of our study was to examine the effect of H on the growth of TSMC from Fisher rats. Cells (1st-5th passage) were plated in 24 well plates (104/ml) and immediately exposed to either normoxia (N), severe H (O21%, CO25% balance N2) or moderate H (O23%) and counted dailly from day 2 to day 4 (Group 1). Another set of cells (Group2), after 2 days growth in DMEM-10%FBS, was growth arrested (48hrs in DMEM-0,5%FBS) then stimulated with PDGF 10ng/ml and exposed for 48 hrs to either N, severe or moderate H. Cell growth was assessed by cell counting with a standard hemacytometer. Cells obtained from at least 6 rats were used for each experiment. Results are expressed as # of cells x10^4($\pm$SE) **= p<.05 H vs N.

Group1	day2	day3	day4	Group2	Control	PDGF
N		30.2(7)	58.5(5)	118(10)	46.2(4)	95.3(10.7)
H1%	21.8(5)	45.3(8)	82.3(11)		43.8(6)	62.8(9)**
H3%	42.3(8.1)	82(6.3)**	170.7(9.1)**		57.5(6)**	108.6(13.2)**

In severe H, TSMC grow at a lower rate and the response to mitogens is slightly but not significantly impaired. In contrast, in moderate Hcell growth is significantly enhanced both under baseline conditions and in the presence of mitogens. Moderate H seems therefore to have a mitogenic effect on TSMC. (Supported by MRC of Canada, Canadian Cystic Fibrosis Foundation and the J.T. Costello Memorial Research Fund).

[1]presented as *Hot Topic in Mountain Medicine*; [2]presented as *Hot Topic in Hypoxia*; [3]*oral poster communication.*

Near Infrared Spectroscopy: A Novel Method For High Altitude Research? [3]

Colier, Willy N.J.M. and Berend Oeseburg. Dept. of Physiology (237), Faculty of Medical Sciences, University of Nijmegen, P.O. Box 9101, 6500 HB Nijmegen, The Netherlands.

The most commonly used method to assess ones level of oxygenation at high altitude is pulse oximetry (POX). This is an easy to use device measuring arterial saturation. However, local differences in oxygenation changes can not be assessed. Using near infrared spectroscopy (NIRS), an optical technique with similarities to POX, this is possible. Using NIRS the oxygenation status and hemodynamics of organs like brain and muscle can be assessed non-invasively. The method is based on the fact that tissues are relatively transparent for light in the near infrared region of the light-spectrum, combined with the fact that tissues contain chromophores, mostly hemoglobin (Hb) and, in muscle, myoglobin (Mb), with oxygenation dependent light absorption characteristics. By using a number of different wavelengths the relative changes in concentrations of the Hb/Mb components can be displayed continuously and with a high temporal resolution. The method employs the use of fiber-optic light guides which are placed over the area of interest. In general, several cubic centimeters of tissue can be monitored. The figure shows an example of a significant increase in frontal brain oxygenation during a reaction time test (between dotted lines) at an altitude of 5200 m in a human subject. In muscle not only changes in oxygenation can be monitored but also the regional oxygen consumption of a muscle or muscle group can be calculated during a period of diminished or even ceased blood flow. This situation can be reached by, externally, applying an inflated cuff or, internally, by applying a workload to the muscle.

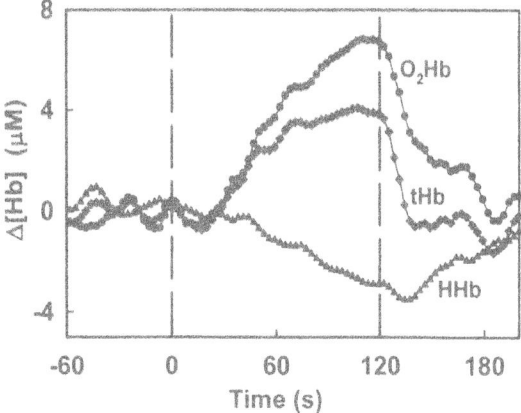

High Altitude Pulmonary Edema At 4559 M: A Population Study. [1]

Cremona G, Asnaghi R, Baderna P, Brunetto A, *Brutsaert T, Cavallaro C, *Clark T, ‡Cogo A, Donis R, Donner C, Lanfranchi P, *Luks A, Mazzuero G, Panzetta S, Perini L, *Putnam M, Spagnolatti L, *Wagner H, & *Wagner P. "S. Maugeri" Foundation IRCCS, Veruno, Italy, *Dept of Physiology, UCSD, USA, ‡Italian Alpine Club.

In order to characterise the functional characteristics of subjects who develop high altitude pulmonary edema (HAPE), 262 subjects (39 female, aged 40±12 yrs range 16-70) were studied at 1200 m (LA) and within an hour of reaching 4559 m (HA) on foot.

---

[1]presented as *Hot Topic in Mountain Medicine*; [2]presented as *Hot Topic in Hypoxia*; [3]*oral poster communication.*

Spirometry, gas transfer, ECG, blood pressure & clinical examinations were performed at LA and again at HA. Chest radiographs, Lake Louise scores and medical history were obtained at HA. Of these, 28 had a previous history of acute mountain sickness, 2 of high altitude cerebral edema and 2 of HAPE. Average FEV1, FVC were normal (103 ± 13 & 104 ± 13% pred) but covered a wide range (66-161%); DLCO was 117 ± 36 % pred. At HA SaO2 fell from 96 ± 2 to 77 ± 6 % with a range of 60 - 93%. ECG changes consisted mainly of right axis deviation and strain which were usually present at LA. DLCO rose to 133 ± 23 % pred but FEV1/FVC were unchanged. Fourteen subjects developed radiological evidence of HAPE while a further 27 exhibited clinical signs of mild HAPE (râles). No differences were found in age, sex, medical history, ECG and blood pressure in those subjects who developed HAPE. Lake Louise scores were marginally higher in subjects who developed HAPE. The data suggest that mild HAPE is not infrequent (15%) in healthy subjects exposed to high altitude for a short period of time when heavy exertion is undertaken.

Effect Of Simulated Altitude Exposure On Speech Motor Control And The Development Of Acute Mountain Sickness (AMS). [3]

Cymerman. A.[1], Lieberman, P.[2], Hochstadt, J.[2], Rock, P.B.1, Butterfield, G.E.[3], and Moore, L.G.[4] [1]U.S. Army Research Institute of Environmental Medicine, Natick, MA 01760, [2]Brown University, Providence, RI, [3]Palo Alto VA Health Care, Palo Alto, CA and [4]University of Colorado, Denver, CO.

Disturbances in cognition and speech motor control have been associated with high-altitude exposure and may involve selective hypoxic vulnerability of specific brain areas. Given the cerebral origin of AMS, we hypothesized that speech motor control as determined by voice onset timing (VOT) would be an objective measure of AMS. Fifteen women (24.7±1.8 yrs) were studied at sea level and after 4 and 39 h of simulated exposure to 4,300 m altitude. AMS was assessed twice daily using the cerebral factors of the Environmental Symptoms Questionnaire (ESQ-C). Speech motor control was determined from digitally recorded timing patterns of 60 monosyllabic words, representing three places of articulation (labial, alveolar, and velar) and further categorized as 'voiced' or 'unvoiced' (i.e., initial consonant timing <20 msec or >20msec, respectively). VOTs, defined as the time between the initial burst of air at the mouth and the beginning of vocal cord resonance for each word, were reduced at the labial site with 4 and 39 hrs of exposure. MD, the minimum timed distance between 'voiced' and 'unvoiced' consonants, was not affected by altitude. Timing differences between the places of articulation were preserved during altitude exposure. ESQ-C scores obtained at 39 h, but not at 4 h, significantly correlated with MDs derived from two places of articulation (labial, r= 0.73, P<0.01; velar, r= 0.63, P<0.02, respectively). VOT may be a promising new tool to objectively assess the severity of AMS.

Components Of Resting Pulmonary Co-Diffusing Capacity In Subjects Susceptible To HAPE.

Dams, C.[1], C. Schirlo[1], M. Maggiorini[2], J. Kohl[1] and E.A. Koller[1]. Institute of Physiology, University of Zurich[1]; Medical Department, University Hospital Zurich[2], Switzerland.

Hemodynamic alterations in the pulmonary capillary bed in subjects susceptible to HAPE (HAPE-S) are still largely unknown. In the present study we aimed to investigate the components of the pulmonary CO-diffusing capacity, membrane conductance and pulmonary capillary blood volume, in HAPE-S in comparison to healthy controls. 7 HAPE-S and 7 controls without a history of HAPE were examined on day 2 after the ascent to 4559 m and

---

[1]presented as *Hot Topic in Mountain Medicine*; [2]presented as *Hot Topic in Hypoxia*; [3]*oral poster communication*.

some of these subjects were additionally tested under normoxic conditions (Zürich, 473 m). Single-breath diffusing capacity for CO (SB-DLCO), membrane conductance (Dm) and pulmonary capillary blood volume (Qc) as well as total lung capacity (TLC) and alveolar volume (VA) were determined in the supine posture according to the method of Roughton and Forster. Particularly under hypoxic conditions, SB-DLCO was lower in HAPE-S compared to controls (35.7±3.9 ml*mmHg^{-1}*min^{-1}, mean±SD vs. 40.9±8.8 ml*mmHg^{-1}*min^{-1}, p=0,19). Moreover, VA was significantly smaller in HAPE-S than in controls (5.6±0.5 liters vs. 6.8 ±0,8 liters, P<0.01). No significant differences in Dm between groups were found either in normoxia or in prolonged hypoxia, whereas the Qc related to body surface area was higher in HAPE-S compared to controls and reached statistical significance at 4559 m (113.8±44.3 ml/m^2 vs. 72.3±15.7 ml/m^2, P<0.05). The results of the present study confirm a lower resting SB-DLCO in HAPE-S compared to C-S mainly related to a smaller VA in terms of a reduced available area for gas exchange. The finding of a higher pulmonary capillary blood volume during prolonged hypoxia is consistent with the overperfusion concept in the development of HAPE with heterogeneous vasoconstriction leading to high flow and high pressure in those capillaries not protected by vasoconstriction.

Pulmonary Co-Diffusing Capacity In Subjects Susceptible To HAPE: Effects Of Positional Changes.

Dams, C.[1], C. Schirlo[1], U. Scherrer[2], J. Kohl[1] and E.A. Koller[1]. Institute of Physiology, University of Zurich[1]; Department of Internal Medicine, University Hospital, Lausanne[2], Switzerland.

Pulmonary artery pressure and arterial oxygen saturation data suggest that body position has more pronounced effects on gas exchange in HAPE susceptible subjects (HAPE-S) than in controls. In 14 HAPE-S and 9 controls we examined posture dependent changes in pulmonary CO-diffusing capacity under normoxic conditions (Zurich, 473 m), and during short-term hypobaric hypoxia (4000 m for 90 min) in a decompression chamber. Single-breath diffusing capacity for CO (SB-DLCO), total lung capacity (TLC, measured by helium dilution), and vital capacity (VC) were determined in the sitting and in the supine position in randomized order. The major new findings were that when changing from the sitting to the supine position, SB-DLCO increased significantly (P<0.05) in controls both during normoxia (+5.9±3.6 ml*mmHg-1*min-1, mean±SD), and short-term hypoxia (+4.7±4.1 ml*mmHg^{-1}*min^{-1}). In contrast, in HAPE-S, SB-DLCO did not increase with positional changes from sitting to lying (normoxia, +1.4±2.6 ml*mmHg^{-1}*min^{-1}; hypoxia, -0.1±2.1 ml*mmHg^{-1}*min^{-1}), resulting in significantly lower SB-DLCO in the supine position compared to controls (P<0.01 for both normoxia and hypoxia). In addition, in comparison to controls, HAPE-S had a smaller TLC (sitting: 6.1±0.9 vs. 6.9±1.1 liters, lying: 5.6±0.9 vs. 6.5±1.1 liters, P<0.01), and smaller VC (sitting: 4.2±0.7 vs. 4.9±0.8 liters, lying: 3.9±0.7 vs. 4.7±0.8 liters). We conclude that in the supine position, HAPE-susceptible subjects have an impairment in pulmonary gas exchange. This impairment appears to be related to a lack of the normal increase in resting SB-DLCO when changing the body position from sitting to lying. We speculate that in HAPE-S this impairment of the pulmonary diffusing capacity in the supine position may be one of the factors contributing to exaggerated nocturnal hypoxic pulmonary vasoconstriction, and augmented incidence of HAPE after a night at high altitude.

[1]presented as *Hot Topic in Mountain Medicine*; [2]presented as *Hot Topic in Hypoxia*; [3]*oral poster communication.*

Peak Blood Lactate And Anaerobic Power After Acute And Chronic Altitude Exposure.
Davis J.E. , R.L. Brands, and J.D. Seelbach. Department of Exercise and Health Science,
Alma College, Alma, MI 48801.

The purpose of this study was to look at the effects of acute and chronic altitude exposure
on maximum anaerobic power and peak blood lactate. Six subjects (mean age = 20.2±0.75 yr,
mean weight = 67.0±5.5 kg) performed Wingate Anaerobic Power Tests at sea level (SL 1),
on acute exposure to 3400 m (ALT 1), two weeks following acclimatization at 3400 m (ALT
2), and upon return to sea level (SL 2). Maximum anaerobic power (MAnP) was considered
the highest power output during a standard 30-second Wingate Anaerobic Power Test. Blood
lactate was measured immediately after the anaerobic power test and periodically after the
test. Peak blood lactate ([BL]p) was taken as the highest blood lactate after the anaerobic
power test. MAnP decreased significantly (p<.05) from SL 1 (4950±733 kg/m/min) to ALT 2
(4718±728 kg/m/min) and from SL 1 to SL 2 (4543±705 kg. m/min). There was a significant
decrease in [BL]p from SL 1 (9.43±1.32 mmol/L) to SL 2 (8.51±91 mmol/L). These data
suggest that chronic exposure to altitude lowers MAnP and that MAnP remains depressed
upon return to sea level for the first two days. In addition, the decline in MAnP is
accompanied by a decline in [BL]p after chronic altitude exposure and upon return to sea
level.

**Pulmonary Artery Pressure Variation Measured By Dopper Echo Cardiography In
Healthy Subjects At 4250m.**
Dubowitz G, AJ Peacock. Pulmonary Vascular Unit, Western Infirmary Glasgow UK.

Hypoxia causes pulmonary vasoconstriction (HPV) which can be estimated using Echo-
Doppler cardiac ultrasound. We documented the prevalence of HPV and its relation to Acute
Mountain sickness (AMS) in a group of normal trekkers at 4250m in the Everest Region of
Nepal. Setting: HRA Pheriche Aid Post (4250m).Subjects: 58 volunteers. Exclusion criteria:
History of cardiopulmonary illness or inter-current illness (excluding AMS).Methods:
Subjects were screened for tricuspid regurgitation (TR), using Doppler echocardiography
(Esaote Biomedica "Challenge" Portable Colour Echo Doppler). Pulmonary artery systolic
pressure (PASP) was estimated from maximum TR velocity (Vmax), in the semi-reclining
position, using the modified Bernouilli equation (PASP=4Vmax2 +CVP). Oxygen saturation
(SaO$_2$) was measured simultaneously, using an oximeter (Nellcor NP20). Oxygen was then
administered via a mask at 4lpm for 15 minutes and PASP estimation repeated. AMS was
assessed using the "Lake Louise" Score. Results/Analysis of Results: 58 subjects: 11F, 47M.
33 had significant TR. There was no relationship of PASP to AMS score (8 subjects had
AMS). Pre-0$_2$ mean Vmax=2.18ms-1 (calculated PASP=25mmHg; range =17.67-
36.43mmHg). Post-0$_2$ mean Vmax = 1.80ms-1 (calculated PASP=19 mmHg; range = 12.97-
30.84mmHg) Using a paired T Test, mean Vmax after 0$_2$ therapy was significantly lower than
pre-0$_2$ at 4250m (p<0.0001). (T = 10.494. DF=32).Conclusions: This was a unique
opportunity to non-invasively determine PASP in healthy subjects at high altitude. A large
variation in the PASP was recorded and no relation between AMS and PASP was evident. (In
part due to the low incidence of AMS). The intervention of 0$_2$ produced a significant decrease
calculated PASP. Thus by comparing subjects with varying HPV, we may further understand
the relationship between pulmonary hemodynamics and those who are at risk of AMS or
HAPE. Funded by The British Heart Foundation. Thanks to Himalayan Rescue Association.

---

[1]presented as *Hot Topic in Mountain Medicine*; [2]presented as *Hot Topic in Hypoxia*; [3]*oral poster
communication.*

Stages Of Cerebral Hypoxia.

Dunn Jeff F., Ellis Rolett*, Depts of Radiology and Medicine*, Dartmouth Medical School Hanover, NH 03755.

Because the brain has an absolute requirement for oxygen, there is considerable interest in determining the role of reduced inspired oxygen (hypoxic hypoxia) on brain metabolism and physiology. In this paper, based on evidence from the literature and our own laboratory, we propose a model of progressively severe acute hypoxic hypoxia which proceeds through a series of physiological and metabolic stages and culminates in suppression of brain electrical activity. These stages are classified on the basis of changes in arteriovenous oxygen difference, blood flow, intracellular pH, phosphocreatine (PCr), ATP and electrical activity. Oxygen delivery is maintained over a broad range of declining values of arterial and tissue pO_2. The first stage is characterized by increased oxygen extraction and the second stage by increased blood flow. Although increased blood flow may be linked to an onset of lactic acidosis in the second stage, this is debatable. We will use, therefore, a fall in pH as the definition of the third stage. The fourth stage is characterized by declining PCr and more profound intracellular acidosis. A fall in ATP concentration and suppression of cerebral electrical activity, corresponding to the final stage, do not occur until hypoxia is very severe.

The Brain CRF During Hypoxia.

Du, Jizeng. Department of Biology, Zhejiang University, Hangzhou 310027, China.

The effects of hypoxia on CRF of hypothalamus were studied in rats and Tibet-Plateau native mammals Pika (Ochotona curzoniae) in simulated altitude chamber acutely and chronically. The acute hypoxia stimulated the release of CRF from Me of hypothalamus of rats, enhancing plasma levels of both CRF and corticostetone, and the release response is intensity-hypoxia dependent and blocked by icv injections of CRF antiserum and CRF receptor blocker. The plateau Pikas are genetically of the adaptation to hypoxia because of without showing noticeable above response in rats, The expressions of CRF mRNA in PVN areas of rats by in situ hybridization of cytochemistry during 2.5d of 10% O_2 hypoxia increased, on the contrary the expressions of AVP mRNA in PVN reduced, and then their expressions levels in both CRF and AVP mRNA returned to control levels 10d and 30d later. However the TRH mRNA expressions kept the suppressed status throughout the whole hypoxia duration, which might be responsible for the suppression of development and growth of neonatal rats. Meantime with changes of mRNA mentioned above, plasma control levels chronically. CRF release from ME was inhibited by endogenous AVP in hypothalamus as its action blocked by AVP V1 receptor blocker. NE stimulated CRF secretion from ME of the hypothalamus of pika during hypoxia. The endogenous b-endorphin inhibited the hypoxia-induced CRF releasing for naloxone reversing the effects of b-endorphin through opiate receptor. In acute hypoxia both cAMP-AC and PKC pathway were activated and involved in the regulation of CRF secretion as second messenger pathway. Hypoxia influences CRF development of rats hypothalamus. During 5 km altitude of hypoxia body growth suppressed with age of neonatal rats was inhibited respectively when hypoxic exposure for 20 and 30d. Meantime anterior potuitary cAMP formation reduced and adrenal corticosterone development was also markedly suppressed at the crucial stage of age. * Supported by NNSFC No. 39770288.

[1]presented as *Hot Topic in Mountain Medicine*; [2]presented as *Hot Topic in Hypoxia*; [3]*oral poster communication.*

The Regulations Between The Neuroendocrine And The Immune System During Hypoxia Stress.

Du, Jizeng, Bai Haibo. Department of Biology, Zhejiang University, Hangzhou 310027, China.

To study the effect of hypoxia on humoral immunity function of rat and Ochotona curzoniae (pika), the specific antibody production to novel antigen IgG and immunoresponse to sheep red blood cell (hemolysin forming HF) were measured. Hypoxia resulted in a decrement in HF in rats. When rats were secondarily immunized and kept at the same hypoxia for 10d, the reduction in HF was present. However those effects were not found in the pikas. When rats were immunized two days before hypoxia, hypoxia failed to supress HF. ICV CRF decreased HF and the production of IgG, but ip CRF had no effect. However, icv. CRF receptor antagonist prior to hypoxia, the effects was partly blocked, suggesting CRF in CNS involved in modulation of immune response. The effects of hypoxia on the cellular immune function as well as levels of Ach and catecholamine in spleen of 14-day old neonatal rats were studied. When the animals were exposed to 5km simulated altitude in hypobaric chamber for 5d which resulted in a 43.4% decrement in DNA contents in spleen lymphocytes and a 13.2% decrease in lymphocyte proliferation. Similar suppression of the immune function (decreased by 39%) and DNA (decreased by 19.8) in baby rats exposed to 7km for 24h was noted. The suppressive effects of hypoxia of 7km 24h on DNA contents were partly blocked when rats were pretreated icv. With DSP-4 one day before hypoxia. The levels of catecholamine in the spleen were increased, meanwhile the levels of Ach were decreased after exposure to 7km 24h. These observations indicate that hypoxia suppresses cellular immune function of neonatal rats and sympathetic-parasympathetic nervous system might be involved. CRF modulates hypoxia-induced suppression of immune function. Stimulated hypoxia suppressed T-lymphocyte proliferation (TP), and similar suppression in response to acute hypoxia was found in ADX rats as well. There is no change to be found in Pika. Icv. CRF resulted in decrease of TP, which was similar to that observed in hypoxia stress. Icv CRF antiserum and blocker, suggesting CRF may play a significant role in modulating hypoxia-induced immune suppression could block the effects. NE Regulation of T-Lymphocyte Proliferation of Rats During Acute Hypoxia The role of NE in the immunoregulation in rats during simulated hypoxia in hypobaric chamber was examined. Hypoxia of 7 km for 24h inhibited TP by 41%. Hypoxia for 7 d and 20 d of 5 km altitude reduces TP by 34% and 60% respectively. Icv. 5 10-4mol/L NE(2ml) decreased TP by 29%. Icv. Phentolamine 25mg/rat prior to hypoxia of 7 km for 10h attenuated hypoxia-induced suppression of TP from 42% to 21%. In addition, hypoxia of 7 km for 10h increased CRF level was also noted after 5 10-6 mol/L NE icv. Rats were exposed to hypoxia at 7 km for 10h, dispersed spleen lymphocytes incubated with certain dose of CRF in vitro, TP decreased dosa-dependently with increasing CRF concentrations. These findings suggest hypoxia inhibits TP through an immune inhibition action by the modulation of CRF-NE system. b-Endorphin Affects Immune Function of Rats during Acute Hypoxia Either acute hypoxia (7 km, 24 h) or icv. b-endorphin (0.01 nmol 2ml) inhibited concanavalin A (Con A)-induced splenic T-cell proliferation and SRBC-sensitized HF. Naltrexone, which per se did not show influence on T-cell proliferation and HF, blocked partly the immunosuppressive effects of acute hypoxia. The results suggest that b-endorphin may modulate the immune response to hypoxia stress by opioid receptor. * Supported by NNSFC No. 39770288 .

[1]presented as *Hot Topic in Mountain Medicine*; [2]presented as *Hot Topic in Hypoxia*; [3]*oral poster communication.*

Acclimatisation And Performance In The 1997 Everest Marathon.

English Brian, Stan Grant, Dr Andrew Peacock, Martin Watt and Ian Young*.
*Correspondence to Dr M Watt, Monklands Hospitals, UK.

A group of runners and their attendants in the 1997 Everest Marathon had their acclimatisation assessed from Kathmandu and at various intervals (1,000, 3,000, 4,000 and 5,000 metres) up until the start of the marathon. Observations which were taken at rest were:
heart rate
respirator rate
end tidal CO_2
SAO_2 (using a NPB 75 capnograph as provided by Eden Medical, Edinburgh.
A note was also made of symptoms of altitude illness using the Hackett score. The subject's most recent personal best marathon time was used as a means of ranking the runners in terms of speed and their consequent performance in the Everest Marathon was recorded. Those subjects who dropped two or more positions in the ranking had their acclimatisation profile reviewed in detail. Of the 14 subjects, two were unable to finish the marathon due to symptoms of altitude illness. Two subjects dropped four positions and a further three dropped two positions in the ranking. All of these athletes showed at one or more observation points, diminished respiratory responses to altitude at rest, as evident by a low respiratory rate and a high end tidal CO_2 compared with the others in the group at that altitude point. These data suggest that performance in the Everest Marathon is likely to be influenced by an individual's ability to make an appropriate respiratory response to hypoxia. This study was supported by Pfizer.

Serum Leptin And Lipid Variations After A Long-Distance Ski-Alpinism Race.

Ermolao A., *Roi G.S., Englaro P., *Giacometti M., Varnier M., Zaccaria M. Sport Medicine Unit - University of Padua and *Peak Performance Project. Via Ospedale Civile, 105, 35128 Padova, Italy.

Leptin inversely correlates with energy expenditure. It has been demonstrated that exercise, when chronically performed, increases energy expenditure influencing Leptin levels, while the effect of acute exercise on serum Leptin is still controversial. We previously observed a significant Leptin decrease in subjects performing an ultramarathon race at sea level and in this study we evaluated whether Leptin levels were influenced also by an endurance race performed at altitude. We studied 11 male subjects (mean age 34.6 ± 2.5 years) before and after the "Mezzalama Trophy", a long-distance ski-alpinism race, starting from Cervinia (2080m) up to 4226 m, and than down to Gressoney (1637m). The race lasted about 6 hours and was 45 km long. Blood samples for Leptin, Insulin, Free Fatty Acids (FFA), Glycerol and Triglycerides (TG) were drawn before the start and 10-30 min. after the arrival. Body mass index (BMI) was also calculated at the same times. During the race athletes reintegrated their water losses drinking ad libitum, and eating energetic bars. Results show that basal Leptin levels were in the range of normal population and well correlated with fat mass (r=0.84; p<.01). The race induced a significant decrease of Leptin (from 1.1±0.28 to 0.62±0.15 µg/L; p<.01) and plasma TG (from 108.1±10.8 to 75.8±6.9 mg/dl; p<.02), while plasma FFA (from 487±55 to 1484±222 µEq/L; p<.002) significantly increased, the former showing a positive correlation with Leptin variations. Also BMI significantly decreased after the race (from 22.04±0.37 to 21.57±0.34 Kg/m^2; p<.002), while Insulin and Glycerol didn't change. In conclusion, we showed that Leptin levels are influenced by a long-distance race at altitude similarly to an ultramarathon race performed at sea level, suggesting that the short exposure to altitude does not influence Leptin variations. Moreover, after the race the increased FFA positively correlate with Leptin, suggesting that its variations match the supply of adipose tissue for the energy expenditure.

[1]presented as *Hot Topic in Mountain Medicine*; [2]presented as *Hot Topic in Hypoxia*; [3]*oral poster communication*.

Morphologically And Electrophysiologically Distinct Smooth Muscle Cells In The Pulmonary Veins Of The Rat.[3]

Evangelos D. Michelakis and Stephen L. Archer. University of Alberta (Cardiology), 2C2 WCM Health Sciences Centre, 8440-112 St, Edmonton, Canada T6G 2B7.

Pulmonary Veins (PV) have been implicated in the mechanism of pulmonary edema due to high altitude or congestive heart failure. PV rings constrict to hypoxia and catecholamines but the cellular electrophysiology of PV smooth muscle cells (PVSMC) has never been studied. In pulmonary arteries (PA), hypoxic vasoconstriction is initiated by the inhibition of an oxygen-sensitive K^+ channel. Similar mechanisms may exist in the PVs. We used the whole-cell patch-clamp technique (amphotericin perforated) and studied freshly isolated rat PVSMC. There are 3 morphologically and electrophysiologically distinct PVSMC types. Type 1 cells are similar in appearance to PASMC (30μ, smooth, perinuclear bulge) and have similar Ik, mostly inhibited by TEA. Type 2a cells are smooth, long (90μ) and spindle shaped. Ik is voltage insensitive and inhibited by Ba but not glyburide. A large inward current is present, mostly inhibited by Ba. Type 2b cells are crenated, long (90μ) and spindle shaped. A large inward current is present, mostly inhibited by Ba. In addition to a voltage insensitive Ik there is a voltage sensitive component, which is inhibited by 4-AP in some cells and TEA in others. Type 3 cells are, long (100μ) and crenated. A rapidly inactivating 4-AP-sensitive current (type A) is present, as well as a Ba-sensitive inward current. Glyburide and TEA have no significant effects. Type 2 and 3 cells are spontaneously beating and are significantly hyperpolarized (-70±4 mV, n=5). We have not previously recorded inward or type A currents in VSMC. These electrophysiologal features might be related to the spontaneous beating of type 2 and 3 cells, which may explain the previously reported spontaneous contractions of PVs. The Ba-sensitive inward currents might be due to Kir channels that have only been reported in the cerebral and coronary microcirculation. Type A currents are present in spontaneously depolarizing cells, like neurons.

The Effects Of Chronic Hypoxia On Calcium Sensitivity In Fetal Coronary Arteries.

Garcia, Felizabel C. , Virginia M. Stiffel, and Raymond D. Gilbert. Div of Perinatal Biol, Loma Linda Univ Sch Med, Loma Linda, CA 92350.

We have previously demonstrated that in response to long-term hypoxia, fetal coronary arteries exhibit decreased contractile responses to K^+ and U46619, a thromboxane A2 agonist. To test the hypothesis that this observed decrease in fetal coronary artery contractility is due to decreased calcium sensitivity of the coronary vessels, pregnant ewes were exposed to high altitude (3,820 m) from days 30 to 141 gestation. Fetal coronary artery rings (3-4 mm) were isolated from the left circumflex (LCx), left anterior descending (LAD) and right coronary artery (RCA) in hypoxic (HYP) and normoxic (CON) fetuses. Coronary artery rings were mechanically denuded, permeabilized with 50 uM β-escin, and depleted of intracellular calcium with 1.0 uM calcium ionophore A23187. Contractile responses of permeabilized artery rings were measured at free calcium concentrations between pCa 8.5 to 3.0 at 25 °C. Maximum Ca^{2+} activated force (Tmax) was lower in the HYP LCx (CON 0.0845 + 0.0007 vs HYP 0.0571 + 0.0055 gm/cm^2, p < 0.05) and HYP LAD (CON 0.0552 + 0.0055 vs HYP 0.0307 + 0.0073 gm/cm^2, p < 0.05). There was no difference in the response of the HYP RCA (0.0352 + 0.0135) compared to the CON RCA (0.0283 + 0.0057 gm/cm^2). There was no change in the pD2 (-log EC50) values between CON and HYP fetal vessels. These results indicate that the Ca2+ responsiveness of the contractile elements of fetal LCx and LAD, but not in RCA, is altered by exposure to long-term hypoxia. This may partially explain the decreased contractile capability of fetal coronary arteries during chronic intrauterine

[1]presented as *Hot Topic in Mountain Medicine*; [2]presented as *Hot Topic in Hypoxia*; [3]*oral poster communication.*

hypoxemia. The mechanisms underlying the regulation of $Ca2^+$ sensitivity in HYP fetal coronary arteries remain to be explored. Supported by USPHS Grant HD 31226.

5-Ht$_1$ Receptor Agonists For Treatment Of High-Altitude Headache.

Greif, R. Research Fellow, Outcomes Research™, Department of Anesthesia and Perioperative Care, University of California — San Francisco, USA. [permanent address: Department of Anesthesiology and Intensive Care Medicine, Donauspital-SMZO, Vienna, Austria].

The International Headache Society classifies high-altitude headache as a metabolic disorder. The symptoms are similar to those resulting from migraines. A similar pathophysiology is believed to underlie each type of headache. A likely common source of the headache is cranial arterial dilatation, which has been observed in patients with migraine attacks and results from hypoxia at high elevation. Preliminary observations suggest that sumatriptan is effective at even higher altitudes, although a randomized, double-blind crossover trial at an altitude of 3480 m failed to confirm the efficacy of this treatment. Sumatryptan reduces the neuropeptide-related inflammatory responses and binds to receptors for 5-HT$_1$, which constricts cerebral and dural arteries. I wish to report the successful treatment of severe high-altitude headaches on four occasions. The 38-year-old author and his 34-year-old wife each developed severe headache after abruptly ascending from 3700 m to 4200 m. We both took sumatriptan 6 mg subcutaneously. Within 15 minutes, the symptoms were fully relieved and we each felt fit and functional. No side effects were observed, and the headaches did not recur. Our AMS-scores, which were 8 and 9 before treatment, decreased to 3 and 2, respectively, after treatment. In a subsequent ascent to 4800 m, which also was associated with severe headache, I treated myself with 100 mg of Sumatriptan orally. My headache dissipated after 45 minutes; there were again no adverse effects and the headache did not recur. My AMS-score was 5 before treatment, and 0 afterwards. On an additional ascent, I treated a severe headache at 3800 m with oral Zolmitriptan 2.5 mg. This time the headache dissipated within 30 minutes. My AMS-scores before and after treatment were 4 and 0, respectively. Again, there were no side effects and the headache did not recur although I remained at altitude. The conventional, and very effective, treatment of acute mountain sickness is descent to lower altitude. However, there are times when rapid descent is impossible. In such situations, 5-HT$_1$ agonists may prove helpful. A placebo-controlled trial should verify, if 5-HT$_1$ agonists were a causative treatment.

Distribution Of Cardiac Output (DCO) In High Altitude Natives (HAN).

Greene ER, M Araoz, H Spielvogel, RC Roach. New Mexico Highlands University, Las Vegas, NM 87701; IBBA, La Paz, Bolivia; CMRC, Copenhagen, DK.

Chronic hypoxia (CH) alters, developmentally or genetically, the human cardiovascular system and the mechanisms of oxygen transport. Although the effects of hypoxia on central hemodynamics and various regional blood flows are well understood, the influence of CH on the global DCO and its convective transport of oxygen has not been reported. Using noninvasive image-guided Doppler flowmetry (95% CI, accuracy $1\pm1\%$, linearity 17%), we studied 8 healthy, lean, echogenic Andean HAN males (27 ± 6yrs) during steady state hypobaric normoxia (HN: $P_IO_2=150$ Torr) and during hypobaric hypoxia (HH: $P_IO_2=80$ Torr, Chacaltaya, Bolivia). We measured supine, resting phasic steady-state blood flows (avg. 6 cycles) in the: ascending aorta (CO, cardiac output); common carotid (CQ, brain); subclavian (SQ, arm); renal (RQ, kidney); superior mesenteric (MQ, gut) and common femoral (FQ, leg) arteries. Mean blood pressure (BP), pulse oximetry (SpO$_2$), heart rate (HR), and total peripheral resistance (PR) were also determined. Results are given as means 1 SD. During

---

[1]presented as *Hot Topic in Mountain Medicine*; [2]presented as *Hot Topic in Hypoxia*; [3]*oral poster communication*.

HN, CO and HR dropped 1216% (p<0.05), and SpO$_2$ rose 16±3% (p<0.05). BP and PR were unchanged. DCO during HH and HN, respectively, given as % of CO, are as follows: CQ 21±4, 19±3; SQ 8±3, 10±4; MQ 13±5, 16±6; RQ 20±6, 23±5; FQ 12±4, 13±6; Other 26±6, 19±5. These observations suggest that: 1) the resting, supine DCO is similar to reported values in healthy normoxic sea level natives; and 2) no major redistribution of the DCO occurs with acute normoxia in Andean HAN. Supported, in part, by Copenhagen Muscle Research Center and NIH R25GM S0110-02, S06GM 08066- 25S3.

Down-Regulation In Muscle Na$^+$-K$^+$ ATPase Concentration Following A 21 Day Expedition To 6200 m. [2]

Green, H.*, B. Roy*, S. Grant*, M. Burnett*, C. Otto+, A. Pipe+ and D. McKenzie^,
*University of Waterloo, Waterloo, ON N2L 3G1, +University of Ottawa, Ottawa, ON, K1Y 4E9 and ^University of British Columbia,Vancouver, BC, V6T 1Z3.

To investigate the hypothesis that acclimatization to altitude would result in a down-regulation in muscle Na$^+$-K$^+$ pump concentration, tissue samples were obtained from the vastus lateralis of 6 volunteers (5 males and 1 female, age 29±2.4 yr; (x±SE) both prior to and within 3 days following a 21 day climb to the summit of Mount Denali, Alaska (6200 m). Na+-K+ ATPase, measured by the [3H] ouabain-binding technique, decreased by 13.8% (348±12 vs 300±7.6 pmol/g wet wt; p<0.05). No changes were found in the maximal activities (mol•kg^{-1} protein•h^{-1}) of the mitochondrial enzymes, succinic dehydrogenase (3.63±0.20 vs 3.25±0.23), citrate synthase (4.76±0.44 vs 4.94±0.44) and malate dehydrogenase (12.6±1.8 vs 12.7±1.2). Maximal aerobic power (VO$_2$peak) (3.76±0.26 vs 3.55±0.29 l/min) was decreased (p<0.05) by the expedition. Body weight was unchanged (74.5±4.3 vs 72.8 ±3.9). It is concluded that acclimatization to altitude results in a down-regulation in muscle cation pump concentration that occurs independently of changes in oxidative potential. Since regular exercise promotes an increase in Na$^+$-K$^+$ ATPase expression, it would appear that sustained hypoxia is a potent inhibitory influence. Supported by the University of Ottawa Heart Institute and the Natural Science and Engineering Research Council (NSERC), Canada.

Respiration After Snow Burial In Humans Using An Avalung™ Breathing Device.

Grissom CK, CH Harmston, MI Radwin, N Beidleman, E Hirshberg, and TJ Crowley.
Pulmonary Division, LDS Hospital, Salt Lake City, Utah, 84143, and the University of Utah, Salt Lake City, Utah, 84132.

Probability of survival after live burial in an avalanche is 90% at 15 min and 30% at 35 min. Unpublished observations suggest that persons buried in snow become hypoxemic and breathe a fraction of inspired CO$_2$ (FICO$_2$) that increases to about 6% within 10 min. The AvaLung increases surface area contact with snow so that a buried person can breathe the air contained in snow. A mouthpiece connects to a plastic mesh air pocket via two one way valves. Expired CO$_2$ is shunted away from the air pocket via another one way valve. The device is built into a vest worn over clothing. We studied ventilation and oxygenation in 5 subjects fully buried in snow breathing through an AvaLung for up to 60 min. We hypothesized that the AvaLung would maintain normal ventilation and oxygenation during snow burial. The study site was at 2500 m elevation (Pb 565 mm Hg). Subjects were buried in compacted snow (30% to 60% density) with the head 30 cm and the AvaLung 100 cm under the surface. Partial pressure of end tidal CO$_2$ (ETCO$_2$) in mm Hg, inspired CO$_2$ (PICO$_2$) in mm Hg, and percent saturation of hemoglobin with oxygen (SpO$_2$ %) were continuously monitored. Baseline measurements were made breathing ambient air. Four subjects remained buried for 60 min and one subject for 45 min. Mean SpO$_2$ at baseline (93%, range 89 to 99)

[1]presented as *Hot Topic in Mountain Medicine*; [2]presented as *Hot Topic in Hypoxia*; [3]*oral poster communication.*

did not change after 45 min of burial (91%, range 87 to 94) or 60 min (92%, range 88 to 94). Mean ETCO$_2$ at baseline was 33 mm Hg (range 29 to 37) and increased after 45 min of burial to 46 mm Hg (range 37 to 50) and after 60 min to 49 mm Hg (range 45 to 53). Mean PICO$_2$ increased after 45 min of burial to 33 mm Hg (range 23 to 41) and after 60 min to 37 mm Hg (range 31 to 44). We conclude that breathing through the AvaLung allows persons buried in snow to maintain adequate oxygenation for up to one hour but an increase in FICO$_2$ of up to 8% results in hypercapnia. The AvaLung may increase chances of survival for avalanche burial victims. Supported by Black Diamond Equipment, Ltd.

Confinement Of Real And Simulated Spaceflight Seems To Depress Plasma ANP And cGMP.

Haditsch B*, Noskov VB**, Roessler A***, Polyakov VV**, Hinghofer-Szalkay HG*, * Austrian Society for Aerospace Medicine: Institute for Adaptive and Spaceflight Physiology, Graz, Austria. ** Institute for Medical-Biological Problems, Moscow, Russia, *** Physiological Institute, School of Medicine, Karl-Franzens-University Graz, Austria.

Rationale: The Austro-Russian project "RLF" (http://www.asm.at/RLF.htm) investigated adaptation to the microgravity confinement of sojourn onboard the space station MIR, and simulated spaceflight with -6 degree head-down tilt confinement (HDTC). Our group studied endocrine components of cardiovascular volume regulation using lower body suction (LBNP) as a stimulus to induce hormonal responses which are indicative of adaptation state. Methods: Venous blood was obtained 3 min into, and 2 min after the LBNP maneuver (-15/-30/-35 mmHg for 15/15/10 minutes) in two cosmonauts preflight supine, inflight (FD=flight day), and postflight supine (landing=L) and in five subjects before, at the end, and after 5 d HDTC. Samples were stored at -20°C. Hormones determined were AVP, PRA, aldosterone, ANP, cGMP. Results: In cosmonaut 1 (10 days in space), plasma cGMP fell from preflight 4.3 to 1.4 mM on FD6, and was 3.0 mM on L+4. In cosmonaut 2 (438 days in space), it fell from preflight 4.9 to 0.5 mM on FD3, and stayed <0.1 mM with 5, 9, and 14 months in space, as well as on L+4; 3 months postflight his plasma cGMP was back to normal (6.4 mM). Cosmonaut 2 displayed low inflight ANP and returned to preflight levels immediately after landing. Other hormones stayed essentially unchanged during the entire flight and after landing. In the ground-based simulation, supine plasma cGMP was reduced by >30% (from 5.4±0.7 to 3.8±0.9 nM) within 5 days HDTC. Conclusion: The data demonstrate lowered plasma cGMP with real (N=2) and simulated (N=5) weightlessness, and a dramatic reduction during, and shortly after, one long-duration (14 months) mission. We are not aware of analogous observations under similar conditions, and believe to be the first to report suppression of plasma cGMP during extended spaceflight. It remains to be seen if confinement and/or weightlessness per se would produce similar results.

Carbon Dioxide Or Oxygen At Altitude? The Effect On Arterial Blood Gases At Sea Level And On Acute Exposure To Altitude.

Hale D, S Walsh, T Clarke, T Harvey, M Cooper S Brearey, A Bradwell, C Imray and the BMRES. Dept. Vascular Surgery, Walsgrave Hospital, Coventry, CV2 2DX, UK.

Objectives: Supplemental oxygen is an important treatment for acute mountain sickness. CO$_2$ has been proposed by some as an alternative treatment. This study was designed to compare the effects of 3% CO$_2$, O$_2$ at 6lmin-1 and a CO$_2$/O$_2$ mix on digital pulse oximetry (SpO$_2$) and arterial blood gases. Methods: Twelve subjects (ten men), aged 24-53, were studied at 150m and one month later, the morning after ascent to 3,450m by cable car. SpO$_2$, inspiratory (PiCO$_2$) and expiratory (PeCO$_2$) CO$_2$ were measured using a Propac Encore. Arterial line blood gases were analyzed on an AVL OPTI I blood gas pH analyzer. Non-

---

[1]presented as *Hot Topic in Mountain Medicine*; [2]presented as *Hot Topic in Hypoxia*; [3]*oral poster communication.*

invasive measurements were made every minute. Blood gases were measured after five minutes of each gas mixture. Results:

	Baseline	3% CO_2	O_2	CO_2/O_2
SpO_2 SL	97.6(.4)	98.4(.3)*	99.4(.4)*	99.5(.2)*
SpO_2 Alt	87.0(2.2)	89.4(2.4)*	97.9(1.2)*	99.1(0.6)*
PaO_2 SL	13.4(.9)	15.4(1.1)*	22.8(4.0)*	24.5(3.4)*
PaO_2 Alt	6.5(0.5)	7.2(0.6)*	14.3(4.3)*	19.0(3.4)*

*$p<0.01$ vs Baseline, Student t test, Mean(SD)

Conclusion: 3%CO_2 has a measurable effect on SpO_2 and PaO_2 at both sea-level and at altitude. Oxygen has a more marked effect at both altitudes, but the gas mix of 3% CO_2/O_2 was the most effective in raising SpO_2 and PaO_2 at both altitudes and this may have important therapeutic implications. Supported by the Arthur Thomson Trust and Mount Everest Foundation.

Changes In Airway Responsiveness Induced By Chronic Exposure To Hypoxia.

Hart ND, Wilson CM, Bakewell SE, McMorrow R, Collier DJ, Williams D, Miller MR, Pollard AJ. Medical Expeditions. 125 Marlborough Park Central, Belfast, BT9 6HP, N. Ireland, UK.

Bronchial responsiveness is increased in asthmatics on acute exposure to hypoxia and cold. This study evaluated changes in bronchial responsiveness in non-asthmatics subjected to hypobaric hypoxia. Fifty subjects were studied at sea level, on arrival at 5000m, and after a minimum of 7 days acclimatization to this altitude. Saline or doubling concentrations of histamine (0.125mg/ml to 8mg/ml) were administered using a previously validated ultrasonic nebuliser. After each dose spirometry was undertaken using a Micromedical Microspirometer. Histamine challenges were stopped if a fall in FEV_1 of >20% occurred. Full and partial flow volume loops were recorded. Changes in FEV_1 after each dose and at each location were analysed. There was no significant difference found in the concentrations of histamine causing a 20% fall in FEV_1 at sea level compared with altitude. However, the fall in FEV_1 at the highest dose for each individual was greater at sea level than with the same dose at altitude, both before (p=0.019) and after acclimatization (p=0.034). Acclimatization did not affect the fall in FEV_1 (p=0.67). In normal subjects, FEV_1 falls less at 5000m following bronchial challenge with histamine than at sea level. Further analysis of partial flow volume loops may provide further insight into bronchial reactivity after exposure to hypobaric hypoxia. We thank the subjects, Medical Expeditions, Liverpool University and Micromedical UK for their support of this work.

Effect Of High-Altitude On The Cognitive Function. Experience At The Gasherbrum 2 (8035m) Japanese Women's Expedition.

Hashimoto Shiori , Rika Ide, Tetsuji Sawada, Mikio Osawa and Makoto Iwata. Department of Neurology, Tokyo Women's Medical University 8-1 Kawata, Shinjuku, Tokyo Japan 162. Department of Otolaryngology, National Children's Hospital, Tokyo Japan. Department of allergy and Rheumatology, University of Tokyo School of Medicine.

Aim: We have experienced cases who developed olfactory disorders at high altitude. The aim of the present study is to examine the effect of high altitude on the cognitive function, based on the neuro-psychological tests, including Kana-hiroi test, Wisconsin card sorting test and Event related potential P300 and an olfactory threshold test. Method: Studies were conducted in eleven female climbers between the age of 22 and 40 (mean 32.8) who summited the Gasherbrum 2 in 1988 expedition. The olfactory threshold test, Kana-hiroi test and WCST were performed at Base camp (BC, 5200m), Camp 1 (C1, 6000m) and Camp 3

[1]presented as *Hot Topic in Mountain Medicine*; [2]presented as *Hot Topic in Hypoxia*; [3]*oral poster communication.*

(C3, 7400m). P300 was recorded at Tokyo before and after the expedition. Results: The prolongation of peak latency as well as the decrease of peak amplitude in P300 test was observed in some members. There was no significant change in CA, PEM and PEN values in WCST. Although higher scores were obtained in kana-hiroi test at C1 and C3 as compared with BC, it was probably as a result of training effects. The olfactory threshold test revealed the loss of olfactory function at high altitude. Conclusion: It is considered that P300 as well as the olfactory threshold test may be useful for evaluating the alteration of cognitive functions at high altitude.

Human Sexual Intercourse Does Not Increase Middle Cerebral Artery Blood Velocity At Moderate Altitude.

Hayward WA, KR Fritz, JA. Montano, MM Gallegos, ER Greene. Lynchburg College, Lynchburg, VA; Mesa State College, Grand Junction, CO; New Mexico Highlands University, Las Vegas, NM.

The dynamic effects of human sexual intercourse on cerebral blood flow are unknown, due, in part, to previous technical limitations. Accordingly, we tested the hypothesis that cerebral blood flow increases during sexual intercourse. We used 2 MHz transcranial Doppler flowmetry to determine phasic middle cerebral blood velocity (BV, an index of hemispheric cerebral flow) in 10 healthy, young, consenting, sexually acquainted adult couples (31±3yr). A modified temporal fossa transducer was securely fixed to appropriate forehead strapping to minimize motion artifacts. Doppler audio spectra and event markers (controlled by the instrumented subject) were recorded on an audio tape recorder. Measurements of BV and heart rate (HR) were made in an isolated and quiet setting (bedroom) with the instrumented subject supine and their partner in the superior missionary position. The altitude was approximately 1650m. HR and BV were determined during rest, pre-excitement, excitement, pre- penetration, penetration, pre-orgasm, orgasm, and resolution phases. By ANOVA, HR increased (p <0.05) by 51±18% at orgasm. Unexpectedly, BV remained unchanged (p <0.10) from its resting, unexcited value of 61±11cm/s. Importantly, there were no significant gender differences in the measured variables. Therefore, we conclude that hemispheric cerebral blood flow does not rise during human sexual intercourse. (NIH: S06GM 08066-25S2).

Mountaineering Oxygen Mask Efficiency At 4572 m.

Hendricks DM, Pollock NW, Natoli MJ, Hobbs GW, Gabrielova I, Vann RD. FG Hall Lab, Box 3823, Duke Univ Med Cen, Durham, NC 27710.

Supplemental O_2 delivered by mask is used to increase arterial O_2 saturation (SaO_2), thereby mitigating physiological and cognitive dysfunction secondary to hypoxemia. O_2 mask efficiency (defined as O_2 flow required to maintain a target SaO_2) is not well documented even though this is a critical factor in determining the O_2 volume an expedition must carry. To compare efficiencies, the SaO_2 achieved with three mountaineering masks used by 10 healthy, non-altitude-acclimatized subjects (8 male, 2 female) was measured. Masks tested were: (ZE) Zvezda Enterprise; (LSEL) Life Support Engineering Ltd.; (FGH) a Hall Lab design. Test conditions were: 0 & 4572 m simulated altitude; rest & 75 watts cycle exercise; 0, 1.1±0.05 & 1.7±0.06 Lpm (±SD) supplemental O_2 flow. All masks with 1.1 & 1.7 Lpm O_2 flow significantly improved SaO_2 at 4572 m versus no O_2 (p<0.0001). Statistical analysis was completed using repeated measures ANOVA (SAS software).

No O_2 flow SaO_2			O_2 flow	1.1 Lpm	1.7 Lpm	
Altitude	0 m	4572 m	Altitude	4572 m	4572 m	Mask
Rest	97.7%	79.0%	Rest	95.9%	97.7%	LSEL

[1]presented as *Hot Topic in Mountain Medicine*; [2]presented as *Hot Topic in Hypoxia*; [3]*oral poster communication.*

				97.8%	98.3%	FGH
				97.0%	98.4%	ZE
75 W	97.6%	74.7%	75 W	83.9%	86.5%	LSEL
				90.1%	92.9%	FGH
				91.1%	93.0%	ZE

The data indicate a greater efficiency of the FGH & ZE masks as compared to the LSEL mask (p<0.0001). The FGH & ZE masks maintained >90% SaO_2 with 1.1 Lpm O_2 flow during light exercise at 4572 m (15000 ft), while the LSEL mask failed to achieve this level of saturation even at 1.7 Lpm. (LSEL mask courtesy of Life Support Engineering Ltd.,West Sussex, UK ; ZE mask, Zvezda Enterprise, Moscow, Russia, courtesy of High Ascent Light O_2, Inc., Seattle, WA).

A Randomised Controlled Trial Of Progesterone In Preventing Acute Mountain Sickness (AMS).
Hillenbrand P., M. Beazley, P.J.G. Forster, J.J. Milles, R.N. Clayton, A.D.Wright, C.H.E. Imray and Members of BMRES. The Medical School, University of Birmingham, Edgbaston, Birmingham B15 2 TJ, U.K.

Our previous studies of acetazolamide and Medroxyprogesterone (MP) were conducted in a small number of subjects and suggested a reduction in AMS scores by MP. We have extended our observations of MP in preventing AMS in a double blind, placebo controlled trial in a larger (n=20) group of subjects ascending to 4680m over three days. Total AMS scores were lower on MP (16.9 SD 9.4) compared with placebo (20.7 SD 8.8) (p<0.05). 7/10 subjects on MP and 9/10 subjects on placebo recorded a score of 3 or more in at least one Lake Louise questionnaire at altitude. Peripheral oxygen saturation (79.9% 6.9SD vs 78.0% 4.2SD NS) and cerebral regional oxygen saturation (65.3% 2.2Sd vs. 63.5% 2.7SD NS) were slightly greater on MP compared with placebo and endtidal CO_2 lower (2.98kPa 0.23 SD vs 3.19kPa 0.21 SD NS). We conclude that MP acts as a respiratory stimulant but clinical benefit is limited. Supported by the Arthur Thomson Trust and Mount Everest Foundation.

Relation Of AMS Symptoms During Normobaric Hypoxia To Personality Traits.
Hildebrandt W, Schuster M, Hartmann* M, Herzog* W, Bärtsch P. Inst. of Sports Medicine, Hospitalstr.3, 69115 Heidelberg, Germany *Dep.of Intern. Medicine, Bergheimerstr.58, 69115 Heidelberg, Germany.

We tested the hypothesis that personality traits like anxiety, stress coping strategies and body evaluation may have an impact on the subjective perception of acute mountain sickness (AMS) symptoms induced by exposure to 4 h hypoxia (12% FiO_2) in a normobaric chamber. Therefore we performed the following standardized psychometric tests in 16 healthy subjects at least one day before hypoxic exposure: Spielberger's state and trait anxiety inventory (STAI and TRAI), the Mainz-Coping-Inventory (MCI), the Neo Five Factor Personality Inventory (NEOFFI); Cook-Medley-Hostility-Scale (CMHS), body image inventory (FKB-20). To assess sympathetic activation, which may be related to anxiety and stress coping strategies, we measured heart rate (HR) before and after 1, 2 and 4 h as well as plasma norepinephrine (NE) levels before and after 4 h of hypoxia. The Lake Louise score (LLS) and peripheral O_2-saturation (pulse oxymetry) were determined before and after 2 and 4 h of hypoxia. LLS after 4 h hypoxia was positively related to TRAI (r=.61, p<.01), FKB-20 body evaluation (r=.48 p<.05), neuroticism subscale of NEOFFI (r=.56, p<.05) as well as to rises in NE (r=.64, p<.01) and mean HR during 4 h hypoxia (r=.46, p<.05). NE increases and mean HR correlated with TRAI (r=.73, p<.01 and r=.49, p<.06, respectively). Multiple stepwise regression analysis proved TRAI to be the main predictor of LLS in hypoxia. These findings

[1]presented as *Hot Topic in Mountain Medicine*; [2]presented as *Hot Topic in Hypoxia*; [3]*oral poster communication*.

demonstrate, that subjects with greater trait anxiety (and related coping strategies and body evaluation) experience accentuated symptoms when exposed to hypoxia in a normobaric chamber and they suggest that HR and NE responses may be markers of greater trait anxiety.

Rise Of Erythropoietin During Acute Normobaric Hypoxia Is Inversely Related To The Hypoxic Ventilatory Response.

Hildebrandt W, Schuster M, Weymann J, and Bärtsch P. Inst. of Sports Medicine, Hospitalstr. 3, 69115 Heidelberg, Germany.

Peripheral chemoreceptor stimulation may have opposing effects on the erythropoietin (EPO) response during hypoxia: while the increase of ventilation and diuresis will attenuate the EPO increase via increases in blood pO_2 and blood O_2-capacity, the accompanying alkalosis will enhance it. The present study examined the overall relationship between the EPO response to 4 h hypoxia (12% FiO_2) in a normobaric chamber and the O_2-chemosensitivity in 20 healthy male subjects (aged 19-40). O_2-chemosensitivity was determined through the isocapnic hypoxic ventilatory response (HVR) at least 2 days before hypoxic exposure. Before and after 2 and 4 h hypoxia we measured ventilation, end-tidal pO_2 ($petO_2$) and pCO_2 ($petCO_2$), capillary blood pO_2, pCO_2 and pH, as well as peripheral O_2-saturation (SaO_2 pulse oxymetry). Plasma EPO levels and percentage plasma volume (PV) changes, calculated from hemoglobin concentration (hb) and hematocrit (hct) changes, were determined before and 0, 1, 2, 4, and 8 h after hypoxia. Normoxic control measurements of EPO, hb, and hct followed an identical time schedule on a different day. EPO increased from 9.7 ±3.9 to maximal 17.8 ±3.9 mU/ml (mean±SD) 1 h after hypoxia. Individual maximal EPO increases, corrected for changes in normoxic control, showed a negative correlation with HVR (r=-.47, p<.05) and ΔpH (r=-.58, p<.01), while correlations with SaO_2, blood O_2-content (considering PV changes between 7.1 and -15.6%), $petO_2$, $petCO_2$, pO_2 or pCO_2 during hypoxia failed to reach statistical significance. Beside HVR, predictors of the EPO response were normoxic baseline $petO_2$ (r=-.59, p<0.01), SaO_2 (r=-.64, p<0.01) and $petCO_2$ (r=.54, p<0.05). These data suggest that HVR may be a more important modifying factor of the acute EPO response to hypoxia than changes in PV or in pH.

Carbon Dioxide Contributes To The Beneficial Effect Of Pressurization In A Portable Hyperbaric Chamber.

Hoar H, C Imray, S Walsh, T Clarke, M Cooper, D Mole, A Wright and BMRES. Dept. Vascular Surgery, Walsgrave Hospital, Coventry CV2 2DX, UK.

Objectives: To measure changes in cerebral oxygenation in subjects in a portable hyperbaric chamber, and to determine the clinical importance of the build up of CO2 within the chamber on digital pulse oximetry and cerebral oxygenation measured by near-infrared cerebral spectroscopy (NIRs). Methods: Ten subjects were studied. Three days after ascent to 3475m subjects were pressurized to 200mB in a Certec chamber. Digital pulse oximetry (SpO_2), inspiratory ($PiCO_2$) and expiratory ($PeCO_2$) CO_2 were measured using a battery powered Propac Encore. Continuous non-invasive NIRs regional saturations (rSO_2) were measured using a Critikon 2020 monitor (Johnson & Johnson Medical, UK). After 5 minutes at 200mB a Waters 'to and fro' soda lime (SLime) canister was inserted into the breathing circuit, and after a further five minutes a dead space (Spacer) tube was inserted. Results:

	SpO_2 %	rSO_2 %	$PiCO_2$	$PeCO_2$
Baseline	91.0(2.8)	63.4(4.5)	0.059(0.18)	3.8(0.33)
200mB	97.8(1.4)*	66.9(4.7)*	1.33(0.18)*	4.17(0.52)*
200mB SLime	96.1(1.4)π	65.7(5.7)π	0.05(0.13)π	4.01(0.41)π

---

[1]presented as *Hot Topic in Mountain Medicine*; [2]presented as *Hot Topic in Hypoxia*; [3]*oral poster communication.*

200mB Spacer 98.2(1.5)   66.1(5.0)   1.63(0.17)μ 4.16(0.53)

* $p<0.01$ vs Baseline, π $p<0.02$ vs 200mB, μ $p<0.001$ vs 200mB. Student t Test. Mean(SD).

Conclusion: SpO_2 and rSO_2 rose rapidly on pressurization reaching a plateau at about three minutes. There was a fall in SpO_2 and rSO_2 when the soda lime was introduced into the breathing circuit. At this altitude the build up of CO_2 within the chamber accounts for up to 1/3 of the beneficial effect of the portable hyperbaric chamber on cerebral oxygenation.

Perinatal Hypoxia Caused Residual Right Ventricular (RV) Hypertrophy And Gender Specific Effects On Left Ventricular (LV) And Septal Dimensions In Young Adult Mice.
Hohimer A.R , L.E. Davis, and G.A. Pantley. Depts. Obstetrics and Medicine, Oregon Health Sciences University, Portland OR.

We sought to investigate the hypothesis that perinatal hypoxic stress can "program" the adult cardiovascular system by causing altered adult ventricular size, shape or performance. Newborn mice (CD-1) were randomized and cross-fostered to litters of 8 and within 24 hours of birth were subjected to ambient hypoxia (12% O_2, HYP) for 16 days while controls breathed air (21% O_2, CON). Following this stress the mice (were returned to room air (weaned at 21 days) and recovered until they were young adults (47 days) when under isoflurane anesthesia, transthoracic ultrasound measurements were made (HP5500, 15 MHz) and the ventricles excised and weighed. There was no difference in body weights (BW) between CON and HYP mice. HYP of both sexes retained significant RV hypertrophy (43% greater RV/BW, $P<.001$) and a slightly lower heart rate (8%, $P<.05$). There appear to be gender specific effects on the both residual LV diastolic dimension with HYP males tending to decrease and females increase ($P<0.03$; gender-treatment interaction, 2-way ANOVA.) relative to CON. The intraventricular septal diastolic and systolic thickness was increased in perinatally HYP males but appeared to decrease in females (interactions; $P<.05$). Similar differences were not seen in the LV posterior wall and no other indices of LV function were altered. While these residual effects are not debilitating in young adults, they may be the basis of more severe pathology that will be seen with increasing age, afterload or when growth stress are applied in adulthood. We speculate that there may be quantitative or even qualitative differences in either the response or the recovery of male and female ventricles to perinatal hypoxic stress and conclude that future studies must be designed with this in mind. (Supported by the Congenital Heart Center of Oregon).

The Effect Of Oral Garlic Administration On Hypoxic Pulmonary Vasoconstriction (HPV) In Normal Subjects.
Hopkins S. R. , M. E. Trump, R.B. Schoene, J. R. Stratton and E. R. Swenson. Depts. of Med. Univ. of Calif. San Diego, La Jolla CA 92093, Univ. Wash. Seattle, WA and Faculty of Med., Univ. British Columbia, Vancouver, BC.

A brisk HPV is associated with increased susceptibility to high altitude pulmonary edema (HAPE). Recently, oral garlic administration has been shown to completely inhibit HPV in rats, presumably via activation of NO synthase, since the effect is largely blocked by L-NAME (AJP 275(19):L283-L287, 1998). We investigated the effect of garlic on HPV in healthy human volunteers. 4 male subjects [age = 33.7±8.4 y, height = 185.7±6.1 cm, weight = 79.4±9.4 kg, means ± SD] had resting measurement of pulmonary arterial systolic pressure (PAP) using 1.9 MHz continuous wave Doppler echocardiography, on room air and after 15 minutes of breathing 12.5% O_2, before (C) and after (G) 48 h of oral ingestion of pure garlic powder (30 mg/kg/day). HPV was calculated as PAP hypoxia - PAP normoxia. No side effects of garlic ingestion were reported. Normoxia mean systemic arterial pressure was

[1]presented as *Hot Topic in Mountain Medicine*; [2]presented as *Hot Topic in Hypoxia*; [3]*oral poster communication.*

lowered by garlic [95 ± 16 mm Hg, (C) v 84 ± 6 (G), p = 0.17] and HPV was reduced [7.9±4.6 mm Hg (C) v 3.2 ± 4.1 (G), P<0.01]. These preliminary data suggest that oral garlic administration reduces HPV and may be beneficial in the prophylaxis of HAPE. Supported by NIH MO1 RR00827, HL 17731 and HL 45571.

The Respiratory Chemosensitivities To Hypoxia And Hypercapnia With Chronic Respiratory Disease Experienced A Near Fatal Episode. [3]
Horie, Y., H.Kimura, M.Niijima, Y.Yoshida, S.Masuyama, K.Tatsumi, T.Kuriyama. Department of Chest Medicine, Chiba University School of Medicine, 1-8-1, Inohana Chuo-ku Chiba 260-8670, Japan.

[Purpose] The aim of this study is to clarify the clinical significance of the respiratory chemosensitivities to hypoxia (HVR) and hypercapnia (HCVR) in patients with chronic respiratory disease who experienced a near fatal episode (NF). [Subjects and Methods] Sixty patients, whose clinical course could be followed up for at least 3 years after the examination, were evaluated as to HVR and HCVR in the stable condition. NF was defined as the case who received mechanical ventilation when falling into acute exacerbation. [Results] There were no significant differences in age, PaO_2, $PaCO_2$, %VC and FEV_1% between 10 NF and 50 non-NF patients. HVR and HCVR in terms of VI response were lower in NF than those in non-NF and healthy subjects (controls). Similarly, HVR and HCVR in terms of occlusion pressure (P0.2) response were lower in NF than those in controls whereas non-NF showed higher values than controls. Effective impedance during HCVR ($\Delta P0.2/\Delta VI$) was not significantly different between NF and non-NF patients. Attenuation of HVR and HCVR was persistently observed when evaluated at different time points in NF patients, suggesting that it might be genetically determined. [Conclusion] We conclude that the persistent decrease in respiratory chemosensitivities, responsible for depressed central outputs but not mechanical impairments, predispose to near fatal episodes in chronic respiratory disease.

Hypoxic Ventilatory Response And Associated Heart Rate Change Predict The Severity Of Acute Mountain Sickness. [3]
Hoefer M., Juhász J., Bauer D., Sybrecht G.W. Innere Medizin V, Universitätskliniken des Saarlandes, 66421 Homburg/Saar, Germany.

Introduction: The hypoxic ventilatory response (HVR) determined at low altitude correlates significantly with the individual risk to develop high altitude pulmonary edema (Hohenhaus et al. 1995, Eur Respir J 8: 1825-33). Its prognostic value regarding symptoms of common acute mountain sickness (AMS) is still unclear and controversially debated. Methods: We studied the poikilocapnic normobaric HVR (10% O_2) and consecutive change of heart rate at low altitude (200 m, 656 ft) in 12 healthy male subjects (age 30-60 years). Subsequently, the individual Lake Louise Score (LLS, acute mountain sickness symptom score) was recorded every morning during a 10 day stay at high altitude. The average sleeping-height elevation was 350 m (1150 ft) per day with a maximum at 5300 m (17390 ft) above sea level. In addition, at 4300 m (14110 ft) a nocturnal cardiorespiratory polygraphy was conducted (PolymesamÔ). Results: The severity of AMS symptoms in terms of cumulative LLS correlated inversely with HVR (r = -0.643, p < 0.05) and the HVR-associated increase of heart rate (r = -0.747, p < 0.01). There was no correlation of LLS with basal oxygen saturation or periodic breathing index at high altitude. Conclusion: HVR determined at low altitude, and especially HVR-associated increase of heart rate allow for estimation of the individual risk to develop acute mountain sickness. This work was partially supported by MAP, Martinsried, Germany.

---

[1]presented as *Hot Topic in Mountain Medicine*; [2]presented as *Hot Topic in Hypoxia*; [3]*oral poster communication*.

Cranial CSF Volume (cCSF) Is Reduced By Altitude Exposure But Is Not Related To Early Acute Mountain Sickness (AMS). [2]

Icenogle M[1], Kilgore D[2], Sanders J[1], Caprihan A[3], Roach R[4]. VA Medical Center[1], Lovelace Respiratory Research Institute[2], New Mexico Resonance[3], 2425 Ridgecrest Dr SE, Albuquerque, NM 87108 and New Mexico Highlands Univ[4], Las Vegas, NM 87701.

With altitude exposure, there is an increase in cerebral blood flow and intracranial pressure, and a global shift of water into the brain, which may reduce cCSF. One hypothesis is that brain fluid shifts are responsible for AMS. Prior studies have demonstrated the accuracy of T2 magnetic resonance imaging (MRI) in quantifying cCSF (Kohn et al., Radiology 178: 115, 1991 and Clarke et al., Mag Res Imag 13: 343, 1995). Regional T2 changes have been described in high altitude cerebral edema (Hackett et al., JAMA 280: 1920, 1998), but little information is available on cCSF changes with acute exposure to altitude or how these changes may relate to early AMS. The goals of our study were to determine 1) if cCSF estimated by T2 MRI decreased with altitude exposure and 2) if cCSF changes correlated with AMS severity. The T2 brain images were acquired on 25 subjects (10 males) after 8-12 hours of simulated altitude (426 mm Hg, ~4800 m) and compared with images taken on the preceding control day. Subjects were resting at altitude and diet was controlled with fluid ad lib on both days. The Lake Louise scoring system (LL) was used to serially evaluate AMS and scores for 6th and last hr were averaged. Results showed a control cCSF of 109 ml and a 10 ml reduction in cCSF ($P<0.0001$) after altitude exposure. Twelve subjects with no AMS (mean LL = 0.7, headache = 0.2) and 13 subjects with severe AMS (mean LL = 6.8, headache = 2.6) had similar reductions in cCSF (10.0 vs. 10.4 ml, respectively). Moreover, for all subjects AMS scores were not correlated with the change in cCSF (r = -0.02, n = 25). Further analyses are necessary to determine if the fall in cCSF during acute altitude exposure was related to regional brain swelling. In summary, T2 MRI detected acute altitude-induced reductions in cCSF, apparently unrelated to the early stages of AMS. Supported by US Army Med Res Materiel Cmd, DAMD17-96-C-6127.

The Utility Of Telemedicine In The Diagnosis Of Altitude Related Illnesses.

Johnson MC, Lynge DC, Burke M, Bezruchka S, Otto CA, Johnson EL, Basnyat B. Virginia Mason Medical Center, Department of Anesthesiology, B2-AN, 1100 Ninth Ave., Seattle, WA. 98101.

The purpose of this investigation was to examine the utility of mobile telemedicine in the diagnosis of altitude related illnesses. 20 patients were studied at the Himalayan Rescue Association Aidpost in Pheriche, Nepal, altitude 14,200 feet. Physiologic data, including heart rate, blood pressure, and oxygen saturation, as well as Lake Louise Scores for Acute Mountain Sickness, limited pertinent medical history, and 7 day altitude profiles were recorded. Physiologic data were recorded directly by Telemedics /IBM laptop computer monitor system, using Vital-link graphic representation software. All other data were entered into a file using Microsoft Word software. Vital link and Word files were compressed (using a Zip program) and sent modem to modem using a Comsat Planet One Satellite Telephone and Inmarsat satellite to a US based physician familiar with altitude related disorders. Files were transmitted in a "store and forward" mode. Laptop computer and satellite phone were powered by a photovoltaic panel. Upon receiving the files, the US based physician attempted to make a diagnosis for each patient. Onsite and remote diagnoses were compared. Files of 18 patients were successfully transmitted from the Himalayan Aidpost to the US physician. Diagnoses made by onsite physicians included 10 cases of AMS, 2 cases of High Altitude Cerebral Edema, 1 case of High Altitude pulmonary Edema, 1 case of HAPE plus myocardial infarction, 1 case of AMS plus bronchitis, 1 case of pneumonia, 1 case of fatigue, and 1

---

[1]presented as *Hot Topic in Mountain Medicine*; [2]presented as *Hot Topic in Hypoxia*; [3]*oral poster communication*.

healthy patient. Diagnoses made by remote physician included 12 cases of AMS, 1 case of HACE, 3 cases of HAPE, 1 case of HAPE plus mild HACE, and 1 case of fatigue. There was exact correlation of diagnoses in 13 cases, strong correlation in 1 case, and no correlation in 4 cases. There is a role for mobile telemedicine in the remote alpine environment for the diagnosis and treatment of altitude related disorders. This study establishes that the technology functions in this extreme setting and suggests that the diagnosis and treatment of altitude related illness can be made from a distance. The technology promises to become more powerful, portable, and easy to use. Future applications include the possibility of a nonclinician entering patient data to be received by a high altitude medicine specialist. Further study needs to be done to design a better model for the obtainment and transmission of data. Supported by Telemedics, Comsat Mobile Communications, and a grant from Virginia Mason Medical Center Department of Anesthesiology.

Gender-Related Differences In The Control Of Breathing In Prepubertal High Altitude Rats: Effect Of The Neonatal Testosterone Secretion. [2]

Joseph, V., J. Soliz, JM. Pequignot, R. Favier, H. Spielvogel. Instituto Boliviano De Biologia De Altura, Embajada De Francia, Casilla 717, La Paz, Bolivia.

Gender differences in hypoxic ventilatory response (HVR) appear before puberty at sea level (SL). Prepubertal females living at high altitude (HA - 3600 m - La Paz, Bolivia) had higher resting ventilatory rate (Ve100, ml/min/100 g) and catecholamine synthesis rate in the carotid body than males. Brainstem noradrenergic cell groups are implicated in cardiorespiratory, neuroendocrine and behavioral regulations under basal condition and in response to the hypoxemic stimulation of the carotid body. We present here, along with the functional and neurochemical description of the maturation of the chemosensitive pathways in male and female, HA and SL rats, the role of the neonatal testosterone (nT) secretion in prepubertal gender ventilatory differences at HA. methods: Tyrosine hydroxylase (TH) activity, the rate limiting enzyme in catecholamine synthesis was assessed in the central noradrenergic cell groups A2 (rostral -A2r- and caudal -A2c-), A5 and A6 of intact male and female, HA and SL rats. One day-old HA female rats were treated with T (1mg), compared with vehicle-treated females and intact males. One day-old HA male rats were castrated, compared with sham-operated males and intact females. results: At SL, TH activity in the brainstem cell groups was gender dependant during growth. At HA there was a drop of TH activity in the brainstem cell groups of male and female rats between the 2nd and the 3rd postnatal week. Between the 1st and the 3rd postnatal weeks at HA, testosterone-treated females exhibited a male developmental pattern whereas neonatal castrated males had a female developmental pattern of Ve100. The nT secretion exerts an inhibitory influence on Ve100 in HA rats during the first weeks of life. Thus a strong interaction between hypoxic environment and gender appeared in a period known to be critical for normal maturation of the rat central nervous system. The ventilatory effect of nT should be a direct consequence of the neurotrophic regulations exerted by testosterone on the brainstem during growth and is likely to be enhanced at HA.

Embryonal Carcinoma P19 Cells Produce Erythropoietin Constitutively But Express Lactate Dehydrogenase In An Oxygen-Dependent Manner.

Kambe T., J. Tada, M. Chikuma, S. Masuda, M. Nagao and R. Sasaki. Division of Applied Life·Sciences, Graduate School of Agriculture, Kyoto University, Kyoto 606-8502, Japan.

ES cells and embryonal carcinoma P19 cells produce erythropoietin (Epo) in an oxygen-independent manner, though lactate dehydrogenase A (LDHA) is hypoxia-inducible. To

---

[1]presented as *Hot Topic in Mountain Medicine*; [2]presented as *Hot Topic in Hypoxia*; [3]*oral poster communication.*

explore this paradox we studied the operation of cis-acting sequences from these genes in P19 and Hep3B cells. The Epo gene promoter and 3Õ enhancer from P19 cells conveyed hypoxia-inducible responses in Hep3B cells but not P19 cells. Together with DNA sequencing and the normal transcription start site of P19 Epo gene, this excluded the possibility that the non-inducibility of Epo gene in P19 cells was due to mutation in these sequences or unusual initiation of transcription. In contrast, reporter constructs containing LDHA enhancer and promoter were hypoxia-inducible in P19 and Hep3B cells, and mutation of a hypoxia inducible factor-1 (HIF-1) binding site abolished the hypoxic inducibility in both cells, indicating that HIF-1 activation operates normally in P19 cells. Neither forced expression of hepatocyte nuclear factor-4 in P19 cells nor deletion of its binding site from the Epo enhancer was effective in restoring Epo enhancer function. P19 cells may lack an unidentified regulator(s) required for interaction of the Epo enhancer with Epo and LDHA promoters. T. Kambe et al., Blood, 91, 1185 (1998).

The Bipolar Effect Of Altitude On Mood State In Women.

Kambis, K.W.*, Rock, P.B.^, Butterfield, G.E.', Muza, S.R.^, Cymerman, A.^, Fulco, C.S.^, and Moore, L.G."", *The College of William and Mary, Williamsburg, VA; ^U.S. Army Research Institute of Environmental Medicine, Natick, MA; 'Palo Alto VA Health Care System, Palo Alto, CA; ""University of Colorado, Denver, CO.

Changes in mood state relative to altitude elevation, rate of ascent, and duration of stay have been well documented in men. However, few studies have examined mood state in women at altitude. Most instruments utilized to measure mood state were developed for clinical settings and thus focus on negative moods such as depression and anxiety. Therefore, it seems inappropriate to use such instruments when testing mood state alterations in normal subjects at altitude. The Profile of Mood States Bipolar Form (POMS-BI) was developed to assess transient mood state in normal subjects. PURPOSE: This study utilized the POMS-BI to evaluate mood alterations in women sojourning for 12 d at high altitude. We hypothesized that the Profile of Mood State Bipolar Form is an instrument sensitive to mood state alterations in women exposed to high altitude and that mood state would change with acclimatization. METHODS: 6 informed women volunteers (25.3 +/- 6.5 yrs) were administered the POMS-BI at sea level and again at 0700 h each day during a 12 d stay at 4300 m. The POMS-BI uses adjectives grouped into positive or negative poles measuring 6 subjective mood states: Composed-Anxious, Agreeable-Hostile, Elated-Depressed, Confident-Unsure, Energetic-Tired, and Clearheaded-Confused. RESULTS: Analysis revealed reduction (P<0.05) of energetic, confident, elated, and composed moods compared to sea level by day 2 at altitude. Most changes returned to sea level values by day 5 at altitude, all by day 11. CONCLUSIONS: The Profile of Mood States Bipolar Form is sensitive to the effect of altitude on mood state in women. Mood state alterations in women exposed to 12 d high altitude revert to normal values after acclimatization, as has been observed in previous studies.

Effects Of Local Cooling On Blood Pressure And P-Catecholamines In Acute And Subacute Hypoxia.

Kanstrup I-L, Poulsen TD, Hansen JM, Andersen LJ, Bestle MH, Christensen NJ, Olsen NV. Dept of Clinical Physiology and Nuclear Medicine, Herlev Hospital, University of Copenhagen, DK-2730 Herlev.

Objective: To elucidate the pressor and catecholamine response to local cooling in acute and more prolonged hypoxia. Methods: 8 healthy males (22-35 yrs) were studied at rest and after 10 and 45 min of local cooling of one hand and forearm at sea level (SL) and again 24

---

[1]presented as *Hot Topic in Mountain Medicine*; [2]presented as *Hot Topic in Hypoxia*; [3]*oral poster communication*.

hours and 5 days, respectively, after rapid passive transport to 4,559m altitude. BP was recorded with a Finapress, and cardiac parameters and thoracic fluid index were measured with bioimpedance. Results: AMS-scores ranged between 5-16 (max attainable 20) on the first day, but were reduced to 0-8 on day 5. On day 1 control blood pressures, especially the systolic pressure, heart rate and p-epinephrine were all increased compared to SL. On day 5 these values had diminished again, while diastolic and mean blood pressures continued to rise in parallel with p-norepinephrine. With local cooling, a marked pressor response, both in magnitude and duration, was seen on the fifth day, whereas the increases in blood pressure and heart rate after local cooling on the first day in hypoxia were similar to those obtained at SL. Heart rate increased twice as much on the fifth day compared to the other two occasions. Thoracic fluid index increased with cooling on day 5 with no changes on the other two days, suggesting an increase in pulmonary vascular resistance. Conclusion: The results confirm a gradual development of increased systemic blood pressure with time in high altitude in parallel with a rise in p-norepinephrine concentration. In susceptible individuals even very high pressures may be seen. Furthermore, an augmented pressor response to an adrenergic stimulus as local cooling was demonstrated in the systemic and most likely also the pulmonary circulation, a mechanism that may be of importance in the development of high altitude pulmonary or cerebral edema.

Carbon Moxoxide Exposure From Cooking In Snow Caves At High Altitude.
Keyes LE, Hamilton RS, Rose JS. Alameda County Medical Center – Highland Campus / UCSD Medical Center; Mailing address: 3833 Lamont St. #2G, San Diego, CA 92109 (Hamilton).

The dangers of carbon monoxide (CO) exposure from cooking inside sealed tents or snow caves are frequently discussed in mountaineering texts and literature. Objective: We sought to determine the significance of acute CO exposure from cooking in snow caves at high altitude. We hypothesized that at high altitude, carbon monoxide exposure from cooking inside snow caves would increase serum carboxyhemoglobin (COHb) and that even low levels of COHb would be associated with symptoms of CO poisoning. Methods: This was a prospective observational study with a paired design. 22 healthy volunteer subjects age 18 or older were recruited from members of a mountain rescue group during a snow cave camping trip at 10,500 feet. Subjects filled out symptom questionnaires and heart rate, oxygen saturation, serum COHb and ambient CO were all measured before and after cooking inside snow caves. Results: Mean age of subjects was 33 and 87% were male. The mean ambient CO level increased from 1.9±0.1 PPM to 15.3±3.6 PPM after cooking. (p=0.002, range=2-38) There was no correlation between cave volume and the ambient CO. Mean serum COHb level rose from 0.35±0.4 % to 1.8±0.3% (range 0.2-5.2%) after cooking (p<0.0001) There were no differences in symptom scores before and after cooking. There was no significant effect on heart rate or oxygen saturation. Conclusion: A single exposure to CO at 10,500 feet may cause a significant rise in COHb, which is not clinically important. Further studies are needed to examine the risks or longer exposures at higher altitudes.

---

[1]presented as *Hot Topic in Mountain Medicine*; [2]presented as *Hot Topic in Hypoxia*; [3]*oral poster communication.*

Spectral Analysis Of Arterial Oxygen Saturation And RR Intervals In Himalayan Sherpas And Sea-Level Residents.

Keyl, Cornelius[2], Annette Schneider[2], Claudio Passino[1], Giammario Spadacini[1], Paul Feil[3], Richard E. Greene[3], Gabriele Bandinelli[4], Maurizio Bonfichi[1], Luca Arcaini[1], Luca Malcovati[1], Amerigo Boiardi[5], Luciano Bernardi[1, 1]Univ. of Pavia and IRCC Ospedale S. Matteo, Pavia, Italy; [2]Univ. of Regensburg, Germany; [3]Highlands Univ., Las Vegas, NM, USA; [4]Ospedale S. Maria Nuova, Florence, Italy; [5]IRCCS Besta, Milan, Italy.

Very low frequency (VLF; 0.0033 to 0.04 Hz) fluctuations in heart rate are of clinical interest, as they have prognostic value in patients with cardiac disease. One phenomenon associated with long wavelenght fluctuations in heart rate is periodic breathing. We analyzed the VLF component of heart rate variability in non-adapted sea-level and adapted high altitude residents and examined whether these fluctuations were related to fluctuations in arterial oxygen saturation, indicating periodic breathing patterns. 14 short-term acclimatized sea-level residents and 14 Himalayan Sherpas were studied during resting conditions at an altitude of 5050 m. Spectral analysis was performed on 15 minute periods of RR intervals and simultaneously recorded oxygen saturation measured by pulse oximetry (SpO_2). There was no difference in mean SpO_2 between sea-level residents and Sherpas (78.5±7.0% vs. 79.4±5.8%). VLF power (logarithmic transformation) of SpO_2 as well as of RR intervals was significantly higher in sea-level residents than in Sherpas (SpO_2: 3.8±1.0 vs. 2.8±0.7, $p<0.01$; RR intervals: 9.5±0.8 vs. 8.7±1.0 ln ms2, $p<0.05$) with a squared coherence>0.5, indicating a significant relationship between both parameters, in 10 sea-level residents and 6 Sherpas. Regression analysis revealed a significant relationship between VLF power of SpO_2 and RR intervals, expressed as normalized units, in sea-level residents (r2 = 0.56, $p<0.01$), but not in Sherpas. Our results demonstrate differences in SpO_2 fluctuations and indicate differences in breathing control between non-adapted lowlanders and Himalayan high altitude residents. Periodic breathing at high altitude seems to affect VLF power of RR intervals, similarly to the effects of chemical instability of breathing control in patients with heart failure.

Corpus Callosum (CC) MRI: Early Altitude Exposure.

Kilgore D[2], Loeppky J[2], Sanders J[1], Caprihan A[3], Icenogle M[1], Roach RC[4]. VA Medical Center[1], Lovelace Respiratory Research Institute[2], New Mexico Resonance[3], Albuquerque, NM 87108 and New Mexico Highlands Univ[4], Las Vegas, NM 87701.

Most patients with clinical high altitude cerebral edema demonstrate T2 magnetic resonance imaging (MRI) signal enhancement in the CC which is qualitatively more evident in the splenium than the genu region (Hackett, JAMA 280: 1920, 1998). This is consistent with tissue edema in the CC. Because of these observations, it was postulated that edema in the CC may occur within the first 12 hr at altitude and account for the symptoms of acute mountain sickness (AMS). The goals of our study were to determine if: 1) calculated MRI T2 values (T2 MRI) of the CC increased with acute exposure to simulated high altitude and 2) changes in T2 MRI of the CC correlated with AMS severity. The T2 MRI of the CC was obtained from 25 men and women exposed to 4800m (426 mm Hg) for 8-12 hr. The T2 values in the splenium and the genu of the CC were measured from MRI's started 20 min following altitude exposure and compared with images taken on the preceding control day. During exposure, the subjects were evaluated for AMS by the Lake Louise scoring system (LL). Twelve of these subjects did not have AMS (mean LL = 0.7, range: 0 - 1.5) and 13 had marked AMS (LL = 6.8, range: 5.0 - 9.0), with severe headache. The T2 MRI from the CC increased overall in AMS and non-AMS subjects by 1.2 ms (P = 0.05) in the genu and 0.6 ms (NS) in the splenium. Although the average difference (altitude exposure minus control) in T2 MRI from the two regions was greater in AMS than non-AMS subjects (1.1 vs. 0.6 ms),

---

[1]presented as *Hot Topic in Mountain Medicine*; [2]presented as *Hot Topic in Hypoxia*; [3]*oral poster communication.*

the difference was not significant (0.5<P<0.8). There was no significant correlation between AMS severity and the change in T2 MRI from either region (genu: r = -0.14, splenium: r = +0.13, n = 25). Although these results show that acute exposure to altitude was associated with a very small but statistically significant increase in T2 MRI in the genu of the CC, there was no evidence that this change corresponded to the development or severity of AMS. Supported by US Army Med Res Materiel Cmd, DAMD17-96-C-6127.

Anthropometry And Body Composition Of Shift Workers In The Chilean Andes (Collahuasi Mine, >4,600 m).

Kirsch K[1]., B. Johannnes[1], E. Koralewski[1], J. Brito[2], D. Jimenez[3], M. Vargas[4], H.-C. Gunga[1, 1] Berlin, Germany; [2] Universidad Arturo Prat, Iquique, Chile; [3] Collahuasi Mining Company, [4]Mutual de Seguridad, Iquique, Chile.

Introduction. Nowadays mining takes place at high altitude between 4000-5000m. In Chile the mining personnel is recruited from all parts of the country especially from the coastal areas and then shifted from the low-lands to high altitude (intermittent hypoxia, 7-day shift cycle). It was the hypothesis that in shift workers changes might occur in body composition and tissue thickness due to fluid shifts along the body axis at high altitude. Methods. 29 miners were studied (25.2 ± 4.6 yrs; body mass 72.5 ± 11.7 kg; height 171.4 ± 5.4 cm). The measurements were taken before (baseline data collection, BDC), during and after high altitude exposure. The subjects were transported by bus to the mining camp located in Collahuasi (3,700 m) and worked for 7 days in the normal high altitude shift. The experiments were done 2 days after the ascent. During daytime the workers were out in the fields at altitudes ranging from 4,000 to 5,000m. After the 7-day shift they returned to sea level and were examined 2 days after the descent. The following measurements were made: anthropometry (body typing), body weight (BW), body mass index (BMI), tissue thickness (TT) at the front and tibia using an ultrasound device. Body composition was determined with a caliper method and the Body Composition Analyzer (Akern-Rcl BIA 101, Germany). From these data the Total Body Water (TBW), the Lean Body Mass (LBM) and the Fat Mass (FM) were calculated. Results. At BDC the following number of subjects (n) fall into the following group: 3 (n) were very leptomorphic/leptomorphic, 13 mesomorphic, 14 pyknomorphic/very pyknomorphic. group (48%). 20 subjects (69%) showed a BMI between 21.2-27.5, 2 cases (7%) were clearly overweight BMI 33.3-34.6. The shift workers had a waist/hip ratio of 0.9 ± 0.1 and a fat mass of 22.5%. At high altitude the body composition data showed a significant BW loss (-2.5%), paralleled by a loss of TBW (p<0.05) and a reduction in the LBM (-1.2%) The TT increased in the front area from 4.47mm to 4.81mm at altitude (+8%, p<0.003, N=21) and remained elevated at 4.74 mm even after the descent (p<0.001). Most impressive was the decrease in TT in the tibial area when returning to sea level. In this case the TT decreased by 50% (p<0.001). Conclusions. In conclusion, the FM of the subjects was at the upper tolerable limits. The TT data show that even 24 to 48 hours after the return from high altitude the fluid distribution along the body axis had not yet reached control level. Further test settings should improve the predictive value to better define preventable risks for subjects working at high altitude. This study was supported by the Fondef D 97 11068.

---

[1]presented as *Hot Topic in Mountain Medicine*; [2]presented as *Hot Topic in Hypoxia*; [3]*oral poster communication.*

Decreased Iodine⁻¹²³-MIBG Lung Uptake In Patients With High-Altitude Pulmonary Edema.

Koizumi, T., Keishi Kubo, Masayuki Hanaoka, Hiroshi Yamamoto, Shinji Yamaguchi, Zenichi Yazaki, Hiroshi Kitabayashi, Ge Ri-Li, Tadashige Fujii, Toshio Kobayashi. The first Department of Internal Medicine, Shinshu University School of Medicine, 3-1-1 Asahi Matsumoto, 390-8621, JAPAN.

Iodine-^{123} metaiodobenzylguanidine (^{123}I-MIBG) has been widely used to assess cardiac adrenergic function. However, MIBG pulmonary uptake is also proposed as a potential marker of endothelial function because MIBG behaves quantitatively similar to norepinephrine in the pulmonary circulation. The present study was designed to characterize the behavior of MIBG lung uptake in patients with an increased permeability edema. ^{123}I-MIBG scintigraphic examinations were performed in two patients with high-altitude pulmonary edema (HAPE) and the results were compared to the findings in subjects with congestive heart failure. MIBG imaging in patients with HAPE was performed at 7 and 10 th days after admission, respectively. The lung to mediastinum ratio of ^{123}I-MIBG uptake (LMR) was calculated in both lungs. The values of LMR in case 1 and 2 with HAPE were 1.33, 1.48 in right lung and 1.12, 1.14 in left lung, respectively. These values were apparently low compared to those in congestive heart failure. (mean LMR;1.45±0.16). Thus, we found decreased lung MIBG uptake at the early recovery stage in HAPE. We speculate that the finding could reflect an impairment in endothelial cell metabolic functions in the development of HAPE. ^{123}I-MIBG may provide a significant implications for interpretation in various pathologic situations in pulmonary edema.

Acetazolamide (Diamox®) Prevents Hypoxic Pulmonary Vasoconstriction In Conscious Beagle Dogs.

Krebs, MO; Boemke W; Swenson E; Seiferheld M; Kaczmarczyk G. AG Exp. Anaesthesie, Klinik fuer Anaesthesiologie u. operative Intensivmedizin; Charite, Campus Virchow Klinikum, 13353 Berlin 65; Augustenburger Platz 1; Germany.

Hypoxic pulmonary vasoconstriction (HPV) is presumably caused by oxygen-sensing potassium channels in pulmonary vascular smooth muscle cells. Many substances (NO. Nifedipine) and conditions (alkalosis, hypercapnia) are known to modify this response. We hypothesized, that Acetazolamide (Acet) would decrease the HPV by increasing hyper-ventilation and thus raised PaO_2 and lower $PaCO_2$ values compared to untreated animals. With approval of the animal protection committee, six conscious beagle dogs, which had been tracheotomized weeks before, were used in two experiments, three weeks apart. In random or-der the dogs received either Acet (250 mg iv bolus, followed by 125 mg/hour iv infusion; [ACET]) or vehicle (D5W; control [CONT]) and breathed spontaneously for five hours. In the first hour all dogs breathed room air, in the following four hours, the FIO_2 was decreased to 0.1. At the end of each hour blood pressure was recorded in the aorta and in the pulmonary artery; in addition, cardiac output (CO) was determined and blood was drawn for blood gas analysis. The data were compared by GLM ANOVA. Significance was assumed at $p<0,05$. Results are given as means±SD; *= compared to 1st hour; § = ACET compared to CON.

Table 1. PAPm = pulmonary artery mean pressure.

	1st h PAPm mm Hg	5th h PAPm	1st h PaO$_2$ mm Hg	5th h PaO$_2$
CON	15±3	23±2 *	93±•6	40±6 *
ACET	15±2	17±2 *§	104±2 §	50±2 *§

PAP and PaO$_2$: mmHg

---

[1]presented as *Hot Topic in Mountain Medicine*; [2]presented as *Hot Topic in Hypoxia*; [3]*oral poster communication*.

CONCLUSION: The rise of PAPm during acute hypoxia was widely prevented by infusion of Acet. The dogs had higher PaO_2 values in the ACET experiments in normoxia and hypoxia as well, compared to CON experiments. Whether the hyperventilation alone or an additional effect of Acet is responsible for the nearly complete blockade of the hypoxic pulmonary vasoconstriction, has to be adressed in further experiments; e. g. with infusion of HCL to produce metabolic acidosis during hypoxia.

Theophylline Prevents Decrease Of Plasma Renin Activity And Angiotensin II Concentration During Acute Hypoxia In Conscious Beagle Dogs. [3]

Krebs MO; Hoehne C; Boemke W; Kaczmarczyk G, AG Exp. Anaesthesie; Charite, Campus Virchow Klinikum, 13353 Berlin; Augustenburger Platz 1; Germany.

Acute hypoxia decreases plasma renin activity (PRA) and angiotensin II (Ang II) concentrations in spite of overt sympathetic stimulation. Adenosine is a potential mediator for this effect, as it is known to decrease renin release from juxtaglomerular cells and is also found increased during ischemia and hypoxia. The aim of the study was to show that Adenosine is involved in the decrease of PRA in acute hypoxia. We used an indirect approach by blockade of adenosine receptors with Theophylline. METHODS: Studies were approved by the animal protection committee. Eight conscious beagle dogs, maintained on a low sodium diet (0.5 mmol kg^{-1} body weight (wt) for five days before the experiments, were used: Each dog was studied twice in randomized order in a three hour (h) experiment: In the first hour, the dogs breathed room air, thereafter they received either a theophylline bolus injection (3 $mgkg^{-1}$ body weight) followed by maintenance infusion (0,5 mg kg^{-1} body weighth^{-1}) = Theophylline experiments (THEO), or vehicle (D5W) = control experiments (CON). In the following two hours, the dogs breathed a hypoxic gas mixture ($FIO_2 = 0.1$). Blood was taken after every hour for measurement of PRA, ANG II and atrial natriuretic peptide (ANP) (radio-immunoassay) and blood gas analysis. The data were compared by GLM ANOVA; significance was considered at $p < 0.05$. The results are given in the table (means ± SEM); * = compared to 1sth; § = THEO compared to CON, in the respective hour. RESULTS:

	CON	THEO
1sth PRA	6,8±0,8	5,9±0,8
2ndh PRA	4,3±0,9 *	6,1±0,9 §
3rdh PRA	3,0±0,9 *	7,1±1,6 §
1sth AngII	13,3±1,9	15,9±2,3
2ndh AngII	8,4±1,8 *	14,8±2,6§
3rdh AngII	7,3±1,9 *	16,4±3,3§

PRA: ng Ang I$ml^{-1}hr^{-1}$; AngII: pgml^{-1}.

ANP did not change throughout the experiment in any group. PaO_2 decreased from 95±2 mm Hg to 38±2 mm Hg (2nd h; CON) and from 96±2 mmHg to 36±1 mm Hg (2nd h; THEO). CONCLUSION: The decrease of PRA and ANG II with acute hypoxia could be prevented by blockade of the adenosine receptors. This suggests, that the downregulation of the renin-angiotensin system is in part modulated by adenosine.

Imaging Ventilation-To-Perfusion Ratios (V̇/Q̇).

Kuethe[1], D. O. , A. Caprihan[2], H. M. Gach[3], I. J. Lowe[3], N. C. Staub[4], J. A. Loeppky[1] & E. Fukushima[2]. [1]Lovelace Respiratory Research Inst., 2425 Ridgecrest Dr. SE, Albuquerque, NM 87108, USA; [2]N.M.R., Albuquerque; [3]U. Pittsburgh; [4]U. San Francisco.

A dozen or so labs that do nuclear magnetic resonance (NMR) imaging have taken up the challenge of imaging lungs in the last decade. With the possible exception of crystalline tissues, lungs are the nastiest things to image with NMR in a mammal. Lungs mess up the

---

[1]presented as *Hot Topic in Mountain Medicine*; [2]presented as *Hot Topic in Hypoxia*; [3]*oral poster communication*.

nice uniform magnetic fields in our magnets and do not contain much to image. There is a good deal of NMR prowess in imaging lungs, which makes one feel accomplished despite the inevitable, "So what?", from most pulmonologists, who already image lungs with X-rays and γ-rays. We have nonetheless persevered to come up with something that is probably useful. If a mammal breaths a high fraction of oxygen, and a low fraction of an insoluble, inert gas that one can image, the imagable gas will concentrate in regions of the lung with low V/Q. Using the theories developed in the 40s and 50s by Canfield, Rahn, Farhi, Fenn, Otis, and Olszowka, codified in computer programs lent to us by Prof. Olszowka, we calculate that by imaging a gas like SF_6, we can achieve good discrimination of V/Qs in the range of 0.2 to 0.01, which are clinically relevant in obstructive lung disease. In addition, one might use this technique to visualize the spatial distribution of the V/Qs that are calculated from all that complicated multiple inert gas elimination stuff, practiced by Wagner, West, Hlastala, and the like. Our NMR technique takes a unique form. While some folk image expensive gases like He^3 and Xe^{129}, and use cool physics tricks to make them give 500,000 times as much NMR signal as normal, and other folks image the water in the lung tissues, we image the fluorine in gases like SF_6 and C_2F_6 using the naturally puny NMR signal.

Prevention Of Acute Mountain Sickness With Theophylline.[1]

Kuepper, Th., MD[1]; Hoefer, M., MD[2]; Gieseler, U., MD[3]; Netzer, N., MD[4]
[1]Dept. for Occupational Medicine, Evangelisches Krankenhaus, D-40591 Duesseldorf, Germany; [2]Dept. for Pneumology, University of Saarland, Homburg, Germany [3]Dept. for Internal Medicine, Diakonissenkrankenhaus, Speyer, Germany [4]Dept. for Sports Medicine, University of Ulm, Germany.

The basis of our investigation was: i. sleep disturbance, i.e. phases of apnoea, is very common at altitude and one symptom of acute mountain sickness (AMS), ii. persons with a low hypoxic ventilatory drive are predisposed to AMS, and iii. theophylline (TH) increases ventilation during sleep. We investigated whether TH decreases the symptoms of AMS at moderate and high altitude in a randomized, placebo-controlled, double blind setting, which was in agreement with the declaration of Helsinki. Each person (n = 20) took verum (300 mg TH (Unilair, 3M Medica Ltd.)) or placebo at 10 p.m. for 5 days at sea level, climbed to Mantova Hut (3440 m) for 2 nights and then to Margherita Hut (4559 m, Monte Rosa) to stay there for 5 other days. Every day the AMS-Score (Lake Louise-Score) was obtained. Blood samples were taken 2 hours after TH intake. Statistics were performed using SPSS (Mann-Whitney-U-test). At sea level there was no difference in the AMS-Score between both groups. At 3440 m the mean score was 1.6 in the placebo group and 0.8 in the verum group (p<0.05). At 4559 m this difference was even more pronounced: 2.7 vs. 1.6 (p<0.02). The analysis of the AMS symptoms showed no difference between both groups in gastrointestinal problems and dizziness/lightheadedness. Headache showed a tendency with less symptoms in the verum group (3440 m: p = 0.069; 4559 m: p = 0.056). Fatigue/weakness was less in verum group at 4559 m (p<0.04). The difference in sleep disturbance was highly significant (3440 m: p<0.005; 4559 m: p<0.0001). The mean serum concentrations of TH were 0.31 vs. 3.41 mg/l (p<0.000001). No drug related side effects were observed. We conclude that TH reduces sleep disturbances and sleep related symptoms and therefore it is of benefit to AMS.

[1]presented as *Hot Topic in Mountain Medicine*; [2]presented as *Hot Topic in Hypoxia*; [3]*oral poster communication.*

Acute Intermittent Exposure To Hypobaric Hypoxta Stimulates Erythropoiesis In Humans And Facilitates Acclimatization.

Leadbetter III, G.W., R.A. Robergs, B.C. Ruby, D.L. Lium, S. McMinn, and C. Mermier. Mesa State College, Box 2647, Grand Junction, Colorado 81502 and University of New Mexico.

To evaluate the erythropoietic response to intermittent altitude exposure, six subjects (3 males, 3 females) were exposed to hypobaric hypoxia (HH) (2.5 hrs per day at 5,488 m for 6 consecutive days. On days 1, 3, and 5 of HH, hemoglobin oxygen saturation was estimated from pulse oximetry (PO). Venous blood samples were obtained at baseline, before and after each day of HH, and at a similar time of day on follow-up days 2, 4, 6, 8, and 10. Baseline, daily pre-exposure, and follow-up blood samples were used for hemoglobin, hematocrit, and reticulocyte count determinations. Blood samples at baseline, pre and post exposure for days 1, 3, and 5 and follow-up day 2 were prepared for the measurement of erythropoietin (EPO). AMS questionnaires (ESQ) were filled out at baseline and the last 10 minutes of HH. Data are expressed as mean + standard error of the mean. Altitude exposure significantly ($P<0.05$) decreased PO from 97.6±0.8 to 62.6±3.3, 66.8±2.4, and 69.3±2.0 % for baseline, and days 1, 3, 5, respectively. Serum EPO remained within normal baseline values throughout the 6 days of exposure and did not increase significantly during any single exposure. Blood reticulocyte counts increased significantly from baseline after 4 days of exposure (0.98±0.12 to 2.51±0.32%, and remained significantly elevated throughout the 10 days follow-up (day 10=1.77±0.09%). A significant difference was found between ESQ scores at baseline, and days 1, 2, and 3 (0.0±0.0, 1.9±0.4, 1.24±0.3, 0.5±0.1 respectively). The results appear to indicate that intermittent HH is effective in stimulating erythropoiesis because of the production of immature reticulocytes after a three day period. Erythropoiesis occurred without significant acute increases in EPO, and the increased reticulocyte counts were not a result of increased hemoglobin or hematocrit levels. Acute HH did result in acclimatization by day three using 0.7 as the cut-off score for a positive AMS-Cerebral determination.

Susceptibility To Acute Mountain Sickness In Spinal Cord Injured And Amputee Populations.

Leadbetter, G.W.III, J. Cordova, S. Trombetta. Mesa State College, Box 2647, Grand Junction, Colorado 81502.

The object of this exploratory study was to determine whether there is a difference in susceptibility to acute mountain sickness-cerebral (AMS) if one is spinal cord injured (SCI) or is missing one or more limbs. Little research has been conducted on disabled populations at altitude, however increasing access to the mountains and high technology sport equipment for the disabled necessitates study on their response to a high altitude environment. Environmental Symptom Questionnaires III (ESQ) were sent one month in advance to the participants (42 SCI, 18 amputees, and 26 able bodied controls) of the VA Winter Sports Clinic in Crested Butte, Colorado. Those subjects whose residency was above 1538m were eliminated from the data. Post questionnaires were completed the morning after their arrival at altitude (2861m). A repeated measures ANOVA was conducted on the pre and post ESQ scores of three groups of participants: spinal cord injured, amputee and the control group. No significant difference was found. Means and standard deviations are presented in the table below.

[1]presented as *Hot Topic in Mountain Medicine*; [2]presented as *Hot Topic in Hypoxia*; [3]*oral poster communication.*

Table 1. Pre and post group score averages Mean(SD).

Group	Pre-ESQ Score	Post-ESQ Score
Spinal Cord Injured	.18(.54)	.45(.61)
Amputee	.16(.20)	.77(1.20)
Control	.04(.14)	.49(.67)

We felt the possibility existed that less blood redistribution to active muscle, especially in the full lower limb amputees and all SCI subjects, may decrease their susceptibility to AMS by decreasing hypoxia at the pulmonary and cerebral level. In addition, both Amputee and SCI may be less active than controls during the day and night leading up to the post ESQ, therefore decreasing the risk of exacerbating AMS symptoms. In conclusion, this data indicates that there is no significant difference between spinal cord injured, amputee, and able-bodied participants. Further investigation is necessary to determine if AMS prevention strategies developed for able-bodied can be generalized to the disabled groups. In addition, controlling for the level of SCI lesion, as well as, the type and reason for amputation would identify, more specifically, susceptibility within each group.

Both Hypoxia And Chronic Norepinephrine Infusion Alter The Protein Kinase C Activity In Rat Ventricles.

Leòn-Velarde F[1,3], Crozatier B[2], Richalet JP[1]. Laboratoire "Réponses cellulaires et fonctionelles à l'hypoxie"[1], U. Paris XIII, Bobigny, INSERM U400[2], Créteil, France. Laboratorio de Transporte de Oxigeno/IIA[3], U. Cayetano Heredia, Lima, Peru.

Chronic hypoxia imposes an additional load to the right heart, and norepinephrine (NE) infusion to left heart, leading to a consequent ventricular hypertrophy. Additionally, hypoxia increases adrenergic activity. Protein kinase C (PKC) plays distinct roles in signaling pathways leading to changes in contractility and hypertrophy. This study examines the differential effect of hypoxia and NE in the subcellular distribution of PKC activity in rat ventricles. We evaluated the activity of cytosolic (C, nmol/min/g) and particulate (P, nmol/min/g) fractions and translocation (P/C+P) of PKC in right (RV) and left (LV) ventricles of rats subjected to 21 days of hypoxia (HX, 380 torr) compared to rats infused with NE HCl (osmotic minipumps, 0.3 mg/kg/h) for 21 days. NE treatment resulted in LV hypertrophy while hypoxia resulted in RV hypertrophy. Rats in normoxia (NX) were used as a control group. NE decreased C and total PKC activity in the LV when compared with NX and HX (C, NE: 1.44±0.29SD; HX: 2.44±0.08, NX: 2.11±0.55; n=6; p<0.05), and P/C+P when compared with HX (NE: 23.57±6.84; HX: 14.12±1.43; NX: 18.73±5.68; p<0.05) without changes in P. HX and NE induced in the RV a decrease in total of PKC activity, when compared with NX (NE: 1.40±0.35; HX: 1.40±0.22, NX: 1.93±0.30; n=7; p<0.01). In conclusion, the decreased PKC activity found in the RV of rats stimulated by NE, is not present in the LV of hypoxic rats. In contrast, both hypertrophied ventricles showed a decrease in PKC activity. The decreased PKC activity in the hypoxic LV may be masked by the hypoxia-induced upregulation of alpha1-adrenergic receptors.

---

[1]presented as *Hot Topic in Mountain Medicine*; [2]presented as *Hot Topic in Hypoxia*; [3]*oral poster communication.*

Time Course Of Cardiovascular Responses To Intermitent Hypoxia (4,600 m) In Conscious Rats.

Leòn-Velarde F[1,3], Soto G[2], de la Barra R[2], Richalet, JP[3]. Laboratoire "Réponses cellulaires et fonctionelles à l'hypoxie"[1], U. Paris XIII, Bobigny, France. Laboratorio de Fisiologia de Altura[2]. U. Arturo Prat, Iquique-Chile. Laboratorio de Transporte de Oxigeno/IIA[3], U. Cayetano Heredia, Lima - Perù.

The objective of this study was to evaluate the effect of two different periods of 2-months intermitent exposure (IH) on time course of mean resting heart rate (HR) and mean systemic blood pressure (MBP). We measured the body weight (BW, g), HR (b/min) and MBP (mm Hg) of rats exposed to 24h HX/24h NX (IH1; n=10) and of rats exposed to 48h HX/24h NX (IH2; n=10). Rats in normoxia NX (n=10) were used as controls (C). HR and MBP were measured, each other day, by a non invasive blood pressure measurement at the tail of the rats. After 15 days of HX exposure (IH1), the HX groups showed a significantly reduced BW (IH1, 356±26; IH2, 331±27; p<0.05), when compared with their own BWs values in NX (IH1, 375±26; IH2, 346±30), but they recovered their weight after two months exposure. HR starts to increase after 1 month, but increased significantly after 2 months of exposure to HX (IH1, 369±21; IH2, 414±52) when compared with C (335±29; p<0.05), and with their own HRs values in NX (IH1, 334±29; IH2, 342±23). MBP start to increase after 15 days of HX (IH1, 153±7; IH2, 152±10) when compared with NX (121±16; p<0.05), and with their own MBPs values in NX (IH1, 121±3; IH2, 121±7). In conclusion, IH induces systemic hypertension and an increase in HR with different time courses, but there is no difference between the two periods of exposure. With grant from FONDEF D97-11050.

Amiloride Sensitive Sodium Transport Dysfunction Augments Susceptibility To Hypoxia-Induced Lung Edema.

Lepori M., E. Hummler, F. Feihl, C. Sartori, P. Nicod, B. Rossier, and U. Scherrer. CHUV, and Institute of Pharmacology, Univ. of Lausanne, Switzerland.

Amiloride-sensitive sodium transport (ENaC) plays an important role in alveolar fluid removal, as evidenced by aENaC(-/-) deficient mice which died shortly after birth due to failure to clear liquid from their lungs. Transgenic expression of aENaC driven by a CMV promoter in aENaC(-/-) mice [aENaC(-/-)Tg] rescues the perinatal lethal pulmonary phenotype (Hummler et al., PNAS 1997;94:11710-5). Adult aENaC(-/-)Tg mice have lower amiloride sensitive Na[+] transport in the lungs than littermate control mice, and offer a model to study effects of infraclinical ENaC dysfunction on alveolar fluid clearance. Hypoxia causes pulmonary vasoconstriction, capillary leakage, and augmented alveolar fluid flooding in vivo, and impairs ENaC function in vitro. We examined, in 10 aENaC(-/-)Tg mice and 10 wild type littermates, effects of hypoxia (FIO$_2$ 0.08 for 72 hrs) on wet/dry (W/D) lung weight ratio, a parameter of lung water content. The major new findings are that at normoxia, W/D ratio was comparable in both groups (5.02±0.01 vs. 5.08±0.8; X±SE, p=NS). In contrast, during hypoxia, W/D lung weight ratio was markedly larger in rescued (transgenic knockout) than in wild type mice (5.56±0.3 vs.5.89±0.3; p<0.05). These findings provide the first evidence, that infraclinical ENaC dysfunction which, under normal conditions (normoxia), was not associated with any detectable fluid accumulation in the lungs, leads to markedly augmented alveolar fluid flooding during hypoxic stress. We speculate that in clinical conditions associated with augmented alveolar fluid flooding, ENaC dysfunction may act as a sensitizer to lung edema. (Supported by FRNS 32.046797 and 31-43384.95).

[1]presented as *Hot Topic in Mountain Medicine*; [2]presented as *Hot Topic in Hypoxia*; [3]*oral poster communication*.

Light And Electron Microscopic Study Of The Long-Term Hypoxic Ovine Fetal Myocardium.

Lewis, A.Malia, Odile Mathieu-Costello and Raymond D. Gilbert. Div of Perinatal Biol, Loma Linda Sch of Medicine, Loma Linda, CA 92350 and Dept of Medicine, UCSD, La Jolla, CA 92093.

Previous experiments from our laboratory have shown a significant reduction in contractility and cardiac output in the heart from the ovine fetus following ~109 days hypoxia. To determine if these adaptations have an anatomical basis we measured fiber cross-sectional area, capillary density and capillary to fiber volume ratios from light micrographs, and mitochondrial and myofibrillar volume densities per volume of fiber from electron micrographs. We hypothesized that an elevated capillary number and attenuated fiber cross-sectional area would facilitate physiologic tissue oxygenation and that decreased mitochondrial and myofibrillar volume densities could explain contraction and cardiac output deficits in hypoxia. Ovine fetal hearts (n=6) from control (sea level) and hypoxia (3820 m altitude from days 30 to 139 of gestation) were fixed by retrograde aortic perfusion with 6.25% glutaraldehyde and processed for light and electron microscopy. No changes were observed in fiber cross-sectional area or capillary density between hypoxic and control, whereas capillary to fiber volume ratio was significantly reduced in hypoxic hearts (12.5±0.5%) compared to controls (14.1±0.5%, p<0.05). Preliminary data (n=4) suggest no differences in mitochondrial or myofibrillar volume densities between control and hypoxia. However, myofibrillar volume density was significantly higher in right (61±2%) than left (55±1%; p<0.05) ventricle in controls. In the hypoxic group the difference between right (58±3%) and left (54±2%) ventricles was not significant. The same trends were observed for mitochondria volume density. Contrary to our hypothesis, these data do not explain the reduced contractility and cardiac output observed in the fetus following altitude exposure. Supported by USPHS grants: HD 31226 and NIH 5POHL 17731.

Effect Of Gender, Altitude And Sleep On Arterial Saturation Of Sea Level Residents Traveling To High Altitude.

Lilly M, T. Harris, S. Wood, K. Yoneda, and M. Eldridge. Summa Health System, Akron, OH 44306, University of California at Davis, Sacramento, CA 95616.

Although periodic breathing and arterial desaturation have been studied at high altitude, relatively little is known concerning gender differences and arterial desaturation during sleep at high altitude. We tested the hypothesis that females, due to the stimulatory effect of progesterone on the hypoxic ventilatory response, would have less arterial desaturation than males during sleep at high altitude. We studied 10 sea level residents (5 male, 5 female) at elevations of 3414 meters, 4541 meters, and 4877 meters in Ladakh, India. Arterial saturation (SaO_2) and heart rate (HR) were measured with pulse oximetry (NPB-40) while awake and 3-4 times during sleep. Acute mountain sickness was assessed using the Lake Louise scoring system. At 3414 m, the decrease in SaO_2 (awake vs. sleep) in women was (91.8-83.2) p=0.015. In men the decrease in SaO_2 was (90.0-84.2) p=0.007. At 4541 m, the decrease in SaO_2 in women was (87.2-66.8) p=0.019. In men the decrease in SaO_2 was (85.0-76.2) p=0.013. At 4877 m, the decrease in SaO_2 in women was (83.8-78.0) p=0.021. In men the decrease in SaO_2 was (84.2-79.0) p=0.083. Contrary to our hypothesis, women had a lower SaO_2 than men at all altitudes. The mechanism of this is unknown. The gender difference in SaO_2 correlated with a significant gender difference in Lake Louise scores. Research supported by the Summa Health System Foundation and the University of California at Davis.

[1]presented as *Hot Topic in Mountain Medicine*; [2]presented as *Hot Topic in Hypoxia*; [3]*oral poster communication.*

Fibrinolysis Is Enhanced In Healthy Young Women Acclimatizing To 4300 m.

Lindenfeld J, S Zamudio, G Butterfield, S Dominick, M Manco-Johnson, P Rock, LG Moore. Univ. CO. Hlth Sci. Ctr. & Denver campuses, Denver CO; Stanford Univ. & Palo Alto VA Med. Ctr. Palo Alto, CA; US Army Research Inst. Env. Med., Natick, MA.

Objective: High altitude exposure is thought to enhance thrombosis. We asked whether altitude exposure is associated with endothelial cell activation, altered fibrinolytic capacity and increased thrombin generation in women. Because the menstrual cycle is thought to alter coagulation, we also asked whether there were cycle-associated differences in coagulation parameters during acclimatization. Methods: 20 women participated. 13 were measured in both the follicular (SL F) and luteal (SL L) phase of their menstrual cycle at sea level. 15 of these 20 women were measured on day 11 of acclimatization to 4300 m (HA F or HA L). Venous blood was drawn through an indwelling catheter without tourniquet after subejcts rested for 30 min. Samples were spun at 4 $^\circ$C at 2500 RPM for 15 min, and plasma was assayed for Euglobulin Clot Lysis Time (ECLT, seconds - an integrated of measure of fibrinolytic activity), Fibrinogen (Fib, mg/dL), Thrombin/Anti-Thrombin complex (TAT, ng/ml), Von Willebrand Factor Antigen (VWF, U/ml), and Pro-thrombin fragment F1+2 (nM/L).

	SL F	SL L	HA F	HA L	ALL SL	ALL HA
ECLT	249±16	302±12*	220±21	265±4•	270±12	235±15†
Fib	269±11	292±22	286±15	309±14	278±11	293±11
TAT	8.0±1.9	8.2±1.3	20.1±6.4	7.7±2.9	8.1±1.3	15.3±4.3
VWF	.71±.08	.62±.08	.76±.12	.94±.22	.67±.06	.82±.11†
F1+2	.85±.06	.73±.04*	1.1±.16	.69±.05	.80±.04	.94±.11

Results: ECLT was increased and F1+2 decreased in the L phase of the menstrual cycle at sea level (Table * p<.05 SL F vs. L). There was no interaction between cycle phase and altitude. ECLT decreased and VWF ag increased at high altitude († p<.05 SL vs HA). Conclusions: Fibrinolysis is influenced by both cycle phase and altitude. Firbinolysis was slower in the luteal phase at both sea level and 4300 but there was an overall enhancement of fibrinolysis at 4300 m. There was evidence of endothelial cell activation at HA (VWF) which was not affected by menstrual cycle phase.

Ventilation Differences Between Men and Women and Response to Acute Simulated Altitude (426 mm Hg).

Loeppky JA[1], Riboni K[1], Maes D[1], Conn C[1], Charlton GA[2], Icenogle M[2], Roach RC[3]. Lovelace Respiratory Research Inst[1] and VA Medical Center[2], Albuquerque NM 87108 and New Mexico Highlands Univ[3], Las Vegas, NM 87701.

It has been reported that women, compared to men, have a greater ventilation (V_E) per CO_2 output (VCO_2) at rest and a lower V_E response to an acute drop in F_IO_2 (HVR), with some variation with menstrual cycle phase (White et al., JAP 54, 874, 1983). We wished to verify these results in more subjects and during early altitude exposure. The V_E and blood gases were measured in 17 men (once) and in 17 women twice, in luteal (L) and follicular (F) phase, before and during simulated altitude of 16,000 ft after 1 hr (A1) and during the 12th hr (A12). At baseline (635 mmHg) the mean $PaCO_2$ (and $P_{ET}CO_2$) were significantly lower in women than men by 3 mmHg, which confirms significantly greater alveolar and effective ventilation relative to VCO_2 in women. Women had the same breathing frequency in L and F, which was significantly higher than in men, resulting in greater deadspace ventilation per V_E in women. At altitude these PCO_2 differences between men and women persisted, with $PaCO_2$ falling by 3 and 7 mmHg at A1 and A12, respectively, in both men and women. The V_E

[1]presented as *Hot Topic in Mountain Medicine*; [2]presented as *Hot Topic in Hypoxia*; [3]*oral poster communication*.

increased by 28 and 19% at A1 and 33 and 24% at A12 for men and women, respectively. The V_E increase in L was significantly greater than in F at A1 only. Relative to metabolic rate (VO_2), the percentage increases in V_E and effective ventilation were the same for men and women (22%). At baseline, A1 and A12, the mean $PaCO_2$ was never more than 2 mmHg above $P_{ET}CO_2$, indicating no V_A/Q variation between gender, menstrual phase or altitude. The mean PaO_2 was between 43-45 mmHg (SaO_2 between 78.3-80.5 %) at altitude for all, indicating equivalent oxygenation. These results show that, relative to metabolic rate, women have a greater V_E and maintain a lower PCO_2 than men at baseline and altitude. However, the early ventilatory response to altitude is the same in women and men. Supported by US Army Med Res Materiel Cmd, DAMD17-96-C-6127.

Impaired Clearing Function Of The Lung For Endothelin-1 In Subjects Susceptible To HAPE.

Löffler, B.-M.[1], C. Schirlo[2], V. Pavlicek[2], S. Gibbs[5], U. Scherrer[3], O. Oelz[4] and E.A. Koller[2]. Hoffmann-La Roche Ltd., Basel[1], Institute of Physiology, University of Zurich[2], Medical Department, University Hospital of Lausanne[3] and Triemlispital Zurich[4], Switzerland and Dept. of Cardiology, Charing Cross Hospital London, London, UK[5].

To investigate whether plasma endothelin-1 (ET-1) values are altered in subjects susceptible to high altitude pulmonary edema (HAPE-S) in relation to pulmonary artery pressure (PAP) and how exercise influences these parameters, 7 HAPE-S and 5 controls (N) were exposed to simulated altitude corresponding to 4000 m in a hypobaric chamber for 22 h. Venous blood samples were collected at Zürich level (450 m, LA) and at 4000 m (HA) both at rest and after a 30 minute period of exercise (Ex; LA: 50% $VO_{2,max}$) HA: 25% $VO_{2,max}$ and ET-1 immunoreactivity was measured with a specific RIA. PAP was determined using a 7F micromanometer tipped catheter (Gaeltec Ltd, UK). Results: In controls ET-1 values are neither increased by Ex nor by HA, while PAP is augmented by Ex at LA and HA. In HAPE-S the increase of PAP after Ex is associated with a significant raise in plasma ET-1. Furthermore, in contrast to controls ET-1 at rest in HA is significantly increased compared to LA. In HAPE-S, plasma ET-1 and PAP values show a linear correlation in contrast to controls (r=0.40, p=0.04). Conclusions: The pronounced increase of PAP values in HAPE-S is correlated with significantly enhanced circulating ET-1 plasma concentrations. Thus, the increased pressure in the pulmonary circulation seems to be due, at least in part, to an activation of the endothelin system. Our data suggest that the increased circulating ET-1 values are a result of an impaired clearing function of the lung for ET-1.

	Parameter	Low Altitude (LA)		High Altitude (HA)	
		Rest	Exercise (Ex)	Rest	Exercise
N	ET-1 [pg/ml]	15.06±4.32	16.22±3.51	17.16±2.33	15.26±2.69
	PAP [mmHg]	7.56±2.60	15.54±3.46	15.52±3.37	22.32±4.62
H	ET-1 [pg/ml]	16.23±3.87	25.31±10.46a	21.82±6.16a	24.23±3.91a,b
	PAP [mmHg]	9.78±1.77	21.19±2.92e	24.75±3.60c,d	34.80±5.38d

N = controls, H = HAPE-S; data are means ± SD and are analyzed by ANOVA and two tailed paired T test: a, p<0.02 vs. RestLAH; b, p<0.002 vs. ExHAN; c, p<0.002 vs. ExLAH; d, p<0.005 vs. HAN; e, p<0.02 vs. ExLAN.

---

[1]presented as *Hot Topic in Mountain Medicine*; [2]presented as *Hot Topic in Hypoxia*; [3]*oral poster communication.*

Decrease in Arterial PO₂ Down To 35 Torr Does Not Influence Muscle Blood Flow, Lactate Release And Performance During Forearm Exercise. [3]

Maassen N., D. Reddingius. Sportsphysiology, Medical School, Carl Neuberg Str. 1, 30625 Hannover FRG.

Introduction: The influence of hypoxia on muscle blood flow and lactate production during exercise is still a matter of debate. Most experiments on humans were performed with large muscle groups. The drawback of those experiments is that one can not differentiate between the systemic effects of exercise and the effects of hypoxia on muscle. Thus we performed handgrip exercise under graded hypoxia. Methods: Seven male subjects performed continuous forearm exercise between 50 and 67 % of the maximal workload reached in an incremental test. Contraction frequency was 24 per min. Subjects were connected to a closed spirometric system. During exercise oxygen concentration was reduced in the inspired gas every 10 min by about 3 % down to about 9%. Contraction velocity and distance were measured continuously. [Lactate], PO₂, and saturation were determined in arterialized blood from an earlobe and from cubital venous blood draining the working forearm. Forearm blood flow was measured plethysmographically. Results: Arterialized PO₂ decreased from 109.6 (±24.7) to 33.3 (±5.2) torr and cubital venous PO₂ from 30.2 (±6.6) to 18.5 (±2.8) torr. Venous [Lactate] and thus lactate release was highest after 5 min exercise with normoxia. Afterwards [Lac] decreased in spite of the decreasing oxygen pressure and the increasing sympathetic drive. Blood flow increased during the first 5 min of exercise under normoxia and remained constant as power did until exercise was stopped. Most of the experiments had to be finished not because of muscular fatigue but because of central problems of the subjects. Conclusions: If there is an influence of PO₂ on the tone of arterioles it might be compensated by the increasing sympathetic drive. But this increasing drive does not influence [Lac] production or release under these conditions.

Hypoxia Influences Lactate Elimination More Than Muscular Lactate Production During Exercise Of Medium Intensity.

Maassen N. , F. Stifft, S. Baerwalde, G. Schneider. Sportsphysiology, Medical School, 30625 Carl Neuberg Str. 1, Hannover, Germany.

Introduction: To distinguish between systemic effects and muscular effects of hypoxia on arterial [Lac] we performed combined handgrip and cycling exercise under normoxia (NO) and hypoxia (HY: 12,5% oxygen). Methods: 13 male subjects took part in the study. The experiment started with forearm exercise (HAND) at 50% of the maximal workload (Wlmax) reached in an incremental test for 15 min, afterwards 10 min cycling exercise at 50 % of Wlmax was added while HAND continued. [Lac], PO₂ and O₂-Saturation were measured in arterialized blood from an hyperaemized earlobe and in cubital venous blood from the exercising forearm. Catecholamine concentration was measured in cubital venous blood (HPLC). Blood flow in the exercising forearm was measured plethysmographically. The experiments were performed twice (under NO and HY). Results: Lactate release from the working forearm was not effected significantly by hypoxia neither during hand nor during comb. [Lac]art was significantly (p<0.001) higher only during comb. There was no relation between PO₂ in venous blood and [Lac] or Lac release. Additionally under both conditions there was no correlation between Lac release and [epinephrine]. But there was almost the same correlation between arterialized [Lac] and [norepinephrine] (NO: [Lac]= 0.29*NE + 0.35, r= 0.739; HY [Lac]=0.27*NE + 0.27, r= 0.726) under both conditions. Conclusions: Lactate production and release from the exercising muscle at medium intensities is not dependent on PO₂ and [Epinephrine]. As [Norepinephrine] reduces blood flow through Lac-

---

[1]presented as *Hot Topic in Mountain Medicine*; [2]presented as *Hot Topic in Hypoxia*; [3]*oral poster communication.*

eliminating organs probably HY reduces the elimination of Lac and by this way results in a higher [Lac]art under hypoxia.

Effects Of High Altitude On Serotonin, Angiotensin And Endothelin-1 Plasma Levels In High Altitude Pulmonary Edema Susceptible And Control Subjects.

Maggiorini[1] M., Zaccaria[2] M., Greve[1] I., Walter[4] R., Pierre[5] S., Bonvincini[2] P, Naeije[5] R., Nussberger[3] J. DIM University Hospital Zürich[1], CHUV[3], Lausanne, Kantonspital Chur[4] Switzerland; University Padova[2], Italy and Erasmus University Hospital[5], Brussels, Belgium.

The mechanism of excessive hypoxic pulmonary vasoconstriction in high altitude pulmonary edema susceptible subjects (HAPE-S) is still unknown. We measured arterial and venous plasma levels of angiotensin (Ang) I and Ang II, serotonin (SE) and enothelin-1 (ET-1) in 14 control (C) and 16 HAPE-S subjects. Mixed-venous (pulmonary artery) and arterial (radial artery) blood samples were taken at low altitude (LA) (490 m) and after rapid ascent to 4559 m (HA). In both subjects groups, acute exposure to HA decreased markedly arterial and venous Ang I and Ang II by 64% to 83%, decreased arterial SE and almost doubled arterial and venous ET-1 ($p < 0.01$). At the same time exposure to HA decreased venous SE in HAPE-S only ($p < 0.05$). At HA HAPE-S subjects had higher arterial SE than venous SE, in contrast to C who had higher venous SE ($p < 0.05$). The arterial-venous gradient in Ang I and Ang II found in both HAPE-S and C at LA, disappeared at HA. Thus, acute exposure to HA suppresses Ang I, Ang II and arterial SE and increases ET-1. HAPE-S may present with an impaired uptake of SE by the lung. This abstract is funded by: Olga-Mayenfisch , EMDO and Lausanne Cardiovascular Research Foundation, Switzerland.

Effects Of Inhaled Nitric Oxide And Inhaled Prosta-Glandin On Pulmonary Hemodynamics In High Altitude Pulmonary Edema Resistant And Susceptible Climbers.

Maggiorini[1] M., Mélot[4] C., Pierre[4] S., Hauser[2] M., Greve[1] I., Sartori[3] C., Lepori[3] M., Scherrer[3] U., Naeije[4] R. Department of Internal Medicine1 and Radiology[2], University Hospital Zürich; CHUV[3], Lausanne, Switzerland, and Erasmus University Hospital[4], Brussels, Belgium.

Aim of the study was to compare the effects of different vasodilators on high altitude associated pulmonary hypertension. We investigated the effects of 33% oxygen breathing, inhaled nitric oxide (NO) and inhaled iloprost (iPG) in 16 high altitude pulmonary edema (HAPE) susceptible (S) and 14 controls (C) subjects at the altitude of 4559 m. Pulmonary hemodynamics were assessed using a Swan-Ganz catheter (SGc). The capillary-venous component (%) of total PVR (cv-PVR) was calculated by analysis of the Ppa curve decay after rapid inflation of the balloon of the SGc. Our results (mean±SE) are shown in the table. (Ppao = pulmonary artery occluded pressure)

	Cardiac index ($l.min^{-1}.m^2$)		Ppa-Ppao (mmHg)		cv-PVR %	
	C	S	C	S	C	S
baseline	3.7±0.2	3.6±0.1	16±1	29±2#	24±2	32±2#
33% O$_2$	3.2±0.1	3.2±0.1	13±1	22±1#*	25±3	31±2(#)
iNO(40ppm)	4.1±0.2f	4.2±0.2f	8±1*f	14±1#*	16±3*f	31±3#
iPG(20µg)	3.9±0.2f	4.0±0.2f	7±1*f	14±1#*	17±4*f	20±3*f†

$p < 0.05$ vs baseline; f vs. 33%O$_2$; † vs. iNO; # vs C; (#) p = 0.11 vs C

At baseline and during all interventions the Ppa-Ppao was always higher (~6 mmHg) in the HAPE-S with HAPE than in those without HAPE ($p < 0.01$). In conclusion pulmonary hypertension in HAPE-S subjects is largely reversible by iNO or iPG, with however a

---

[1]presented as *Hot Topic in Mountain Medicine*; [2]presented as *Hot Topic in Hypoxia*; [3]*oral poster communication*.

decrease in the cv-PVR only after iPG. This abstract is funded by: Olga-Mayenfisch and EMDO Stiftung, Switzerland.

Altered Ion Transport Of Mononuclear Leukocytes From HAPE Susceptibles.

Mairbäurl,H., M.Scheerer, W.Hildebrandt and P.Bärtsch. Dept.Sports Medicine, Med.Clin.Univ.Heidelberg, Germany.

Susceptibles to HAPE differ in various vital functions and show diminished ventilatory response and increased PAP in hypoxia. Yet predictions of the susceptibility to HAPE from these measures is not possible. Chemoreceptor and pulmonary artery responses to hypoxia are linked to ion transport procedures in the respective cell types. Based on the idea that the divergent hypoxic responses of HAPE susceptibles might be a consequence of a generalized "defect" of certain ion transport pathways we studied cation transport in mononuclear leukocytes (MNLs) and platelets from HAPE susceptibles and non susceptibles in normoxia and hypoxia in search of a possible "HAPE marker". Cells were prepared by differential sedimentation. Na/K-pump and Na/K/Cl-cotransport activity were measured as unidirectional 86Rb uptake components sensitive to ouabain and bumetanide, respectively. ATP and ADP concentrations were measured by HPLC. The results show that in MNLs from non-susceptibles total 86Rb uptake and Na/K pump activity were decreased after 3½ hour exposure of subjects to hypoxia, whereas in HAPE susceptibles hypoxia had no effect. No difference was found with other transporters nor was there a difference in transport of platelets. ATP and ADP levels were not affected by hypoxia. These results show a difference in cation uptake by MNLs between HAPE susceptibles and controls. They indicate further that the difference in transport of MNLs is not expressed in other types of blood cells. The significance for MNL function is not clear. Nevertheless this result adds to the above mentioned idea of an altered ion transport activity in a variety of cell types that might characterize HAPE susceptibles.

Signaling By ROS And CAI Does Not Mediate The Transport Inhibition Of Alveolar Epithelial Cells By Hypoxia.

Mairbäurl,H., W.Heberlein, M.Papen, R.Wodopia, P.Bärtsch. Dept.Sports Medicine, Med.Clin.Univ.Heidelberg, Germany.

An inhibition of ion transport by hypoxia of alveolar epithelial cells was discussed as one possible mechanism causing high altitude pulmonary edema (Planes et al. AJP 271: L70, 1996; Mairbäurl et al. AJP 273:L797, 1997). It is not known yet which mechanisms trigger the hypoxia induced inhibition of transport. In many oxygen sensitive tissues responses to hypoxia are probably initiated by a decrease in reactive oxygen species (ROS) that causes closing of K channels and an increase in CAI that triggers cell-specific responses. We tested whether a similar reaction sequence might mediate the inhibition of ion transport of alveolar epithelial cells by hypoxia. Transport was measured as 86Rb and 22Na uptake by A549 cells exposed to normoxia and hypoxia, ROS was varied by adding H_2O_2 and scavengers, membrane potential was altered with extracellular K. CAI in A549 cells and primary cultured rat AII cells was measured as fura-2 fluorescence. The results show that membrane depolarization reduces 86Rb uptake by about 40%. Ca depletion inhibits 86Rb uptake whereas increased CAI activates. H_2O_2 (1mM H_2O_2), a concentration causing partial disintegration of the cell layer, activates 22Na uptake (+200%) but inhibits 86Rb uptake (-30%). N-acetyl-cysteine and diphenyleneiodonium used to reduce ROS both inhibit 86Rb uptake. Neither hypoxia nor membrane depolarization change CAI. H_2O_2 did not increase CAI. These results indicate that ion transport of alveolar epithelial cells is modulated by ROS,

---

[1]presented as *Hot Topic in Mountain Medicine*; [2]presented as *Hot Topic in Hypoxia*; [3]*oral poster communication.*

membrane potential and CAI. However, ROS and CAI appear not to be involved in mediating the inhibition of transport by hypoxia.

Determinants Of Oxygen Transport In Skeletal Muscle Under Adaptation To Moderate Altitude.

Mankovskaya I.N.[1] , Lyabakh K.G.[2], Serebrovskaya T.V.[1] Bogomolets Institute of Physiology, Kiev 252024, Ukraine[1] Institute of Cybernetics, Kiev 252022, Ukraine[2].

This study was designed to examine the changes in local determinants of muscle PO_2 such as capillary bed structure, blood-tissue barrier thickness, muscle fiber size, myoglobin concentration and mitochondria location in the myocytes in the course of adaptation to moderate altitude. Experiments were carried out on 60 adult male Wistar rats weighing 180-220g in Kiev at sea level (control) and in Terskol near Mt Elbrus at 3,100 m above sea level. It was found that after 4-month versus 1-week adaptation period in the mountains there occurred a marked increase of muscle capillarity. It was noted a rise in the number of capillaries per mm^2 in cross-sectional area of the gastrocnemius muscle fibers as well as capillary diameters, capillary / fiber and capillary surface / fiber surface ratios, and the number of intercapillary anastomoses. It was also noted a decrease in mean capillary length, fiber size, and capillary-tissue diffusion distances. After 4-month adaptation to moderate altitude there occurred an increase in myoglobin content in the medial gastrocnemius: from 2.39±0.15 (control) to 3.22±0.10 mg/g tissue, p<0.001. The blood-tissue barrier thickness was found to expand after a short-term stay at 3,100 m (0.92±0.05 vs. 0.35±0.02 μm in control, p<0.001), and to be almost the same as that of control following a long-term stay at this altitude. We have also registered qualitatively that mitochondria are most frequently located near capillaries and in the subsarcolemmal space in the myocytes of adapted rats. In conclusion, due to the above-mentioned shifts the conditions for oxygen delivery from capillary blood to muscle mitochondria improved under adaptation to moderate altitude.

Lung Diffusion During Hypobaric-Hypoxic Excercise In Sherpa Highlanders.

Masuyama, S, Horie Y, S. Hasako K, Mizoo A., Hamaoka T., Arai Y., Kimura H., N. Furuyama*, Y. Honda**, T. Kuriyama. Department of Chest Medicine, Central Operation Center* and Physiology** of Chiba University, 2600856 Japan

Oxygen diffusion in lung capillaries is one of the determinants that limit exercise performance in hypoxic condition. Lung diffusion is reported to become worse at hypobaric-hypoxic exercise. Among lowlander subjects, the degree of deterioration in lung diffusion is correlated with altitude performance. Then, a question arises how about in the case of Sherpa who showed an excellent performance at altitude. Changes in lung diffusion capacity for carbon monoxide (DLCO) and effective pulmonary capillary flow (Qc) were compared during exercise testing at PB=760mmHg and 418mmHg in 4 Sherpa mountain guides and 22 Japanese trekkers as control. After measuring maximum work rate, steady state exercise testing for three minutes at 0%, 25%, 50%, 62.5% and 75% of the maximum work rate were conducted at PB=760mmHg and in a hypobaric chamber (PB=418mmHg) on a separate day. During the last minute of each exercise period, DLCO, Qc, CvO_2 and VO_2 were measured. Magnitude of diffusion limitation during exercise was assessed by diffusion limitation (e(-DLCO/βQc)) vs. VO_2. While no difference in lung diffusion was detected at rest and during exercise at normobaric condition, the degree of deterioration in lung diffusion was smaller in Sherpa than control at heavier exercise than 50%Max work rate at hypobaric-hypoxic condition. It was suggested that Sherpa who showed excellent high altitude climbing performed well with less lung diffusion limit.

[1]presented as *Hot Topic in Mountain Medicine*; [2]presented as *Hot Topic in Hypoxia*; [3]*oral poster communication.*

Serial Changes In Spirometry During An Ascent To 5300m.

Mason NP, PW Barry, AJ Pollard, DJ Collier, N Taub, MR Miller, JS Milledge. British Mount Everest Medical Expedition 1994, Département d'Anesthésie- Réanimation, Hôpital Tenon, 75020 Paris, France.

INTRODUCTION: Exposure to high altitude leads to changes in spirometry including a fall in FVC. Interpretation of previous studies is difficult because of small numbers and a failure to distinguish between the effects of acute and chronic hypoxia. To clarify some of the aetiological factors involved in these changes we made serial spirometric measurements during an ascent to 5300m in the Nepalese Himalayas. METHODS: Forced expiratory volume in 1 second (FEV1); Forced vital capacity (FVC) and peak expiratory flow (PEF) were measured, using a turbine spirometer, in 46 subjects at sea level, and then twice daily during the walk in to Everest Base Camp at 5300m. Oxygen saturation and AMS scores were also recorded. Statistical analysis was carried out using multi-level modelling. RESULTS: FVC fell with altitude, by a mean of 4% from sea level values (95% CI 0.9% to 7.4%) at 2,800m, and 8.6% (95% CI 5.8% to 11.4%) at 5,300m. FEV1 did not change with increasing altitude. PEF increased with altitude by a mean of 8.9% (95% CI 2.7% to 15.1%) at 2,800m, and 16% (95% CI 9% to 23%) at 5,300m. These changes were not significantly related to SpO_2 or AMS scores. The measured increase in PEF was less than predicted by changes in gas density with altitude. CONCLUSION: These results confirm a fall in FVC and increase in PEF with increasing altitude. FEV1 remained unchanged. The fall in FVC may be due to reduced inspiratory force reducing total lung capacity (TLC); sub-clinical pulmonary oedema; an increase in pulmonary blood volume or changes in airway closure. Further studies are required to define the effects of altitude on TLC, residual volume and maximum inspiratory and expiratory pressures in an attempt to obtain a unifying explanation for these changes.

The Effect Of Hypoxia And Its Gender Difference On Ventilatory Response And Respiratory Sensation To Carbon Dioxide In Humans.

Masuda, Atsuko[1], Yoshio Ohyabu[2], Chikako Yoshino[3], Teisuke Komatsu[3], and Yoshiyuki Honda[4] Department of Science, School of Allied Health Sciences, Tokyo Medical and Dental University1, 1-5-45 Yushima Bunkyo-ku, Tokyo 113-8519; Kogakuin University[2]; Chiba College of Allied Medical Sciences[3]; Chiba University[4].

To investigate the effect of hypoxia on ventilatory response and respiratory sensation to carbon dioxide, 25 young adults (9 males and 16 females) were exposed to progressive hypercapnia by modified Read's method. The conventional Read's method has been used to obtain CO_2 response in hyperoxic background. However, we used a different gas mixture with different oxygen content: A. 7% CO_2+ 93% O_2 for hyperoxia run, B. 7% CO_2+19% O_2 for normoxia run, C. 7% CO_2+13% O_2 for light hypoxia run and 7%CO_2+11%O_2 for moderate hypoxia run. By introducing a small amount O_2 or N_2 gas via a small tubing inserted to the inspiratory portion of the respiratory valve, we were able to adjust $PETO_2$ at >300 for A run, 100 for B run, 80 for C run and 60mmHg for D run, respectively. Respiratory sensation was continuously recorded by visual analog scale (VAS). The slope of CO_2-ventilation response curve tended to increase in hypoxia as expected whereas CO_2-VAS curve exhibited parallel upward-shift with intensifying the degree of hypoxia. The amount of the VAS elicited from a given ventilation decreased with advancing hypoxia. Thus, the degree of dyspneic sensation was effectively mitigated by hypoxia. CO_2-ventilation curve was lower in female than male, contrarily, CO_2-VAS curve was higher in female than male.

---

[1]presented as *Hot Topic in Mountain Medicine*; [2]presented as *Hot Topic in Hypoxia*; [3]*oral poster communication*.

Menstrual Cycle Abnormalities And The Oral Contraceptive Pill At High Altitude.

Miller D. Himalayan Rescue Association (HRA), Pheriche, Nepal. Correspondence: 25 Middleton Rd., London, NW11 7NR, U.K.

Background: The combined oral contraceptive pill (COC) is commonly used at high altitude, not only as a contraceptive, but also for controlling symptoms of menstruation. The female hormones estrogen and progesterone have been shown to augment ventilation and it is possible that use of the oral contraceptives may improve acclimatisation. It has been suggested that breakthrough bleeding may be a problem with COC use at high altitude due to poor absorption, diarrhea, or antibiotic use. There are theoretical risks of thromboembolic events, which may be exacerbated by the raised hematocrit associated with high altitude. To date, there is no data to support this theoretical risk. Aim of Study: To investigate the incidence of menstrual irregularities in women using COC at high altitude. Setting: The HRA Clinic at Pheriche, Nepal (4250m). Subjects and Methods: Men and women attending lectures given by the staff of the clinic on altitude sickness were asked to complete a questionnaire (as part of a larger study on altitude sickness). Results: Approximately 1200 people attended lectures, 926 filled in questionnaires, 66% (610) males and 34% (316) females. Females ranged in age from 12 to 71 years (mean=33.5yrs). Of the females 14% (44) were post-menopausal, 2% (5) were using contraceptives containing only progesterone, 28% (87) were using the COC, and 54% (172) had periods and did not take hormones. Of women using the COC, 5% (4) reported heavy periods and 5% (4) reported light periods in comparison to their normal periods. 5% (4) of COC users had breakthrough bleeding or an earlier then expected period was reported, but 3 of the 4 had not taken their pills regularly. Of those not taking hormones, the menstrual abnormalities described were: heavy 2% (n=3), light 12% (n=21), late 2% (n=4), early 2% (n=4), spotting or breakthrough bleeding 5% (n=8). No cases of arterial or venous thromboembolism were seen in the clinic during the time of the study. Conclusion: COC use at high altitude is an effective method of controlling menstrual periods at altitude. However, irregularities may occur, especially if pills are not taken regularly. Although no cases of medical complications of COC use were seen, no conclusion can be drawn about the safety of COC use at altitude as the increased risk, if any, would be very small. Thanks to Himalayan Rescue Association for permission to undertake this study.

Pulmonary Interstitial Pressure And Matrix Structure After Acute Hypoxia Exposure.

Miserocchi* G, D.Negrini*, A.Passi° and G. De Luca°. * Istituto di Fisiologia Umana, Via Mangiagalli 32 , 20133 Milano, ° Centro di Servizi Interdipartimentali, Università di Varese, Italy.

Previous studies have clarified some aspects of pulmonary interstitial fluid dynamics in the transition from physiological condition towards the development of lung edema induced by saline infusion [hydrostatic edema (1,2)] or by intravenous injection of pancreatic elastase [lesional edema (3,4)]. The present study addresses the condition of acute hypoxia exposure, a possible cause of pulmonary edema due both to increased hydraulic capillary pressure and to increased microvascular permeability. Experiments were performed in three groups of anesthetized, spontaneously breathing rabbits (n=24): control (C), 3 and 6 hours of hypoxia (3H, 6H), induced by 12 % O_2 breathing. Arterial PO_2 averaged 88 ± 2 (SD) in C and 39 ± 16 torr in the hypoxic group. Pulmonary interstitial pressure (Pip) was measured in in-situ lungs through the intact parietal pleura using the micropuncture technique. Pip was -10 ± 2 cmH2O in C and significantly (p< 0.05) increased to -1.7 ± 1.9 and 1.6 ± 2.8 cmH$_2$O in 3H and 6H, respectively. The wet weight to dry weight lung ratio was 4.9 ± 0.1, 4.9 ± 0.2 and 5 ± 0.2 in C, 3H and 6H, respectively. Plasma protein concentration was 5.1 ± 0.4 gr/dl in C and decreased to 4.5 ± 0.6 in 6H (p<0.05). Colloidosmotic pressure of fluid sampled through the

[1]presented as *Hot Topic in Mountain Medicine*; [2]presented as *Hot Topic in Hypoxia*; [3]*oral poster communication.*

wick technique from connective interstitial tissue was 11.6 cmH$_2$O in C and increased to 13 cmH$_2$O in 6H. Lung tissue samples were examined for gelatinase activity through zimography and specific antibody using Western blotting technique. Results from zymography showed a progressive increase of gelatinolytic activity going from C to 3H and 6H. Western blotting technique demonstrated that such an increase of the gelatinolytic activity was due to gelatinase A (72 kDa) and B (92 kDa). Furthermore, we could demonstrate that hypoxia exposure caused activation of plasminogen that acts as an activator of metalloproteinases.

1. Miserocchi, G. et al. J.Appl.Physiol. 74: 1171-1177, 1993. 2. Negrini, D. et al. Am. J. Physiol. 270 (Heart Circ. Physiol. 39): H2000-H2007, 1996. 3. Negrini, D. et al. Am. J. Physiol. 274 (Lung Cell. Mol.Physiol. 18) : L203-L211, 1996. 4. Passi, A. et al. Am.J. Physiol. 275 (Lung Cell. Mol. Physiol. 19): L631-L635, 1998.

Near-Infrared Cerebral Spectroscopy To Assess Cerebral Oxygenation At High Altitude.

Morgan J, A Wright, H Hoar, D Hale, C Imray and the Birmingham Medical Research and Expeditional Society. Dept. Vascular Surgery, Walsgrave Hospital, Coventry CV2 2DX, UK.

Objectives: Oxygen delivery to the brain is critical in determining performance and illness at altitude. The aim of this study was to assess cerebral oxygenation on ascent to altitude using non-invasive near-infrared cerebral spectroscopy (NIRs). Methods: Twenty subjects, aged 24-59, were studied. Baseline measurements were made at 150m one month prior to departure. Daily studies were made at sea level, 2770m, 3560m and 4680m. Travel was by minibus. Digital pulse oximetry (SpO$_2$) was measured using an Ohmeda 3770. Expiratory CO$_2$ (PeCO$_2$) was measured using an HP capnograph 78356. NIRs cerebral spectroscopy was performed using a Critikon 2020 monitor, measuring regional saturation (rSO$_2$), and oxygenated (HbO$_2$) and deoxygenated (HDO$_2$) haemoglobin (Johnson & Johnson Medical, UK). Results:

	150m	0m	2770m	3650m	4680m
SpO$_2$	98.1(0.9)	97.3(1.1)	92.0(1.5)	88.3(2.7)	75.1(5.9)
HbO$_2$	79.3(9.2)	73.8(9)	78.9(13)	70.3(11)	72.3(11)
HDO$_2$	33.4(3.8)	32.0(4.2)	37.3(5.1)	36.8(4.8)	42.7(6.3)
rSO$_2$	70.2(2.4)	69.5(2.4)	67.3(3.4)	65.4(2.7)	63.6(2.3)
PeCO$_2$		5.9(0.6)	3.7(0.3)	3.5(0.3)	3.4(0.3)

There were significant differences (p<0.05-0.001) in all altitude measurements vs sea level. Mean(sd). Paired t test. Conclusion: NIRs provided a simple, reliable and robust non-invasive assessment of cerebral oxygenation. Falls in SpO$_2$, rSO$_2$, and HbO$_2$ were observed. The technique provides a useful tool to investigate cerebral oxygenation in the field. Supported by the Arthur Thomson Trust and Mount Everest Foundation.

Magnetic Resonance Angiography Of Human Pulmonary Arteries During Hypoxia And Light Exercise. [2]

Moon RE , PL Watke, BB Hart, BW Stolp, G deL Dear, PW Robertson, PO Doar, DA Vote, C Charles, CE Spritzer. Depts. of Anesthesiology and Radiology, Duke University, Durham, NC 27710.

It has been hypothesized that HAPE is precipitated by non-uniform HPV or accelerated flow during hypoxia. To examine this we performed MR angiography using a 1.5T magnet in 6 healthy volunteers (mean age = 36y, M=4, F=2). Subjects were instrumented with arterial

[1]presented as *Hot Topic in Mountain Medicine*; [2]presented as *Hot Topic in Hypoxia*; [3]*oral poster communication*.

and PA catheters and studied supine under normobaric conditions during normoxia (FiO_2 = 0.21) and hypoxia (FiO_2 = 0.11). During rest and light exercise, individual vessel flows were measured at several points within a cardiac cycle in the main PA and lobar branches (see Fig. 1). Despite some variability in HPV among vessels, peak instantaneous flow was not higher during hypoxia (see Fig. 2). This study does not support higher peak pulmonary vessel flow during acute hypoxia as a major mechanism for HAPE.

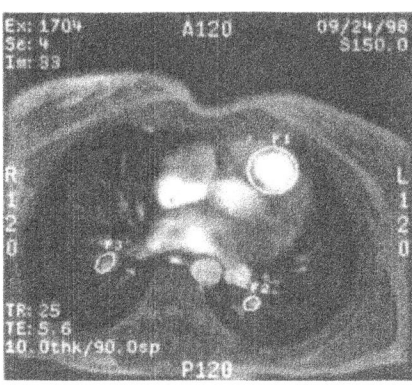
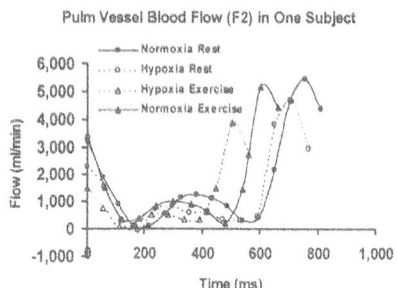

Pulm Vessel Blood Flow (F2) in One Subject

Effect Of Altitude Exposure On Brain Volume And Development Of Acute Mountain Sickness (AMS). [3]

Muza S.R. , T.P. Lyons, P.B. Rock, C.S. Fulco, B.A. Beidleman, S. Smith, I.A. Morocz[1], G.P. Zientara1, and A. Cymerman. U.S. Army Research Institute of Environmental Medicine, Natick, MA, USA, and Brigham & Women's Hospital, Harvard Medical School, Boston, MA, USA[1].

The objective of this study was to assess whether AMS was associated with increased brain tissue volume hypothesized to increase due to cerebral edema. Eleven male volunteers were exposed to simulated altitude (PB =430 torr) in a hypobaric chamber for ~32 h. AMS symptoms were assessed using the Environmental Symptoms Questionnaire. Twenty-four h before and within 4 h after exiting the chamber, brain volume was measured using a magnetic resonance imaging (MRI) brain tissue coronal volumetric series (FA 45 deg, TE 5 ms, TR 35 ms, 24 cm FOV, 1.5 mm thick, 256X192 matrix, 1 NEX, 124 slices). Post-processing segmentation of the image data into white and gray matter volumes was performed on a supercomputer using a method of adaptive 3D segmentation based on tissue properties. Measurements were successfully completed on 7 subjects. SL brain volume differed by less than 0.5% (1287.7 ± 78.6 ml vs 1279.8 ± 89.6 ml) between 2 SL measurements separated by ~2 weeks. After high altitude exposure, brain volume expanded in all subjects. Whole brain volume increased ($p < 0.001$) 2.2% (26.1 ± 7.1 ml) at high altitude above SL values. Gray matter volume increased ($p < 0.05$) more than white matter volume. The magnitude of the brain volume increase was inversely related to the resting arterial oxygen saturation, but the relationship was not statistically significant. There was no significant relationship between the presence or severity of AMS and the magnitude of the brain volume increase. In conclusion, the MRI results revealed a consistent and reproducible increase in brain volume consistent with development of diffuse cerebral edema at high altitude. However, the increase in brain volume per se did not relate to the presence or severity of AMS. This suggests that other

[1]presented as *Hot Topic in Mountain Medicine*; [2]presented as *Hot Topic in Hypoxia*; [3]*oral poster communication.*

factors, such as cranium or spinal column volumes, are contributing variables which determine whether a given increase in brain volume results in AMS.

Women At Altitude: Effect Of Alpha-Blockade On The Ventilatory And Systemic Arterial Pressor Responses To Hypoxia And Hypercapnia. [2]

Muza S.R. , P.B. Rock, G.E. Butterfield[1], E.E. Wolfel[2] and L.G. Moore[2]. U.S. Army Research Institute of Environmental Medicine, Natick, MA, USA, Palo Alto VA Health Care System, Palo Alto, CA, USA[1] and University of Colorado, Denver, CO, USA[2].

Hypoxia activates the adrenergic nervous system which may mediate or enhance the ventilatory and systemic arterial blood pressure responses to high altitude. Alpha-adrenergic vasoconstriction may decrease carotid body blood flow, hence augmenting chemosensitivity. The purpose of this study was to determine the relationship between ventilatory chemosensitivity and pressor chemosensitivity and to assess the role of α -adrenergic receptor activation in the ventilatory and pressor responses to hypoxia and hypercapnia. Ventilatory and mean arterial pressure (MAP) responses to progressive isocapnic hypoxia and progressive hyperoxic hypercapnia were measured in 12 women at sea level (SL) and during 40 h at simulated high altitude (HA: PB 445 mmHg) once on placebo and on an α 1-adrenergic blocker (prazosin: 3mg/d). Results: The magnitude of the arterial pressor response to progressive hypoxia (HPR) was positively correlated to the hypoxic ventilatory response (HVR). However, the magnitude of the arterial pressor response to progressive hypercapnia (HCPR) was not correlated to the hypercapnic ventilatory response (HCVR). Alpha[1]-adrenergic blockade: 1) did not reduce resting MAP at SL nor diminish the resting MAP pressor esponse to HA, 2) did not reduce the HVR, nor diminish the rise in resting V_E at HA, 3) did reduce the magnitude of the HPR at SL and HA, and 4) did not effect the magnitude of the HCPR nor the magnitude of the HCVR. These results suggest that in humans α -adrenergic activation does not appear to augment HVR at HA by vasoconstriction of the carotid body vasculature. Furthermore, whereas the HPR is mediated by α 1-adrenergic activation, the HCPR may not be. Elevated $PaCO_2$ has direct vasodilatory effects, which may mask the action of the alpha blocker. Thus, the HCPR may rely more upon increased cardiac output than vasoconstriction. Supported in part by DOD grant #DAMD 17-95-C5110

Upregulation Of Nitric Oxide Synthase In The Ovine Placenta By Sustained Hypoxemia.[3]

Myatt L., T. Zarlingo, A.L.W. Eis, H. Asano[1], B. Richardson[1]. Departments of Ob/Gyn, University of Cincinnati College of Medicine, Cincinnati, OH and Lawson Research Institute, University of Western Ontario, London, Ontario[1].

Nitric oxide (NO) synthesized by endothelial nitric oxide synthase (eNOS) may play a crucial role in the regulation of placental blood flows. With a compromise in oxygenation, maternal and/or fetal blood flows within the placenta may be altered to enhance fetal oxygen delivery. We determined whether placental eNOS expression is upregulated in response to induced hypoxemia as a mechanism to protect the fetus. Chronically instrumented fetal sheep (130-134 days gestation) were subjected to a reduction in maternal inspired O_2 to 12% (hypoxia, n=6) or 10% (hypoxia plus metabolic acidosis, n=9) for 8 hrs. followed by a 72 hr. recovery period. Instrumented normoxic animals (21% O_2, n=6) were controls. Maternal and fetal pO_2, pH, base excess, O_2 content, and hemoglobin were recorded prior to and at 8 hrs. of experimental treatment, and at 2, 24, and 72 hrs. of recovery. At 8 hrs., fetal O_2 contents (mmol/L mean ± SD) were 3.58±0.31, 1.80±0.50 and 1.09±0.32 and pH was 7.39±0.02,

---

[1]presented as *Hot Topic in Mountain Medicine*; [2]presented as *Hot Topic in Hypoxia*; [3]*oral poster communication.*

7.35±0.02, and 7.12±0.10 in the control, hypoxic and acidotic groups, respectively. At 72 hrs. animals were euthanized and placentomes removed and snap frozen for immunohistochemistry. Villus tissue sections were immunostained for eNOS using the vectastain ABC method. No eNOS immuno-staining was seen in trophoblasts, but was apparent in the endothelial cells of fetal, and maternal, vasculatures of the placentomes. Densitometric analysis showed a significant difference (p<0.05) in the density of eNOS immunostaining between the three groups; 10.5±2.7, 12.4±2.2 and 13.6±2.3 units for the control, hypoxic and acidotic groups, respectively. For all animals, fetal O_2 content and pH at 8 hrs. of experimental treatment correlated with density of eNOS immunostaining (r = -0.49 and r = -0.47, respectively, both p<0.05). Sustained moderate to severe hypoxemia of 8 hrs. duration thus results in an apparent upregulation of eNOS expression in the ovine placenta, suggesting an adaptive response to increase placental blood flows and hence oxygen delivery to the fetus.

Refractive Changes Due To Hypoxia Following Lasik Corneal Surgery.

Nelson ML, Mader TH, Brady S, Winkle RK, White L. Madigan Army Medical Center, Fort Lewis, WA 98431.

Objective: To observe changes in corneal shape, thickness, and visual acuity that may take place in patients whose corneas are exposed to hypoxia following Laser in Situ Keratomileusis (LASIK) corneal surgery. Methods: Twenty LASIK patients and twenty myopic control patients were exposed to ocular surface hypoxia in one eye by filtering humidified, compressed 100% nitrogen (0% oxygen) through an air-tight goggle system at sea level for 2 hours. The other eye was exposed to humidified, compressed air (21% oxygen) simultaneously through the air-tight goggle system. Video keratography, cycloplegic refraction, and pachymetry were evaluated using repeated measures analysis of variance. Results: There was no significant change in corneal topography or cycloplegic refraction in either the myopic control group or the LASIK group after 2 hours exposure to hypoxia. There was a significant increase in central corneal thickness in both control and LASIK eyes exposed to hypoxia, and no change in eyes exposed to compressed air. Conclusions: These results suggest that corneal hypoxia does not cause significant refractive changes in LASIK patients, unlike patients who have had radial keratotomy (RK) corneal surgery. These findings are important for patients involved in high-altitude activities who are considering having refractive surgery in the future.

Theophylline Reduces Periodic Breathing During Sleep In High Altitude- A Placebo Controlled Study.

Netzer N, Hoefer M, Netzer C, Steinacker J, Lehmann M, Gieseler U, Kuepper Th. Dept. Sportsmedicine , University Hospitals Ulm, Steinhoevelstr. 9, D- 89070 Ulm, Germany.

Objective: Periodic breathing accompanied by oxygen desaturations is a physiologic reaction of humans to hypoxia during sleep at high and extreme altitude. Several drugs were studied in the past if they are able to normalize ventilation at high altitude but so far there is no data to show if theophylline as a known central stimulator of ventilation is able to improve ventilation at high altitude. The aim of this double blind placebo controlled randomised study was to obtain information about the effect of theophylline at high altitude. Methods: 18 healthy male volunteers were studied with full 12 channel polysomnography (Respironics Sidas GS) in the first night and again in the third night during their stay at the hut after hiking to 4554m altitude (C.Margherita). 9 randomised subjects had begun to take

---

[1]presented as *Hot Topic in Mountain Medicine*; [2]presented as *Hot Topic in Hypoxia*; [3]*oral poster communication.*

400mg theophylline (verum group) and 9 placebo (placebo group) each evening at 8pm three days before starting the hike and during their stay to reach sufficient theophylline plasma levels. Blood was drawn and theophylline plasma levels were controlled in each individual befor each polysomnographic night. The respiratory polysomnographic data was analized manually breath by breath and sleep was staged manually according RK- criteria for each individual. Statistical evaluation was done using student-t test for significance and descriptive data analysis. Results: Sufficient theophylline plasma levels vere reached in the verum group in each subject. The average respiratory disturbance index (RDI, periodic breath ,ie. central apneas and hypopneas per hour in bed) in the verum group was 50.5 and 107.5 in the placebo group ($p = 0.02$). The oxygen desaturation index was 66.0 in the verum group and 117.6 in the placebo group ($p < 0.01$). Mean oxygen saturation during the night was 68.6 %SaO_2 in the verum and 65.7 %SaO_2 in the placebo group (n.s.). Sleep sufficiency (total sleep time / total time in bed in %) was 74.8 with verum and 85.3 with placebo (n.s.). Conclusions: We conclude that theophylline seems to be effective to normalize ventilation at night in high altitude but may not change sleep and mean SaO_2.

The Ventilatory Response To Timed Inspiratory Pulses Of CO_2 During Acclimatisation To Hypoxia.

Nickol, A.H.*, Collier D.J., Milledge J.S., van-Ruiten H., Williams D. and Wolff C.B. British Kangchenjunga Medical Expedition, c/o *Division of Basic Medical Sciences and Pharmacology, St Bartholomew's and the Royal London School of Medicine, London EC1M 6BQ, United Kingdom.

OBJECTIVES: To investigate changes in the ventilatory response to timed inhaled CO_2 pulses during acclimatisation. Subjects were studied whilst cycling at 60 watts. After a run in period of 51/2 minutes small inspiratory pulses of CO_2 were delivered either early or late in every inspiration, (0-300 and 300-600ms after the onset of inspiration respectively). Two-minute collections of expirate into Douglas bags were made for determination of ventilation. During normoxia at sea level ventilation in response to pulses of CO_2 delivered early was significantly greater than with pulses delivered late, (33.7 ± 0.9 l/min and 31.6 ± 1.0 l/min respectively, n =20, $p = 0.004$). In contrast under conditions of acute hypoxia at sea level (FiO_2 =12%) this response to the timing of CO_2 pulses was abolished (ventilations: 36.4 ± 2.0 and 36.3 ± 2.0 l/min for early and late pulses respectively, n=10, $p =0.89$). Within 3 days of arrival at Kangchenjunga base camp at 5000m there was still no significant ventilatory response to the timing of inspiratory CO_2 pulses (ventilations 68.8 ± 4.3l/min and 65.8 ± 3.8l/min for early and late pulses respectively, n =19, $p = 0.13$). After an acclimatisation period of 4-28 days, however, ventilation in response to early pulses became significantly greater than that in response to late pulses, the magnitude of this response being even greater than at sea level, (ventilations 63.8 ± 5.7 and 57.0 ± 4.9 l/min, n=11, $p =0.006$). We conclude that ventilatory responsiveness to the timing of inspiratory CO_2 pulses is eliminated by acute hypoxia but augmented by hypoxia after acclimatisation.

Impaired Cardiopulmonary Transition at High Altitude.

Niermeyer S, Moore LG, Shaffer E. University of Colorado Health Sciences Center and Denver Campus; Denver, CO, USA.

Infants born at high altitude experience low baseline arterial oxygen saturations and may develop acute or subacute pulmonary hypertension. Unknown are the contributions that irregular respiratory patterns, arterial oxygen desaturations and pulmonary hypertension make to impaired cardiopulmonary transition in the growing numbers of infants living at high altitude. Thirty-five infants $\geq$ 37 weeks gestation born in Leadville, CO (10,152 ft.) were

---

[1]presented as *Hot Topic in Mountain Medicine*; [2]presented as *Hot Topic in Hypoxia*; [3]*oral poster communication.*

studied within 48 hours of birth, at one week, one and 3 months with respiratory inductive plethysmography (Respitrace), pulse oximetry (Nellcor N-200) and echocardiography. Six infants (17%) exhibited impaired cardiopulmonary transition, defined as elevated pulmonary artery pressures or respiratory distress necessitating supplemental oxygen and/or positive pressure ventilation. One infant immediately developed hypoxemia and pulmonary hypertension which required mechanical ventilation at 27 hours. Four others had periodic, apneic respirations with repetitive desaturations < 60% (N = 2) or < 70% (N = 2) and were treated with supplemental oxygen beginning in the first 10 days of life. In these infants, the frequency of apnea/hypopnea (< 25% baseline Vt) episodes ≥ 4 sec increased from 41 ± 9/hr at 24-48 hours to 119 ± 47/hr at 1 week and the percent time in periodic apnea rose correspondingly from 7 ± 2% to 16 ± 4% (both p <.05). The remaining one infant had mean saturations of 82-87% and normal echocardiographic findings until 15 weeks when he developed systemic pulmonary artery pressures. Thus, a substantial proportion of infants at high altitude demonstrate impaired cardiopulmonary transition, often due to periodic, apneic respiratory patterns resulting in desaturation in the first week of life. Acute and late-onset pulmonary hypertension suggest that the infant pulmonary vascular bed retains reactivity for a prolonged period following birth at high altitude. Awareness of the several clinical manifestations of impaired cardiopulmonary transition and time points at which they occur will aid in preventing morbidity in infants living at high altitude.

Nifedipine Prophylaxis Of Pulmonary Edema After Intense Exercise At Altitude.[3]

Novak[1] CP, P Friedman[4], J Bourne[3], JD Anholm.[1,2] Loma Linda University[1] & Jerry L. Pettis VA Medical Center[2], Loma Linda, CA 92357, Mammoth Hospital[3], Mammoth Lakes, CA 93546, University of California, San Diego[4], CA 92130.

High intensity exercise alters the alveolar-capillary blood-gas barrier and produces radiographic changes of interstitial pulmonary edema, both at sea level and at altitude. Nifedipine is useful in the treatment and prophylaxis of high-altitude pulmonary edema. This study examined whether nifedipine would change the radiographic findings of interstitial pulmonary edema after intense exercise at altitude. A randomized, double-blind, placebo-controlled, cross-over trial of 60 mg/day nifedipine was performed. Ten highly-trained, unacclimatized runners (6 male, 4 female) aged 38 ± 9 (mean ± SD) took either nifedipine (N) or a placebo (P) for 6 days prior to ascent to 2440 m. After 36 hours of altitude acclimatization, the subjects competed over a 20 km course at 2400-2600 m. Chest radiographs were obtained prior to exercise and immediately post-exercise (within 10 min). After descent to low altitude and following a 15-day drug washout, subjects crossed over to the alternate regimen (N or P). Subjects then returned to altitude to repeat the initial exercise and testing. A chest radiologist interpreted all films in random order without knowledge of the exercise or medication condition. Films were scored for signs of edema (e.g. hilar blurring, peribronchial cuffing) using a 3-point scale. An edema score was calculated for each subject by summing the scores for the radiographic signs. The edema score for the N and P trials increased from 1.6 ± 2.1 before exercise to 2.6 ± 2.2 after exercise, p < 0.05 by ANOVA (1.2 ± 1.4 to 2.3 ± 1.8 on P; 2.0 ± 2.7 to 2.8 ± 2.6 on N, p = NS for a nifedipine effect). The results indicate that high intensity exercise at altitude causes interstitial pulmonary edema, but prophylactic treatment with nifedipine does not reduce the radiographic signs of edema.

---

[1]presented as *Hot Topic in Mountain Medicine*; [2]presented as *Hot Topic in Hypoxia*; [3]*oral poster communication.*

Hypoxic Vasoconstriction In The Lamprey Dorsal Aorta (DA) Is Calcium-Dependent.

Packer C.S. ,N.J. Pelaez, M.J. Russell and K.R. Olson. Indiana University School of Medicine, Indianapolis, IN. 46202.

The lamprey is a modern-day representative of the ancient vertebrates of the Class Agnatha or jawless fish. The DA of these fish carry oxygenated blood from the gills to the rest of the body. Interestingly, the DA constricts rigorously in response to low PO_2 as do mammalian pulmonary vessels. The current study was designed to test the hypothesis that lamprey DA hypoxic vasoconstriction is $Ca2^+$-dependent as has previously been reported for hypoxic pulmonary vasoconstriction (HPV). Specifically, lamprey DA rings were attached to force transducers in muscle baths of HEPES solution at about 19°C, bubbled with air and stimulated with 90 mM KCl. Following washout and complete relaxation, the rings were made hypoxic by switching from air to N_2 gas. Once the hypoxic contractions had reached a plateau the gas was switched back to air which resulted in complete relaxation. Then the bath was changed to a 0 $Ca2^+$/EGTA solution and intracellular $Ca2^+$ was depleted by a series of repetitive NE (5 x 10-5M)contractions until NE could no longer elicit a response. Ionomycin (40 mM) was added to the bath to ensure removal of any residual $Ca2^+$. Finally, the DA rings were made hypoxic in this very low $Ca2^+$ environment. In another series of experiments, changes in free [$Ca2^+$] and active force were measured simultaneously as functions of time using the $Ca2^+$ indicator FURA and a tissue fluorometer system. Reducing $Ca2^+$ with EGTA andionomycin also reduced the hypoxic contractile response. However, these methods of pharmacological could not completely abolish the hypoxic response of the lamprey DA. The $Ca2^+$ signal and active force production correlated very closely in response to hypoxia. In conclusion: 1. The lamprey DA appears to have a well-developed intracellular $Ca2^+$ store that is difficult to deplete completely and, 2. The lamprey dorsalaortic hypoxic contraction is $Ca2^+$-dependent as is HPV in mammals. Supported by an American Lung Association Career Investigator Award and NSF Grant #IBN 9723306.

Arterial Baroreflex Control Of Cerebral Blood Flow Is Maintained At Simulated High Altitude.

Passino C., Cencetti S., Spadacini G., Quintana R., Parker D., Robergs R., Appenzeller O., Bernardi L. Univ. of Pavia and IRCCS S.Matteo, Pavia, Ospedale S. Maria Nuova, Florence, Italy, Univ. of New Mexico and NMHEMC Found., NM, USA.

To assess the importance of arterial baroreflex control in determining altitude-induced changes in cerebral blood flow (CBF) we compared beat-to-beat changes in RR interval (RR), arterial blood pressure (BP, by Colin tonometry), CBF (by transcranial Doppler velocimetry in the middle cerebral artery), end-tidal CO_2, oxygen saturation (SaO_2) and respiration in 19 subjects at baseline (Albuquerque, 1500m, BL), after acute exposure to simulated high altitude (HA) in a hypobaric chamber (barometric pressure as at 5000m) and after O_2 administration (in order to achieve 100% SaO_2) at similar barometric pressure (HOX). Arterial baroreflex control on each signal was assessed by power spectral analysis (low- and high-frequency oscillations, LF and HF) performed on time series obtained with the subjects in sitting position during controlled (CB, 15br/min.) breathing, before and during carotid baroreflex modulation induced by 0.1Hz sinusoidal neck suction (NS). At BL, NS was able to induce, compared to CB alone, an evident increase in LF power in CBF ($p<0.001$) as well as in RR and BP, with a mild but significant ($p<0.05$) increase in CBF total variability and no changes in HF power. At HA and during HOX, CBF, as well as RR and BP, was still able to respond to NS, significantly increasing LF power ($p<0.001$ and $p<0.01$, respectively), compared to CB alone, despite marked decreases in end-tidal CO_2 and SsO_2 during HA.

[1]presented as *Hot Topic in Mountain Medicine*; [2]presented as *Hot Topic in Hypoxia*; [3]*oral poster communication.*

These data indicate that during acute exposure to simulated high altitude CBF is still modulated by the autonomic nervous system through the baroreflex and that the CBF response to arterial baroreceptor stimulation is not affected by changes in carbon dioxide and SaO_2 levels.

Effects Of Moderate Altitude On Motor Skills In Elite Figure Roller Skaters.
Ponchia A.*, Sarto P., Bigon L., Locandro S., Andreatini R., Pelli C., Merlo A., Giunta P., Noventa D. *Medical Commission of Italian Alpine Club - Italian Roller Skater Federation.

The aim of our study was to assess the effects of moderate altitude (2,600 m) on motor skills in a group of elite figure roller skaters. Eight figure skaters of the Italian national team, 4 males and 4 females (mean age 17 yrs, range 16-18) were studied at sea level and on the third day after arrival at moderate altitude (Bogota, Colombia). Video tape recordings were made on each occasion for the following 3 exercises: 1) five consecutive jumps, without skates, taking off and landing in a 54 cm circle; 2) six consecutive jumps alternatively with single and double pirouette in a 54 cm circle, ending in ""arabesque position""; 3) three consecutive pirouettes with skates in a 54 cm circle, followed by a jump landing on one skate. Three coaches blindly evaluated the recordings, giving a score of the errors in landing for each exercise and, for the last two exercises, an evaluation of technical merit. Oxyhemoglobin saturation was measured in the three conditions using a percutaneous pulse oximetry. At moderate altitude oxyhemoglobin saturation was significantly lower than at sea level (93±2 % vs. 98±1 %, p< 0.004), and we observed a significant reduction in the score and technical evaluation for exercise 2. Thus only unusual complex motor tasks seem to be influenced during the first days at moderate altitude, but not simple (exercise 1) or habitual ones (like jumps with skates for a figure skater). Probably these unusual exercises, differently from habitual ones driven by specific engrams, demand a greater involvement of central nervous system, particularly of structures involved in the control of balance, and consequently are more sensitive to mild hypoxia of moderate altitude.

Is The Coronary Risk Increased During Physical Activity At Moderate Altitude?[3]
Ponchia A., Egloff C., Miraglia G. Division of Cardiology - University of Padua – Italy.

The aim of our study was to investigate if acute exposure to moderate altitude could induce any ECG changes suggestive of myocardial ischemia during physical activity in patients with coronary artery disease (CAD). The study group consisted of 12 patients with documented CAD (11 with a history of myocardial infarction and 1 of coronary artery by-pass surgery), without symptoms and ECG changes suggestive of myocardial ischemia (ST depression > 1.0 mV, flat, downsloping or slowly upsloping persisting > 80 ms after the J point) during a maximal symptom-limited bicycle stress test at sea level in the month before the study. Seven patients were receiving medication (4 ß-blockers, 1 calcium-antagonist, 2 ACE-inhibitors). All the patients underwent two separate 24-hour Holter recordings: the first one completely at sea level; the second one started at sea level and included an excursion at moderate altitude (1300-2900 m) for 4 hours climbing up for a 500 m - difference in altitude. The patients did not report symptoms either at sea level nor at moderate altitude and ECG changes suggestive of myocardial ischemia were absent during all the two recordings. No significant differences were observed in arrhythmias between the two recordings, except for a short run (8 complexes) of ventricular tachycardia in a patient at sea level after the excursion. In conclusion recreational physical activity at moderate altitude appears to be safe and without additional risk of myocardial ischemia in patients with stable CAD.

---

[1]presented as *Hot Topic in Mountain Medicine*; [2]presented as *Hot Topic in Hypoxia*; [3]*oral poster communication.*

Muscle Blood Flow And Myoglobin Saturation During Sleep Apnea In Elephant Seals.

Ponganis[1], P.J., Knower[1], A.T., Kreutzer[3], U., Sailasuta[2], N., Hurd[2], R., Tran[2], T.K., and Jue[3] T, [1]Scripps Inst. of Oceanography, UCSD, La Jolla, Ca. 92093, [2]GE Medical Systems, Inc., Fremont, Ca., and [3]Dept. of Biological Chemistry, UC Davis, Davis, Ca. 95616.

Laser-Doppler flowmetry and 1H nuclear magnetic resonance spectroscopy (NMR) were utilized to evaluate sleep apnea in elephant seals (Mirounga angustirostris) as a model to investigate muscle oxygen consumption and blood-to-muscle oxygen transfer during progressive hypoxemia/ischemia. During six spontaneous 8-12 min apneas of an unrestrained, juvenile seal, apneic muscle blood flow (MBF) averaged 7.9 (+ 1.3) perfusion units, 52% of eupneic blood flow. Apneic MBF decreased progressively; MBF during first 20% of apneic period: 11.7 (+ 1.7) perfusion units; MBF during final 10% of apnea: 4.9 (+ 0.7) perfusion units. However, occasional transient increases in MBF did occur during apnea. NMR records revealed that 1) myoglobin (Mb) desaturation could begin prior to the last breath of the eupneic period, 2) Mb desaturation was nonlinear and fluctuated during apnea, and 3) two-thirds of Mb resaturation occurred within the first min of eupnea; complete resaturation required about six min. This pilot study demonstrated that muscle ischemia during sleep apnea is less severe than that during forced submersions, and that Mb resaturation can occur during apnea, presumably, secondary to transient increases in MBF. We conclude that these techniques will allow us to use the elephant seal to investigate regulation of muscle oxygen consumption and mechanisms of blood-to-muscle oxygen transfer, topics relevant to both diving physiology and end organ tolerance of ischemia. Supported by UCSD Academic Senate Grant RY253S, and a UC MRIF Award.

Ventilatory Acclimatization To Intermittent Hypoxia In Humans.

Powell F.L. , N. Garcia and S.R. Hopkins. Dept. of Medicine and White Mountain Research Station, Univ. of California, San Diego, La Jolla, CA 92093-0689.

Previously, we showed that intermittent hypoxia at sea level (IH, 13% O_2 for 2 hours per day for 12 days) induces ventilatory acclimatization in adult males (FASEB J., 12: A637, 1998). Here we compare those results with the isocapnic hypoxic ventilatory response (HVR) measured in two groups of adult males exposed to an equivalent level of continuous hypoxia (CH, 3,800m altitude). Four of the same subjects from the IH study were exposed to CH for 3 days (CH3d), and four different subjects were exposed to CH for 8 weeks (CH56d). End-tidal PCO_2 was set to produce VI ≈ 155 ml/(min kg) with PiO_2 =200 Torr. In matched IH and CH3d subjects, HVR was not significantly different before hypoxic exposures one year apart (0.06±0.03 and 0.19±0.07 L/(min %SaO_2), respectively). HVR increased to similar levels after 3 days in IH or CH3d (0.51±0.21 and 0.42±0.26 L/(min %SaO_2), respectively). HVR continued to increase in IH, peaking at 0.78±0.15 L/(min %SaO_2) after 5 days and returning to the 0.51±0.34 L/(min %SaO_2) at 12 days. In CH56d, HVR increased from 1.93±0.11 to 3.49±0.36 L/(min %SaO_2) between 2 and 14 days, and did not significantly change over the next 6 weeks. Hence, the maximum HVR measured in CH is 180% of the value measured after 2 days. The maximum HVR observed during IH was 190% of the value measured after 2 days of IH. The results suggest that maximum changes in the HVR can be achieved with intermittent hypoxia faster than with continuous hypoxia, but these changes may not be sustained. Supported by U.C. White Mountain. Research Station, NIH HL17731, RR00827, and Wilderness Medical Society.

[1]presented as *Hot Topic in Mountain Medicine*; [2]presented as *Hot Topic in Hypoxia*; [3]*oral poster communication.*

Ventilatory Responses During Maximal Exercise With Hypobaric Hypoxia In Well Trained Male And Female Cyclists.

Quintana R[1,2], D. Parker[2], A Gibson[2], M.V. Icenogle[2], R. Robergs[2,] The Center for Exercise and Applied Human Physiology, University of New Mexico[1] and Human Performance Laboratory, California State University, Sacramento[2], 6000 J Street, Sacramento, CA 95819-6073.

The purpose of this study was to investigate changes in exercise ventilatory responses with moderate to severe hypobaric hypoxia (HH) in a group of well-trained cyclists. The hypo/hyperbaric conditions consisted of 760, 566, and 486 mmHg. Male (N=14) and female (N=14) competitive cyclists, mean age = 28.79±5.6 yrs, with normal lung function, FEV_1/FVC=81.43±4.34, residential altitude (1640 - 2,460 m), and at least one year of competitive experience completed 3 cycle ergometry VO_2 max tests in a hypo/hyperbaric chamber under randomized single blind conditions. The males and females differed in hematological parameters, hematocrit = 46.21±2.13 vs 42.55±2.65 %, and hemoglobin = 16.97±0.99 vs 14.75±0.98 gm Hb/dl, respectively. VE for both males and females increased similarly from 147.61±29.10 L/min at 760mmHg to 159.99±32.35 L/min at 566 mmHg. No further increases in VE occurred at 486 mmHg, 160.66±30.89. SaO_2 decreased linearly from 93.51+2.80% at 760mmHg to 82.36±5.01% at 566 mmHg and 70.48±5.52% at 486mmHg. VO_2 decreased significantly with HH for both genders from 67.38±5.77 ml•kg^{-1}•min^{-1} at 760 mmHg to 58.34+3.4 ml•kg^{-1}•min^{-1} at 566 mmHg, and 50.87±5.03 ml•kg^{-1}•min^{-1} at 486 mmHg. The maximal exercise VE response with HH increases by approximately 8% at 566 mmHg versus 760 mmHg further increases in VE are blunted due to hypoxia and/or limitations in VE capacity in well trained cyclists.

The Effect Of Hypoxia On Tissue Vascularization.

Rakusan K. , I.V. Ehrenburg, N.V. Gulyaeva, E.N. Tkatchouk. Department of Cellular and Molecular Medicine, University of Ottawa, Ottawa, Canada and Clinical Research Laboratory of Hypoxia Medical Academy, Moscow, Russia.

The effect of intermittent normobaric hypoxia on tissue restructuring was studied in two different organs and species. In the first project, the effect of 20 sessions of hypoxia on vascularization of human myometrium was examined in samples of uterus from patients undergoing myomectomy or ovarial cystectomy. Patients with a preceding course of intermittent hypoxia training were compared with control patients without any pretreatment. The percentage of cross-sectional area of myometrial tissue occupied by vessels increased from 7.9 to 11.9% (p<0.001) in that hypoxia-trained group, while the percentage of tissue occupied by myocytes and interstitial space was proportionally lower (76.8 vs 79.3% and 11.4 vs 12.8% respectively). An increase in the vascular component was due to the significantly higher vascular density (3664 vs 2880/mm2) as well as a larger average vessel size (31.9 μm2 vs 27.6 μm2). These changes in tissue vascularization were accompanied by a significant decrease in the density of mast cells (1.33 vs 1.72/mm2), especially of the mast cells located close to the vessels (there were 53.7% of mast cells close to vessels in samples from hypoxia groups versus 64.0% in control tissue). The decrease in the density of recognized mast cells was probably due to degranulation of these cells during the process of angiogenesis. In the second project, we studied the effect of comparable hypoxia training on myocardial structure in rats. Twenty sessions of hypoxia did not influence myocardial mass or capillary and myocyte densities. In contrast, hypoxia induced the expression of PCNA in cardiac myocytes, especially in the right ventricle, indicating enhanced proportion of cardiac myocytes entering the cell cycle in this experimental situation. Thus, exposure to intermittent normobaric hypoxia results in distinct tissue remodelling, as illustrated by the morphometric analysis of human myometrium and rat myocardium.

Women At Altitude: No Gender Or Menstrual Cycle Effects On Acute Mountain Sickness (AMS).[3]

Riboni K.[1], Maes, D.P.[1], J.A. Loeppky, M. Icenogle[2], R.C. Roach[3]. [1]Lovelace Respiratory Research Institute and [2]VA Med Ctr, Albuquerque, NM, 87108; [3]NM Highlands University, Las Vegas, NM, 87701.

The incidence of AMS in women (W) is not clear from previous studies. For example, one study reported the same incidence between genders (Hackett, Lancet 2: 1149, 1976), while another reported a higher AMS incidence for W (Honigman, Ann Intern Med 118: 587, 1983). Furthermore, the effects on AMS of the luteal (L) and follicular (F) phase of the menstrual cycle are unknown. We compared symptoms of AMS (Lake Louise score) and arterial oxygen saturation by pulse oximetry (S_pO_2; Criticare 503) at baseline (635 mmHg) and near the end of 12 hr at a simulated altitude of 4800 m (426 mmHg; A12). Volunteers were 17 W (27 ± 4 yr, BSA 1.78 ± 0.32m^2) and 17 men (M: 27 ± 3 yr, BSA 1.96 ± 0.18 m^2). The W were studied twice in random order near the mid-point of F and L, confirmed by serum progesterone levels on the day of study (F = 0.3 ± 0.1 and L = 10.4 ± 3.9 ng/ml, $P<0.0001$). The mid-follicular phase was used for comparison of AMS and SPO$_2$ between genders. At altitude, the AMS incidence (Lake Louise score ≥ 3, with headache) was 59% in W and 59% in M (P=NS). Mean AMS scores were 4.1 ± 0.9 and 3.9 ± 0.9 for M and W, respectively. The S_pO_2 was not different between genders (80 ± 7 at A12). In F and L the AMS incidence was 59% and 63%, respectively. Mean AMS scores were also similar between F and L. At baseline and A12, the S_pO_2 was not different between F and L. In conclusion, in a controlled altitude exposure, women and men, and women in the F and L phases of the menstrual cycle had an equivalent incidence and severity of AMS symptoms. Furthermore, S_pO_2 was similar among groups. Supported by US Army Med Res Material Cmd, DAMD 17-96-C-6127.

Miners Exposed To Intermittent High Altitude Hypoxia: A Prospective Study.[3]

Richalet JP, Vargas M, Jiménez D, Moraga F, Osorio J, Antezana AM, Cauchy E, Hudson C, León A, Cortés G, Brito J.
Centro de Investigación en Medicina de Altura (CIMA), Mutual de Seguridad, C.CH.C., Universidad Arturo Prat, Compañía Minera Doña Inés de Collahuasi, Iquique, Chile. A.R.P.E. Faculté de Médecine, Bobigny, France.

The development of mining activities in North Chile involves a great number of workers intermittently exposed to high altitude (HA). This is a new model of hypoxic exposure, distinct from acute (alpinism) or chronic (permanent residence) exposure. A 3-year prospective study was started in February 1998 to characterize this model of intermittent exposure to hypoxia and to know if this condition is progressively leading to a chronic pattern or to an intermediate status between acute and chronic exposure. Some specific features may also appear. Thirty miners, working 7 days at HA (4300 - 4600 m) and resting 7 days at sea level (SL) will be compared to a control group (n=15), living permanently at SL. A complete clinical and physiological evaluation will be performed, including physical examination, EKG, thorax X-ray, spirometry, VO$_2$max, body composition, ventilatory and cardiac response to hypoxia (FiO$_2$=0.114) at rest and exercise, pulmonary vascular response to hypoxia by echocardiography in normoxia and hypoxia (FiO$_2$=0.114), 24-h monitoring of EKG and arterial pressure, renal function evaluated by creatinin, para-amino-hippuric acid and lithium

[1]presented as *Hot Topic in Mountain Medicine*; [2]presented as *Hot Topic in Hypoxia*; [3]*oral poster communication*.

clearances, hormonal status at rest and exercise (IGF-1, insulin, GH, cortisol, aldosterone, renin, ANP, catecholamines), hematological status, nutritional status by daily food questionnaire. Basal evaluations were performed at SL before the first exposure to hypoxia. HA measurements were done during the first ascent: daily Lake Louise AMS score, questionnaire on physical, mental and sleep status, 24-h monitoring of EKG and arterial pressure, hormonal status on the 6th day, hypoxic test and body composition on 2nd and 6th day. These measurements will be repeated every 8 months for 3 years to evaluate, for the first time, the impact of intermittent hypoxic challenge on the health status of miners. This is part of a project financed by FONDEF n° D-9711068.

The Use Of Acupuncture In The Prophylaxis And Treatment Of Altitude Induced Headache And Nausea.[3]

Richards, P. Medical Expeditions Kangchenjunga Expedition 1998, 71 Meadow Rise, Billericay, Essex, UK.

Several studies have demonstrated effectiveness of Acupuncture in migraine, prophylaxis of migraine, and general headache. Furthermore, nausea is clearly amenable to Acupuncture, being more effective than placebo and in some studies, equally effective as drugs. Objective: To show a reduction in mild AMS symptoms with regular prophylactic Acupuncture and that Acupuncture is effective in treating altitude induced mild headache and nausea. Setting: Expedition of 65 people trekked to Kangchenjunga base camp in Nepal (5000m) in self contained groups of 10. Method: One trek group of 7 received Acupuncture at 4 points (Gall Bladder 20, Pericardium 6, Large Intestine 4 and Stomach 36) for 15 minutes twice a week during the ascent phase. Lake Louise AMS scores recorded twice daily for all expedition members with additional questionnaire for those with headache. These scores of the prophylactic Acupuncture group were compared against the rest of the expedition (non acupuncture) as control. Comparison was also made between the groups for other altitude associated symptoms such as sleep and incidence of infective symptoms as some of the chosen Acupuncture points had sedative or immune stimulating properties. Those presenting with mild headache or nausea were offered Acupuncture as a treatment modality and effect monitored by AMS/ headache questionnaire score. Results should be available by April 1999. Preliminary results suggest reduced headache scores and reduced infection incidence. Study numbers are small but if this pilot study suggests Acupuncture may have a role in AMS/altitude related illness then larger studies would be required using conventional needle Acupuncture. Further studies of non-invasive external electoacupuncture stimulation which is possible by the lay person may follow. This latter may prove a useful non-invasive non-chemical adjunct to usual AMS prophylaxis methods.

Effects Of Acute Hypoxia On Myocardial Contractility In Pikas And Rats At High Altitude.

Ri-Li, Ge, K. Kubo, M. Hanaoka, S. Yamaguchi, T. Koizumi, M. Takeoka, Y. Matsuzawa, T. Kobayashi. Department of Internal Medicine, Shinshu University School of Medicine, 3-1-1 Asahi, Matsumoto 390-8621, Japan.

To clarify the mechanism of adaptation to high altitude on cardiac function, we had measurement of pulmonary arterial pressure (Ppa) and right ventricular contractility in pressure with respect to time (dp/dt) in 10 awake pikas (which were transported to Xining after being captured at 4,300m) in 10 Wistar rats in a decompression chamber (simulated 4,300m and 5,000m) in Xining (2,260m).The dp/dt which expressed as peak both negative and positive dp/dt (-dp/dtmax vs +dp/dtmax) was obtained from the blood pressure waveform (p) and the processed waveform (dp/dt)/ p by RM-6000 Series Polygraph System. The

[1]presented as *Hot Topic in Mountain Medicine*; [2]presented as *Hot Topic in Hypoxia*; [3]*oral poster communication.*

dp/dtmax and Ppa were obtained after one hour at each simulated altitude while the animals were in the conscious state and still in the chamber.It was found that the dp/dtmax either negative or positive in pikas after 4,300m and 5,000m altitude exposures increased progressively, whereas in the rats dp/dtmax rose significantly at 4,300m and dropped at 5,000m but still higher baseline values. Mean values of increases in dp/dtmax from baseline values were 56% at 4,300m, 89% at 5,000m in pikas, and 126 % at 4,300m and 73% at 5,000m in rats. Ppa in pikas with altitude exposures did not significantly increase, but in the rats it rose significantly. It is concluded that the compensative ability of myocardial contractility to extreme hypoxia in pikas was much better than that of the rats.

PO$_2$ Changes In Hypoxic Skeletal Muscle.

Lyabakh K.G.[1] , Mankovskaya I.N.[2]
Institute of Cybernetics, Kiev 252022, Ukraine[1] Bogomolets Institute of Physiology, Kiev 252024, Ukraine[2].

The distribution of pO$_2$ values in mammalian skeletal muscle under prolonged hypoxia represents an area of research that has received little attention up till now. The aim of this study was to obtain and investigate the pO$_2$ histograms in rat skeletal muscle under adaptation to moderate altitude. O$_2$ transport parameters and O$_2$ consumption were measured in normally perfused resting gastrocnemius muscle at sea level in Kiev (control) and in Caucasus (3,100 m) at 1-week and 4-month adaptation terms. pO$_2$ distribution was investigated by means of the mathematical model of O$_2$ diffusion-reaction in skeletal muscle. This model deals with the parameters of O$_2$ supply to tissue, oxygen demand qO$_2$ and capillarity, and permits to calculate the pO$_2$ histogram in different muscle fiber regions. The mathematical model includes following assumptions: muscle tissue consists of 40 % white fibers (1)and 60% red and intermediate ones (2). Muscle blood flow F= 4 ml/min/100g in (1) and 33 ml/min/100g in (2),qO$_2$O$_2$=0.2 ml/min/100g and 2 ml/min/100g in (1) and (2), respectively. We supposed that transarteriolar O$_2$ diffusion exists only in (1) due to its slow F. It was found that after 4-month versus 1-week adaptation period there occurred an increase in O$_2$ binding properties of the blood as well as pO$_2$ and O$_2$ content in the arterial and venous blood, and regional arterio-venous oxygen difference. After 4-month adaptation period it was also noted a significant decrease in intercapillary distances. Calculations showed that the lowest pO$_2$ values approach 4-6 Torr and the highest ones - 58-60 Torr in control. On the early terms of adaptation the pO$_2$ histogram shifted to the left and situated within a range of 2-50 Torr. On the later terms the pO$_2$ histogram shows a distinct shift to the right as compared to the pO$_2$ histogram achieved at 1-week adaptation period, and had a very similar configuration to the control one. The important factors of improvement of O$_2$ transport in skeletal muscle during adaptation to hypoxia were found to be an increase in O$_2$ binding properties of the blood and rearrangements of the capillary network geometry.

Operation Everest III (Comex '97): Effect Of Plasma Volume Changes On $\dot{V}O_2$,max And Fluid Regulating Hormones During And After High Altitude Exposure.[2]

Robach P., Déchaux M., Jarrot S., Marfaing R., Herry J.-P., Gardette B., Richalet J.P.
E.N.S.A., BP 24 74401 Chamonix; A.R.P.E., 93017 Bobigny; Laboratoire de Physiologie, Hôp. Necker, 75015 Paris; COMEX S.A., 13275 Marseille, France.

Plasma volume (PV) is decreased both by high altitude (HA) exposure and by intense exercise. We hypothetize that PV decrease (PV) is involved in the limitation of maximal O$_2$ transport (VO$_{2,max}$) at HA. Eight male subjects reached the equivalent altitude of Mt Everest (8,848 m) after a 30-day gradual decompression. This study was carried at sea-level (SL), at 370 mmHg, or 6,000 m (HA, days 10-12 in the hypobaric chamber), and 1-3 days after return

---

[1]presented as *Hot Topic in Mountain Medicine*; [2]presented as *Hot Topic in Hypoxia*; [3]*oral poster communication.*

to SL (RSL). Exercise until exhaustion was performed at SL, HA, and RSL, without (CTL) and with (INF) plasma expander (6% hydroxyethyl starch) infusion during exercise. PV was determined at rest at SL, HA, and RSL by Evan's blue dilution, and exercise-induced PV by hematocrit and hemoglobin changes. Plasma renin ([Ren]), aldosterone ([Aldo]) and atrial natriuretic factor ([ANF]) were measured at rest and at exhaustion. PV was decreased by 26% ($P<0.01$) at HA and was 10% higher (n.s.) at RSL than at SL. Exercise-induced PV was reduced both by INF ($P<0.05$) and by HA ($P<0.05$). Compared to SL, $VO_{2,max}$ decreased by 58% at HA and 11% at RSL. The changes in $VO_{2,max}$ were related to the corresponding changes in resting PV (HA vs SL: $r=0.72$; $P<0.05$, and RSL vs SL: $r=0.74$; $P<0.05$). VO2,max was enhanced by INF at HA (9%, $P<0.05$), but not at SL or RSL. The more PV was decreased at HA, the more $VO_{2,max}$ was improved by INF ($r=0.89$; $P<0.005$). At exhaustion, in comparison to SL, [Ren] and [Aldo] were not modified at HA, but were higher at RSL, whereas [ANF] was lower at HA. INF increased [ANF] response to exercise in SL and HA, and blunted [Ren] and [Aldo] at exhaustion only in RSL. The present results therefore suggest that PV contributes to the limitation of $VO_{2,max}$ during acclimatization to high altitude. PV expansion in RSL, which may be due to an increased activity of renin-aldosterone system, would also influence the recovery of $VO_{2,max}$. With grants from Région PACA and Ministère Jeunesse et Sports, France.

Impairment Of Amiloride-Sensitive Sodium Transport In Individuals Susceptible To High Altitude Pulmonary Edema.
Sartori C., M. Lepori, M. Maggiorini, Y. Allemann, P. Nicod, and U. Scherrer. CHUV Lausanne, USZ Zurich and Inselspital Berne, Switzerland.

The mechanisms predisposing individuals to augmented susceptibility to high altitude pulmonary edema (HAPE) are unknown. In the respiratory tract, sodium (and water) are transported across the epithelium both by amiloride-sensitive sodium channels (ENaC), and an amiloride-insensitive Na/K-ATPase pump. The importance of alveolar sodium transport and fluid removal by ENaC has recently been evidenced by ENaC deficient mice which developed pulmonary edema shortly after birth. In vivo, measurement of the nasal transepithelial potential difference (PD) allows to assess the transport of sodium across the respiratory epithelium of the lower respiratory tract. To test whether an impairment of sodium transport may contribute to HAPE susceptibility, we measured, at low altitude, basal nasal PD in 7 HAPE-prone and 18 HAPE-resistant mountaineers. To assess specifically the contribution of ENaC to sodium transport, we also measured PD during a superfusion of amiloride (10-4 M for 3 minutes). The major new findings are that, at low altitude, nasal PD was roughly 30 percent lower in HAPE-prone than in HAPE-resistant subjects (19.7 ± 0.8 vs. 26.6 ± 1.9 mV, X+SE, $p<.01$). Moreover, amiloride superfusion induced a significantly smaller ($p<.05$) decrease in nasal PD in HAPE-prone than in HAPE-resistant subjects (-10.1 ± 0.5 vs. -14.5 ± 1.9 mV, respectively). These findings provide the first evidence for an impairment of respiratory transepithelial sodium and water transport in HAPE-prone subjects. This defect appears to be related specifically to ENaC dysfunction. We speculate that a defect in respiratory transepithelial sodium transport may play an important role in the pathogenesis of high altitude pulmonary edema. (Supported by FNRS 32.046797).

---

[1]presented as *Hot Topic in Mountain Medicine*; [2]presented as *Hot Topic in Hypoxia*; [3]*oral poster communication*.

Transitory Perinatal Hypoxic Pulmonary Hypertension Predisposes To Exaggerated Pulmonary Vasoconstriction In Young Adults Exposed To High Altitude. [2]

Sartori C., L. Trueb, Y. Allemann, P. Nicod and U. Scherrer. CHUV, Lausanne, and Univ. of Berne, Berne, Switzerland.

Pulmonary hypertension is a hallmark of high altitude pulmonary edema (HAPE), but predisposing factors are unknown. In rats, transitory exposure to hypoxia during the first days of life predisposes to exaggerated hypoxic pulmonary vasoconstriction in adulthood. We measured systolic pulmonary artery pressure (PAP, Doppler echocardiography) at high altitude (4559 m) in 10 healthy young adults (age 21±1 y, X±SE) who had suffered from transitory hypoxic pulmonary hypertension during their first week of life, and 10 age and sex-matched control subjects. To gain further insight we also examined effects of nitric oxide inhalation (NO, 40 ppm for 20 min) on PAP at high altitude. The major new findings are that a) subjects with a positive perinatal history, while having normal PAP at low altitude, had markedly more pronounced pulmonary hypertension at high altitude than subjects with a negative perinatal history (62.3±2.3 vs 49.7±3.6 mmHg, p<0.01); b) NO inhalation led to 2-fold larger decreases in PAP in subjects with a positive than in those with a negative history (-28.2±2.2 vs -13.2±1.9 mmHg, p<0.01); and c) despite such large increases in PAP at high altitude none of the subjects developed HAPE. In conclusion, transitory perinatal hypoxic pulmonary hypertension predisposes to exaggerated pulmonary vasoconstriction at high altitude that could be related in part to a defect in NO synthesis. Exaggerated pulmonary hypertension alone does not appear to be sufficient to trigger HAPE, suggesting that additional mechanisms play a role. We speculate that in disease states characterized by chronic hypoxia, transitory perinatal pulmonary hypertension could represent a risk factor for the development of chronic pulmonary hypertension.

In Vivo Evidence That Hypoxia-Inducible Brain Erythropoietin Protects Neurons From Ischemic Damage. [2]

Sasaki R., S. Masuda , M. Nagao and M. Sakanaka*, Division of Applied Life Sciences, Graduate School of Agriculture, Kyoto Univ. Kyoto 606-8502 and *Department of Anatomy, Ehime Univ. School of Medicine, Shigenobu, Ehime 791-0295, Japan.

Erythropoietin (EPO) produced by the kidney and the liver (in fetuses) stimulates erythropoiesis. In the central nervous system, neurons express EPO receptor (EPOR) and astrocytes produce EPO. EPO has been shown to protect primary cultured neurons from N-methyl-D-aspartate (NMDA) receptor-mediated glutamate toxicity. Here we report in vivo evidence that EPO protects neurons against ischemia-induced cell death. Infusion of EPO into the lateral ventricles of gerbils prevented ischemia-induced learning disability and rescued hippocampal CA1 neurons from lethal ischemic damage. The neuroprotective action of exogenous EPO was also confirmed by counting synapses in the hippocampal CA1 region. Infusion of soluble EPOR (sEPOR, an extracellular domain capable of binding with the ligand) into animals given a mild ischemic treatment that did not produce neuronal damage, caused neuronal degeneration and impaired learning ability, whereas infusion of the heat-denatured sEPOR was not detrimental, demonstrating that the endogenous brain EPO is crucial for neuronal survival. The presence of EPO in neuron cultures did not repress a NMDA receptor-mediated increase in intracellular Ca2', but rescued the neurons from nitric oxide-induced death. Taken together EPO may exert its neuroprotective effect by reducing the nitric oxide-mediated formation of free radicals or antagonizing their toxicity. EPO supports survival of cortical neurons of rats with occlusion of the middle cerebral artery. M. Sakanaka et al., Proc. Natl. Acad. Sci. USA, 95, 4635 (1998). Y. Sadamoto et al., Biochem. Biophys. Res. Commun. in press.

---

[1]presented as *Hot Topic in Mountain Medicine*; [2]presented as *Hot Topic in Hypoxia*; [3]*oral poster communication.*

Acute Mountain Sickness In The Himalaya.

Savard, G.K, K. Zafren and B. Basnyat. Dept. Physiology and Biophysics, University of Calgary, Calgary, AB; Himalayan Rescue Association, Kathmandu, Nepal.

This retrospective study examined the incidence of acute mountain sickness (AMS), high altitude pulmonary edema (HAPE) and high altitude cerebral edema (HACE) in Nepali (n=4792) and trekkers (n=4655) visiting Himalayan Rescue Association (HRA) Aid Posts in Pheriche (4243 m, Everest region) and Manang (3499 m, Annapurna region), from 1986 to 1995. There was a linear increase over time in the number of trekkers entering both regions, as assessed by entrance visas. The incidence of AMS, HAPE and HACE in all Aid Post visitors (Nepali, trekkers) was greater in Pheriche than in Manang. The incidence of AMS increased between 1986 and 1995 in Pheriche, from 14.8% to 24.8% (mean values); there was no change in the incidence of HAPE or HACE over time (mean 2.1% and 1.9%, respectively). No change in incidence in either AMS, HAPE or HACE was found over time in Manang (mean 5.8%, 0.3% and 0.3%, respectively). The rising incidence of AMS between 1986 and 1995 in Pheriche was observed alongside unchanged proportions of trekkers (mean 61.4%) and Nepali (mean 38.6%) visiting this Aid Post. These findings suggest that altitude illness awareness drives by organizations like the HRA may be effective in stabilizing the incidence of the more life-threatening forms of AMS (HAPE, HACE) in Nepali and trekkers going to higher altitudes. Efforts are continuing to halt the rising incidence of AMS amongst these visitors.

Postischemic Blood Flow Response At High Altitude: A Comparison Of Himalayan Sherpas And Sea-Level Residents. [3]

Schneider Annette[2], Richard E. Greene[3], Cornelius Keyl[2], Gabriele Bandinelli[4], Claudio Passino[1], Giammario Spadacini[1], Maurizio Bonfichi[1], Luca Arcaini[1], Luca Malcovati[1], Amerigo Boiardi[5], Paul Feil[3], Luciano Bernardi[1], [1]Univ. of Pavia and IRCC Ospedale S. Matteo, Pavia, Italy; [2]Univ. of Regensburg, Germany; [3]Highlands Univ., Las Vegas, NM, USA; [4]Ospedale S. Maria Nuova, Florence, Italy; [5]IRCCS Besta, Milan, Italy.

In order to investigate whether the regulation of the vascular system may be a factor contributing to the adaptation to high altitude, we compared conduit artery function between 10 Himalayan Sherpas living at an altitude above 4000 m and 10 recently acclimatized sea-level residents. We recorded ECG, blood flow velocity in the femoral artery and arterial blood pressure in the radial artery by noninvasive methods under baseline conditions and during maximal vasodilatation after a 2 minute leg occlusion. Vascular function was characterized by calculation of the pulse wave velocity and by computation of the input impedance modulus and phase. Pulse wave velocity and input impedance of the femoral vascular bed did not differ between groups under baseline conditions. In the postischemic period, leg vascular reserve, defined as the ratio between maximal hyperemic and baseline flow velocity and normalized for the estimated leg volume, was significantly higher in Sherpas than in sea-level residents ($0.386 \pm 0.13 \ 10^{-3}cm^{-3}$ vs. $0.707 \pm 0.41 \ 10^{-3}cm^{-3}$, $p<0.05$). Leg vascular resistance decreased markedly in all subjects. Analysis of input impedance indicated a different postischemic response of conduit vessels between groups: the postischemic decrease in input impedance modulus at low frequencies was, when related to the leg volume, more marked in Sherpas than in control subjects ($28\pm12\%$ vs. $6\pm19\%$, $p<0.05$, compared to baseline conditions at 2 Hz). Our results demonstrate a superior ability to increase blood flow as a response to muscle ischemia in Sherpas compared to sea-level residents, which is at least partly caused by a different function of conduit vessels.

---

[1]presented as *Hot Topic in Mountain Medicine*; [2]presented as *Hot Topic in Hypoxia*; [3]*oral poster communication.*

Preservation Of Distinct Cognitive Function During Acute Exposure To Hypobaric Hypoxia.

Schirlo, C.[1], P. Brugger[2], A. Nebel[1], M. Regard[2], J. Kohl[1], E.A. Koller[1] and V. Pavlicek[1].
Institute of Physiology, University of Zurich[1]; Department of Neurology, University Hospital of Zurich[2], Switzerland.

Recent experimental data from our group showed, that the regional pattern of cerebral blood flow changes with acute hypoxia in men (1). To investigate distinct cognitive functions during short-term adjustment to acute hypobaric hypoxia in terms of a characterisation of regional cerebral functional alterations, three groups of 7 healthy male right handed volunteers were exposed to different altitude profiles in a hypobaric chamber using a single-blind design. All altitude profiles consisted of three periods each lasting 30 min and started at Zürich (450 m) with an ascent time amounting to 10 min between each period. In altitude profile 1 (AP1) maximum altitude was 4500 m and in altitude profile 2 (AP2) the target altitude was 3000 m both including the intermediate altitude of 1500 m. The third profile served as control (CP) with a maximum exposure to 650 m. The neuropsychological tests performed during each period consisted of a word fluency and three word association tasks investigating processes of cognitive flexibility. A lateralized tachistoscopic lexical decision task was also administered in order to assess hemispheric processing. The cardiovascular and respiratory parameters measured included arterial blood pressure (BP), endtidal PO_2 ($PETO_2$) and arterial oxygen saturation (SaO_2). No significant differences in cognitive and hemisphere-specific processing were found between the three groups, although at maximum altitude in the AP1 and AP2 group SaO_2 (80.1 ± 4.9 % and 91.4 ± 3.8 %, mean$\pm$SD, respectively) and $PETO_2$ (44.8 ± 2.2 mmHg and 62.0 ± 5.50, resp.) were significantly lower ($P < 0.005$ for all data) compared to the control group (98.6 ± 1.4 % and 99.6 ± 5.1 mmHg). Furthermore, in the AP1 group diastolic BP tended to decrease and correlated significantly with SaO_2 at 4500 m (r = 0.53; $P < 0.05$). We conclude that during acute exposure to hypobaric hypoxia equivalent to 3000 m and 4500 m, frontal lobe function as well as hemispheric processing are maintained despite the drop in diastolic blood pressure at 4500 m indicating beginning central hypoxia in terms of a functional impairment of the vasomotor centre. (1) Buck et al. J Cereb Blood Flow Metab (1998) 18(8):906-10.

Body Weight And Body Composition Changes At 3400 Meters.

Seelbach, D., Schaefer M., H. Alverson, J. Davis. Exercise and Health Science Department, Alma College, Alma, MI 48801.

Prolonged exposure to very high altitude results in decreases in total body weight and both fat and lean body mass. At very high altitudes these losses are attributed to hypoxia but are also explained, in part, by decreased caloric intake and altered physical activity patterns. The threshold for significant change in these parameters with chronic exposure has not been established. Therefore the present study was designed to examine the effect of acute and chronic moderate altitude exposure (3400 m) on body weight, body composition, caloric intake and energy expenditure in individuals living in comfortable accommodations. Fifteen subjects, 10 males and 5 females (23.5±8.2 (SD) yr.) participated in this study. Body weight, skinfold measurements, caloric intake, estimated energy expenditure and resting metabolic rate were measured at sea level (SL1), after one day at altitude (ALT1), after 14 days at altitude (ALT2) and upon return to sea level (SL2). Hydrostatic weighing was performed at SL1 and SL2. Body weight at SL1 was 163±7.4 lbs and was significantly lower at all other conditions: ALT1 159±7.0 lbs, ALT2 157±6.9 lbs, SL2 159±6.9 lbs (p<.05). Percent body fat via skinfolds decreased significantly from SL1 17.3±1.3% to ALT2 15.3±1.2% and SL2 16.1±1.3% (p<.05). Hydrostatic weighing confirmed a decrease in body fat from SL1

16.3±1.3% to SL2 14.7±1.5% (p<.05). Lean weight was not significantly different from SL1 136.6±5.0 to SL2 135.8±4.8 lb (p<.05). Estimates of caloric intake and activity level did not differ between conditions. Resting oxygen consumption was significantly lower at ALT2 0.16±.006 l/min compared to SL1 0.19±.014 (p<.05) but was unchanged at ALT1 and SL2. Body weight and percent body fat decreased with chronic moderate altitude exposure but were not explained by changes in caloric intake or resting metabolic rate.

Old Men And Patients With Parkinson's Disease (PD) Under Intermittent Hypoxic Training (IHT): 1) Hypoxic Ventilatory Response (HVR).
Serebrovskaya TV[1], Karaban IN[2], Kolesnikova EE[1], and Safronova OS[1, 1]Bogomoletz Institute of Physiology, Kiev 252024, Ukraine; [2]Institute of Gerontology, Kiev 252114, Ukraine.

Aging is accompanied by the weakening of hypoxic ventilatory sensitivity, and PD aggravates this process. We tested the hypothesis that IHT enhances HVRs and improves the breathing function in old men and PD patients. Eighteen healthy young (23±1.5 yr: Gr1), 9 healthy old (58±0.4 yr: Gr2) males, 6 PD patients (58±0.8 yr: Gr3) which have never been under DOPA treatment, and 12 PD patients (59±0.4 yr: Gr4) which have been using DOPA-contained drugs during two years, were tested before and after a 2-week course of IHT. HVRs to isocapnic, progressive, hypoxic rebreathing were recorded. Before training, some decrease in HVR to minor hypoxia (S1, $PETO_2$ from 110 to 70-80 mm Hg) was found in Gr2, 3, and 4 compared to Gr1 (by 21%, 32%, and 11%, respectively), but more distinct reduction was registered in responses to severe hypoxia (S2, from 70-80 to 50-40 mm Hg) - by 43%, 70%, and 53%, respectively. The hyperbolic shape of the curve was flattened in PD patients, approximating to the straight line. IHT enhanced hypoxic sensitivity in all subjects: S1 increased in Gr1-4 by 79%, 32%, 63%, and 48%, S2 - by 107%, 75%, 41 %, and 119%, respectively. The distinction between S1 and S2 increased in PD patients giving back the hyperbolic shape of the curves. The spirometric indices were also improved. The patients felt better, the clinical symptoms of muscular rigidity and akinesia decreased both in Gr3 and Gr4. We conclude that IHT has a beneficial effect on old men and PD patients. The fact that Gr4 showed primarily higher HVRs compared to Gr3 and higher increasing in HVRs under IHT indicates that DOPA-contained drugs partly improves hypoxic sensitivity and promotes better adaptation to hypoxia.

Old Men And Patients With Parkinson's Disease (PD) Under Intermittent Hypoxic Training (IHT): 2) Blood Dopamine (DA) And DOPA Content.
Serebrovskaya TV[1], Karaban IN[2], Kolesnikova EE[1], Mishunina TM[3], and Mankovskaya IN[1], [1]Bogomoletz Institute of Physiology, Kiev 252024, Ukraine; [2]Institute of Gerontology, Kiev 252114, Ukraine; [3]Institute of Endocrinology , Kiev.

IHT enhanced HVR in healthy humans and PD patients. DA is implicated as a neurotransmitter in the carotid body (CB) chemoreceptor cell response. Because of extensive capillary network, microenvironmental conditions in CB tissue are comparable to those in the blood. Continuous infusion of DA affected ventilation in animals and humans. So, naturally occurring oscillations in blood DA levels may modulate peripheral chemoreflexes. Therefore we have measured HVRs relative to blood DA concentration and it's precursor DOPA. Eighteen healthy young (23±1.5 yr: Gr1), 9 healthy old (58±0.4 yr: Gr2) males, 6 PD patients (58±0.8 yr: Gr3) which have never been under DOPA treatment, and 12 PD patients (59±0.4 yr: Gr4) which have been using DOPA-contained drugs during two years, were tested before and after a 2-week course of IHT. Venous blood was sampled from the ulnar vein to measure DA & DOPA content. Before training, blood DA and DOPA contents were higher (compared

---

[1]presented as *Hot Topic in Mountain Medicine*; [2]presented as *Hot Topic in Hypoxia*; [3]*oral poster communication.*

to Gr1) by 57% and 367% (Gr2), 27% and 244% (Gr3), 289% and 551% (Gr4), respectively, showed strong positive correlation with age (r=0.68 and 0.75; p<0.01, respectively) and negative correlation with HVR (r = -0.71 and -0.65, respectively; p<0.01). IHT increased blood DA level in Gr1 by 13%, did not alter it in Gr2, and lowered it by 13% in Gr3 and 19% in Gr4. DOPA content increased by 74% in Gr1 and decreased in Gr2-4 by 39%, 23%, and 31%, respectively. Thus, the weakening of hypoxic ventilatory sensitivity with aging is accompanied by an increase in venous blood DA & DOPA content. In PD patients this relationship is more pronounced. IHT normalizes the hypoxic ventilatory sensitivity as well as blood DA & DOPA level in PD patients.

TIA After Climbing Down A Mountain Of The 8000m Class.

Shiga, Naoko, Akira Yoshida. Department of Emergency Medicine, Chugoku Rosai Hospital, Hirotagaya 1-5-1, Kure, Hiroshima, Japan.

A 34-year-old man developed dysarthria and hemiparesis as soon as returning home after stay in Himalaya and climbing Mt.Makalu. His symptoms improved within a few hours, and he was normal in cerebral MRI, Xe-CT, angiography and EEG. But increase in RBC, hemoglobin, hematocrit and decrease in platelet and AT-III were observed. It suggests that coagulation system had been accelerated due to the stay in the low pressure and hypoxic environment. Thus we need to pay attention to the occurrence of coagulopathies not only during climbing but also after climbing until the coagulation and fibrinolytic system return to normal.

Evaluation Of A Closed Circuit Breathing System For Treatment Of High Altitude Related Disease.

Steiner*, U., *Fischer, R., Voll, K., *Huber, R.M. *Pneumology, Medizinische Klinik, Klinikum Innenstadt, University of Munich and EMS Inc., Erlangen, Germany. Mail to: Fischer, R., Ziemssenst. 1, D-80336 Munich.

Background: The closed circuit breathing system (CCBS) is primarily used for diving accident rescues. It is comprised of a tight fitting face mask, adaptable overpressure valve, breathing bag, CO_2-absorber, venturi-ventile (V–V) and carbonfibre oxygen cylinder. With an 2l oxygen cylinder, the system achieves continuous oxygen concentrations of more than 95% for 6 hours in normobaric conditions. On the 2nd British Medical Expedition 1998 the system was tested at 5100m looking at the following criteria: -tolerability and efficacy of facial and nasal mask; -increase of SaO_2 with different flow rates and use of V-V (FiO_2 0.82); -feasibility of active descent; -durability under extreme climate conditions. Methods: The CCBS was tested on 10 healthy volunteers. We monitored oxygen saturation, heart rate and breathing frequency. After testing the subjects without any movement in the back position, an active descent was then simulated by walking around in basecamp. Results: At rest, using the face mask under a flow of 1.1 l/min with the V-V (total flow 1.48 l/min) SaO_2 increased from 87.1% to 98.7%, heart rate decreased from 82/min to 72/min and breathing frequency decreased from 17/min to 11/min (mean values, p< 0.05). The nose mask (standard nCPAP) gave similar results but 3 of 10 subjects suffered from a blocked nose due to respiratory infection. The nose mask could not be used in these subjects. The remaining subjects found the nose mask much more comfortable than the face mask and less invasive. During exercise, the subjects complained of headache, probably due to insufficient flow rate. Durability: parts of the light-weight plastic material deteriorated in the extreme climatic conditions. Conclusions: The CCBS is a safe and practical way to deliver high oxygen saturations to patients suffering from hypoxia at high altitude. The main advantages compared to hyperbaric chambers (HC) are weight (4.5kg) and delivery of long-term high oxygen concentration, especially in unconscious patients, when the use of "portable" HC is contraindicated. The durability of some of the plastic components of the system has to be modified. Further tests will be necessary to determine the role of the CCBS during an active descent.

Correction Of Erythro - And Immunopoiesis Abnormalities In Experimental Secondary Immunodeficiency By Hypoxia.

Sukhenko T.G., Kolesnikova O.P., Kozlov V.A. Institute of Clinical Immunology, Jadrintcevskaja Str.14, Novosibirsk, 630099, Russia.

It was shown, that immuno- and erythropoiesis systems interact when erythropoiesis is stimulated (hypoxia) in intact mice. Purpose of this work was the study of interaction of erythro- and immuno-poiesis on the model of acquired immunodeficiency and their correction with the hypoxic hypoxia. As the model of secondary immunodeficiency we used the mice (B57Bl/6 x DBA/2)F1, which were induced chronic graft-v-host by inoculation of the lymphoid cells of DBA/2 mice. On 6 month of illness in animal we observed decrease of primary humoral immune response. The hemolitical anaemia with reticulocytosis and stimulation erythropoiesis in bone marrow indicated by the increase of the quantity nucleated erythroid precursors in the bone marrow smears, the elevation of number BFU-e, CFUs-5 and CFUs-8 was developed in mice. The development of the anaemia in mice is accompanied by increased production of the IL-1 and TNF by peritoneal macrophages. It seem likely, that elevation of the number of erythroblasts in bone marrow in BDF mice is one of the causative factors of the down-regulation of primary humoral immune response. We have tried to correct the immunodeficiency using the modulation of erythropoiesis. It was found that chronical hypoxia (using altitude chamber) increased the IgM-response, abolished the signs haemolytic anemia including diminishing of reticulocytosis, number of early erythroid progenitors in the bone marrow and CFUs-5 and CFUs-8. In mice the correction of immunodeficiency and anaemia were not accompanied with changes in IL-1 and TNF production. So, the immunostimulatory effect of chronical hypoxia in mice with immuno-deficiency, probably, is in connection with the removal of immunosuppressing effects of erythroblasts.

Changes In SpO$_2$ And Pulse Rate At The Time Of A Sleep In The Japanese Alps.

Suzuki T., Y. Goriya, S. Takizawa, Y. Yasuda and K. Kumano. Department of General Medicine, Kanazawa Medical University, Daigaku 1-1, Kahokugun, Ishikawa, 920-0293, Japan: and Kanazawa Red Cross Hospital, 2-251, Minma, Kanazawa City, Ishikawa, 921-8162, Japan.

Arterial oxygen saturation (SpO$_2$) and pulse rate (PR) were monitored using with a pulse oximeter in 5 newcomer subjects (3M, 2F, age 22-39) and one trained climber (M, age 47) to determine the change at the time of a sleep. SpO$_2$ was mean 82.8% in newcomers at the time of sleeps for 2 days to an altitude of 2,500 m. That of trained climber was 85.9% and as for the numerical value did not recognize a more significant difference in comparison with newcomers. The change of SpO$_2$ each of one hour was examined about two groups. SpO$_2$ 4% desaturation per hour (ODI) appeared most frequently in after sleep 2 hours in trained climber and in after 4 hours in newcomer subjects. While ODI did not appear from the sleep 4th time in trained climber as for a group of newcomers ODI was constantly appearing during a sleep. Similarly analysis was attempted regarding PR in a sleep. A PR value decreased in the 4th time most from the 3rd time in newcomer subjects, while a most high price of a curve was recognized in the 3rd time from the 2nd time after a sleep in trained climber. The aforementioned matter more, trained climber sleeps comparatively faster and takes a sleep sounder than newcomers, and is reasoned as the one that is increasing cardiac output, by increasing pulse rate significantly, when SpO$_2$ decreased.

---

[1]presented as *Hot Topic in Mountain Medicine*; [2]presented as *Hot Topic in Hypoxia*; [3]*oral poster communication.*

Women At Altitude: Alpha-Adrenergic Blockade Does Not Impair Cardiac Output Response During Exercise.

Tamhane RM, RE McCullough, EE Wolfel, CCW Hsia, LG Moore. Univ. of Texas at Southwestern Med. Ctr., Dallas, TX 75235 and Univ. of Colorado at Health Sci. Ctr., Denver, CO 80262.

To study the role of alpha-adrenergic blockade in cardiac output response (Qc) response during acclimatization to high altitude in women, Qc was measured by an acetylene rebreathing technique in healthy women (n=16, age 23±4) at rest and during graded ergometer exercise at sea level (SL) and on different days at Pikes Peak (4,300m, HA). Eight subjects received Prazosin (1.0-2.0mg q8h p.o) and the remaining eight received placebo. In both groups cardiac index decreased and heart rate increased at rest ($p<0.05$) between SL and day 9 at HA. During peak exercise there was no statistically significant difference between groups or days. These data suggest that alpha-adrenergic blockade does not impair cardiac response during acclimatization to high altitude in women. Study supported by US Army DAMD 17-95-C-5110, NIH RR-00051, NH, LBI HL-14985.

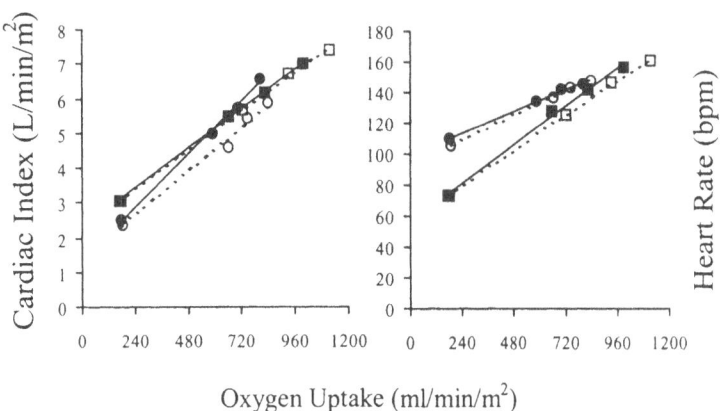

Oxygen Uptake (ml/min/m^2)

Carbon Dioxide And Cerebral Blood Flow At Sea Level And On Acute Exposure To Altitude.

Tiivas C , D Williams, T Harvey, S Brearey, I Chesner, H Hoar, C Imray and the BMRES. Dept. of Vascular Surgery, Walsgrave Hospital, Coventry, CV2 2DX, UK.

Objectives: Oxygen delivery to the brain is in part flow dependent. The aim of this study was to compare the effects of 3%CO_2, O_2 and a CO_2/O_2 mix on middle cerebral artery velocity (MCAV), as measured by transcranial doppler (TCD), at sea-level and at 3450m. Methods: Twelve subjects (ten men), aged 24-53, were studied at 150m and one month later, the morning after ascent to 3,450m by cable car. Expiratory CO_2 (PeCO_2) was measured on a Propac Encore monitor. TCD studies were performed by a single trained observer with subjects lying supine. A 2mhz pulsed TCD probe (Sci-Med Logidop 3) was used to record MCAV (cms/sec) every minute. Results:

	Baseline	3%CO_2	O_2	O_2/CO_2
150m MCAV	58.8(14.2)	68.1(13.7)*	54.0(16.5)*	64.8(13.4)*
3450m MCAV	63.1(18.6)	68.6(19.2)*	58.1(21)*	62.0(20.8)
150m PeCO2	5.3(0.28)	5.9(0.41)*	5.1(0.49)	5.6(0.59)*

[1]presented as *Hot Topic in Mountain Medicine*; [2]presented as *Hot Topic in Hypoxia*; [3]*oral poster communication.*

3450m PeCO2   4.3(0.2)   4.6(0.28)*   4.34(0.24)   4.5(0.24)*

*p<0.01 compared to Baseline. Paired t test. Mean(SD).

Conclusion:At altitude baseline MCAV is increased. At 150m and at 3450m, 3%CO_2 increased MCAV further, whilst O_2 reduced MCAV to below baseline. The addition of CO_2 prevented the fall in MCAV observed with O_2 alone. CO_2 has been proposed in the past and this study appears to support further investigation into its possible therapeutic use. Supported by the Arthur Thomson Trust and Mount Everest Foundation.

Uteroplacental Artery Structure In Term Placentas From High (3100 M) And Low (1500 M) Altitude Human Pregnancies.[3]

Tissot van Patot, M., Ph.D., Crystal Blanford, BS, Andrea Grilli, BS, Polly Lee, CVT, #Alan Tucker, Ph.D., Stacy Zamudio, Ph.D., #Dept. of Physiology, Colorado State University, and Dept. of Anesthesiology, B-113, University of Colorado Health Sciences Center, 4200 E. 9th Ave, Denver, CO 80262.

Uteroplacental arteries (UPA) are remodeled during pregnancy. Smooth muscles cells (SMC) are lost and endothelium (EC) is replaced by invading trophoblasts (Tr). Resistance vessels are converted to conduit vessels, increasing blood flow to the placenta. While some investigators report that remodeling is an all or none phenomenon, others report that remodeling occurs in only a portion of UPA. Tr invasion of UPA in preeclamptic or intrauterine growth retarded (IUGR) term placentas has been reported as reduced or significantly limited. Preeclampsia and IUGR are more prevalent in high altitude communities (3100 m) than low altitude communities (1500 m). Recent in vitro evidence suggests that Tr invasion is reduced under hypoxic conditions. We hypothesized that high altitude placentas from normal pregnancies exhibit decreased Tr invasion. Objective: To examine the extent of remodeling in term UPA from high (HA) and low (LA) altitude normal pregnancies by simultaneously analyzing for the presence of EC, SMC and Tr. Methods: We obtained placentas from 4 high altitude (3100 m) and 6 low altitude (1500 m) normal pregnancies. Four randomly chosen sites containing basal plate were obtained from each placenta and were snap frozen in liquid N_2 without fixation. Four sections (10 μ thick) were obtained from each site. Triple-antibody immunocytochemistry was used to stain for SMC - alpha-actin, EC - von Willebrand's Factor and Tr - cytokeratin. Results: A total of 21 UPA were examined in the high altitude placentas and 20 in the low altitude placentas.

	Tr	EC	Tr + EC	EC + SMC
LA	55%	30%	10%	5%
HA	43%	43%	0%	14%

Conclusions: Our data support the hypothesis that remodeling may occur in only a portion of the UPA in a single placenta. A higher percent of vessels are lined with Tr than EC in low altitude placentas, whereas the opposite is true of high altitude placentas. We speculate that hypoxia of high altitude reduces, but does not prevent, remodeling of UPA.

Oxygen Transport In Persons Adapted To Hypoxia During Acute Hypobaric Hypoxia.

Tkatchouk E.N., Gritsenko P.V., Tsvetkova A.M., Zhou Zhau-Nian*, Wu Xiu Feng*. Clinical Research Laboratory "Hypoxia Medical Academy", Moscow, Russia; *Institute of Physiology, Chinese Academy of Sciences, Shanghai, China.

Two types of adaptation to hypoxia were studied - prolonged residing in mountains and interval hypoxic training (IHT) course. Acute hypoxia was performed during the "ascent" of volunteers in the altitude chamber at a rate of 5 m/s. Oxygen transport was evaluated using the PaO_2, $Pa\text{-}vO_2$, and SaO_2. In the study performed in Shanghai, O_2 transport in Tibetan residents and lowlanders was compared. Ten male Tibetan residents, born on the Tibet

---

[1]presented as *Hot Topic in Mountain Medicine*; [2]presented as *Hot Topic in Hypoxia*; [3]*oral poster communication.*

plateau (3700 m), migrated to Shanghai where they lived for 4 years (average age 17 years). The control group was formed from 8 young men born in Shanghai. The values of PaO_2, Pa-vO_2, and SaO_2 measured at the sea level were similar in both groups. In the altitude chamber (3700 m) the values of these parameters were higher in Tibetan residents: PaO_2 54.1±1.5 vs 41.4±1.5 mm Hg, Pa-vO2 30.1±5.3 vs. 19.5±3.8 mm hg, SaO_2 87.9±3.3. vs. 78.2±1.6%, suggesting their better adaptation to acute hypoxia. In a collaborative research IHT was performed increasing the total time of hypoxic treatment in successive sessions (20 sessions, one a day). Effects IHT on O_2 transport in healthy volunteers residing in Shanghai (n=15, average age 21 years) were studied. Volunteers of the placebo group (n=15) inhaled atmospheric air through the mask. Parameters of O_2 transport in all groups were studied at sea level and during "ascent" in the chamber (3000 m) before and after IHT course. IHT resulted in significant increase of PaO_2 from 53.6±1.4 to 62.4±1.6 mm Hg; Pa-vO_2 from 22.0±2.5 to 31.2±1.1 mm Hg; SaO_2 from 87.1 to 91.3%. The analysis of the results suggests that high altitude residents as well as IHT-treated persons display more prominent adaptational ability towards hypoxia.

Transient Improvement Of High Altitude Headache By Sumatriptan In A Placebo Controlled Trial. [3]

Utiger D, Bernasch D, Eichenberger U, Bärtsch P. University Hospital, Institute of Sports Medicine, Hospitalstr. 3, D-69115 Heidelberg, Germany.

Headache at high altitude often fulfills the criteria of migraine. Therefore we hypothesized that sumatriptan, a drug specifically effective for treatment of migraine, would also alleviate high altitude headache. A placebo-controlled double blind trial was performed in 29 mountaineers with a headache on the day of arrival at 4559 m and no intake of analgesics for the last 4 hours. 14 subjects received 100 mg sumatriptan po and 15 subjects identically looking placebo. The mean age was slightly lower in the placebo vs. sumatriptan group (31 vs. 38 y, p < 0.03) and all 6 women were in the placebo group (p< 0.01). There were no significant differences between groups regarding rate of ascent, duration and severity of headache and acute mountain sickness score. The following headache scores (range 0 – 4) were observed:

	Placebo		Verum	
	n=6	n=9	n = 14	p[1)]
before	2.2 ± 0.4	2.5 ± 0.5	2.3 ± 0.5	0.32
after 1 h	1.5 ± 0.5*	2.3 ± 0.5	1.7 ± 0.7	0.025
after 3 hrs	0.8 ± 1.1**	2.2 ± 0.8	1.5 ± 0.9	0.054
after 12 hrs	1.3 ± 1.3	2.0 ± 0.6	1.5 ± 1.1	0.32

p < 0.005, ** p < 0.025 compared to men of placebo group 1) comparison between verum group and men of placebo group. Analyzing all subjects together, there are no significant effects for sumatriptan vs. placebo at 1, 3 or 12 hours after medication. Improvement with sumatriptan after 1 or 3 hours occurred in 11 individuals of the verum and in 7 of the placebo group (p=0.06). Considering only male mountaineers, there was significant improvement after one hour and headache was reduced by at least 1 score point within the first 3 hours of treatment in 12 subjects with sumatriptan and in 4 subjects with placebo (p=0.04). We conclude that there is a gender difference regarding the effects of placebo in this study and that sumatriptan transiently improves headache at high altitude in male mountaineers.

[1]presented as *Hot Topic in Mountain Medicine*; [2]presented as *Hot Topic in Hypoxia*; [3]*oral poster communication.*

Cold Induced Vasodilation At Altitude.[3]
Van Ruiten H.J.A.*, Dr. H.A.M. Daanen**, * Fac. Human Movement Sciences Amsterdam, The Netherlands ** TNO Human Factors Research Institute, Soesterberg, The Netherlands Kangchenjunga Medical Expedition.

Cold induced vasodilation (CIVD) is seen as an important protective mechanism for the occurrence of local cold injuries. A significant reduction in CIVD is found during exposure to high altitude, where cold co-exists with systemic hypoxia (Mathew et al., 1977). Takeoka et al. (1993) showed that the finger skin temperature during CIVD was lower in seven Japanese men at an altitude of 4860 m (ambient temperature 9°C) as compared to 2260 m (ambient temperature 12°C). Therefore, it seems that systemic hypoxia reduces the magnitude of CIVD and that the risk for local cold injuries may be enhanced at altitude. However, the core temperature is known to reduce the magnitude of CIVD (Daanen et al., 1997) and this core temperature was not measured in these studies. Therefore, a study was performed in which CIVD is simultaneously measured with core temperature during the Kangchenjunga Medical Expedition 1998. 17 Subjects participated in the study (13 M / 4 F). The male subjects were divided in two groups: climbers (n=5) and non-climbers (n=8). The climbers were exposed to high altitude for 45 days, the non-climbers only for three days. All subjects immersed the middle finger of the non-dominant hand in water of 0°C for 30 minutes. Finger skin temperature was measured every minute, oral temperature was measured every other minute in the sublingual pocket. The subjects were asked to assess pain in the finger every other minute on a scale ranging from 1 (no pain) to 11 (unbareable pain). Each subject performed a control test at sea-level and a test at altitude (over 5000 m). A post test at sea level is planned with the oral temperature controlled to simular values as measured at altitude. The minimum (Tmin) and maximum (Tmax) finger skin temperatures were derived from the data, as well as the onset time (time to Tmin) and peak time (time between Tmax and Tmin). The test at sea level was performed at an ambient temperature of 21.5°C and the test at altitude at 17.8°C. However, the oral temperature at altitude (37.2°C) was significantly higher than at sea level (36.9°C). Despite the increased core temperature at altitude, mean Tmax was significantly lower (4.8°C as compared to 7.1°C) and peak time was longer (11.3 versus 5.6 minutes). Tmin (0.7°C) and onset time (7.4 min) did not differ between sea level and altitude. Pain was more pronounced at altitude (4.5) than at sea level (3.5). These results confirm the reduced magnitude of the CIVD reaction at altitude, but indicate that the core temperature is not the cause of this reduction. It is likely that baroreceptors and chemoreceptors reduce skin blood flow at altitude. This is confirmed by the reduced finger skin temperature at altitude as compared to sea level just prior to immersion (22.1°C versus 30.9 °C). Although mean Tmax showed no difference between the climbers and non-climbers at sea level, the differences were striking at altitude. For the climbers, Tmax rose to 6.0°C at altitude, which is rather similar to sea level values. For the non-climbers, however, who just arrived at altitude, mean Tmax only rose to 3.7°C. The differences are probably related to the lack of acclimatization of the latter group. In summary, the CIVD-reaction is reduced at altitude, not due to the cold, but to the hypobaric/hypoxic condition. Acclimatization seems to partially restore the CIVD reaction.

No Lactate Paradox After Prolonged Acclimatization To Severe Hypoxia In Sea Level Subjects.[1]
Van Hall G, Søndergaard H, Saltin B, Calbet JAL, CMRC, Rigshospitalet section 7652, 20 Tagensvej, DK-2200, Copenhagen N, Denmark.

Lactate concentration during graded incremental cycle exercise after chronic exposure to hypoxia has been shown to be reduced compared to acute hypoxia approaching sea level, a phenomenon referred to as the 'lactate paradox'. The aim of the present investigation was to

---

[1]presented as *Hot Topic in Mountain Medicine*; [2]presented as *Hot Topic in Hypoxia*; [3]*oral poster communication.*

describe the lactate paradox by quantifying leg lactate production during graded incremental cycle exercise in six Danish lowlanders 25 ± 2 years after ~9 weeks of acclimatization to chronic hypoxia (~5200 m) while breathing ambient air (Chronic) and Normoxia (47% oxygen in nitrogen).

Power (watt), arterial lactate concentration (mmol·l^{-1}) and leg lactate release (mmol·min^{-1}) in Chronic hypoxia and Normoxia (means ± SE).

Chronic			Normoxia		
Intensity	[lactate]	lact release	Intensity	[lactate]	lact release
0	1.4±0.2	0.0±0.1	0	1.3±0.2	0.0±0.0
80	2.3±0.4	1.9±0.5	80	1.8±0.3*	1.0±0.6*
160	4.5±0.7	6.9±0.8	160	2.7±0.5*	3.6±1.3*
236	8.6±1.2	14.3±1.3	240	4.8±0.7*	8.7±1.9*
248	13.3±2.3	20.5±3.9	306	8.5±1.1*	14.2±3.4
			340	11.0±2.0	18.2±6.3

Arterial lactate concentration and leg lactate release were higher for each given workload under Chronic compared to Normoxia conditions. Peak lactate concentration and release were not either. Furthermore, peak arterial lactate concentration reached during Chronic exercise was far higher than peak venous lactate concentration at sea level with acute hypoxia (7.2 ± 0.7 mmol·l^{-1}) or normoxia (9.2 ± 0.7 mmol·l^{-1}). In conclusion, ~9 weeks of chronic exposure to altitude (5260 m) does not reduce peak lactate concentration and leg lactate production during exercise and thus no lactate paradox exists in well acclimitized healthy, active and well motivated lowlanders.

Periodic Breathing At High Altitude. Effect Of Time Of Exposure To Intermittent Hypoxia And Supplementary Oxygen.

Vargas M., Moraga F., Osorio J., Jiménez D., Hudson C., León A., Cortés G, Richalet JP. Centro de Investigación en Medicina de Altura (CIMA), Mutual de Seguridad, C.CH.C., Compañía Minera Doña Inés de Collahuasi, Iquique, Chile. A.R.P.E. Faculté de Médecine, Bobigny, France.

Our objective was to characterize the effects of oxygen supplementation on the nocturnal ventilatory pattern of miners exposed to intermittent hypobaric hypoxia at 4200 m. Nine acclimatized miners (at less 1 year of intermittent exposure to 4200 m) were studied at high altitude. Nocturnal ventilatory pattern was studied by plethysmographic inductance (Respitrace plus), oxygen saturation and heart rate by pulse oximetry. All measurements were performed during at least 7 hours of sleep. Subjects were studied while sleeping at high altitude without (control, C) and with (treated, T) supplementary oxygen (FiO$_2$= 0.25). Statistical analysis was performed by paired t-test, between both conditions. Data presented are mean±SD, * : P<0.05 or better. The number of events of periodic breathing during sleep were 209±161 in group C, and 55±48* in group T. Time spent in periodic breathing (as % of total sleeping time) was 24±19 in group C and 6.4±5.8* in group T. Higher oxygen saturation (%) was observed in group T (92.5±1.3) than in group C (85.8±1.3*). Heart rate (bpm) was lower in group T (68.8±8) than in group C (75.2±6.9*). A significant inverse correlation was observed in the control group (r=0.75) and in the treated group (r=0.95) between total time spent in apneas and previous experience of exposure to high altitude. In conclusion, apneas and periodic breathing were still present in miners exposed to high altitude for 1 to 5 years, but were reduced by treatment with supplementary oxygen.

---

[1]presented as *Hot Topic in Mountain Medicine*; [2]presented as *Hot Topic in Hypoxia*; [3]*oral poster communication.*

Determinants Of Maximal Exercise At 5200m In Aymaran Natives And Acclimatized Danish Lowlanders.
Wagner, P.D., M. Arroz, R. Boushel, J.A.L. Calbet, G. Rådegran, H. Søndergaard, H. Spielvogel, H. Wagner, B. Saltin. Department of Medicine, University of California, San Diego, La Jolla, CA 92093-0623A, and Copenhagen Muscle Research Center, Denmark.

At 5200m, 7 Aymaran natives (AN) (resident 3600-4100m) and 9 acclimatized Danish lowlanders (DL) exercised to maximal capacity breathing air and 55% O_2 on both 2-leg cycle (CYCLE) and 1-leg kick (KICK) ergometers. Expired gas analysis, and arterial and femoral venous (FV) samples coupled to FV blood flow measurements allowed both pulmonary and muscle O_2 transport to be studied for small (KICK) and large (CYCLE) muscle mass exercise. On 55% O_2 neither group significantly increased peak power during KICK, despite a 30% increase in O_2 delivery, but DL and not AN increased power 25% during CYCLE. Peak KICK and CYCLE leg VO_2 in AN were slightly higher on 55% O_2 than air, in proportion to FV PO_2, suggesting O_2 supply limitation of VO_2. Arterial PO_2 was similar in AN and DL but arterial PCO_2 was 8 Torr lower in DL, indicating in AN: 1) similar arterial oxygenation due to a much smaller $AaPO_2$, and 2) a lower ventilatory cost. Maximal heart rate was significantly reduced by altitude in DL but not in AN. Parasympathetic blockade in both groups had no effect on exercise capacity or gas exchange despite raising maximal heart rate in DL. These data extend observations on the inability of AN to use significantly more O_2 than ambiently available at 4000m, and on more efficient pulmonary gas exchange maintaining arterial oxygenation at lower ventilatory cost. They point collectively to down-regulation of the O_2 sensing and utilization systems in AN in response to lifelong hypoxia, yet to pulmonary gas exchange improvement probably due to larger lungs and thus diffusing capacity.

Cerebral Oxygenation At High Altitude And The Response To Carbon Dioxide, Hyperventilation And Oxygen.
Walsh S, C Imray, T Clarke, D Mole, D Hale, J Morgan, A Wright and the BMRES. Dept. Vascular Surgery, Walsgrave Hospital, Coventry CV2 2DX, UK.

Objectives: Cerebral oxygenation is dependent upon various factors, including arterial oxygenation, oxyhaemoglobin dissociation, haemoglobin concentration and cerebral blood flow. Aims: to assess the effect of 3%CO_2, hyperventilation (HV) and O_2 6lmin-1 on cerebral oxygenation at altitude using near-infrared cerebral spectroscopy (NIRs). Methods: Twenty subjects, aged 24-59, were studied. Baseline measurements were made at sea level. Daily studies were made at 2770m, 3650m and 4680m. Digital pulse oximetry (SpO_2) was measured with an Ohmeda 3770. Baseline expiratory CO_2 (PeCO_2 BL) was measured on an HP capnograph 78356. Non-invasive NIRs regional saturation (rSO_2) was measured using a Critikon 2020 monitor (Johnson & Johnson Medical, UK).

Results:	0m	2770m	3650m	4680m
SpO_2	97.3(1.1)	92.0(1.5)	88.3(2.7)	75.1(5.9)
SpO_2CO_2	98.3(0.6)			83.5(4.0)
SpO_2 HV	98.9(0.4)	96.5(2.5)	96.0(3.5)	95.2(4.0)
SpO_2 O_2				98.2(1.4)
rSO_2	69.5(2.4)	67.3(3.4)	65.4(2.7)	63.6(2.3)
rSO_2 CO_2	71.2(2.3)			65.9(2.1)
rSO_2 HV	68.1(0.6)	66.8(0.9)	65.9(0.7)	66.3(0.7)
rSO_2 O_2				70.6(2.9)
PeCO_2 BL	5.9(0.6)	3.7(0.3)	3.5(0.3)	3.4(0.3)

[1]presented as *Hot Topic in Mountain Medicine*; [2]presented as *Hot Topic in Hypoxia*; [3]*oral poster communication.*

There were significant differences (p<0.05-0.001) at all altitudes vs sea level. Paired t test. Mean (sd) Conclusion: NIRs allowed multiple non-invasive measurements to be made. CO_2, hyperventilation and O_2 all rapidly improved peripheral and cerebral oxygenation. O_2 had the greatest effect. Supported by the Arthur Thomson Trust and Mount Everest Foundation.

Altitude Acclimatisation By Intermittent Hypobaric Chamber Exposure.

Watt, S.J., Jutley, R.,Johnson, D, Johnston, R, Fraser, J and Dick, F. Department of Environmental and Occupational Medicine, University of Aberdeen, Foresterhill, Aberdeen AB25 2ZD, UK.

Aims. To determine whether intermittent hypobaric chamber exposure would provide useful improvement in performance and reduction in symptoms during a short ascent to moderate altitude in addition to that obtained from prophylactic acetazolamide. Methods. Two groups of 5 volunteers matched for VO_2max. ascended Kilimanjaro (5895m) moderately quickly (17hrs climbing spread over 56 hours). Six days before starting the climb group A commenced a series of 5 consecutive overnight chamber exposures, 1 at 2700m, 1 at 3300m and then 3 at 4000m - group B acted as controls. On the 6th night both groups flew overnight to E. Africa (cabin altitude 1700m) and started climbing the following evening. Self reported symptoms of AMS were recorded using the Lake Louise questionnaire (scores above 4 considered significant) and resting SaO_2 was measured by pulse oximeter during chamber exposures and the ascent. All subjects took acetazolamide 250mg bid. starting 24 hours before the climb. Results. Overnight chamber exposures were well tolerated and permitted subjects to continue normal work. AMS scores increased with chamber altitude (max score 6) but decreased with successive nights at 4000m. During the climb SaO_2 was lower in group A at all altitudes, markedly above 4700m (p<0.01). All 5 in group A vs 3/5 of group B reached the summit. One control subject retreated from 4700m with suspected HAPE. 1/5 in group A had significant AMS symptoms on the summit ridge compared to 4/4 in group B. (p<0.05). Conclusion. Intermittent hypobaric exposure was well tolerated and appeared to improve performance, SaO_2 and reduce AMS symptoms. The best regime and mechanisms require further investigation.

Increased Susceptibility To Acute Mountain Sickness In Individuals With Migraine At Low Altitude.

Weyman J. , D. Bernasch, S. Maggi, P. Bärtsch. University Hospital, Institute of Sports Medicine, Hospitalstr. 3, D-69115 Heidelberg, Germany.

To examine the relationship between a history of migraine at low altitude and susceptibility to acute mountain sickness (AMS) 759 male and 167 female mountaineers were evaluated by questionnaire at an altitude of 4559 m. We obtained AMS-C scores, rate of ascent, symptoms of AMS on previous exposures to high altitude and the history of headache at low altitude. Migraine was diagnosed according to the criteria of the Kieler Headache Questionnaire. Overall prevalence of migraine at low altitude was 11.4%. It was higher in women than men (15.5% vs. 10.5%, p=0.05). AMS-C scores (0.41 ± 0.51(SD) vs. 0.33 ± 0.46, p=0.11) and the number of individuals with AMS-C > 0.7 were not significantly different between mountaineers with (M+) and without (M-) a history of migraine while the rate of ascent was slower in M+ (3.1 ± 1.8 vs. 2.7 ± 1.6 days, p=0.02). At high altitude headache was more frequent (58% vs. 43%, p < 0.01), more severe (p < 0.04) and fulfilled more often (33% vs. 21%, p = 0.07) the criteria of migraine in M+ vs. M-. A score composed of the major symptoms of AMS like headache, loss of appetite, nausea, vomiting, dizziness, insomnia and peripheral edema (each graded from 0 to 4) on previous exposures was higher in M+ (4.9 ± 2.8 vs. 3.6 ± 2.6, p=0.001). We conclude that individuals with a history of

[1]presented as *Hot Topic in Mountain Medicine*; [2]presented as *Hot Topic in Hypoxia*; [3]*oral poster communication.*

migraine were somewhat more susceptible to AMS on previous exposures. A significantly slower rate of ascent most likely accounts for the similar incidence of AMS in individuals with and without a history of migraine in the present study.

Impairment Of Nasal Mucociliary Clearance At Altitude May Be Reduced By Intermittent Moistening Of The Nasal Passages.

Wilson CM, Bakewell SE, McMorrow RCN, Hart ND, Collier DJ, Williams D, Barry PW. 19 Cambridge Road, Girton, Cambridge, CB3 0PN.

The upper respiratory tract conditions inspired air, and recovers heat and water during expiration. It has previously been shown that subjective feelings of nasal blockage and nasal mucociliary transport times are increased at altitude, possibly due to the inhalation of large volumes of air drying out the nasal mucosa. We have investigated the effect of intermittent nasal moistening on the saccharin time, an established method of assessing nasal mucociliary function, in a group of subjects at sea level and after ascent over two weeks to 5,000m in the Kangchenjunga region of Eastern Nepal. Fifteen subjects were randomised to self administer a buffered saline nasal spray (Blairex Laboratories, Inc, Indianapolis, USA), instilling 0.5mls into each nostril at least four times a day. The 25 control subjects had no intervention. Saccharin times were increased significantly in the control group on arrival at 5,000m by a median of 8.2 minutes (95% confidence intervals 3.0 to 23, p=0.002), but there was no statistically significant change in the treatment group (median difference 7.4 minutes, 95% CI -4.3 to 27.3, p=0.3). A smaller number than expected of the treatment group had prolonged saccharin times when compared with the control group, but this did not reach statistical significance (p=0.073). This study has again demonstrated impairment of nasal mucociliary transport on ascent to altitude, and is supportive of the hypothesis that nasal moistening may prevent this. Further studies are planned to determine the optimum method of nasal moistening, and the effect of nasal mucociliary dysfunction on activity at altitude. We thank the subjects, Medical Expeditions, Liverpool University and Blairex Laboratories for their support of this work.

Reduction In Cerebrovascular Reserve Capacity In Normal Individuals At Altitude.

Williams D, C Tiivas, D Hale, S Walsh, T Clarke, C Imray and the BMRES. Dept. Vascular Surgery, Walsgrave Hospital, Coventry, CV2 2DX, UK.

Objectives: The cerebrovascular reserve capacity (CVRC) is a measure of the capacity of the cerebral circulation to increase it's blood flow to a vasodilatory stimulus. This study aimed to investigate CVRC in normal individuals at sea level and on acute exposure to altitude. Methods: Twelve subjects (ten men), aged 24-53, were studied at 150m and one month later, the morning after ascent to 3,450m by cable car. A 2mhz pulsed TCD probe (Sci Med Logidop 3) was used by a single trained observer to record the middle cerebral artery time averaged mean velocity (MCAV) (cms sec-1) and pulsatility index (PI) every minute. 3% CO_2 was used as the cerebral vasodilatory stimulus. End tidal CO_2 (PeCO$_2$) was measured using a Propac Encore Monitor. CVRC= MCAV$_{CO2}$-MCAV$_{BL}$/ Δ PeCO$_2$. Results:Mean(SD)

		Baseline	3%CO$_2$		
MCAV	SL	58.8(14.2)	68.1(13.6)*		
MCAV	Alt	63.1(18.6)$^\pi$	68.6(19.2)*		
PI	SL	0.93(0.11)	0.83(0.01) $^\#$		
PI	Alt	0.9(0.15)	0.84(0.15) $^\#$		
CVRC	SL	2.9(1.5)	CVRC	Alt	1.6(0.9)**

Paired t test: $^\pi$ p<0.01 vs sea level, * p<0.005 vs baseline, #p<0.02 vs baseline.
Wilcoxin signed rank: ** p<0.034 vs sea level

---

[1]presented as *Hot Topic in Mountain Medicine*; [2]presented as *Hot Topic in Hypoxia*; [3]*oral poster communication.*

Conclusion: Cerebral haemodynamics in normal subjects are altered by hypoxia. There is a rise in baseline MCA velocity at at 3450m. The response to $3\%CO_2$ is further rise in MCA velocity, but the CVRC is lower than that seen at sea level, suggesting the cerebrovascular bed is approaching maximal vasodilation. The PI which reflects cerebro-vascular resistance falls by a similar amount at both altitudes.

Diminished Sympathetic And Preserved Para-Sympathetic Activity With Alpha-Adrenergic Blockade In Women At High Altitude.

Wolfel E.E. , M. Meertens, J. Tokeshi, R. E. McCullough, R. G. McCullough, P. Rock, G.E, Butterfield, B. Braun. and L.G. Moore. Univ. Colorado Health Sciences Ctr., Denver, CO. 80262, Palo Alto VA Health Care System, Palo Alto, CA. 94304, and USARIEM, Natick, MA. 01760.

Prior studies in women at high altitude using heart rate variability (HRV) analysis have shown an initial increase in sympathetic (SNS) activity and a dimunition in parasympathetic activity (PNS) with a return toward normoxic values with more prolonged exposure. To determine the role of the alpha-adrenergic limb of the SNS on autonomic balance at altitude, we studied 16 women (23±1yr) on days 4 and 11 of the same phase of their menstrual cycle at sea level and 4,300m (Pikes Peak). Subjects were randomized to receive either placebo (P) or prazosin (D), an alpha-adrenergic blocker at 6 mg/day. Spectral analysis of HRV was determined from recordings obtained during metronome-guided breathing at 12 breaths/min in both supine and upright positions. Heart rates were greater at 4,300m compared to sea level in both groups with a greater response to upright posture in D. SNS activity was greatly attenuated in the supine but not upright position with D at sea level and 4,300m. PNS activity was greater in D than P and alpha-adrenergic blockade prevented the decrease in PNS with altitude exposure in the upright position. (* $p < 0.05$, P vs D).

	Sea Level	PP-4	PP-11
SNS -supine (nu)			
placebo	0.88±0.35	1.35±0.49	1.01±0.27
prazosin	0.31±0.07*	0.42±0.14*	0.30±0.07*
PNS -upright (nu)			
placebo	0.41±0.07	0.26±0.07	0.29±0.08
prazosin	0.35±0.03	0.35±0.11*	0.41±0.09*

Thus, the alpha-adrenergic limb of the SNS appears to play a role in regulation of heart rate with altitude exposure.

Diminished Vascular Response To Phenylephrine Infusion In Women After Nine Days At 4,300m Altitude.

Wolfel E.E., P. Rock, R.E. McCullough, R.G. McCullough, S. Zamudio, B. Braun, G.E. Butterfield, and L.G. Moore. Univ. Colorado Health Sciences Ctr., Denver, CO. 80262, Palo Alto VA Health Care System, Palo Alto, CA. 94304, and USARIEM, Natick MA. 01760.

Prior studies in men at altitude have demonstrated a decrease in the cardiac response to beta-adrenergic stimulation with prolonged hypoxia secondary to receptor down-regulation from increased sympathetic activity. To determine if a similar response can occur with alpha-adrenergic stimulation, 16 young women (23±1 yr) were given progressive doses of phenylephrine, an alpha agonist, on day 9 of the same phase of their menstrual cycle both at sea level and at 4,300m (Pikes Peak). Subjects were also randomized to receive placebo (P) or prazosin (D), an alpha-adrenergic blocker. The dose of phenylephrine required to produce a 20 mmHg increase in systolic blood pressure (PD20) was evaluated in both groups at sea level and altitude. The PD20 for D was greater than P both at sea level and 4,300m indicating

---

[1]presented as *Hot Topic in Mountain Medicine*; [2]presented as *Hot Topic in Hypoxia*; [3]*oral poster communication.*

significant alpha-adrenergic blockade with prazosin. There was a significant increase in the PD20 (ug/kg/min) in both the P and D groups at 4,300m (* p < 0.05, sea level vs altitude; § p < 0.05 P vs D).

	Sea Level	Altitude
P-Placebo (n=7)	1.23±0.28	3.83±0.61*
D-Prazosin (n=8)	6.87±0.90 §	15.05±2.78*§

Diastolic and mean BP were lower in D than in P at the peak dose of phenylephrine at 4,300m. Thus, a hypoxia-related attenuated response of alpha-adrenergic receptors to exogenous stimulation was found in young women at 4,300m, even in the presence of alpha-adrenergic blockade. Down-regulation of vascular alpha-adrenergic receptors may occur with prolonged hypoxia as a result of persistently elevated sympathetic activity.

Women Of Ladakh: Effect Of Age And Pregnancy On Arterial Saturation, Hemoglobin, And Heart Rate.
Wood S., T. Harris, M. Lilly, T. Norboo and M. Eldridge. Summa Health System, Akron, OH 44306, NIEHS, Research Triangle Park, NC and S.N.M. Hospital, Leh, Ladakh 194101.

We examined effects of age, gender, and reproductive state on hematology of 346 residents of Leh, Ladakh (3523 m) and 89 highlanders at Nyoma Changthang (4347 m). A primary hypothesis was that pregnancy would result in significant increase in arterial saturation (SaO_2) due to known effect of progesterone. SaO_2 and heart rate (HR) were measured with pulse oximetry (NPB-40); Hemoglobin (Hb) using the azide method (HemoCue AB, Sweden). **At 3523 m**, SaO_2 of non-pregnant females was significantly higher than that of males (92.6 vs. 91.0%). As predicted, pregnant females had significantly higher SaO_2 than control females (94.0 vs. 92.6%). Hb levels of women were 10.8 ± 1.8 g/dL (N=69) and 11.5± 3.5 for pregnant and non-pregnant subjects respectively. SaO_2 of females in menopause did not differ significantly from males. SaO2 in control females and males was not dependent on age (range; 5-75; mean 18.5 y) or, for females, stage of menstrual period. HR varied significantly with age in females (y = 115.9 ± 3.014 -0.9373 ± 0.1429; r^2 = .2; p = 0.0001) but not in males. **At 4347 m**, there was no gender difference in SaO2 between control females and men (89.5 vs. 88.8%). SaO2 of pregnant females (N=6) was significantly elevated (93%). HR was significantly lower in all groups at 4347 m vs. 3523 m. Hb of control females at 4347 m was significantly less than males (14.3 vs. 16.8 g/dl). The basis for this difference may, part, be CMS (Monge's Disease) in some of the men (Hb > 20 g/dl). Research supported by the Summa Health System Foundation and the University of California at Davis.

The Effect Of Angiotensin II On Secretion Of CRF And AVP During Acute Hypoxia.
Yan, Wu and Du Jizeng. Department of Biological Science and Technology Zhejiang University, Hangzhou 310027, China.

Using the method of stimulated hypopressure hypoxia, radioimmunoassay (RIA) and i.c.v. administration we studied the effect of angiotensin II (AII) on corticotropin-releasing factor (CRF) and arginine vasopressin (AVP) secretion from hypothalamus in Wistar rat during acute hypoxia. CRF content in median eminence (ME) significantly decreased after exposed to 7000m altitude for 2h and the level of plasma corticosterone rose, but AVP content in ME unchanged. After i.c.v. administration 0.1nM AII and exposed to 7000m altitude for 2h, the content of CRF in ME unchanged, AVP in ME significantly decreased and the level of plasma corticosterone significantly enhanced, comparing with control group of i.c.v. saline. Whereas i.c.v. together A¢ò with its antibody could attenuate or block the effect of AII on AVP and plasma corticosterone partly. These results suggest that AII can augment activation of hypothalamo-pituitary-adrenalcortex(HPA) axis activated by hypoxia through

---

[1]presented as *Hot Topic in Mountain Medicine*; [2]presented as *Hot Topic in Hypoxia*; [3]*oral poster communication.*

increasing AVP secretion from ME. The mechanism of AVP to increase level of plasma corticosterone is unclear. * Supported by NSFC. No: 39770288

The Response Of Neonatal Rat To Hypoxia And The Regulation Of Angiotensin II and β-endorphin.

Yan, Wu and Du Jizeng. Department of Biological Science and Technology Zhejiang University, Hangzhou 310027, China.

We studied the response to acute hypoxia and the regulation of angiotensin II (AII) and β-endorphin(β-EP) to the response. Using Wistar rat of 20d after birth at 2300m altitude. After exposed to hypoxia of altitude 5000m and 7000m for 2h, the CRF content in ME decreased and the level of plasma corticosterone increased, but AVP content in ME unchanged. Rat of 20d was given AII and β-EP by i.c.v. and was exposed to 7000m altitude for 2h the change of CRF and AVP content in ME was the same as that induced by hypoxia itself. AII did not change the enhancement of plasma corticosterone induced by hypoxia, but β-EP decreased it. The study showed that hypoxia can activate hypothalamo-pituitary-adrenalcortex (HPA) axis in 20 days old rat and 20 days old rat has had ability of response to acute hypoxia. AII and β-EP had no effects on secretion of CRF and AVP from hypothalamus induced by hypoxia.

Effect Of Acute Intermittent Hypoxia On Apoptosis Of Cerebral Cells In Rats.

Yinzhi Xie, Yin Zhaoyun, Jiang Lixian and Lui Yunda. Department of Hypoxia Biology, Institute of Health & Environmental Medicine, Tianjin 300050.

This study aimed to examine the effect of acute intermittent hypoxia on apoptosis of cerebral cells in rats, and the relationship between the apoptosis and free radical scavenging ability. The rats in hypoxia group were put into hypobaric chamber at a simulated altitude of 7,000m for 5h each day for 2, 4, 6, 8 days, respectively. Ultrastructure examination showed that the condensation of both the nucleus and cytoplasm following 2-day hypoxia, the fragments and pinches off at the surface protuberances, and the apoptotic bodies were observed. TUNEL-stain positive cells emerged as early as at the second day after hypoxia in cerebral cortex, at 4th-day in thalamus and hippocampus. However, the ladder-like pattern of DNA was not observed until 6th or 8th day after hypoxia. It was also found that the number of the apoptotic cells increased with the increase of hypoxic exposure duration, the ratio of GSH/GSSG and the activity of SOD decreased. The regression analysis showed that there was a negative exponential relationship between the number of apoptotic cells and the activity of SOD in a limited range. These studies demonstrate that hypobaric hypoxia can induce apoptosis of cerebral cells and there would be an intrinsic relationship between apoptosis and free radical scavenging in brain.

Forearm Hemodynamics During Acclimatization To 4300 m With And Without α[1]-Adrenergic Blockade.

Zamudio Ph.D. S., M Douglas MSIV, RR Rathod, RE McCullough BS, RG McCullough RN, S Muza Ph.D., P Rock DO, Ph.D., G Butterfield Ph.D., LG Moore Ph.D., Univ. of Colo. Denver & Hth Sci.Ctr. Denver CO; Stanford Univ. & Palo Alto VA Medical Ctr., Palo Alto, CA; US Army Research Inst, Environ. Medicine, Natick, MA.

Objective: We asked whether the α-adrenergic branch of the SNS mediates peripheral vascular changes associated with acclimatization. Methods: Eight women taking an α1 receptor blocker (prazosin, 2 mg TID) were compared with 8 women on placebo at sea level (SL) and 3 and 10 days after ascending to 4300 m (Pikes Peak, CO - PP 3, PP 10). Forearm blood flow (FBF - ml/100 ml tissue/min.) and venous compliance (VV30 – Δ venous volume

---

[1]presented as *Hot Topic in Mountain Medicine*; [2]presented as *Hot Topic in Hypoxia*; [3]*oral poster communication.*

from BL to 30 mmHg venous pressure/100 ml tissue) were measured by plethysmography. Data were analyzed with a repeated measures ANOVA and are presented as means ± SEM (Figure: solid=drug, shaded=placebo * = p<.05 vs. sea level, † = p<.05 drug vs. placebo at a

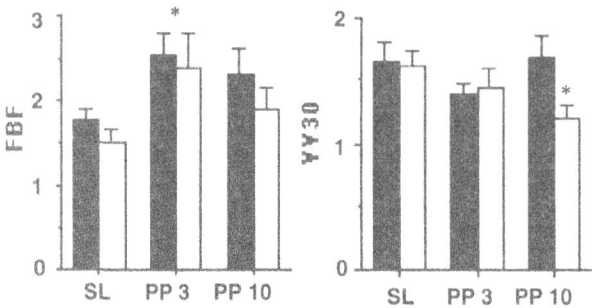

given time). Results: FBF was greater at high altitude on day 3 (p<0.005, drug and placebo), but not on day 10 (p=0.10 drug, p=NS placebo). There was no interaction between drug treatment and changes in FBF, but a borderline interaction between VV30 and drug treatment was observed (p=0.09). VV30 fell by PP 10 in women on placebo, (p<.05) but not in those taking drug. Conclusion: α^1 receptors are likely mediators of the peripheral venous response to high altitude.

Healthy Subjects Develop Mild Pulmonary Hypertension > 3 Weeks At 3800-4200 m.
Zieliński J. [1], G. Palasiewicz [1], R. Plywaczewski [1], D.A. Usupbajeva [2], H. Le Roux [3], A.Sh. Sarybajev [2], M.M. Mirrakhimov [2]. [1] Institute TB and Lung Diseases, Warsaw, Poland; [2] National Centre of Cardiology and Internal Medicine, Bishkek, Kyrgyzstan; [3] Medical Service, Kumtor Operating Company. Department of Respiratory Medicine, 01-138 Warsaw, Plocka 26, Poland.

It was found that healthy male subjects submitted to simulated ascent to Mount Everest developed moderate pulmonary hypertension during 6 weeks exposure to increasing hypoxia (Groves AM, JAP 1987, 63, 521). We were interested in effects of 3 week exposure to the altitude of 3800-4200 m on pulmonary circulation. We studied 27 healthy caucasian subjects aged 24 to 59 yrs, mean 41.6 +/- 9 y. They are working on 4 week shifts at the Kumtor gold mines in Kyrghyzstan. Pulmonary circulaton was studied twice by Echo-Doppler using Toshiba SSD-160. The first investigation (1) was performed at 730 m at the end of 4 week holiday spent in the lowland. On the same day all subjects were transported by air to the mine site. Majority (19) worked 12 h/day at 4200 m, the others worked at 3800 m. All were spending the rest of the day and night at 3800 m. The second investigation (2) took place at the 23rd day at altitude. The results are shown on the Table:

	BMI	CO L/min	RVD cm	AcT ms	PAPc mmHg	EF %	HR bs/min
1.	26±3	5.1±0.8	1.6±0.4	131±14	15.1+/-2	66.4±7	66.6±11
2.		5.8±1.1	1.7±0.4	105±14	25.4±8	66.1±6	75.9±12
P		<0.02	NS	<0.001	<0.001	NS	<0.001

BMI - body mass index, CO - cardiac output, RVD right ventricular dimension, AcT – acceleration.

[1]presented as *Hot Topic in Mountain Medicine*; [2]presented as *Hot Topic in Hypoxia*; [3]*oral poster communication.*

SUBJECT INDEX

AUTHOR INDEX

The manufacturer's authorised representative in the EU is Springer
Nature Customer Service Centre GmbH, Europaplatz 3, 69115 Heidelberg,
Germany. If you have any concerns regarding our products, please
contact ProductSafety@springernature.com

Printed and bound by CPI Group (UK) Ltd, Croydon, CR0 4YY
26/04/2026
02097340-0002